Handbook of Nutraceuticals and Natural Products

Handbook of Nutraceuticals and Natural Products

Biological, Medicinal, and Nutritional Properties and Applications

Volume 1

Edited by

Sreerag Gopi

Preetha Balakrishnan
ADSO Naturals Private Limited,
Bangalore, India

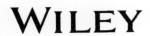

Registered Office
John Wiley & Sons, Inc., 111 River Street, Hoboken, NJ 07030, USA

Editorial Office
111 River Street, Hoboken, NJ 07030, USA

For details of our global editorial offices, customer services, and more information about Wiley products visit us at www.wiley.com.

Wiley also publishes its books in a variety of electronic formats and by print-on-demand. Some content that appears in standard print versions of this book may not be available in other formats.

Library of Congress Cataloging-in-Publication Data applied for:

9781119746805[hard back]
9781119746799[set]

Cover Design: Wiley
Cover Images: © Kseniya Tatarnikova/Shutterstock; Anna-Ok/Getty Images

Set in 9.5/12.5pt STIXTwoText by Straive, Pondicherry, India

Contents

List of Contributors

Shreya C. Adangale
Shobhaben Pratapbhai Patel School of
Pharmacy & Technology Management,
SVKM's NMIMS, Mumbai, Maharashtra, India

Saima Afzal
Soft Matter Research Group, Department of
Chemistry, University of Kashmir, Srinagar,
Jammu and Kashmir, India

Himanshu Agrawal
Molecular Endocrinology Laboratory,
Department of Biotechnology, Indian Institute
of Technology Roorkee, Roorkee, Uttarakhand,
India

Firdous Ahmad Ahanger
Soft Matter Research Group, Department of
Chemistry, University of Kashmir, Srinagar,
Jammu and Kashmir, India

R.S. Arvind Bharani
Department of Biotechnology, Sathyabama
Institute of Science and Technology, Chennai,
Tamil Nadu, India

Iffath Badsha
Department of Nanotechnology, Anna
University, Chennai, Tamil Nadu, India

Sunil Bishnoi
Department of Food Technology, Guru
Jambheshwar University of Science and
Technology, Hisar, Haryana, India

Natalia Angelo da Silva Miyaguti
Laboratory of Cancer and Nutrition,
Department of Structural and Functional
Biology, Institute of Biology, University of
Campinas – UNICAMP, Campinas, São Paulo,
Brazil

Maria Daglia
Department of Pharmacy, School of Medicine
and Surgery, University of Naples Federico II,
Naples, Italy

Aijaz Ahmad Dar
Soft Matter Research Group, Department of
Chemistry, University of Kashmir, Srinagar,
Jammu and Kashmir, India

Quintanar-Guerrero David
Laboratorio de Posgrado en Tecnología
Farmacéutica, Facultad de Estudios Superiores
Cuautitlán, Universidad Nacional Autónoma
de México, Estado de México, Mexico

Zambrano-Zaragoza María de la Luz
Laboratorio de Procesos de Transformación
y Tecnologías Emergentes de Alimentos,
Facultad de Estudios Superiores Cuautitlán,
Universidad Nacional Autónoma de México,
Estado de Mexico, Mexico

Gabriela de Matuoka e Chiocchetti
Laboratory of Cancer and Nutrition, Department
of Structural and Functional Biology, Institute of
Biology, University of Campinas – UNICAMP,
Campinas, São Paulo, Brazil

Giuseppe Derosa
Department of Internal Medicine and
Therapeutics, University of Pavia, Pavia, Italy
Laboratory of Molecular Medicine, University
of Pavia, Pavia, Italy

Debasmita Dutta
Department of Biotechnology, National
Institute of Technology Durgapur, Durgapur,
West Bengal, India

Debjani Dutta
Department of Biotechnology, National
Institute of Technology Durgapur, Durgapur,
West Bengal, India

Leyva-Goméz Gerardo
Departamento de Farmacia, Facultad de
Química, Universidad Nacional Autónoma de
México, Ciudad de México, Mexico

Chandrachur Ghosh
Molecular Endocrinology Laboratory,
Department of Biotechnology, Indian Institute
of Technology Roorkee, Roorkee, Uttarakhand,
India

Ritushree Ghosh
Shobhaben Pratapbhai Patel School of
Pharmacy & Technology Management, SVKM's
NMIMS, Mumbai, Maharashtra, India

Souvik Ghosh
Molecular Endocrinology Laboratory,
Department of Biotechnology, Indian Institute
of Technology Roorkee, Roorkee, Uttarakhand,
India
Plant Molecular Biology Laboratory,
Department of Biotechnology, Indian Institute
of Technology Roorkee, Roorkee, Uttarakhand,
India

Maria Cristina Cintra Gomes-Marcondes
Laboratory of Cancer and Nutrition,
Department of Structural and Functional
Biology, Institute of Biology, University of
Campinas – UNICAMP, Campinas, São Paulo,
Brazil

C. Jayaprakash
Defense Food Research Laboratories (DFRL),
Mysore, Karnataka, India

S. Karthick Raja Namasivayam
Department of Biotechnology, Sathyabama
Institute of Science and Technology, Chennai,
Tamil Nadu, India

Parul Katiyar
Molecular Endocrinology Laboratory,
Department of Biotechnology, Indian Institute
of Technology Roorkee, Roorkee, Uttarakhand,
India

Pawandeep Kaur
Soft Matter Research Group, Department of
Chemistry, University of Kashmir, Srinagar,
Jammu and Kashmir, India

Haroon Khan
Department of Pharmacy, Faculty of Chemical
& Life Sciences, Abdul Wali Khan University,
Mardan, Pakistan

Shalvi Sinai Kunde
Shobhaben Pratapbhai Patel School of
Pharmacy & Technology Management, SVKM's
NMIMS, Mumbai, Maharashtra, India

Mohd. Sajid Lone
Soft Matter Research Group, Department of
Chemistry, University of Kashmir, Srinagar,
Jammu and Kashmir, India

Leisa Lopes-Aguiar
Laboratory of Cancer and Nutrition,
Department of Structural and Functional
Biology, Institute of Biology, University of
Campinas – UNICAMP, Campinas, São Paulo,
Brazil

Pamela Maffioli
Department of Internal Medicine and
Therapeutics, University of Pavia, Pavia,
Italy

N. Mendoza-Muñoz
Laboratorio de Farmacia, Facultad de
Ciencias Químicas, Universidad de Colima,
Coquimatlan, Mexico

Deepak Mudgil
Department of Dairy & Food Technology,
Mansinhbhai Institute of Dairy & Food
Technology, Mehsana, Gujarat, India

Aparna S. Narayan
Department of Biotechnology, Sathyabama
Institute of Science and Technology, Chennai,
Tamil Nadu, India

Nighat Nazir
Department of Chemistry, Islamia College of
Science and Commerce, Hawal, Jammu and
Kashmir, India

Jayshree Nellore
Department of Biotechnology, Sathyabama
Institute of Science and Technology, Chennai,
Tamil Nadu, India

A.Y. Onaolapo
Behavioural Neuroscience Unit, Neurobiology
Subdivision, Department of Anatomy,
Ladoke Akintola University of Technology,
Ogbomosho, Oyo State, Nigeria

O.J. Onaolapo
Behavioural Neuroscience Unit,
Neuropharmacology Subdivision,
Department of Pharmacology, Ladoke
Akintola University of Technology,
Ogbomosho, Oyo State, Nigeria

K. Renugadevi
Department of Biotechnology, Sathyabama
Institute of Science and Technology, Chennai,
Tamil Nadu, India

Partha Roy
Molecular Endocrinology Laboratory,
Department of Biotechnology, Indian Institute
of Technology Roorkee, Roorkee, Uttarakhand,
India

Saakshi Saini
Molecular Endocrinology Laboratory,
Department of Biotechnology, Indian Institute
of Technology Roorkee, Roorkee, Uttarakhand,
India

Narges Shahgholian
Food Machinery Division, Department of
Biosystems Engineering, Shahid Chamran
University of Ahvaz, Ahvaz, Iran

Debabrata Sircar
Plant Molecular Biology Laboratory, Department
of Biotechnology, Indian Institute of Technology
Roorkee, Roorkee, Uttarakhand, India

Swetha Sunkar
Department of Bioinformatics, Sathyabama
Institute of Science and Technology, Chennai,
Tamil Nadu, India

Varunesh Sanjay Tambe
Shobhaben Pratapbhai Patel School of
Pharmacy & Technology Management,
SVKM's NMIMS, Mumbai, Maharashtra,
India

Jaya Krishna Tippabathani
Department of Biotechnology, Sathyabama
Institute of Science and Technology, Chennai,
Tamil Nadu, India

Hammad Ullah
Department of Pharmacy, School of Medicine
and Surgery, University of Naples Federico II,
Naples, Italy

C. Valli Nachiyar
Department of Biotechnology, Sathyabama Institute of Science and Technology, Chennai, Tamil Nadu, India

Laís Rosa Viana
Laboratory of Cancer and Nutrition, Department of Structural and Functional Biology, Institute of Biology, University of Campinas – UNICAMP, Campinas, São Paulo, Brazil

Sarika Wairkar
Shobhaben Pratapbhai Patel School of Pharmacy & Technology Management, SVKM's NMIMS, Mumbai, Maharashtra, India

Preface of Volume 1

Handbook of Nutraceuticals and Natural Products: Biological, Medicinal, and Nutritional Properties and Applications

Handbook of Nutraceuticals and Natural Products: Biological, Medicinal, and Nutritional Properties and Applications – Volume 1 presents logical data on the significance of nutraceuticals and natural food sources to human well-being and the likely mechanisms of nutraceuticals in the anticipation, treatment, and the executives of illnesses. This book comes when there is a pressing need to address the rising instances of metabolic illnesses and high rates of death coming about because of the absence of appropriate information or deviation from great dietary patterns. The overall population ought to comprehend what and why they ought to eat specific food sources or utilize specific dietary enhancements. This book fills this need while adjusting the confirmations of their well-being, advancing advantages and the related dangers. The worldwide interest for natural products and nutraceuticals has persistently advanced during that time with a projected worldwide nutraceutical market increasing from \$241 billion market in 2019 to \$373 billion out of 2025 at a build yearly development pace of 7.5%. The main section of this book has a bottom to top approach on nutraceuticals and functional foods, types, technology, mode of action and delivery, etc. Proof-based medical advantages of natural products as well as nutraceuticals are likewise introduced that are additionally examined in the succeeding sections. The accompanying sections are conversations of the various natural products and nutraceuticals, their sources, bioactive parts, medical advantages, and dangers. Additionally included are the rising regions of the business. Subjects on guidelines and security were likewise thought about. The contributors of this book are pioneers and experts in this area.

Handbook of Nutraceuticals and Natural Products, volume 1, compiles the data from experts in the field that potentiates the already established credibility of the earlier editions. In its two-volume format, it provides an authoritative summary of the types, varieties, and medicinal benefits of natural foods and nutraceuticals and their constituents that are linked to favorable health outcomes. Beginning with an overview of the field and associated regulations, each chapter describes the chemical properties, bioactivities, dietary sources, and evidence of these health-promoting dietary constituents.

Features:

- Bottom to top approach of various nutraceutical and natural products
- Chapters on bioavailability, delivery mechanisms, encapsulation of nutraceuticals, and natural products
- Includes current prospects of herbal nutrition

- Discusses antioxidant and anti-inflammatory activities of nutraceuticals and natural products
- Provides an update on the health benefits and requirements of protein and performance and therapeutic application and safety of products

The primary target of this book includes academicians, scientists working on natural product chemistry and nutraceuticals, research scholars, nutritionists, phytochemistry students, etc. Also, the general public will find this book valuable. The sections are all around considered and created utilizing basic English so that even the general public (not from scientific background) will be able to understand. Our sincere appreciation goes to the chapter contributors for their great contributions, patience, and cooperation during the editorial process. Their hard work and dedication have significantly contributed to the completion of this book.

1

Introduction to Nutraceuticals and Natural Products

Narges Shahgholian

Food Machinery Division, Department of Biosystems Engineering, Shahid Chamran University of Ahvaz, Ahvaz, Iran

1.1 Introduction

Actually, foods have important bioactive compounds and are the most powerful drugs. According to the old belief of Iranian physicians like Avicenna "Nutrients in small amounts are medicine, in the usual amounts are food and in large quantities are considered toxins for us."

"Focus on prevention rather than cure," which has also been considered in ancient texts, is the key point in the new trend of health considerations. This consciously driven point of view made intense desire to consume dietary supplements, functional food, multifunctional food, etc. Hippocrates (known as the father of medicines) said, "Let food be your medicine and let medicine be your food." (Kalra 2003). There is an ancient Chinese saying, "medicine and food are isogenic."

These foods could delay, manage, or prevent the premature onset of chronic diseases. Research indicates that diets high in fat may increase the risk of cardiovascular disease (CVDs), whereas diets containing plant sterols, omega-3 fatty acids, soluble fibers, or antioxidants may help in preventing these diseases (Shimizu 2003).

What is certain is that food and medicine can have both preventive and curative properties.

Many basic science and clinical researchers focus their research on using naturally occurring chemicals as drugs to treat disease and mitigating chronic inflammation by dietary means, with the goal to prevent the early stages of a pathological condition from progressing into disease (Ullah and Ahmad 2019).

It should be noted that there might be a lot of similar confusing words related to the term "nutraceuticals," such as phytochemicals, pharma foods, medical foods, functional foods, dietary supplements, designer foods, etc. There is a thin dividing line in their interchangeable usage by different people on different occasions. Pharmaceuticals are considered as medications used mainly to treat diseases, while nutraceuticals are the substances that are mostly considered to prevent diseases (Zhao 2007).

The nutraceuticals' revolution is becoming part of the mainstream medical discovery process.

Practitioners are now accepting nutraceuticals as part of the clinical treatment because of more and more scientific medical research.

Handbook of Nutraceuticals and Natural Products: Biological, Medicinal, and Nutritional Properties and Applications, Volume 1, First Edition. Edited by Sreerag Gopi and Preetha Balakrishnan.

1.2 Confrontation of Different Definitions of Nutraceuticals

It is better to ask first what "nutraceuticals" are?

The term "nutraceuticals" may be relatively unfamiliar and new, while people have been trusted with their ingredients for hundreds of years. The term "nutraceuticals" was coined by Stephen Defelice MD, founder and chairman of the foundation for innovation in medicine (FIM) Cranford, New Jersy, in 1989 (Brower 1998). According to terminology, "nutraceutical" is a hybrid word composed of "nutrition" (nourishing food) and "pharmaceutical" (component and a medical drug). According to Defelice, "Nutraceuticals are food or part of a food that provide(s) medical or health benefits including the prevention and/or treatment of a disease" (Chauhan et al. 2013). Since then, different definitions of nutraceuticals have been presented.

Health Canada defines a nutraceutical as "a product isolated or purified from foods, that is generally sold in medicinal forms not usually associated with food, is demonstrated to have a physiological benefit or provide protection against chronic disease" (Singh and Orsat 2014).

We come across different definitions of the term "nutraceuticals," each of which defines/interprets it to some extent. Here you can consider some definitions of nutraceuticals (which has nothing to do with the year of its expression):

1) A nutraceutical is something that has both nutritional and medical benefit. To this point, all foods could be considered nutraceuticals (Cao and Sutherland 2018).
2) Nutraceuticals are dietary supplements present in a nonfood matrix that deliver a concentrated form of NBCs from food and used for enhancing health in excess dosages that could be obtained from normal foods (Shahidi 2009; Zeisal 1999).
3) Nutraceuticals are dietary supplements utilized to ameliorate health, delay senescence, prevent diseases, and support the proper functioning of the human body (Sachdeva et al. 2020).
4) A nutraceutical is "a medicinal or nutritional component that includes a food, plant, purified or concentrated naturally occurring material that is used for the improvement of health, by preventing or treating a disease." (Lockwood 2007).
5) Nutraceuticals are food or part of food that provide(s) medical or health benefits including the prevention and/or treatment of a disease, maintaining health and acting against nutritionally induced acute and chronic diseases. Nutraceuticals, on the basis of their natural source, unlike medicine, have no side effects while consumed in certain doses (within their acceptable Recommended Dietary Intakes, thereby promoting optimal health, longevity, and quality of life) (Chauhan et al. 2013).
6) Karla proposed to redefine functional foods and nutraceuticals as the sole item of a meal or diet. While functional foods provides the body with the required amount of nutrients needed for its healthy survival (vitamins, fats, proteins, carbohydrates, etc.), nutraceuticals must not only supplement the diet but should also aid in the prevention and/or treatment of disease and/or disorder. Nutraceuticals are the same as functional foods used with specific-purpose aids in the prevention and/or treatment of disease(s) and/or disorder(s) other than anemia. Thus, functional food for one consumer can act as a nutraceutical for another one (Kalra 2003).
7) Modified in the definition of nutraceuticals: "Nutraceuticals developed from food, dietary substance, traditional herbal or mineral substance or their synthetic derivatives, which are delivered according to the pharmaceutical principles. They are prepared in dosage forms and manufactured under pharmaceutical principles and process controls to ensure the reproducibility and therapeutic efficacy of the product" (Pathak 2009).

What is clear is that most definitions refer to a specific dosage. Pharmaceutical dosage forms mean any forms of pills, tablets, capsules, liquid orals, lotions, delivery systems, as well as dermal preparations. What is certain is that nutraceuticals have gained attention due to nutrition and therapeutic potentials.

To cut a long story short, a general term for nutraceuticals is "food supplements." Another closely related term is "functional foods." It is a difference between nutraceuticals and functional foods. When a bioactive compound is added into a food formulation, it results into a new potential functional food, whereas the equivalent amount of the same substance in a tablet or capsule is considered a nutraceutical (Espín et al. 2007).

1.3 Natural Bioactive Compounds (NBCs)

"Natural bioactive compounds (NBCs)" refer to chemical substances found in nature and represent pharmacologically active agents with distinctive abilities to serve as novel lead compounds or pharmacophores in drug discovery. Some of the most effective drugs in clinical practice are derivatives of natural products (Ullah and Ahmad 2019).

NBCs include pigments (anthocyanins, carotenoids, lycopene, and chlorophyll), herbal polyphenols and flavonoids extract (ginger, garlic, tea, turmeric, etc.), essential oils and omegas, flavors, enzymes, vitamins and minerals, dietary compounds, bioactive peptides and different natural antioxidants. Fruits, vegetables, medicinal plants and other plant-based foods are rich in bioactive phytochemicals that may provide desirable health benefits beyond basic nutrition to decrease or delay the risk of chronic diseases. These compounds have different or similar properties to prevent, delay, or fight against different diseases in our bodies most of them related to inflammation.

NBCs with a broad diversity of chemically active agents and functionalities provide a marvelous collection of molecules for the production of nutraceuticals, functional foods, and food additives.

NBCs have the potential for the treatment and prevention of human diseases. In new researches, NBCs are still more important than ever. It is clear that NBCs are the future in the field of nutraceuticals. Dietary supplements, functional food, multifunctional food, with specific medicinal or health benefit, moreover nutritional effect, fall into this category.

1.3.1 Classification of NBCs (Focusing on a Few Applications)

Nutraceuticals can be classified on the basis of their natural sources (as the products obtained from plants, animals, minerals, or microbial sources), mechanism of action and pharmacological conditions, or as per the chemical constitution of the products.

Bioactive compounds are categorized into the herbal source and dietary supplements. Carbohydrates, proteins, minerals, vitamins, lipids, omegas, fibers, prebiotics and probiotics (synbiotics) and also mushrooms are put in the dietary supplements' group. Mushrooms themselves contain β-glucans, terpenes, and high bioavailable ergothioneine, selenium, vitamin B_1 and D_2 (Sachdeva et al. 2020). On the other hand, herbal sources and medicinal plants (as another group), contain important bioactive compounds like alkaloids, tannins, carotenoids, flavonoids, coumarins, lignans, phthalates, plant sterols, polyphenols, saponins, sulphides, and terpenoids (Sachdeva et al. 2020). In another classification, NBCs are classified on the basis of origin to plants, animals, and microbial groups (Singh and Orsat 2014) or the biological origins of the major nutraceuticals divided into three groups of human metabolites, plant constituents, and animal constituents (Lockwood 2015). Actually, phytochemicals and zoochemicals are the two most constituents derived from plants and animals, respectively. We will discuss some of these in the following sections.

1.3.1.1 Natural Products from Plants (NPFPs)

Plant-based diets confer considerable health benefits, partly attributable to their abundant micronutrient content (e.g. polyphenol) (Rodríguez-García et al. 2019). The bioactive phytochemicals have become a very significant source for nutraceutical ingredients (Espín et al. 2007). Different parts of seed, fruit, stem, and root or rhizomes of plants can be the source of NPFPs.

Some sources of NPFPs including different types of spices (turmeric, pepper, cinnamon), the premium ones are widely grown in India. Pomegranate, Saffron, Jujube, fig, and barberry have different kinds of NBCs, widely cultivated in Iran. Grape, date, nuts (walnut almond, hazelnut), oat, barley, cereals, legumes, olive, onion, garlic, ginger, tomato, algae, aloe vera, tea, coffee, different kind of medicinal plants (milk thistle, chamomile, thyme, clove, caraway, fennel flower, roselle,. . .), gums, and mucilages are among other products.

Polyphenolic compounds are classified into groups (their subcategory) such as stilbenes, flavonoids, phenolic acids, lignans, and others, which are present available in almost all plants. Polyphenols are characterized by high structural diversity and, consequently, a very broad spectrum of biological activities and have been proved to inhibit early stages of carcinogenesis in experimental models (Lewandowska et al. 2014).

Many bioactive compounds have been discovered. These compounds vary widely in chemical structure and function and are grouped accordingly. These include substances such as carotenoids, vitamin C, vitamin E, selenium, dietary fiber (and its components), dithiolthiones, isothiocyanates, indoles, phenols, protease inhibitors, allium compounds, plant sterols, and limonene (Kris-Etherton et al. 2002).

Various phytoestrogens are not only present in soy, but also in flaxseed oil, whole grains, fruits, and vegetables. However, phytoestrogens act both as partial estrogen agonists and antagonists; so, their effects on cancer are likely complex. Hydroxytyrosol is one of many phenolics found in olives and olive oil. Resveratrol is found in nuts, grape wine and red wine, lycopene in tomato, isothiocyanates in cruciferous vegetables, monoterpenes in citrus fruits, cherries, and herbs, and organosulfur compounds in onion and garlic.

Lignans, which possess a steroid-like chemical structure and are defined as phytoestrogens, are of particular interest to researchers (Rodríguez-García et al. 2019).

1.3.1.2 Natural Products from Animals (NPFAs)

Animal-based nutraceuticals nowadays have received great attention. Some sources of NPFAs include honey, royal gel, propolis (actually containing plant-derived compounds), bee or snake venom, camel milk, quail egg, meat, poultry, fish and sea products.

These include substances such as conjugated linoleic acids (CLA), n-3-Polyunsaturated fatty acids (PUFAs), chondroitin, glucosamine, vitamin B_{12}, minerals (Zn, Ca, and Se), coenzyme Q10, melatonin, creatine, taurine, carnitine, choline, glucosamine, chondroitin, sphingolipids, chondroitin, methylsulfonylmethane, and S-adenosyl methionine (Singh and Orsat 2014). Collagen and gelatin gained from bone and skin (of cow, fish, and poultry), lecithin from eggs, branched-chain amino acids from milk and meat, and conjugated fatty acids from the fish liver are limited examples of bioactive compounds originated from animal sources. It is worth mentioning that minerals can be extracted from animal or mine sources.

Fish oil is known as a source of omega-3 fatty acids, docosahexaenoic acid (DHA), and eicosapentaenoic acid (EPA). EPA- and DHA-specific diets are good dietary options for an anti-inflammatory disease like different types of lung disease progressions (Hwang and Ho 2018).

NPFAs could be considered as important functional foods for patients with respiratory diseases (such as omega-3 fatty acids and heparin) because of their potential in disrupting procollagen or extracellular matrix deposition (Hwang and Ho 2018).

1.3.1.3 Microbial-based Products

Different kinds of edible yeast and lactic acid bacteria, like *Saccharomyces, Bifidobacterium, Lactobacillus, and Bacillus* fall into this group (Lockwood 2015). Microbial source are used directly as nutraceuticals or target products obtained by fermentation or biotechnological processing of them.

Microbes are used in the production of food flavors, bacteriocins, carotenoids, flavonoids and terpenoids, xylitol and other polyols, prebiotic oligosaccharides, polyunsaturated fatty acids, enzymes, organic acids for use in food, viable probiotic cells, and amino acids and their derivatives for use in foods, nutraceuticals, and medications (Gupta et al. 2011).

Bacteriocins are heat-stable antimicrobial peptides and produced by various bacteria such as food-grade lactic acid bacteria (LAB). They have a huge potential of not only being used as food preservatives but also as next-generation antibiotics targeting drug-resistant pathogens (Perez et al. 2014).

LAB produces and enhances the uptake of folic acid, increases iron absorption by optimization of pH in the digestive tract and activates enzyme phytases. Some LAB species are antidiabetic, antiobesity, antiallergy, anticancer and have the property of improving the immune system. Diterpenoid of taxol and glutaminase, known as anticancer agents, are produced as a result of microbial fermentation. Bacterial cells are also genetically modified to produce large quantities of human insulin (Gupta et al. 2011).

Microbial Xanthan, Levan, Gellan, and Curdlan classified as food additives are another example of microbial production (Ateş and Oner 2017).

Fibrinolytic enzymes are a special type of proteases that can degrade the fibrin mesh of blood clots. These are used in cardiovascular diseases. Fibrinolytics have bacterial strain origins such as *B. subtilis*. Fibrinolytic enzymes are accessible from Japanese food (natto), salt-fermented Japanese food (Skipjack), Asian fermented shrimp paste, Chinese soybean-fermented food (Douchi), Indonesian fermented-soybean food (tempeh), Korean fermented food (Doen-jang), Korean salty fermented fish (Jeot-gal), parboiled wheat and milk (kishk), traditional fermented pickled vegetables (kimchi) and edible mushrooms (Kotb 2017).

1.3.2 Extraction of NBCs

Bioactive compounds are often synthesized in small quantities in fruits, vegetables, whole grains, etc. They are present as conjugates or mixtures in extracts that need labor-intensive and time-consuming purification procedures (Lam 2007). The processing of nutraceuticals can be divided into four steps, namely pretreatment, extraction, isolation/purification, and encapsulation (Routray and Orsat 2012).

New technologies for the extraction of NBCs could provide an innovative approach to increase the production of intended compounds for use as nutraceuticals or as ingredients in the design of functional foods. These advanced technologies include pressurized-liquid extraction, subcritical and supercritical extractions, microwave- and ultrasound-assisted extractions, which are even efficient for extracting materials in low concentrations (Joana Gil-Chávez et al. 2013).

1.4 Nutraceuticals and Their Role in Human Health

It has been known for years the health-promoting effects of foods, natural products in foods, and their derivatives. The existence of specific NBCs and biologically active compounds in phytochemical and animal or microbial extracts gives them specific properties from strengthening the immune system to cure and prevent life-threatening diseases like cerebral stroke, cancers, hypertension, heart diseases, and neurodegenerative disorders. Other properties which are attributed to this compound include antibacterial, antidiabetic, antitumor, antifungal, antithrombotic, and antiviral activities.

The most important factors causing different types of diseases are related to inflammation and those directly related to the accumulation of free radicals and toxic substances in the body. The buildup of free radicals damages over one's lifetime.

Although a diet rich in fruits and vegetables helps maintain health, but little information is available about the biological effects of individual food components and the effects of their metabolites and derivatives (Ullah and Ahmad 2019).

Factors affecting the formation of free radicals within the body include radiation, environmental stress, or the normal process of mitochondria and cells. As you grow older, your body's ability to fight against oxidative damage decreases and subsequently neutralization of the effect of generated free radicals decreases (Cao and Sutherland 2018).

Antioxidants can protect the living cells from oxidative damage usually due to free radicals. Antioxidants are divided into two groups: enzymatic (endogenous) and nonenzymatic (exogenous), counteracting the adverse effects of age-associated diseases (Garg et al. 2018).

Within the body, there exist a number of enzymatic antioxidants, such as superoxide dismutase (SOD), glutathione peroxidase (GPx), peroxidase glutathione reductase (GR), and catalase (CAT), most of which have the ability to directly scavenge the superoxide radicals and hydrogen peroxide, convert them into hydrogen peroxide, and then into water/less reactive species (Garg et al. 2018).

However, another interested group of antioxidant are nonenzymatic antioxidants. Many of these have large phenolic groups to engage the effect of the free electrons in the radicals. Different types of vitamins, minerals, or enzymes can fall into this category. These exogenous antioxidants include dietary antioxidants such as polyphenols, lipoic acid, acetylcarnitine, and sulfur-containing amino acids such as L-cysteine and N-acetylcysteine (NAC). Vitamin E, vitamin C, flavonoids, glutathione, CoQ_{10}, and beta-carotene are other examples of nutraceutical antioxidants. These molecules can help clear the body of these oxygen radical waste products (Cao and Sutherland 2018; Garg et al. 2018).

Here are a few limited examples of using dietary supplements originated from natural compounds.

A dietary supplement is believed to supply nutrients that may not be consumed in sufficient quantities.

Some of the well-known antioxidants in grains and fruits are chocolate and derivatives from the cocoa bean, pomegranates, berries, such as blueberries and cranberries, which contain the highest concentrations of phenolic antioxidants. Plants produce these molecules to protect themselves against their forms of oxidative damages. These phenolic compounds, such as catechin and procyanidin (in the group of flavonoids) are composed of tricyclic structures that act as free radical scavengers during periods of oxidative stress (Cao and Sutherland 2018). Both catechin and epicatechin have shown an increase in nitric oxide production, impacting the vascular endothelium, and these polyphenols have also shown an anti-inflammatory function (Cao and Sutherland 2018).

Products such as green tea and omega-3 fatty acids are taken for weight loss and cardiovascular health (Perez et al. 2018).

Quercetin belongs to the flavonols group, is a popular dietary antioxidant present in tea, fruits, and vegetables, exhibits significant heart-related benefits as inhibition of LDL oxidation, reduction of adhesion molecules and other inflammatory markers, and prevents neuronal oxidative and inflammatory damage, and platelet anti-aggregant effects. Experimental *in vivo* evidence in human has validated the cardioprotective effects of quercetin (Patel et al. 2018).

Dietary intake of lignan-rich foods could be a useful way to bolster the prevention of chronic illness, such as certain types of cancers and cardiovascular disease (Rodríguez-García et al. 2019).

Stress is quite common in a person's life nowadays and may occur repeatedly. You may either allow the stress to cause suffering to your body or you may opt to do something about it. An adequately balanced diet plan to our routine will help us conquer any challenges offered by stress that we may come across. Stress and poor eating habits can be accompanied by relations to nutritional deficiencies. Magnesium deficiencies are associated with stress personality problems. If you are undergoing a surge of stress for a long span, then it is suggested to consume plentiful of magnesium- and calcium-rich foods or diet. Bone-strengthening nutrients, in particular, are calcium, magnesium, and vitamins D and K (Bagchi et al. 2015).

In China, licorice is the second most prescribed herb. Compounds of this plant root are effective against forms of LDL oxidation. LDL oxidation is a key factor in the early formation of atherosclerotic lesions and licorice may be used to curb or prevent such processes (Cao and Sutherland 2018).

Sulfur-containing amino acids not only act as precursors of protein but also are antioxidant compounds and important to maintain physiological redox conditions inside or outside of the cell. The thiol group of methionine chelates lead from tissues and protects the brain from oxidative stress. Cysteine, methionine, reduced glutathione, and whey protein contains sulfur in its structure (Garg et al. 2018).

Flaxseed, sesame, rye, barley, prunus, and butterbur have lignin. They were found to have antioxidant, anticancer, antiatherosclerosis, anti-inflammatory, and neuroprotective activities in animal experiments, although extensive studies to prove the clinical efficacy remain to be carried out. Among the lignan, hydroxypinoresinol displays more powerful antioxidant activity than pinoresinol glucoside or pinoresinol with respect to more hydroxyl groups (Sok et al. 2009).

Recently, the use of zinc in the prevention and treatment of flu and colds has gained great attention as its importance in maintaining the health of the immune system is well established (Haase and Rink 2014).

The recent coronavirus disease 2019 (COVID-19) outbreak, cause mild to severe symptoms such as flu-like disease, and acute respiratory syndrome. Researchers have shown the importance of the role of micronutrients (zinc, folate, vitamin D) as complementary components of treatment regimens and boosting immune system. Akhtar et al. (2021), have presented a systematic literature review to identify nutritional interventions for preventing or helping in the recovery from COVID-19.

1.5 Types of Formulated Nutraceuticals

Many formulated nutraceutical supplements can be found in a widely broad range (different dosages) in most commercial nutraceutical products on the market.

The formulated nutraceuticals are basically available in the market in two types of general formulations:

1) Non-specified constituents: containing a complex constituent profile, non-fractionated extracts (may contain up to 70%, neither fully elucidated by the manufacturer, nor evaluated for biological activity). Nutraceuticals can be whole food products such as *spirulina* in tablet form.

2) Specified constituents: containing any single-constituent can be found in widely varying labelled ranges of contents (for example, the resveratrol content may be claimed to be present from 10 to 500 mg in different products). The nutraceutical compound(s) in the dietary supplements may be concentrated to provide the claimed health benefits put into this group (e.g., pigment extracted from microalgae) (Espín et al. 2007; Islam et al. 2017).

Reports have shown varying quality or poor compliance in both mentioned groups. Lack of label compliance is even more pronounced for complex materials such as soy, containing substandard levels of isoflavones. This may have occurred as a result of improper manufacturing or breakdown of the constituents like creatine (Singh and Orsat 2014).

1.6 Combination of NBCs

Buckminster Fuller (1968) said, "*Universe is synergetic. Life is synergetic*" (Pezzani et al. 2019).

Synergy is broadly defined as the interaction of two or more substances to produce a combined effect greater than the sum of their separate portions. Contrary to synergy, antagonistic effects of two compounds are less than the simple sum of the single effects. They can be considered a straight strategy that has evolved by nature to obtain more efficacy at a low cost.

The question is whether combination therapies are more effective and safe in comparison to a single therapy in controlling severe inflammation or not?

Different methodologies have been developed to study plant–drug interactions, such as the isobologram method of Berenbaum and Loewe, the fractional product method of Webb and the combination index method of Chou and Talalay. Interactions are derived from physiological and pathological individual differences, such as age, gender, inter-individual variances in drug metabolism and the presence of comorbidities in elderly patients (Pezzani et al. 2019).

1.6.1 Synergism and Beneficial Products

It has been assumed that a combination of antioxidants acting at multiple levels is more effective than any single antioxidant. For example, sulfur-containing amino acids along with other antioxidants have pronounced and synergistic protective effects against various metabolic and age-related neurological disorders (Garg et al. 2018).

It has been shown clear that effectiveness of natural polyphenols as cancer-preventive and therapeutic agents resulting from their synergy with synthetic or semisynthetic anticancer drugs as well as with other phenolic compounds of plant origin (Lewandowska et al. 2014).

It is confirmed that the hypothesis of whole grain fiber consumption is associated with a reduced mortality risk in comparison to a similar amount of refined grain fiber (Jacobs et al. 2000).

Evidence shows that piperine enhances the technological or physiological performance of curcumin (found in turmeric). These properties attributed to a decrease in lipid peroxidation in meat and enhancement of the anticancer or neuroprotective effect of curcumin (Abdul Manap et al. 2019; Bolat et al. 2020; Zhang et al. 2015).

The experimental studies in a rat have shown that extracts from Indian celery seed and the NZ green-lipped mussel are powerful nutraceuticals that amplify the potency of salicylates and prednisone for treating pre-established chronic inflammation of arthritis and brosis (Whitehouse and Butters 2003).

1.6.2 Antagonism and Detrimental Products

Despite their food and health applications, plant-based bioactive compounds contain different level of phytotoxic compounds. For example flaxseeds contain linatine, phytic acids, protease inhibitors, and cyanogenic glycosides. Epidemiological studies have shown that poor bioavailability of coessential nutrients containing these compounds can lead to health complications. These components must be removed or inactivated to render flaxseeds safe for consumption (Dzuvor et al. 2018).

Some key issues such as bioavailability, metabolism, dose/response, and toxicity of food bioactive compounds and nutraceuticals have not been well established yet (Espín et al. 2007).

1.7 Quality of Nutraceuticals and Manufacturing Process

Growing worldwide demand for plant-derived medicines in developing countries for their primary healthcare is related to inexpensive process economics and the lack of stringent product governance associated with the exploitation of traditional plant. The hurdles of large-scale application of traditional plant medicines related to lack of traceability in the supply chain, lack of effective quality assurance in the manufacturing processes and inefficient identification of molecular species that affect the therapeutic efficacy of the final product. To overcome these challenges, the implementation of hazards analysis and critical control point in the manufacturing process has been suggested (Pan et al. 2013).

Better and more effective execution of the good manufacturing process/plants (GMP) norms in the long-term is accessible and applicable by incorporating Quality by Design (QbD) which can be an impetus for industries to gradually make their manufacturing facilities compliant with cGMPs, hazard analysis critical control point (HACCP), and process analytical technology (PAT) tools. The FDA defines PAT as a system for the analysis and control of manufacturing processes based on timely measurements of critical quality parameters and performance attributes of raw materials and in-process materials, involving the application of process analytical chemistry tools, feedback process-control strategies, information management tools, and/or product-process optimization strategies for the manufacturing of pharmaceuticals (Pan et al. 2013).

In countries where control is less effective, patients may be at risk through the production of inadequate quality drugs. The application of the total quality system for the production of pharmaceuticals was proposed as a process for a probable integration of "Six Sigma methodology" to large-scale production. (Nandi et al. 2014).

1.8 Biorefinery and Sustainable Source of Nutraceuticals

There is an increasing need and growing demand for green, sustainable and eco-friendly products. Phenolic compounds are easily accessible low-cost sources like wastes from agri-food processing. Natural phenolic compounds have become increasingly attractive from the technological point of view (Panzella et al. 2020). As an example, the effective utilization of sesame and other byproducts in food supplements and the nutraceuticals industry could provide a way of valorization in the transition to becoming more sustainable (Mekky et al. 2019). Microalgae and Seaweed pigments and microbial gums are limited example of sustainable sources of nutraceuticals.

1.9 Encapsulation of Nutraceuticals

The matter of solubility, oxidation, odor and organoleptic issues are the major obstacles to use some NBCs, especially herbal medicines. The design of the delivery systems depends on the physicochemical properties of the nutraceuticals and functional food components. Ingredients prone to deterioration, unpleasant odor and lack of compatibility to their specific medium must be properly formulated (Le and Pathak 2011).

Seeking new methods of formulation has aided the growth of the nutraceuticals industry.

Microencapsulation is an inclusion technique for confining a bioactive substance (such as phytochemicals) into a polymeric matrix by virtue of which the encapsulated compound becomes more stable and protected than its isolated or free form (Shahgholian and Rajabzadeh 2016). Encapsulation of ingredients is one promising way to improve the solubilization of compounds with low solubility, to mask some bitter taste or unpleasant smell, or even formulation of slow-release supplement with edible cross-linking agents such as genipin (Shahgholian et al. 2017) or even stabilization of sensitive materials.

Delivery systems that will maintain their bioavailability and efficacy of NBCs during processing until they are delivered to the physiological target within humans are important in both the food and pharmaceutical industries. Meanwhile, the use of natural and biocompatible materials for encapsulating and preventing their deterioration, their uptake in the organism, and their controlled release are another important issue (Bochicchio et al. 2016).

The new generation of nutraceuticals in the form of micro- and nanocapsules has overcome the barriers to consumption of these products. Biopolymers have been used commonly for safe and efficient transport and release of drug at the intended site. The most widely used encapsulation methods include preparation either from preformed polymers (methods such as nanoprecipitation, salting-out, solvent evaporation, ionotropic gelation) or from the polymerization of monomers (radical polymerization, interfacial polymerization,. . .) (George et al. 2019). Various techniques are employed to form the capsules, including extrusion coating, fluidized bed coating, liposome entrapment, coacervation, spray drying, spray chilling or spray cooling, inclusion complexation, centrifugal extrusion, and rotational suspension separation (Gibbs et al. 1999).

As a new approach in nanoformulation of nutraceuticals, an ultrasonic oscillator to generate aerosols of less than 1 μm is recommended. Researchers successively prepared nanopowder in a one-step procedure using an ultrasonic oscillator without need for surfactant. In this work, CN was incorporated into the spherical albumin-based nanocarrier. This method offers priorities over the other methods, due to its relative simplicity, low cost, and ease of collecting the produced product. The strategy is applicable to a vast range of low-viscose biopolymers, allows the design of more sophisticated structures with control over their composition and size (Shahgholian and Rajabzadeh 2019).

The nanoformulations can overcome the problems that persisted in the old-style herbal remedies. These formulated doses have a higher therapeutic index compared to the earlier phytochemicals and herbal remedies (Kumar and Sharma 2018). Size reduction offers several advantages over larger particles, comprising larger surface area, which may affect dissolution rate and mass transfer from the particles into the surrounding medium. Bioavailability, pharmacokinetics, pharmacodynamics, and therapeutic index of nano-formulated nutraceuticals have been improved and enhanced in comparison with common commercial formulation.

1.10 Nutraceuticals – Global Market Scenario

It is challenging to predict the size of the nutraceuticals market. For a long time, every country had its own system of products, that had both nutritional and medicinal values (Le and Pathak 2011). A different definition of nutraceuticals creates confusion of accurate statistics of the global market. In some scientific documents terms, such as nutraceutical food, nutraceutical beverages, and nutraceutical supplements are used together and no distinction is made between them.

Some of the most common compounds in nutraceuticals available in the market are lignan extract flax, fenugreek galactomannan, green tea extract, ω-3 FA, DHA, EPA, carotenoids, soybean phytoestrogen, lutein esters, and probiotics (Bagchi et al. 2015).

In a larger perspective, it has been estimated that more than 80% of people in Africa and Asia and 60–70% of the American population are using herbal medicines, together with an increasing number in developed countries (Zhao 2007).

According to the markets report from "Transparency Market Research" the global nutraceuticals market has increased so significantly that it is predicted to reach a value of US\$278.96 billion by 2021 as stated (Nutraceuticals Market 2015).

The global market for nutraceutical is huge i.e. approximately USD 117 billion (Sachdeva et al. 2020).

1.11 Regulations and Health Claims

Nutraceuticals, in contrast to pharmaceuticals, are substances, which usually have not patent protection and generally do not need testing documents, while pharmaceutical compounds need expensive testing documents and have governmental sanction (Chauhan et al. 2013).

The common false perception that "all natural medicines are good" creates the wrong image of "cure preference" in the mind of common patients around nutraceuticals (Kalra 2003). However, according to research results, caution should be exercised in the excessive use of supplements and nutraceuticals.

1.12 Conclusion

The trend toward eating all-natural ingredients promotes the use of healthful products such as natural functional foods and nutraceuticals. *"Nutraceuticals"* and *"functional foods"* are two new terms used to describe health-promoting foods or their extracted components. *Functional foods* are products that are consumed as foods and not in dosage form while *nutraceuticals* are formulated and taken in dosage form (capsules, tinctures, or tablets). Nutraceutical efficacy depends on source, dose, and the right combination of ingredients. These benefits have been associated, at least partially, due to some of the phytochemical constituents, and, in particular, to polyphenols (Espín et al. 2007). The prevention of various chronic diseases, cardiovascular diseases, and cancer is attributed to their antioxidant activity (Rodríguez-García et al. 2019).

Microencapsulation is a promising approach to overcome the limiting factors and removes barriers to the effective consumption of bioactive compounds. Bioavailability, pharmacokinetics, pharmacodynamics, and therapeutic index of encapsulated bioactive compounds or supplements have been improved and enhanced in comparison with common commercial formulations. Formulators should be aware of the target consumer of different types. Currently, dozens of physiologically active components are under investigation for their potential role in disease prevention and health promotion.

References

Abdul Manap, A.S., Tan, A.C.W., Leong, W.H. et al. (2019). Synergistic effects of curcumin and piperine as potent acetylcholine and amyloidogenic inhibitors with significant neuroprotective activity in SH-SY5Y cells via computational molecular modeling and in vitro assay. *Frontiers in Aging Neuroscience* 11: 206.

Akhtar, S., Das, J.K., Ismail, T. et al. (2021). Nutritional perspectives for the prevention and mitigation of COVID-19. *Nutrition Reviews* 79 (3): 289–300.

Ateş, O. and Oner, E.T. (2017). Microbial xanthan, levan, gellan, and curdlan as food additives. In: *Microbial Functional Foods and Nutraceuticals* (eds. V.K. Gupta, H. Treichel, V. Shapaval, et al.), 149–174. Hoboken, NJ: Wiley.

Bagchi, D., Preuss, H.G., and Swaroop, A. (2015). *Nutraceuticals and Functional Foods in Human Health and Disease Prevention*. CRC Press.

Bochicchio, S., Barba, A.A., Grassi, G., and Lamberti, G. (2016). Vitamin delivery: carriers based on nanoliposomes produced via ultrasonic irradiation. *LWT-Food Science and Technology* 69: 9–16.

Bolat, Z.B., Islek, Z., Demir, B.N. et al. (2020). Curcumin-and piperine-loaded emulsomes as combinational treatment approach enhance the anticancer activity of Curcumin on HCT116 colorectal cancer model. *Frontiers in Bioengineering and Biotechnology* 8: 50.

Brower, V. (1998). Nutraceuticals: poised for a healthy slice of the healthcare market? *Nature Biotechnology* 16 (8): 728–731.

Cao, C. and Sutherland, K. (2018). *Antioxidant Nutraceuticals: Historical Perspective and Applications in Various Traditional Systems Worldwide Antioxidant Nutraceuticals*, 1–24. CRC Press.

Chauhan, B., Kumar, G., Kalam, N., and Ansari, S.H. (2013). Current concepts and prospects of herbal nutraceutical: a review. *Journal of Advanced Pharmaceutical Technology & Research* 4 (1): 4.

Dzuvor, C.K.O., Taylor, J.T., Acquah, C. et al. (2018). Bioprocessing of functional ingredients from flaxseed. *Molecules* 23 (10): 2444.

Espín, J.C., García-Conesa, M.T., and Tomás-Barberán, F.A. (2007). Nutraceuticals: facts and fiction. *Phytochemistry* 68 (22–24): 2986–3008.

Garg, G., Singh, A.K., Singh, S., and Rizvi, S.I. (2018). Anti-aging effects of sulfur-containing amino acids and nutraceuticals. In: *Nutraceuticals and Natural Product Derivatives: Disease Prevention & Drug Discovery* (eds. M.F. Ullah and A. Ahmad), 25–38. Hoboken, NJ: Wiley.

George, A., Shah, P.A., and Shrivastav, P.S. (2019). Natural biodegradable polymers based nanoformulations for drug delivery: a review. *International Journal of Pharmaceutics* 561: 244–264.

Gibbs, F., Kermasha, S., Alli, I. et al. (1999). Encapsulation in the food industry: a review. *International Journal of Food Sciences and Nutrition* 50 (3): 213–224.

Gupta, C., Garg, A.P., Prakash, D. et al. (2011). Microbes as potential source of biocolours. *Pharmacologyonline* 2: 1309–1318.

Haase, H. and Rink, L. (2014). Multiple impacts of zinc on immune function. *Metallomics* 6 (7): 1175–1180.

Hwang, Y.-Y. and Ho, Y.-S. (2018). Nutraceutical support for respiratory diseases. *Food Science and Human Wellness* 7 (3): 205–208.

Islam, M.N., Alsenani, F., and Schenk, P.M. (2017). Microalgae as a sustainable source of nutraceuticals. In: *Microbial Functional Foods and Nutraceuticals* (eds. V.K. Gupta, H. Treichel, V. Shapaval, et al.), 1–19. Hoboken, NJ: Wiley.

Jacobs, D.R. Jr., Pereira, M.A., Meyer, K.A., and Kushi, L.H. (2000). Fiber from whole grains, but not refined grains, is inversely associated with all-cause mortality in older women: the Iowa women's health study. *Journal of the American College of Nutrition* 19 (sup3): 326S–330S.

Joana Gil-Chávez, G., Villa, J.A., Fernando Ayala-Zavala, J. et al. (2013). Technologies for extraction and production of bioactive compounds to be used as nutraceuticals and food ingredients: an overview. *Comprehensive Reviews in Food Science and Food Safety* 12 (1): 5–23.

Kalra, E.K. (2003). Nutraceutical-definition and introduction. *AAPS Pharmscience* 5 (3): 27–28.

Kotb, E. (2017). Microbial fibrinolytic enzyme production and applications. *Microbial Functional Foods and Nutraceuticals* 13: 175.

Kris-Etherton, P.M., Hecker, K.D., Bonanome, A. et al. (2002). Bioactive compounds in foods: their role in the prevention of cardiovascular disease and cancer. *The American Journal of Medicine* 113 (9): 71–88.

Kumar, R. and Sharma, M. (2018). Herbal nanomedicine interactions to enhance pharmacokinetics, pharmacodynamics, and therapeutic index for better bioavailability and biocompatibility of herbal formulations. *Journal of Materials NanoScience* 5 (1): 35–60.

Lam, K.S. (2007). New aspects of natural products in drug discovery. *Trends in Microbiology* 15 (6): 279–289.

Le, U. and Pathak, Y. (2011). Nutraceuticals. In: *Handbook of Nutraceuticals Volume II: Scale-Up, Processing and Automation*, vol. 2 (ed. Y. Pathak), 1. CRC Press.

Lewandowska, U., Gorlach, S., Owczarek, K. et al. (2014). Synergistic interactions between anticancer chemotherapeutics and phenolic compounds and anticancer synergy between polyphenols. *Postepy Higieny i Medycyny Doswiadczalnej (Online)* 68: 528–540.

Lockwood, B. (2007). *Nutraceuticals: A Guide for Healthcare Professionals*. London; Grayslake, Ill: Pharmaceutical Press.

Lockwood, G.B. (2015). Quality evaluation and safety of commercially available nutraceutical and formulated products. In: *Nutraceutical and Functional Food Processing Technology* (ed. J.I. Boye), 113–150. Wiley. ISBN 978-1-118-50494-9.

Mekky, R.H., Abdel-Sattar, E., Segura-Carretero, A., and Contreras, M.d.M. (2019). Phenolic compounds from sesame cake and antioxidant activity: a new insight for agri-food residues' significance for sustainable development. *Foods* 8 (10): 432.

Nandi, A., Pan, S., Potumarthi, R. et al. (2014). A proposal for six sigma integration for large-scale production of penicillin g and subsequent conversion to 6-APA. *Journal of Analytical Methods in Chemistry* 2014: 1–10.

Pan, S., Neeraj, A., Srivastava, K.S. et al. (2013). A proposal for a quality system for herbal products. *Journal of Pharmaceutical Sciences* 102 (12): 4230–4241.

Panzella, L., Moccia, F., Nasti, R. et al. (2020). Bioactive phenolic compounds from agri-food wastes: an update on green and sustainable extraction methodologies. *Frontiers in Nutrition* 7: 1–27.

Patel, R.V., Mistry, B.M., Shinde, S.K. et al. (2018). Therapeutic potential of quercetin as a cardiovascular agent. *European Journal of Medicinal Chemistry* 155: 889–904.

Pathak, Y.V. (2009). *Handbook of Nutraceuticals Volume I: Ingredients, Formulations, and Applications*, vol. 1. CRC Press.

Perez, R.H., Zendo, T., and Sonomoto, K. (2014). Novel bacteriocins from lactic acid bacteria (LAB): various structures and applications. Paper presented at the Microbial cell factories.

Perez, A., Nguyen, R., Valladares, A., and Pathak, S. (2018). *Antioxidant Nutraceuticals: Present Market and Future Trends*, 25–35. CRC Press.

Pezzani, R., Salehi, B., Vitalini, S. et al. (2019). Synergistic effects of plant derivatives and conventional chemotherapeutic agents: an update on the cancer perspective. *Medicina* 55 (4): 110.

Reportlinker (2015). Nutraceuticals market – global industry analysis, size, share, growth and forecast 2015–2021. https://www.reportlinker.com/p03989925/Nutraceuticals-Market-Global-Industry-Analysis-Size-Share-Growth-and-Forecast.html.

Rodríguez-García, C., Sánchez-Quesada, C., Toledo, E. et al. (2019). Naturally lignan-rich foods: a dietary tool for health promotion? *Molecules* 24 (5): 917.

Routray, W. and Orsat, V. (2012). Microwave-assisted extraction of flavonoids: a review. *Food and Bioprocess Technology* 5 (2): 409–424.

Sachdeva, V., Roy, A., and Bharadvaja, N. (2020). Current prospects of nutraceuticals: a review. *Current Pharmaceutical Biotechnology* 21: 1–13.

Shahgholian, N. and Rajabzadeh, G. (2016). Fabrication and characterization of curcumin-loaded albumin/gum arabic coacervate. *Food Hydrocolloids* 59: 17–25.

Shahgholian, N. and Rajabzadeh, G. (2019). Preparation of BSA nanoparticles and its binary compounds via ultrasonic piezoelectric oscillator for curcumin encapsulation. *Journal of Drug Delivery Science and Technology* 54: 101323.

Shahgholian, N., Rajabzadeh, G., and Malaekeh-Nikouei, B. (2017). Preparation and evaluation of BSA-based hydrosol nanoparticles cross-linked with genipin for oral administration of poorly water-soluble curcumin. *International Journal of Biological Macromolecules* 104: 788–798.

Shahidi, F. (2009). Nutraceuticals and functional foods: whole versus processed foods. *Trends in Food Science & Technology* 20 (9): 376–387.

Shimizu, T. (2003). Health claims on functional foods: the Japanese regulations and an international comparison. *Nutrition Research Reviews* 16 (2): 241–252.

Singh, A. and Orsat, V. (2014). Key considerations in the selection of ingredients and processing technologies for functional foods and nutraceutical products. In: *Nutraceutical and Functional Food Processing Technology* (ed. J.I. Boye), 79–111. Wiley.

Sok, D.-E., Cui, H.S., and Kim, M.R. (2009). Isolation and boactivities of furfuran type lignan compounds from edible plants. *Recent Patents on Food, Nutrition & Agriculture* 1 (1): 87–95.

Ullah, M.F. and Ahmad, A. (2019). *Nutraceuticals and Natural Product Derivatives: Disease Prevention & Drug Discovery*. Wiley.

Whitehouse, M. and Butters, D. (2003). Combination anti-inflammatory therapy: synergism in rats of NSAIDs/corticosteroids with some herbal/animal products. *Inflammopharmacology* 11 (4–6): 453–464.

Zeisal, S.H. (1999). Regulation of Nutraceuticals. *Science* 285: 1853–1855.

Zhang, Y., Henning, S.M., Lee, R.-P. et al. (2015). Turmeric and black pepper spices decrease lipid peroxidation in meat patties during cooking. *International Journal of Food Sciences and Nutrition* 66 (3): 260–265.

Zhao, J. (2007). Nutraceuticals, nutritional therapy, phytonutrients, and phytotherapy for improvement of human health: a perspective on plant biotechnology application. *Recent Patents on Biotechnology* 1 (1): 75–97.

2

Functional Nutraceuticals: Past, Present, and Future

A.Y. Onaolapo[1] and O.J. Onaolapo[2]

[1] *Behavioural Neuroscience Unit, Neurobiology Subdivision, Department of Anatomy, Ladoke Akintola University of Technology, Ogbomosho, Oyo State, Nigeria*
[2] *Behavioural Neuroscience Unit, Neuropharmacology Subdivision, Department of Pharmacology, Ladoke Akintola University of Technology, Ogbomosho, Oyo State, Nigeria*

2.1 Introduction

In the twenty-first century, a rapidly increasing knowledge on the complex relationships that link nutrition, health and disease is revolutionizing how people think about food, food production, and food consumption (McGrattan et al. 2019; Venter et al. 2020). From time immemorial, plants have been very important sources of human food and medicines. In recent years, the awareness that diet and dietary practices not only impact the development of single-nutrient deficiencies but are also linked to the epidemic of chronic diseases that are now occurring globally is causing a paradigm shift leading to the emergence of concepts such as functional foods and nutraceuticals (Ramadan and Al-Ghamdi 2012; Ramalingum and Mahomoodally 2014; Kumar et al. 2018). There is strong evidence of the health benefits as well as increasing advocacy for adopting dietary patterns such as the Mediterranean diet, in addition to dietary approaches to stop chronic disorders such as hypertension. The benefits are not limited to the ability of such dietary patterns to prevent/reduce the incidence of hypertension, obesity and metabolic diseases, but also extend to their effects on the immune system, the brain, and the prevention of aging-related body systems decline (Zhao 2007; Onaolapo et al. 2011, 2012; Onaolapo and Onaolapo 2012, 2019, 2020; Nasri et al. 2014; Mollica et al. 2017a, b, 2018; Solfrizzi et al. 2017; Onaolapo et al. 2017, 2019a, b, 2020a, b; Abbatecola et al. 2018; Chen et al. 2019; McGrattan et al. 2019; Román et al. 2019; Ezra-Nevo et al. 2020; Venter et al. 2020).

Since the term "nutraceuticals" was coined (Brower 1998; Kalra 2003) to emphasize the potential of food as both nutrition and drug, the need to consume natural plant-based foods and the use of phytotherapy/nutritional therapy in the improvement of health and prevention/treatment of diseases (Raskin et al. 2002; Zhao 2007; Trottier et al. 2010; Nasri et al. 2014) have become globally popular trends (Melina et al. 2016).

Nutraceuticals have been defined as food or parts of food that provide(s) medical and/or health benefits including the prevention and/or treatment of disease (Brower 1998; Kalra 2003; Chauhan et al. 2013; Onaolapo et al. 2019a) and functional foods are described as ordinary foods with components or ingredients that have specific medicinal or health benefits in addition to a nutritional

Handbook of Nutraceuticals and Natural Products: Biological, Medicinal, and Nutritional Properties and Applications,
Volume 1, First Edition. Edited by Sreerag Gopi and Preetha Balakrishnan.
© 2022 John Wiley & Sons, Inc. Published 2022 by John Wiley & Sons, Inc.

effects (Kalra 2003). However, till date, the term "nutraceutical" has no regular or consistent definition (Zeisel 1999; Cencic and Chingwaru 2010; Aronson 2017) and has sometimes been used interchangeably with functional foods, medicinal foods, and dietary supplements, despite the fact that these terminologies have been reported to differ in many regards (Cencic and Chingwaru 2010).

In addition to being conventional foods or sole items of a meal, nutraceuticals can be consumed in a nonfood matrix forms (as capsules, pills, or tablets), while functional foods are taken as part of normal food (Kalra 2003; Bernal et al. 2011; Ramalingum and Mahomoodally 2014). Also, there have been suggestions that a functional food becomes classified as nutraceutical when that food or food product aids in the prevention and/or treatment of diseases other than anaemia (Cencic and Chingwaru 2010). Regardless of the definitions, there are reports that what works as a nutraceutical for one person could be a functional food for another (Cencic and Chingwaru 2010). Classified as nutraceuticals or functional foods are fortified dairy products, omega-3, lutein, vitamins, fruits, ginseng, green tea, cod liver oil, and plant/herbs that have a dietary component (Kalra 2003; Schmidt et al. 2008; Cencic and Chingwaru 2010). In this chapter, we explore the origins of functional foods and nutraceuticals, how it all began, the challenges and successes associated with their use, as well as future projections regarding the possibility of nutraceuticals as adjuncts and/or alternative therapies.

2.1.1 Historical Perspective

2.1.1.1 History of Food and Sickness

Although the twentieth century heralded the theories about diseases such as scurvy, pellagra, and rickets (at the time considered deficiency diseases) and their relationship with the "accessory food factors" it took to research and observations from renowned researchers and physicians in the nineteenth century (Table 2.1) to get to that point. Despite these theories, the generally believed and accepted concept of food was that there were five proximate principles of food, including three

Table 2.1 History of food and diseases and food as medicine.

Date	Disease	Benefit/treatment	Reference
1809	*Beriberi*	A need for a nourishing diet	Christie (1804) and Carpenter (2000)
1830	Scurvy	Can be remedied with fresh food	Carpenter (2003)
1842	Scurvy, pellagra, and rickets	Classified as diseases of defective nutriment	
3500 BCE	Diabetes	Ancient Egyptian scripts reported the use of diet in the treatment of metabolic diseases	Frank (1957)
865–925 CE	All diseases	Rhazes wrote about the importance of food and nutrition in the maintenance of health and the treatment of diseases	Cannon (2005) and Nikaein et al. (2012)
1753	Great sea plague (Scurvy)	James Lind (1716–1794) discovered the importance of a diet rich in fresh fruits in the prevention and management of scurvy	Krehl (1953) and Stewart and Guthrie (1953)
1912	*Beriberi*	Antiberiberi factor	Funk (1912, 1922)
1912, 1922	Scurvy, pellagra and rickets	Linked to deficiencies of "vitamins"	Funk (1912, 1922)

organic (proteins, fats, and carbohydrates) and two inorganic (salts and water). Little regard was given to the curative principle of fresh fruits, despite years of their use in scurvy (Drummond and Wilbraham 1957, 1991; Hughes 1973). At that time, science seemed focused on developing an artificial diet that could fulfil a man's need for food (Singer and Underwood 1962; Hughes 1973) and the problem of nutritional deficiency or how the diet would impact its cure was secondary.

Prior to the twentieth century, physicians suggested a possible link between diet and the development of some very common diseases. While working in Sri Lanka in 1809, Thomas Christie suggested that the main culprit in the development of *beriberi* was definitely a need for a nourishing diet (Christie 1804; Carpenter 2000). However, at that time, *beriberi* now known to be due to thiamine deficiency was assumed to be caused either by miasmas or an infectious agent. In 1830, John Elliotson shared the opinion that scurvy which he believed was a chemical disease can be remedied with fresh food (Carpenter 2003, 2012). In 1842, George Budd classified a number of conditions including scurvy, pellagra, and rickets as diseases of defective nutriment (Hughes 1973; Carpenter 2003). This is believed to be the beginning of a man's search for food and food products to solve health problems.

2.1.1.2 History of Food as Medicine

The phrase "Let food be thy medicine and let medicine be thy food" has long been credited to the father of modern medicine, Hippocrates, although opinions are beginning to differ as to its origin (Caderas 2013). Irrespective of its origin, the meaning of this phrase has become clearer in the last century, with strides in our understanding of the complex relationship that exists between good food and well-being. Globally, people now understand that trends in food production methods, quality of food, and eating habits strongly impact body health and disease prevention (Cencic and Chingwaru 2010).

It has been one hundred and eight years since Casimir Funk described the antiberiberi factor, and suggested that a number of the common diseases of the time (including scurvy, pellagra, and rickets) could be linked to deficiencies of then yet-to-be-identified factors for which he coined the name "vitamins" (Funk 1912, 1922). Today, vitamins have been identified and isolated and the knowledge of single nutrient deficiencies has improved astronomically. Our understanding of the role of vitamins, consumption of fruits/vegetables, and vitamin supplementation in the maintenance of health and prevention of diseases has also increased (Carpenter 2003; Mozaffarian et al. 2018).

However, the science of the links between food and medicine dates back several centuries (Cannon 2005; Nikaein et al. 2012). Ancient Egyptian scripts dating back to 3500 BCE, reported the use of diet in the treatment of metabolic diseases such as diabetes mellitus (Frank 1957). Information regarding the dietary traditions of ancient Greece which had been garnered from writings attributed to Hippocrates suggested that food was considered by the Greeks as the most important way of preventing and curing diseases. In Hippocratic medicine, it is believed that food quality was analogous to the four bodily humors (blood, phlegm, choler, and black bile) (Hippocrates et al. 1983; Wilkins et al. 1995). The Greeks also believed that too much of any kind of food was bad; so, they considered the consumption of well-balanced foods as being crucial to the maintenance of sound health and treatment of disease. They also created an allopathic system whereby foods with opposite virtues, for example, cucumbers, which were considered cold and moist, were used to correct contrasting humours (Hippocrates et al. 1983; Wilkins et al. 1995; Anderson 1997; Fieldhouse 1998; Albala 2019).

Galen was another great scientist and physician (who was central to ancient Roman medicine) who also shared the opinion that the humors are linked to food (Conrad 1998). Galen was said to have characterized sicknesses as cold, hot, moist or dry, attributing their causes to the consumption of certain types of foods (Anderson 1997; Fieldhouse 1998; Grant 2000). Galen also linked the quality of physicians to their ability to cook well, and his dietary treatise included recipes with information on best-suited culinary practices (Grant 2000), further elucidating his firm beliefs in the complex relationship between food and health.

In the middle East, excerpts from the books (*manfe' al aghzie va mazareha* (benefits of food and its harmfulness)) and *Ata'me al marza* (food for patients) written by Rhazes (865–925 CE), the great Persian chemist and physician, draw attention to the importance of food and nutrition in the maintenance of health and the treatment of diseases. His writing also gave detailed directives regarding the consumption of fruits and good-quality food (Cannon 2005; Nikaein et al. 2012).

In India, where the Ayurveda is a system of medicine and lifestyle, the Charaka Samhita is a compendium of Charaka's treatises (Meulenbeld 1999; Agarwal 2002), which is believed to have originated in the first millennium BCE, but was put into writing years later (Meulenbeld 1999; Agarwal 2002). The Charaka Samhita also includes a dietary system that continues to be practiced judiciously in the twenty-first century. This system, which is somewhat similar to the Greek and Roman system, is based on five elements (air, fire, water, earth, and space) which combine to form a *dosha* (a basic life force) that governs body functions. Also as in the Greek and Roman traditional medicine systems, food can increase or decrease the power of any of the *doshas* (Meulenbeld 1999; Agarwal 2002; Albala 2019). Also, in China, ancient texts such as *The Yellow Emperor's Classic of Internal Medicine* (Su 1972; Ilza Veith and Potts 2016), believed to have been composed by Huang-ti (a celestial emperor), in accordance with other cultures demonstrate the importance of diet in maintaining the flow of the *qi* (energy force of life) as well as the balance of the *yin* and *yang* (two basic universal forces). Also, in Asia, the Okinawan tribe, who are found on the Ryukyu islands (located between Japan and China) and considered one of the longest living persons in the world harbor strong beliefs and dietary practices, and consider certain foods to have many medicinal attributes linked to longevity. Okinawans also believe that "food maketh the man" and this food is "medicine for life" (Food as Medicine 2020).

In old traditional Europe, diets rich in wild greens were considered very important for the maintenance of health and the treatment of disease. Young leaves from a variety of plants including dandelion, stinging nettle, and purslane were eaten raw (Food as Medicine 2020). Overall, it is apparent that across human cultures and civilizations, the importance of food and dietary patterns in the prevention and treatment of diseases cannot be over emphasized (Su 1972; Ilza Veith and Potts 2016; Albala 2019). One very important discovery that best demonstrates the relationship between diet and the treatment of diseases, and also revolutionized naval medicine was the discovery by James Lind (1716–1794) of the importance of a diet rich in fresh fruits in the prevention and management of scurvy (the great sea plague) amongst sailors (Krehl 1953; Stewart and Guthrie 1953).

2.1.1.3 The History of Functional Foods and Nutraceuticals

Modernization and advances in medical and pharmaceutical practices did not completely deter human perception and beliefs that food and dietary practices are important in the maintenance of health and the treatment of diseases. In the early decades of the twentieth century, the attention of scientists and researchers was focused on the identification of essential elements, particularly vitamins, and their role in the prevention of various dietary deficiency diseases and undernutrition (Hasler 2002; Mozaffarian et al. 2018). However, in the later decades of the twentieth century, there was a dramatic shift in this emphasis when diseases linked to obesity became a major public health concern (Hasler 2002; Mozaffarian et al. 2018).

This problem could have arisen because at this time, the "modern" concept that food was consumed only to satisfy hunger (which differed significantly from ancient systems) was gradually beginning to gain ground (Albala 2019). Also, based on the observation of two pioneers of sports physiology and nutrition, namely Antoine-Laurent Lavoisier and Justus von Liebig (Carpenter 1994), the human body began to be considered as an engine; with food being the fuel needed to run it, and food requirements began to be calculated in calories and energy expended (Albala 2019). However, the emergence of the epidemic of obesity led to major changes in dietary guidelines and regulations, emphasizing the importance of consuming food rich in vegetables/fruits and low in saturated fat to decrease the risk of chronic diseases including cardiovascular disease, diabetes mellitus, and stroke (Hasler 2002; Mozaffarian et al. 2018). There was also the identification of physiologically active compounds (in foods) called phytochemicals (plants) and zoochemicals (animals) that could potentially reduce chronic disease risk (Hassler 2002).

Also, in the later part of the twentieth century (1980s), escalating healthcare costs, drug toxicities, allergies, and the desire to meet the growing demands of a booming health-improvement food market (Swinbacks and O'Brien 1993; Swinbanks 1993) may have prompted the Japanese Ministry of Health and Welfare to rethink ancient oriental philosophy relating to the common origins of medicine and food in a bid to find cheaper and safer ways of meeting the healthcare needs of their aging population. This led to the development of a regulatory system used to approve foods with documented health benefits and an ad-hoc committee to explore the links between food and medicine (Arai 1996; Hasler 2002; Ohama et al. 2006).

The term "physiologically-functional food" was first used in 1993 in a news magazine to depict a new trend in Japan which was the marketing of common foods such as rice as health products (Swinbanks and O'Brien 1993). Since then, "functional food" has been used globally, although not recognized by law. While no universal definition for functional food exists, different health regulation authorities have tried to proffer definitions for the term. In the United states of America, functional food was defined by the National Academy of Sciences' Food and Nutrition Board as "any modified food or food ingredient that may provide a health benefit beyond the traditional nutrients it contains" (Committee on Opportunities in the Nutrition and Food Sciences 1994). While the American Dietetic Association defined it as "food which is whole, fortified, enriched, or enhanced," and must be consumed as "part of a varied diet on a regular basis, at effective levels" for their potential health benefits to be reaped. In Canada, Health Canada defined it as food "similar in appearance to conventional food, consumed as part of the usual diet, with demonstrated physiological benefits, and/or to reduce the risk of chronic disease beyond basic nutritional functions" (Health Canada 2000). In Europe, the European Commission Concerted Action on Functional Food Science defined functional food as a food whose benefits affect one or more target functions in the body beyond adequate nutritional effects in a way that is relevant to either an improved state of health and well-being and/or reduction of risk of disease (Consensus Document 1999; Bagchi 2008).

Till date, Japan which has the most advanced functional food market was the first country to consider functional foods as a distinct category, known as foods for specified health use (FOSHU) (Iwatani and Yamamoto 2019). In 2015, Japan established a more flexible Foods with Function Claims (FFC) regulation based on the Dietary Supplement Health and Education Act system of the United states of America. In that year, more than 400 foods were approved compared to 1271 approvals under the FOSHU scheme since 1991 (Scattergood 2018; Iwatani and Yamamot 2019).

The term "nutraceutical" has also been used interchangeably with functional foods. This term was coined by Stephen De Felice of the Foundation for Innovation in Medicine (more than three decades ago) from two words nutrition and pharmaceutical (Brower 1998; Maddi et al. 2007; DaS et al. 2012). Stephen De Felice defined nutraceuticals as food (or a part of food) that provides medical or health benefits, including the prevention and or treatment of a disease. However, over the years, several definitions have been used to characterize products or foods that should be considered as nutraceuticals. Nutraceuticals have also been defined as products prepared from foods, but sold as pills, powder, or other medicinal forms, not usually associated with foods (Das et al. 2012). Generally, nutraceuticals include nutrients, herbal products, dietary supplements, and genetically engineered foods (Dureja et al. 2003; Malik 2008; Das et al. 2012).

2.1.2 Functional Food and Nutraceutical Categories

The classification or categorization (Table 2.2) of nutraceuticals/functional food varies severally depending on the application (clinical trial design, academic instruction, dietary recommendations, or functional food development), food sources, chemical nature, and mechanism of action (Das et al. 2012). Broadly, nutraceuticals and functional foods have been classified based on components into three groups including (i) Nutrients: which are products with defined nutritional function including vitamins, amino acids, minerals, and fatty acids, (ii) Herbal products: which include botanical products, extracts, or concentrates, and (iii) Phytochemicals: which are bioactive compounds derived from different plant sources and having well-specified functions or benefits (Verma and Mishra 2016; Chanda et al. 2019). Based on food sources, nutraceuticals and functional foods can be classified as dietary fibers, polyunsaturated fatty acid, pre- and probiotics, antioxidants, polyphenols, and spices (Kokate et al. 2002; Das et al. 2012; Verma and Mishra 2016). Nutraceuticals/functional foods have also been classified as enriched foods, fortified foods, or enhanced foods based on the use of biotechnological methods or engineered bioactive components which have the ability to boost the beneficial effects on the body (Lau et al. 2013; Chanda et al. 2019). Classification with regard to specific therapeutic properties has been used to group nutraceuticals into antimicrobial agents, immunomodulatory agents, antioxidant, anti-inflammatory, antihyperglycaemic, cytoprotective, anti-parasitic, antifungal, and many other therapeutic classes. Classification of nutraceuticals and functional food can also be based on chemical

Table 2.2 Classification and categorization of functional foods and nutraceuticals.

Categories	Classes
Nutrients	Vitamins, amino acids, minerals and fatty acids,
Herbal products	Botanical products, extracts or concentrates
Phytochemicals	Bioactive compounds
Based on food sources	Dietary fibers, polyunsaturated fatty acid, pre- and probiotics, antioxidants, polyphenols, and spices
Based on the use of biotechnological methods or engineered bioactive components	Enriched foods, fortified foods, or enhanced foods
Specific therapeutic properties	Antimicrobial agents, immunomodulatory agents, antioxidant, anti-inflammatory, antihyperglycaemic, cytoprotective, antiparasitic, antifungal
Based on chemical constituent	Fatty acids, amino acid carbohydrates, flavonoids, tannins, phenols, and isoprenoid derivatives

constituents into fatty acids, amino acid carbohydrates, flavonoids, tannins, phenols, and isoprenoid derivatives (Chanda et al. 2019).

2.2 Functional Food and Nutraceuticals: Where Are We Now?

2.2.1 The Functional Food and Nutraceutical Market

At the beginning of the twenty-first century, there was a rapid explosion in the use of nutraceuticals for the maintenance of health and well-being, with the market value of the nutraceutical industry exceeding $250 billion per year as at 2012. Between 2019 and 2023 (according to Technavio Research Report), the nutraceutical industry would experience regional growths in Europe, Asia, and the Americas, reaching about $149.89 billion (Technavio Research 2019). Also, globally, there have been suggestions that the size of the global nutraceutical market would reach approximately $722.49 billion by the year 2027 (Grand View Research 2020). This growth potential has been attributed to the rising awareness of the world's population to the beneficial effects of nutraceuticals. Initial growth trends in the nutraceutical industry were due to the effects of available nutraceuticals in caloric reduction and weight loss; however, there is increasing awareness at a global level of the ability of nutraceuticals to boost immunity and enhance cognitive behavior (Grand View Research 2020). The growing trend among consumers to alter dietary habits in order to treat diseases, and the use of prebiotics and probiotics by food-manufacturing industries to provide improved nourishment and reduce health problems have also been suggested as likely boosts to the demand for nutraceuticals (Grand View Research 2020). There have also been projections that a significant percentage of the global nutraceutical market growth would arise from the sale of hemp (legal marijuana) and cannabinoid containing nutraceutical products. Global legal marijuana sales are projected to attain a market value of about $73.6 billion by the year 2027, with the increasing legalization of cannabis for medical and adult-use expected to promote growth (Grand View Research 2020).

The passage and signing into law of the 2018 Farm Bill in the United States of America gave a significant boost to the nutraceutical industry, because it not only established a new federal hemp regulatory system that facilitated the commercial cultivation, processing, and marketing of cannabis (hemp and hemp seeds), it also allowed the possible exploitation of its nutraceutical value for the management and prevention of diseases (Romero 2018). The medicinal value of cannabis had been known for centuries; a seventeenth-century author documented the antiseptic, antispasmodic, anti-inflammatory and analgesic properties of cannabis (Straumietis 2014). Also, in the nineteenth century, evidence from written documentation revealed that amongst medicinal practitioners, cannabis was considered as food medicine or inhaled medicine that was valuable for the alleviation of symptoms of fatigue, dysmenorrhoea, headache, nausea, loss of appetite, and convulsions (Straumietis 2014). Since the legalization of medicinal marijuana the market value of the medicinal marijuana industry has increased considerably to an estimated $13.6 billion in 2019, creating over 340 000 jobs that are devoted to plant handling (New Frontier Data 2019; the United States Drug Enforcement Agency 2019).

2.2.2 Functional Food and Nutraceuticals: Current Challenges

The driving force of the global functional food/nutraceutical market is the increasing awareness of the health benefits of food and food supplements in disease prevention and health maintenance. In the last decade or more, several studies and projects have examined the possible mechanisms by which functional foods and nutraceuticals improve health and well-being. In trying to understand the mechanisms of action of functional foods and nutraceuticals as well as the ways to improve on the health-beneficial effects of functional foods; extensive research has shown that while the food matrix determines the bioavailability of nutrients within any given food or food product, the interactions between nutrients and non-nutrients in the food matrix could be synergistic, additive, or neutralizing (Crowe and Francis 2013). Therein lies one of the major challenges that may be associated with optimal use of functional foods and nutraceuticals, as a detailed understanding of these diverse interactions is crucial to the development of nutraceuticals and functional foods with the greatest potential of synergistically impacting human health (Crowe and Francis 2013).

Another important challenge to the global success of nutraceuticals and functional foods is the reliability of the qualified health claims (which communicate to the consumers the potential health benefit of a product). There have been questions regarding the possibly deceptive or misleading nature of the QHCs. While these QHCs are used to describe the relationship between the consumption of functional food or nutraceutical and the reduced risk or ability to prevent a disease or health condition, the claims by the respective companies could be nuanced (Berhaupt-Glickstein et al. 2019). The value of a QHC is in the degree to which a company can convince the consumers to purchase their products; hence, consumers need to be well informed as to how to correctly interpret QHCs so that they are not misled (Moors 2012; Berhaupt-Glickstein et al. 2019). Because the level of evidence that backs a QHC is measured by regulatory bodies, regulations must ensure that food labeling is precise so that consumers are able to make well-informed choices in selecting appropriate functional foods and nutraceuticals (Moors 2012; Berhaupt-Glickstein et al. 2019). However, the absence of a unified global definition for functional foods and nutraceuticals means that there exist wide variations between countries on what food or food product can be classified as such, and this creates problems for companies that have to tailor their products to the legislative framework of the different regions or countries in which their product is consumed.

2.3 Functional Foods and Nutraceuticals: Future Perspectives

In 1903, the great inventor and business man Thomas Edison wrote that "The doctor of the future will give no medicine, but will interest his patient in the care of the human frame, in diet and in the cause and prevention of disease." In the last century, while orthodox medical practice is yet to attain the level predicted by Thomas Edison, an increase in personalized healthcare and the search for safer ways to improve general health and well-being has continued to raise the awareness of humans to the health benefits of nutraceuticals and functional foods. Also, the gradual shift in the concentration of healthcare providers from the treatment of disease toward its prevention is likely to increase the use and dependence on functional foods and nutraceuticals for the prevention of disease and the maintenance of body health. A number of the companies that make up the nutraceutical and functional food industry now have a better understanding of the relationship between good nutrition and healthy living, and are looking for better ways to integrate disease prevention/treatment and nutrition so that holistic medical care is provided. That being said, in 2020, conventional medicine is still limited to the use of drugs to treat diseases; however, there are suggestions that in the not-too-distant future, there would be significant improvements in our understanding of how medicine and nutrition can better interact and complement one another.

The availability of new technology including the application of genetics in the food industry would assist in creating functional foods and nutraceuticals that are safe and can better deliver on their QHCs. The use of converging technologies such as nutrigenomics and nanotechnology could enhance the development of foods with better delivery systems and for targeted population groups (Singh 2016; Sampathkumar et al. 2020; Perrone et al. 2020).

2.4 Conclusion

From the era of philosophical concept to the current age of scientific understanding of the details of biochemical contents of foods and their specific roles in health and well-being, the idea of nutraceuticals and functional foods has come a long way. However, it is still a ship on a voyage and is yet to arrive at its destination. A lot has to be learned, relearned, and unlearned for nutraceuticals and functional foods to be able to sit side by side with orthodox medications in the quest to prevent and cure human diseases. Finally, as we continue to change the way we look at food, we shall be able to reap all the benefits that our foods can offer.

References

Abbatecola, A.M., Russo, M., and Barbieri, M. (2018). Dietary patterns and cognition in older persons. *Curr. Opin. Clin. Nutr. Metab. Care* 21 (1): 10–13. https://doi.org/10.1097/MCO.0000000000000434.

Agarwal, D.P. (2002). About the date of caraka, the famous ancient physician. www.infinityfoundation.com (accessed 1 July 2020).

Albala, K. (2019). Dietary systems: a historical perspective in encyclopedia of food and culture. Encyclopedia.com (accessed 1 July 2020)

Anderson, E.N. (1997). Traditional medical values of food. In: *Food and Culture: A Reader* (eds. C. Counihan and P. Van Esterik). New York: Routledge.

Arai, S. (1996). Studies on functional foods in Japan. *Biosc. Biotechnol. Biochem.* 60: 9–15.

Aronson, J.K. (2017). Defining "nutraceuticals": neither nutritious nor pharmaceutical. *Br. J. Clin. Pharmacol.* 83 (1): 8–19. https://doi.org/10.1111/bcp.12935.

Bagchi, D. (2008). *Nutraceutical and Functional Food Regulations*. New York: Elsevier.

Berhaupt-Glickstein, A., Hooker, N.H., and Hallman, W.K. (2019). Qualified health claim language affects purchase intentions for green tea products in the United States. *Nutrients* 11 (4): 921. https://doi.org/10.3390/nu11040921.

Bernal, J., Mendiola, J.A., Ibáñez, E. et al. (2011). Advanced analysis of nutraceuticals. *J. Pharm. Biomed. Anal.* 55 (4): 758–774.

Brower, V. (1998). Nutraceuticals: poised for a healthy slice of the healthcare market? *Nat. Biotechnol.* 16 (8): 728–731.

Canada, H. (2000). Standards of evidence for evaluating foods with health claims. *Fact Sheet* 1: 1–47. November 2000.

Cannon, G. (2005). The rise and fall of dietetics and of nutrition science, 4000 BCE–2000 CE. *Publ. Health Nutr.* 8 (6A): 701–705. https://doi.org/10.1079/phn2005766.

Cardenas, D. (2013). Let not thy food be confused with thy medicine: the hippocratic misquotation e-SPEN J. 8: e260–e226.

Carpenter, K. (1994). *Protein and Energy; A Study of Changing Ideas in Nutrition*. London: Cambridge University Press.

Carpenter, K.J. (2000). *Beriberi, White Rice and Vitamin B:26*. Berkeley: University of California Press.

Carpenter, K.J. (2003). A short history of nutritional science: part 4 (1945–1985). *J. Nutr.* 133 (11): 3331–3342. https://doi.org/10.1093/jn/133.11.3331.

Carpenter, K.J. (2012). The discovery of thiamin. *Ann. Nutr. Metab.* 61 (3): 219–223. https://doi. org/10.1159/000343109.

Cencic, A. and Chingwaru, W. (2010). The role of functional foods, nutraceuticals, and food supplements in intestinal health. *Nutrients* 2 (6): 611–625. https://doi.org/10.3390/nu2060611.

Chanda, S., Tiwari, R.K., Kumar, A., and Singh, K. (2019). Nutraceuticals inspiring the current therapy for lifestyle diseases. *Adv. Pharmacol. Sci.* 2019 (1–5): 6908716. https://doi.org/10.1155/2019/6908716.

Chauhan, B., Kumar, G., Kalam, N., and Ansari, S.H. (2013). Current concepts and prospects of herbal nutraceutical: a review. *J. Adv. Pharm. Technol. Res.* 4 (1): 4–8.

Chen, X., Maguire, B., Brodaty, H., and O'Leary, F. (2019). Dietary patterns and cognitive health in older adults: a systematic review. *J. Alzheimer's Dis.* 67 (2): 583–619. https://doi.org/10.3233/JAD-180468.

Christie, T. (1804). Letter on *beriberi*. In: *An Essay on the Diseases Incident to Indian Seamen* (ed. W. Hunter), 77–87. Calcutta: Honorable E. India Co.

Committee on Opportunities in the Nutrition and Food Sciences, Food and Nutrition Board, Institute of Medicine (1994). Enhancing the food supply. In: *Opportunities in the Nutrition and Food Sciences: Research Challenges and the Next Generation of Investigators* (eds. P.R. Thomas and R. Earl), 98–142. Washington, DC: National Academy Press.

Conrad, L.I. (1998). *The Western medical tradition, 800 BC to AD 1800 (Reprinted. ed.)*, 58–70. Cambridge: Cambridge University Press. ISBN: 0-521-47564-3.

Crowe, K.M. and Francis, C. (2013). Academy of nutrition and dietetics. Position of the academy of nutrition and dietetics: functional foods. *J. Acad. Nutr. Diet.* 113 (8): 1096–1103. https://doi.org/10.1016/j.jand.2013.06.002.

Das, L., Bhaumik, E., Raychaudhuri, U., and Chakraborty, R. (2012). Role of nutraceuticals in human health. *J. Food Sci. Technol.* 49 (2): 173–183. https://doi.org/10.1007/s13197-011-0269-4.

Document, C. (1999). Scientific concepts of functional foods in Europe consensus document. *Br. J. Nutr.* 81: S1–S27.

Drummond, J.C. and Wilbraham, A. (1957). *The Englishman's Food*, 361. London: Rev. by D.F. Hollingsworth.

Drummond, J. and Wilbraham, A. (1991). *The Englishman's Food. Five Centuries of English Diet*. London: Pimlico (first published in London: Jonathan Cape, 1939).

Dureja, H., Kaushik, D., and Kumar, V. (2003). Developments in nutraceuticals. *Indian J. Pharmacol.* 35: 363–372.

Ezra-Nevo, G., Henriques, S.F., and Ribeiro, C. (2020). The diet-microbiome tango: how nutrients lead the gut brain axis. *Curr. Opin. Neurobiol.* 62: 122–132. https://doi.org/10.1016/j.conb.2020.02.005.

Fieldhouse, P. (1998). *Food and Nutrition: Customs and Culture*, 2e. London: Stanley Thornes.

Frank, L.L. (1957). Diabetes mellitus in text of old hindu medicine (Charaka, Susruta, Vaghabata). *Am. J. Gastroenterol.* 27: 76.

Funk, C. (1912). The etiology of the deficiency diseases. *J. State Med.* 20: 341–368.

Funk, C. (1922). *The Vitamines*, 2e. Baltimore: Williams & Wilkins.

Grand View Research (2020). Nutraceutical market size. https://www.grandviewresearch.com/industry-analysis/nutraceuticals-market (assessed June 2020).

Grant, M. (2000). *Galen on Food and Diet*, 1–224. London and New York: Routledge, information gotten from, pp. ix, 214.

Hasler, C.M. (2002). Functional foods: benefits, concerns and challenges-a position paper from the American Council on Science and Health. *J. Nutr.* 132 (12): 3772–3781. https://doi.org/10.1093/jn/132.12.3772.

Hippocrates, Chadwick, J., Lloyd, G.E.R., and Mann, W.N. (1983). *Hippocratic Writings.* Harmondswerth Penguin Books.

Hughes, R.E. (1973). George Budd (1808–1882) and nutritional deficiency diseases. *Med. Hist.* 17 (2): 127–135. https://doi.org/10.1017/s002572730001841x.

Iwatani, S. and Yamamot, N. (2019). Functional food products in Japan: a review. *Food Sci. Human Welln.* 8 (2): 96–101.

Kalra, E.K. (2003). Nutraceutical – definition and introduction. *AAPS PharmSci.* 5: E25.

Kokate, C.K., Purohit, A.P., and Gokhale, S.B. (2002). *Nutraceutical and Cosmaceutical. Pharmacognosy,* 21e, 542–549. Pune, India: Nirali Prakashan.

Krehl, W.A. (1953). James Lind, October 4, 1716–July 18, 1794. *J. Nutr.* 50 (1): 3–11. https://doi.org/10.1093/jn/50.1.1.

Kumar, A., Mosa, K.A., Ji, L. et al. (2018). Metabolomics-assisted biotechnological interventions for developing plant-based functional foods and nutraceuticals. *Crit. Rev. Food Sci. Nutr.* 58 (11): 1791–1807. https://doi.org/10.1080/10408398.2017.1285752.

Lau, T.-C., Chan, M.-W., Tan, H.-P., and Kwek, C.-L. (2013). Functional food: a growing trend among the health conscious. *Asian Soc. Sci.* 9 (1). ISSN 1911-2017 E-ISSN 1911-2025.

Maddi, V.S., Aragade, P.D., Digge, V.G., and Nitaliker, M.N. (2007). Importance of nutraceuticals in health management. *Phcog. Rev.* 1: 377–379.

Malik, A. (2008). The potentials of nutraceuticals. Pharmainfo.net 6 (assessed July 2020).

McGrattan, A.M., McGuinness, B., McKinley, M.C. et al. (2019). Diet and inflammation in cognitive ageing and Alzheimer's disease. *Curr. Nutr. Rep.* 8 (2): 53–65. https://doi.org/10.1007/s13668-019-0271-4.

Food as Medicine (2020) Monash University CRICOS No. 00008C

Melina, V., Craig, W., and Levin, S. (2016). Position of the academy of nutrition and dietetics: vegetarian diets. *J. Acad. Nutr. Diet.* 116 (12): 1970–1980. https://doi.org/10.1016/j.jand.2016.09.025.

Meulenbeld, G.J. (1999). Caraka, his identity and date. In: *A History of Indian Medical Literature, Part 1,* vol. 1A. Groningen: E. Forsten. ISBN: 9069801248. Bp. 114. OCLC 4220745.

Mollica, A., Zengin, G., Locatelli, M. et al. (2017a). An assessment of the nutraceutical potential of *Juglans regia* L. leaf powder in diabetic rats. *Food Chem. Toxicol.* 107: 554–564. https://doi.org/10.1016/j.fct.2017.03.056.

Mollica, A., Zengin, G., Locatelli, M. et al. (2017b). Anti-diabetic and anti-hyperlipidemic properties of *Capparis spinosa* L.: in vivo and in vitro evaluation of its nutraceutical potential. *J. Funct. Foods* 35: 32. https://doi.org/10.1016/j.jff.2017.05.001.

Mollica, A., Zengin, G., Stefanucci, A. et al. (2018). Nutraceutical potential of *Corylus avellana* daily supplements for obesity and related dysmetabolism. *J. Funct. Foods* 47: 562–574.

Moors, E.H.M. (2012). Functional foods: regulation and innovations in theEU, innovation. *Eur. J. Soc. Sci. Res.* 25 (4): 424–440.

Mozaffarian, D., Rosenberg, I., and Uauy, R. (2018). History of modern nutrition science-implications for current research, dietary guidelines, and food policy. *BMJ* 361: k2392.

Nasri, H., Baradaran, A., Shirzad, H., and Rafieian-Kopaei, M. (2014). New concepts in nutraceuticals as alternative for pharmaceuticals. *Int. J. Prev. Med.* 5 (12): 1487–1499.

New Frontier Data. (2019). Potential cannabis market job growth. Fronteirs Financial Group, Inc. https://newfrontierdata.com/cannabis-insights/potential-cannabis-market-job-growth/# (accessed May 2020).

Nikaein, F., Zargaran, A., and Mehdizadeh, A. (2012). Rhazes' concepts and manuscripts on nutrition in treatment and health care. *Anc. Sci. Life.* 31 (4): 160–163. https://doi.org/10.4103/025 7-7941.107357.

Ohama, H., Ikeda, H., and Moriyama, H. (2006). Health foods and foods with health claims. *Toxicology* 221: 95–111.

Onaolapo, A.Y. and Onaolapo, O.J. (2012). *Ocimum Gratissimum* Linn causes dose dependent hepatotoxicity in streptozotocin-induced diabetic Wistar rats. *Maced. J. Med. Sci.* 5: 17–25.

Onaolapo, A.Y. and Onaolapo, O.J. (2019). Nutraceuticals and diet-based phytochemicals in type 2 diabetes mellitus: from whole food to components with defined roles and mechanisms. *Curr. Diabet. Rev.* 216 (1): 12–25. https://doi.org/10.2174/1573399814666181031103930.

Onaolapo, A.Y. and Onaolapo, O.J. (2020). African plants with antidiabetic potentials: beyond glycaemic control to central nervous system benefits. *Curr. Diabet. Rev.* 16 (5): 419–437. https://doi. org/10.2174/1573399815666191106104941.

Onaolapo, A.Y., Onaolapo, O.J., and Adewole, S.O. (2011). Ethanolic extract of *Ocimum grattissimum* leaves (Linn.) rapidly lowers blood glucose levels in diabetic Wistar rats. *Maced. J. Med. Sci.* 4: 351–357.

Onaolapo, A.Y., Onaolapo, O.J., and Adewole, S.O. (2012). *Ocimum gratissimum* linn worsens streptozotocin-induced nephrotoxicity in diabetic Wistar rats. *Maced. J. Med. Sci.* 5: 382–388.

Onaolapo, A.Y., Abdusalam, S.Z., and Onaolapo, O.J. (2017). Silymarin attenuates aspartame-induced variation in mouse behaviour, cerebrocortical morphology and oxidative stress markers. *Pathophysiology* 24 (2): 51–62. https://doi.org/10.1016/j.pathophys.2017.01.002.

Onaolapo, A.Y., Obelawo, A.Y., and Onaolapo, O.J. (2019a). Brain ageing, cognition and diet: a review of the emerging roles of food-based nootropics in mitigating age-related memory decline. *Curr. Aging Sci.* 12 (1): 2–14. https://doi.org/10.2174/1874609812666190311160754.

Onaolapo, O.J., Odeniyi, A.O., Jonathan, S.O. et al. (2019b). An investigation of the anti-Parkinsonism potential of co-enzyme Q10 and co-enzyme Q10 /levodopa-carbidopa combination in mice. *Curr. Aging Sci.* https://doi.org/10.2174/1874609812666191023153724. Online ahead of print.

Onaolapo, A.Y., Adebisi, E.O., Adeleye, A.E. et al. (2020a). Dietary melatonin protects against behavioural, metabolic, oxidative, and organ morphological changes in mice that are fed high-fat, high-sugar diet. *Endocr. Metab. Immune Disord. Drug Targets* 20 (4): 570–583. https://doi.org/10.217 4/1871530319666191009161228.

Onaolapo, O.J., Jegede, O.R., Adegoke, O. et al. (2020b). Dietary zinc supplement militates against ketamine-induced behaviours by age-dependent modulation of oxidative stress and acetylcholinesterase activity in mice. *Pharmacol. Rep.* 72: 55–66. https://doi.org/10.1007/s43440-019-00003-2.

Perrone, L., Sampaolo, S., and Melone, M.A.B. (2020). Bioactive phenolic compounds in the modulation of central and peripheral nervous system cancers: facts and misdeeds. *Cancers (Basel)* 12 (2): 454. https://doi.org/10.3390/cancers12020454.

Ramadan, M.F. and Al-Ghamdi, A. (2012). Bioactive compounds and health-promoting properties of royal jelly: a review. *J. Funct. Foods* 4 (1): 39–52.

Ramalingum, N. and Mahomoodally, M.F. (2014). The therapeutic potential of medicinal foods. *Adv. Pharmacol. Sci.* 2014: 354264. https://doi.org/10.1155/2014/354264.

Raskin, I., Ribnicky, D.M., Komarnytsky, S. et al. (2002). Plants and human health in the twenty-first century. *Trends Biotechnol.* 20 (12): 522–531. https://doi.org/10.1016/s0167-7799(02)02080-2.

Román, G.C., Jackson, R.E., Gadhia, R. et al. (2019). Mediterranean diet: the role of long-chain ω-3 fatty acids in fish; polyphenols in fruits, vegetables, cereals, coffee, tea, cacao and wine; probiotics and vitamins in prevention of stroke, age-related cognitive decline, and Alzheimer disease. *Rev. Neurol. (Paris)* 175 (10): 724–741. https://doi.org/10.1016/j.neurol.2019.08.005.

Romero, D. (2018). *Hemp Industry Expected to Blossom Under New Farm Bill*. NBC.

Sampathkumar, K., Tan, K.X., and Loo, S.C.J. (2020). Developing nano-delivery systems for agriculture and food applications with nature-derived polymers. *Science* 23 (5): 101055. https://doi.org/10.1016/j.isci.2020.101055.

Scattergood, G. (2018) Japan moves beyond FOSHU: Over 400 products approved under new health claims regime in last year. https://www.nutraingredients-asia.com/article/2016/10/10/japan-moves-beyond-foshu-over-400-products-approved-under-new-health-claims-regime-in-last-yeaR (assessed July 2020).

Schmidt, B., Ribnicky, D.M., Poulev, A. et al. (2008). A natural history of botanical therapeutics. *Metabolism* 57 (7): S3–S9. https://doi.org/10.1016/j.metabol.2008.03.001.

Singer, C. and Underwood, E.A. (1962). A short history of medicine. *Oxford* 1962: 610.

Singh, H. (2016). Nanotechnology applications in functional foods; opportunities and challenges. *Prev. Nutr. Food Sci.* 21 (1): 1–8. https://doi.org/10.3746/pnf.2016.21.1.1.

Solfrizzi, V., Custodero, C., Lozupone, M. et al. (2017). Relationships of dietary patterns, foods, and micro- and macronutrients with alzheimer's disease and late-life cognitive disorders: a systematic review. *J. Alzheimers Dis.* 59 (3): 815–849. https://doi.org/10.3233/JAD-170248.

Stewart, C.P. and Guthrie, D. (1953). *Lind's Treatise on Scurvy. A Bicentenary Volume Containing a Reprint of the First Edition of A Treatise of the Scurvy by James Lind, M.D., with Additional Notes.* Edinburgh: University Press.

Straumietis, M. (2014). *Cannabis: The world's Most Promising Nutraceutical.* HPCI Media: Nutraceutical Business Review.

Su, C. (1972). *The Yellow Emperor's Classic of Internal Medicine.* University of California Press.

Swinbanks, D. (1993). Fish-oil miracle additive brings benefits to some. *Nature* 364 (6434): 180. https://doi.org/10.1038/364180b0.

Swinbanks, D. and O'Brien, J. (1993). Japan explores the boundary between food and medicine. *Nature* 364: 180.

Technavio Research. (2019). Global nutraceuticals market: industry developments https://www.technavio.com/talk-to-us?report=IRTNTR30566 (assessed July 2020).

Trottier, G., Boström, P.J., Lawrentschuk, N., and Fleshner, N.E. (2010). Nutraceuticals and prostate cancer prevention: a current review. *Nat. Rev. Urol.* 7 (1): 21–30.

Veith, I. and Potts, E. (2016). *Huang ti nei su wen. The Yellow Emperor's Classic of Internal Medicine.* Berkeley: University of California Press.

Venter, C., Eyerich, S., Sarin, T., and Klatt, K.C. (2020). Nutrition and the immune system: a complicated tango. *Nutrients* 12 (3): 818. https://doi.org/10.3390/nu12030818.

Verma, G. and Mishra, M.K. (2016). A review on nutraceuticals: classification and its role in various disease. *Int. J. Pharmacy Therap.* 7 (4): 152–160.

Wilkins, J., Harvey, D., and Dobson, M. (1995). *Food in Antiquity*, 345. University of Exeter Press. ISBN: 0-85989-418-5.

Zeisel, S.H. (1999). Regulation of "nutraceuticals". *Science* 285: 185–186.

Zhao, J. (2007). Nutraceuticals, nutritional therapy, phytonutrients, and phytotherapy for improvement of human health: a perspective on plant biotechnology application. *Recent Pat. Biotechnol.* 1 (1): 75–97. https://doi.org/10.2174/187220807779813893.

3

Liposomal Nanotechnology in Nutraceuticals

Quintanar-Guerrero David[1], Zambrano-Zaragoza María de la Luz[2], Leyva-Goméz Gerardo[3], and N. Mendoza-Muñoz[4]

[1] *Laboratorio de Posgrado en Tecnología Farmacéutica, Facultad de Estudios Superiores Cuautitlán, Universidad Nacional Autónoma de México, Estado de México, Mexico*
[2] *Laboratorio de Procesos de Transformación y Tecnologías Emergentes de Alimentos, Facultad de Estudios Superiores Cuautitlán, Universidad Nacional Autónoma de México, Estado de Mexico, Mexico*
[3] *Departamento de Farmacia, Facultad de Química, Universidad Nacional Autónoma de México, Ciudad de México, Mexico*
[4] *Laboratorio de Farmacia, Facultad de Ciencias Químicas, Universidad de Colima, Coquimatlan, Mexico*

3.1 Introduction

Today, bioactive substances with nutraceutical potential capable of aiding in, and supporting, treatments for chronic or degenerative diseases and different types of cancer are gaining importance because consumers are interested in including them in their daily diet as a way to prevent disease development (Vergallo 2020). Bioactives have various beneficial properties like antioxidants, antimicrobials, anti-inflammatories, anticarcinogens, and antidiabetics, among others, and also serve as cardiovascular protectors. However, most of the substances with nutraceutical potential derived from natural extracts with antioxidant properties present a challenge; namely, they are unstable under environmental conditions and deteriorate rapidly. For these reasons, their use requires protective systems based on encapsulation. One option in this regard consists in using nanoliposomes (Subramani and Ganapathyswamy 2020). These nanometric structures are advantageous because some of their characteristics are similar to those of cell membranes, so they are compatible with human body tissues and can easily traverse the gastrointestinal tract (GIT), possibly achieving a greater plasmatic concentration of the active ingredient in the bloodstream, which distributes it to the organ(s) where it performs its preventive and/or curative function (Assadpour and Mahdi Jafari 2019). Compounds derived from plants are called phytochemicals. They may come from the seeds, leaves, stems, roots, fruits, or flowers, and can be extracted by various methods to obtain aqueous and/or lipophilic substances. Many compounds with nutraceutical properties, however, have a high antioxidant capacity. So, they are vulnerable to natural conditions like light, oxygen, temperature, pH, and ions. But they also have low solubility in water. So, nanotechnology represents an efficacious tool for encapsulating and protecting them. Nanoliposomes thus provide a system with several important advantages and potentialities that make implementing them in the nutraceutical industry viable, as we discuss below (Rodriguez et al. 2019).

Nanoliposomes are now being used to develop products for preventing or treating cancer. Examples include research on such various phenolic compounds as quercetin, gallic acid,

Handbook of Nutraceuticals and Natural Products: Biological, Medicinal, and Nutritional Properties and Applications,
Volume 1, First Edition. Edited by Sreerag Gopi and Preetha Balakrishnan.

resveratrol, and curcumin, among others (Khorasani et al. 2018). Nutraceuticals capable of impeding the formation of cancer cells act by preventing their formation and differentiation and inhibiting flow transporters, among other mechanisms that await future study. Moreover, these substances can also mitigate the toxic effects of chemotherapy (Dutta et al. 2018). Nanoliposome technology is an excellent means of encapsulating these substances because it stabilizes them, has good encapsulation efficiency, and increases the bioavailability and compatibility of substrates. Reducing the use of toxic solvents and increasing the feasibility of the use of nanoliposome in the alimentary and nutraceutical industries are subjects of intensive research that seeks to develop new and improved methods that employ sustainable, environmentally friendly solvents (e.g. liquefied gases or polyalcohols) to aid in dissolving and trapping specific bioactives (e.g. peptides, anthocyanins, phenols, betalains, and carotenoids) (Chi et al. 2019; Rehman et al. 2020; Sarabandi and Jafari 2020).

Several properties are deemed critical in the development of liposome formulations, for their assessment is important in ensuring adequate nutraceutical activity and future quality control. These properties include: (i) average particle size and distribution; (ii) zeta potential as an indicator of the stability of colloidal systems since recent studies show this to be a key property of the compatibility, interaction, absorption, and bioaccessibility of nutraceutical encapsulation systems, and a key parameter in designing release systems; (iii) encapsulation percentage, which depends greatly on the characteristics of the bioactive (i.e. molecular weight, structure, origin, etc.) and the materials used in preparation; (iv) release kinetics; and (v) system behavior in the GIT.

3.2 Definitions

The word "liposome" is derived from the Greek *lipos* (fat) and *soma* (structure). So, it refers to a structure in which a fat encompasses an internal aqueous compartment (Weissing 2017). Liposomes measure 0.025–2.5 microns and their structure may contain one or more bilayers (Akbarzadeh et al. 2013); hence, they can be classified as (i) unilamellar vesicles; or (ii) multilamellar vesicles. The former contains two subcategories: large and small unilamellar vesicles. These have a single phospholipid bilayer membrane that encloses the aqueous solution. Multilamellar vesicles, in contrast, have an onion-like structure (Akbarzadeh et al. 2013). The application will define the type of liposome required and, therefore, the excipients and manufacturing processes that can be used. In conventional liposomes, the load can be placed either in the central aqueous core or between the layers of the lipid bilayer (Schwendener and Schott 2010). The surface characteristics can be modified to confer targeting properties by adding PEG, or through specific receptor ligands (Crommelin et al. 2020). Another option involves working with stimuli-sensitive cationic liposomes that modify the membrane's fluidity in response to changes in pH or temperature. The foundations of phospholipids and cholesterol make a highly acceptable, biocompatible formulation. Liposomes marked a revolution in cancer drugs and FDA records for modified-release drugs (Allen and Cullis 2013). Records in *Scopus* present 85 188 documents that mention liposomes, with the main areas of application being biochemistry, genetics, and molecular biology, followed by pharmacology, toxicology, and pharmaceutics. This shows the huge impact of these formulations. In 2019 alone, 3674 published documents used the term "liposome," while the patent registry has 325 833 documents that mention it.

Nutraceutical refers to "a food that has the required nutrients along with therapeutic effect" (Ali et al. 2019); thus, most nutraceuticals are products that provide components that are essential for the body and help prevent disease. Nutraceuticals include varied products: dietary supplements, products of plant origin, genetically engineered foods, and nutrients added to prepared beverages, cereals, and soups, among others. Recent lifestyle changes have raised people's awareness that consuming nutraceuticals can compensate for nutrient deficiencies in fast-food products. The increase in cancer cases is another reason to consume more nutraceuticals since they can help prevent chronic diseases. People's longer life expectancy is another reason to ingest highly nutritional products, including nutraceuticals. This is reflected in substantial increases in the sales of nutraceuticals worldwide. These products, however, have some technological limitations – poor aqueous solubility, low oral bioavailability, degradation, and oxidation – that result in low efficacy in vivo (Ali et al. 2019). This lack of efficacy is sometimes solved through excessive consumption, but this can put people's health at risk. Fortunately, these limitations correlate well with the physical and chemical properties of candidate molecules for incorporation into nanotechnology tools, including liposomes (Liu et al. 2019). The development of liposomes that contain nutraceuticals is very recent, dating back only six years. A search of *Scopus*' records found 50 documents that contained the terms "liposomes" and "nutraceuticals."

3.3 Challenges of Nutraceutical Formulations

Achieving high functionality of nutraceuticals depends mainly on the formulation, but elaborating nutraceuticals presents diverse challenges, making preformulating studies essential to obtain useful information on the physicochemical characteristics of the bioactive and the optimum characteristic formulations that prevent the loss of functional properties but provide or maintain, key organoleptic properties. One challenge is conserving the physicochemical stability of the nutraceutical throughout the processes it will undergo during its life-cycle including, at least, extraction, purification, interaction in the formulation or matrix, incorporation into foods, storage, and ingestion (Mehta 2010). The structural diversity of nutraceuticals impedes establishing general rules of behavior, but regarding stability during the development of a nutraceutical, formulators must consider the following issues: the effects of pH, light, temperature, humidity, and oxygen; susceptibility to enzyme inactivation; the functional groups present that can interact with other components through known reactions; reports of different crystalline polymorphs; and the operations to which it will be subjected during manufacture. Their responses to these issues will largely determine the final formulation (e.g. liquid, powder, emulsion, etc.), the kind of container-closure system, and the protective technology (encapsulation, lyophilization, etc.) in each case.

Another challenge in formulating nutraceuticals is to devise strategies to ensure high bioavailability; that is, the amount of the nutraceutical that is effectively absorbed by the body, an aspect also related to delivery speed. Dima et al. (2020) define oral bioavailability as a unifying concept that integrates all the stages through which a bioactive compound (nutraceutical or pharmaceutical) will pass, from swallowing to excretion. Several factors affect the oral bioavailability of nutraceuticals when released from the food matrix: dosage, matrix composition, interaction, and/or degradation with components of the GIT, and the microbiome and permeability of the intestinal epithelium (Cassidy and Minihane 2017; Dima et al. 2020; McClements et al. 2015; Rubió et al. 2014). For pharmaceutical actives Amidon et al. (1995) proposed a biopharmaceutical classification system which have proven to be a useful tool for predicting the bioavailability of drugs, at least for relatively simple molecules. For more complex substances, like peptides, minerals, and microorganisms, in relation to nutraceuticals, the BCS considers two key parameters of active ingredients: solubility and permeability. McClements et al. (2015) proposed the nutraceutical bioavailability classification scheme as a new approach to classifying the factors that affect the bioavailability of nutraceuticals. Nutraceutical bioavailability classification scheme categorizes these factors in three broad groups based on bioaccessibility, absorption, and transformation inside the GIT. Each class has subclasses: bioaccessibility includes liberation, solubilization, and interaction; absorption has a mucous layer, tight junction transport, bilayer permeability, active transporters, and passive transporters; and transformation measures chemical degradation and metabolism. Categorizing the factors that limit the bioavailability of specific nutraceuticals supports the design of effective delivery systems, or food matrices, that enhance bioavailability. Subclass: soluble, for example, says that a nutraceutical must be soluble at the absorption site. So, solubility may be one physicochemical property that formulators need to know in advance to determine the best formulation route. Several techniques exist to increase the solubility of solutes (salt formation, solvency, complexation, etc.). So, formulators must ponder their use if low bioavailability is due to low solubility. Obtaining a soluble nutraceutical, however, does not guarantee high bioavailability if permeability is also low (class: absorption) since even rapid dissolution can lead to problems of degradation at the absorption site (determined by class: transformation). It is, therefore, necessary to analyze the information on stability in the previous section. Here, the release rate is important. So, formulators must evaluate the use of controlled-release technologies, such as matrix systems or encapsulation to adjust the release rate of the nutraceutical. Permeability can be increased by adding promoters, but these need to be formulated in conjunction with the nutraceutical. Guidelines suggest that formulators ask themselves the following questions: is the nutraceutical soluble in TGI fluids?; what is the nutraceutical's permeability in the GIT?; and, is it feasible to add absorption promoters? Figure 3.1 schematizes the issues to consider during the development process of a nutraceuticals.

Encapsulation has emerged as one of the most efficient technologies for overcoming many of these challenges. Both micro- and nanoencapsulation resolve numerous issues for a wide range of

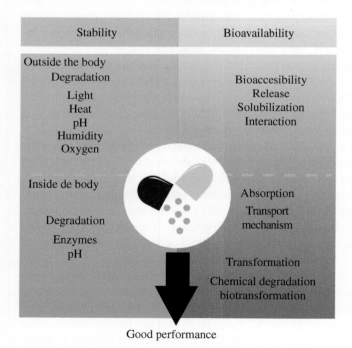

Figure 3.1   Formulation and pre-formulation challenges to consider during the rational design of a nutraceutical dosage form.

nutraceuticals. Encapsulation can, for example, substantially improve the stability of nutraceuticals in the presence of external agents and is useful in the oxidation of lipids and for impeding the degradation of peptides in the GIT. Encapsulation also allows low-solubility nutraceuticals to remain soluble for a longer time and can increase bioavailability through solubilization (Mohan et al. 2015; Ruiz Canizales et al. 2019; Torres-Giner et al. 2010). Finally, encapsulation can mask odors and flavors, a property highly appreciated when minerals and vitamins are involved and makes systems with multiple nutraceuticals viable by preventing interaction among components (Coupland and Hayes 2014; Nedovic et al. 2011).

3.4 Nanoencapsulated Systems for the Food Industry

The late twentieth century saw the formalization of studies that correlated the beneficial effects of food with the absorption and bioavailability of certain natural and functional bioactives presented through nanostructured systems. This advance revealed the need to analyze and develop ways to protect nutraceutical substances using encapsulation technologies, considering desirable properties and compatibility with different systems (Akbari-Alavijeh et al. 2020; Assadpour and Mahdi Jafari 2019). Research in this field over the past three decades has made great strides in implementing systems that can supply natural, functional components with nutraceutical properties necessary for maintaining health, especially nanometric formulations. Figure 3.2 shows the submicronic-size systems now most often used in nanoencapsulation to trap, protect, release, and modify the bioavailability and bioaccessibility of functional nutraceutical substances derived from vegetable sources, including essential oils, peptides, polyphenolic proteins, and other extracts now known to be essential for human diets (Keivani Nahr et al. 2019; Mazloomi et al. 2020). The various systems developed to date in the field of nutraceuticals differ little from those elaborated earlier in the pharmaceutical industry. The main distinction is that because nutraceuticals are derived from foods and are consumed as daily protection systems at various doses, preparation may require stabilizers, polymers, active ingredients, solvents, and other complementary substances, all of which must be "Generally Recognized as Safe" (GRAS) and have FDA authorization for use in foods and nutraceuticals (Akbarzadeh et al. 2013).

An ideal alimentary system of nanometric size must (i) protect the bioactive substances during the formulation and preparation of foods, enteral alimentation systems, and/or dosing systems; (ii) provide stability during storage, distribution, and consumption; (iii) improve bioavailability and bioaccessibility as the nutraceutical passes through the GIT; (iv) remain stable while passing through the GIT so it can be absorbed at the specific site where it is required; and (v) offer controlled release and/or placement in the food to take full advantage of the active's benefits.

A broad range of materials (natural and synthetic polymers, lipids, inorganic materials, phospholipids, etc.) are available for the nanoencapsulation of components with nutraceutical capacity, but a major tendency is to use materials with supplementary activities that function as dietetic fiber and/or provide some other antioxidant and/or antimicrobial effect. These may include pectins, inulin, agave fructans, and chitosan, among others (Akhavan et al. 2018; Sarabandi and Jafari 2020; Wang et al. 2017).

The designers of controlled-release, nanostructure systems must also assess the compatibility of various components: coating materials, surfactants, polymeric stabilizers, solvents, and the nutraceutical to be encapsulated, while also ascertaining the possible effects of the components of the food itself, the environment, and the enzymes in the GIT, on the bioavailability of nutraceutical substances (Durazzo et al. 2020). Table 3.1 illustrates various nanometric structures for protecting

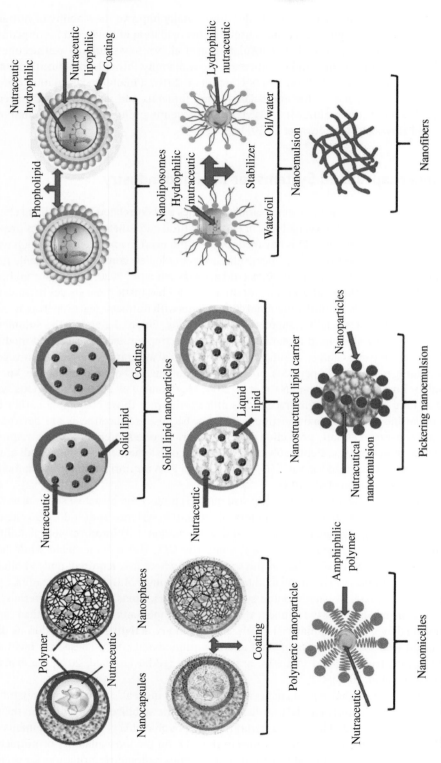

Figure 3.2 Nanosystems used in the development of nutraceutical products, schematic representation.

Table 3.1 Various nanosystems for encapsulating natural nutraceuticals.

Nanostructure type	Entrapment nutraceutical	Wall polymer and preparation method	Functions of entrapment bioactive	Nutraceutical characteristics
Polymeric nanoparticles	Resveratrol	Zein Desolvation method	Anti-inflammatory, antioxidant, and anti-atherosclerosis abilities.	Increase the concentration of resveratrol in plasm using zein as solid wall (Brotons-Canto et al. 2020).
Polymeric nanoparticles	Cyanidin-3-O-glucoside from Crabapple (*Malus prunifolia* Willd. Borkh)	Chitosan Ionic gelation	Anti-cancer, anti-cronic diseases.	Increase aqueous solubility, loading efficiency (5.11%), encapsulation efficiency (53.8%) and good blood compatibility (Sun et al. 2020).
Nanostructured lipid carrier	Vitamin D$_3$	Monegyl Caprylic-/capric triglyceride (CCTG)	Milk beverage fortification	A stable system with zeta potentials between -13.5 to -17 mV, with 20% of CCTG, 30% of Kalliphor and 50% of water, was possible to obtain highest encapsulation efficiency and release or vit D3 with minimal changes in the stability of nano-structured lipid carrier (Maurya and Aggarwal 2019).
Nanoemulsion	Quercetin	High-speed homogenization	Rice bran oil	Nanoemulsion reduce the cytotoxicity and increase cell permeability of quercetin (Chen et al. 2020)
Nanocapsules	Curcumin	Poly-ε-caprolactone/ethyl cellulose Emulsification-diffusion method	Anti-inflammatory, anti-cancer disease	The particle size was of 157 nm from ethyl cellulose nanoparticles and 110 nm from PCL nanoparticles and encapsulation efficiency of 27.7% for both systems (Galindo-Pérez et al. 2018).
Solid lipid nanoparticles	β-carotene	Cocoa butter/tristarin Hot high-pressure homogenization method	Pro-vitamin A, and antioxidant	The particle size was < 170 nm. Shown that cocoa butter contributes to stabilizer the polymorphic transitions. However its necessary the realization of studies to determine antioxidant capacity (Salminen et al. 2020).

several bioactives, vitamins, and micronutrients, considering their composition, structure, function, and application.

Nanosystems can be prepared with natural and/or synthetic polymers – biodegradable or not – proteins, lipids, or polysaccharides, among other materials. This diversity provides paths for designing and developing protection and release systems tailored specifically to a certain application in accordance with the properties of the bioactive encapsulated, the pH into which it will be released, changes in the surface charge, and the composition of the surroundings, and so allow it to interact with cellular membranes and structures. Polysaccharides that can be used are chitosan, pectin, alginate, and starch, among others, while these proteins are also apt: grenadine, albumin, and zein, or synthetic polymers like Eudragit®, poly-ε-caprolactone, and polylactic acid, etc. Nanostructures with lipid walls can utilize wax, solid lipids, lipids that are liquid at room temperature, and nanofibers. Polymeric particles can also be prepared with polysaccharides and/or proteins, while molecular inclusion may utilize cyclodextrins, nanoemulsions stabilized by various tensoactives, and vesicular systems formed with amphiphilic lipids, which is the focus of this chapter. These are just some of the nanosystems that have been developed and applied to protect and administer nutraceuticals (Ali et al. 2019).

Currently, to achieve the goal of enhancing the compatibility, stability, and controlled release of compounds beneficial for health, nanosystems have been coated with natural and/or biodegradable polymers, including polysaccharides and proteins that improve biological functioning and have potential nutraceutical properties; for example, grenadine, zein, and gums extracted from plants rich in polyphenols and other components (Zamani Ghaleshahi and Rajabzadeh 2020). Design systems to protect bioactive compounds must consider all the stages through which the nutraceutical product will pass in order to perform its function at the target site: (i) the origin and form of extraction; (ii) encapsulation method; (iii) components of the formulation and their interaction; (iv) stability and storage; and (v) digestion, absorption, and bioavailability. The latter is the most important aspect in designing release systems, for it requires assessing all the changes associated with the nutraceutical's transit through the GIT. These changes include: enzymatic action, pH, interaction with other components of the alimentary bolus, particle size, and zeta potential, among others. This marks the difference among the various formulations available in the market. Obviously, no design will be of much use if the bioactive encapsulated is unable to cross all the barriers it encounters in the digestive tract before it is absorbed.

3.5 A Brief History of Liposomes

The development of liposomes emerged through a series of events intertwined in nature and later discovered by advances in technology. So, they have an uncertain, unofficial history. The first official records describe the pioneering work of Bangham and Horne in an article in the Journal of Molecular Biology (1964) that displayed the first electron microscope images of multilamellar phospholipid vesicles, informally called "banghasomes" in honor of Alec Bangham. Gerald Weissmann proposed the name "liposomes" due to their structure, based on one or more lipid bilayers (Deamer 2010). The official establishment of liposome research corresponds to a researcher motivated by simple curiosity, not some ambitious expert in a pretentious laboratory. The incipient phenomenon, identified by fortuitous observation, was described as follows: "it was the odd pattern of a well-drawn drop of blood that initiated my curiosity. in the physical chemistry of cell surfaces." From the beginning, liposomes were conceived as models of cell membranes and various aspects of the interaction of substrates with lipid layers are being explored today in greater detail. Bangham was interested in liposomes as a model of lipid membranes that simulate prebiotic conditions, inspired by the first forms of cellular life. His research can be summarized as "membranes came first" (Weissing 2017). In the ensuing years, he examined the application of liposomes as a model for analyzing such membrane properties as permeation, adhesion, and fusion, as well as an action mechanism for drugs. The history of observations of the interaction between oil and water as an approach to the study of lipid membrane models dates from B.C., but Benjamin Franklin's appropriation of the study models in 1774 with an experiment in which he sprinkled oil droplets on pond water until it "was smooth as a looking glass" ended the first crucial stage of research. The second critical stage in the history of liposomes – called *liposomology* by some authors – came in 1995 with the approval of Doxil, the first FDA-approved, injectable liposomal drug composed of doxorubicin-loaded liposomes coated with a layer of PEG chains. Doxil's properties include a prolonged circulation time and the ability to avoid uptake by RES due to the PEG coating on its surface (Barenholz 2012). It is a stable formulation with the capacity to target tumors by passively releasing doxorubicin to exert its effect on tumor cells.

The history of liposomes has not always been marked by success, but has had significant ups and downs, including an inadequate interpretation of results in the 1980s that led various researchers to lose interest (Barenholz 2012). This phenomenon has occurred in other areas of research, where a subsequent, prolific stage of investigation is required to renew interest in the topic. The Doxil story is one of success in medicine, but it also set an important precedent in the FDA's processes of registering and approving future nanoformulations that utilize this technology. Interestingly, the search for generic alternatives to the Doxil prototype has spawned a new line of products for the generic drug industry.

3.6 Uses of Liposomes in Food Products

As vesicular structures are made up of a bipolar layer, liposomes have the ability to encapsulate both hydrophilic and lipidic substances. So, they are attractive for developing new functional systems that contain natural bioactive substances that permit sustained release, improve bioavailability, and can protect encapsulated substances from oxidation, in addition to being biocompatible, biodegradable, and having low toxicity. Recent advances in functional food and nutraceutical research demonstrate that it is important not only to protect substances from the environmental conditions in the GIT and facilitate their digestibility, but also to maintain their therapeutic properties during administration (Singh et al. 2012).

Producing liposomes requires amphiphilic lipids derived from natural sources like egg or soya lecithin, or marine phospholipids, all of which are known to have beneficial effects for health, such as protecting the liver and cerebral protection that aids memory. Cholesterol is used to improve the stability of these systems which are thermodynamically unstable, resulting in short storage times, and the rapid release of the encapsulated substance (Dutta et al. 2018; Lordan et al. 2017). Another drawback of liposome formulations is that the phospholipids used are susceptible to oxidation. So, an antioxidant component must be added or a coating that reduces interaction with oxygen and other pro-oxidants to increase system stability (Zamani Ghaleshahi and Rajabzadeh 2020).

Liposomes have been used in foods and nutraceuticals, including dairy products, juices, energy drinks, and meats, among many others. As mentioned above, their incorporation required a thorough evaluation of the stages through which products pass, from ingestion to breakdown inside the human GIT. Their stability depends largely on the action of digestive enzymes in the mouth, stomach, small intestine, and colon. Findings show that many of these enzymes interact with, and modify, the digestibility of the liposome's wall, thus affecting their later absorption (Subramani and Ganapathyswamy 2020). Observations show that even slight variations in pH or the composition and concentration of ions modify the electrostatic interactions in the GIT, forming bridges or surface changes that alter interactions with the lipid membrane and the digestion profile (Chi et al. 2019). The main substances used to form the lipid membrane are phospholipids and sphingolipids, groups differentiated by the types of fatty acids bonded to the chain (Rasti et al. 2017). Phospholipids can vary in stability and transition temperature from solid to gel according to their origin. So, it is important to obtain precise characterizations of the properties of the liposomes used in their formulation (Luo et al. 2020; Singh et al. 2012). Table 3.2 shows some of the applications of liposomes in the encapsulation of nutraceuticals and their incorporation into distinct formulations.

3.7 Nanoliposome Technology

3.7.1 Background

Liposomes can vary in size depending on the function they are manufactured to perform. Today, there are various types of structures with different layers for distinct functions but controlling particle size is always crucial for sensitive applications. Because nanoliposomes are the nanometric version of traditional liposomes (Khorasani et al. 2018), they share the same chemical, structural, and thermodynamic properties (Dahiya and Dureja 2018). The difference resides in that their small size gives nanoliposomes a greater surface area, increases solubility and bioavailability, improves the controlled release of active substances, and facilitates the targeting of encapsulated drugs (Vahabi and Eatemadi 2017). Their nanometric size and strict control of vesicle size distribution ensure permeation in cell membranes, tissues, and organs. As well, the combination with the active functionalization of the surface offers high efficiency in the transport of active substances; hence, they are a more precise, nanometric version of liposomes. The main chemical composition of phospholipid and cholesterol-based nanoliposomes is bioinspired in a cell membrane. Phospholipids are amphiphilic with a triglyceride-like backbone and a modified, negatively charged polar phosphate-containing group instead of a fatty acid (Wagner and Vorauer-Uhl 2011). Their amphiphilic character favors the formation of lipid bilayers. Cholesterol cannot form lipid bilayers but can be incorporated into phospholipid membranes at high concentrations to increase the lipid bilayer's fluidity and stability. The mechanism for forming nanoliposomes depends on Van-der-Waals forces and hydrophilic-hydrophobic interactions between the phospholipids and water molecules (Khorasani et al. 2018).

Nanoliposomes can incorporate a wide variety of molecules for applications in diverse fields: pharmaceuticals, cosmetics, nutraceuticals, and agriculture. In recent years especially, their use in drug-targeting systems has spurred interest. So, formulations now include proteins and polymers combined with phospholipids. The dynamism of their structure and greater surface area can, however, cause the formation of micrometric vesicles during storage. The strategy of increasing their zeta potential promotes stability in the formulation by incorporating cationic or anionic phospholipids. A common passive strategy consists in adding cholesterol as a lipid to the intercalation of phospholipids to increase the stability of the bilayer vesicles (Khorasani et al. 2018). Cholesterol modulates the fluidity of the phospholipid bilayer, impedes the crystallization of acyl chains of phospholipid molecules, and provides steric impedance to their movement. Metastability is an important aspect of nanoliposomes because, unlike micrometric vesicles, they can be diluted in

Table 3.2 Some examples of bioactive with nutraceutical properties in liposomes.

Nutraceutical	Lipid structures and stabilizers	Nutraceutical beneficial effect	Method	Application
Tyrosol, hydroxytyrosol and oleuropein from olive tree	1,2-dioleoyl-sn-glycero-3-phosphoethanolamine and 1,2-dioleoyl-sn-glycero-3-phosphocholine. 1:1 molar ration	Antioxidants in the osteoarthritic pathologies	Thin-film hydration method	Food supplement. The liposomes were not cytotoxic at any concentration. The zwitterionic liposomes loaded with natural compounds increase the bioavailability of antioxidants in the osteoarthritic pathologies and to reduce the collateral effect of classical drugs (Bonechi et al. 2019).
Procyandins from lychee pericarp (Oligomeric procyanidins)	Yolk lechitin/Cholesterol, Tween®80 Solvent: Ethanol	Antioxidant	Film dispersion method	Food supplement. Best antioxidant capacity (FRAP, ORAC, and CAA) with respect to oligomeric procyanidins alone (Luo et al. 2020).
Carotenoids: lutein, carotene, lycopene, canthaxanthin.	Egg yolk phospholipid (EYP)/ Tween® 80 EYP/lechitin. Solvent: Ethanol	Antioxidant, anti-inflammatory, photoprotective effect.	Thin-film evaporation method	The use of EYP·Tween® 80 had different encapsulation ability for different carotenoids. The stability showed that carotenoids can be load in liposomes (Xia et al. 2015).
Lutein	EYP/Tween® 80 Solvent: Ethanol	Prevention of cardiovascular disease,3 parameters, especially the liposomal formulations. Varying the stroke,4 and lung cancer	Ethanol injection method	The authors evidenced that encapsulation efficiencies (from 82.64 to 91.98) and particle sizes (from 76.46 to 134.82 nm) increased as function of lutein concentration. Fluorescence probes and Raman spectra showed that the stabilization of lutein was correlated with its capacity to affect the lipid membrane dynamics and structure (Tan et al. 2013).
Flavonoids: Quercetina, kampferol, luteolin	EYP/Tween® 80 Solvent: Ethanol	Anti-inflammatory, antioxidant, cardiovascular diseases	Thin-film evaporation method	The encapsulation efficiency was dependent from flavonoid type. The liposomes obtained were stable and antioxidant assays revealed a mutual protective relationship between flavonoid type and liposome structure (Huang et al. 2017).
Vitamin E/ polyphenols: lutein, quercetin, apigenin, proanthocyanidins	Lecithin/Cholesterol/Tween®80 Solvent: Ethanol	Antibacterial, antioxidant, antiviral, anti-inflammatory, anti-allergic, antithrombotic, anti-cancer, and vaso-dilative effects	Thin-layer dispersion method	The load capacity depended on polyphenol loaded. Liposomes loaded with quercetin and proanthocyanidins were smaller in size and disperse more uniformly than those loaded with luteolin and apigenin. The interaction between the polyphenolic compound and the liposome shown that the polyphenolic compounds regulated the fluidity of the lipid bilayer (Zhang et al. 2020).

water without changing the distribution of vesicle size or structure (Khorasani et al. 2018). There are three studies of clinical trials, two on the *Recruiting* status targeting cancer, and one under *Withdrawn* status that targets metastatic colorectal cancer. The *Scopus* publication record has 846 publications in the following – descending – order of subject area: pharmacology, toxicology and pharmaceutics, biochemistry, genetics and molecular biology, chemistry, medicine, chemical engineering, materials science, engineering, and agricultural and biological sciences, among others, as well as 639 patents, predominantly by the US Patent & Trademark Office. The largest boom in nanoliposome development has occurred in the past five years at an exponential growth rate of 200%, a clear reflection of great interest in new applications for this type of formulation.

3.7.2 Advantages and Drawbacks: Liposomes *vs.* Nanoliposomes

The number of nutraceuticals that can be incorporated into liposomal technology is large due to the numerous advantages of encapsulation systems and the particularities of liposome encapsulation. Since their discovery, liposomes have shown a great ability to protect actives from external factors that promote chemical degradation. In this sense, they function as protective agents against the oxidation and photo-oxidation of nutraceuticals (Tan et al. 2013). The materials used to make liposomes are neutral in terms of taste and odor. So, they can also efficiently mask unpleasant organoleptic properties. Other key aspects of the raw materials used to form liposomes are high biocompatibility and biodegradability, coupled with null or low immunogenicity. Moreover, the lipids used are virtually identical to those found in cell membranes, which aids in obtaining the aforementioned properties. However, because most formulations are developed for parenteral applications of liposomes, the oral administration route presents challenges that need to be overcome; among them, improving liposome stability in the GIT, and increasing permeability in the intestinal epithelium (He et al. 2019).

Another advantage of liposomes over other encapsulation systems is their exceptional ability to encapsulate hydrophilic, lipophilic, and amphiphilic actives (Nii and Ishii 2005). This capacity is greatest for hydrophilic actives due to the nature of the aqueous cavity, but the intercalation of lipophilic or amphiphilic nutraceuticals in the phospholipid bilayers is also feasible. This gives liposomes the ability to release two or more functional materials. Some researchers have explored this ability using two nutraceuticals with distinct solubility properties in systems called bifunctional vesicles (Erami et al. 2019). In addition, the methods for incorporating bioactives into liposomes do not demand advanced techniques. So, incorporation can be quite simple but still offer relatively high encapsulation efficiencies, depending mainly on the solubilization of the molecule to be encapsulated (Raslan 2013). Encapsulation efficiencies express the percentage of the bioactive that is actually incorporated into the liposome during preparation; one of the properties of liposomes that can be optimized.

Using liposomes in nutraceuticals requires developing preparation methods that can be raised to an industrial scale. One disadvantage of this technology is that while numerous methods for laboratory-scale preparation of liposomes exist, few can be scaled up to industrial levels. Some of the laboratory methods developed cannot be used by industry because they require potentially toxic organic solvents that would limit their commercialization. In other cases, the methods and processing conditions cause degradation of nutraceuticals due to mechanical, thermal, or pH stress (Subramani and Ganapathyswamy 2020).

Recently, a categorization of liposomal systems has been elaborated that classifies distinct preparation methods by their ability to produce systems with narrow particle size distribution. Here, the category of nanoliposomes refers to liposomes with a particle size below one micron. Generally speaking, liposomes and nanoliposomes have the same composition, but differ in their architecture and certain properties (Mozafari et al. 2008a). Several advantages can be attributed to the small particle size of nanoliposomes compared to micron-sized liposomes, but a particularly important one is their greater physical stability in dispersions. We know that nanodispersions are metastable systems due to the balance between the phenomena of sedimentation or cremation and dispersion related to Brownian movement, which allows nanoliposomes to remain in dispersion longer than conventional micrometer-sized liposomes, which tend to separate (Khorasani et al. 2018). A second key advantage is that the inherent effect of miniaturization gives nanoliposomes a larger surface area that improves bioavailability by increasing permeation, solubility, and the ability to target-specific sites. Miniaturization also allows nanoliposomes to go unnoticed by the human eye. So, they are attractive candidates for including nutraceuticals in clear beverages, a feature highly appreciated by consumers (Khorasani et al. 2018). In contrast, a limitation of nanoliposomes compared to conventional liposomes is the manufacturing process since miniaturization usually demands applying additional energy or high concentrations of stabilizers that can, respectively, promote the degradation of nutraceuticals, and produce incompatibility with foods. At present, more innocuous methods are being developed for elaborating nanoliposomes (Colas et al. 2007; Huang et al. 2014; Mozafari 2010).

3.7.3 Formulation and Specific Food Designs

Liposomes, or artificial phospholipid-trapping vesicles, are attractive, biocompatible encapsulation systems that are useful in food design thanks to their vesicular architecture that provides a protective bi-compartmental structure where food actives (hydrophilic substances) can be encapsulated in a central aqueous cavity or trapped in a bilayer membrane (Mozafari 2010; Rehman et al. 2020). Liposomes can protect sensitive food components from degradation due to exposure to the GIT environment or during digestive processes (Hassane Hamadou et al. 2020) and increase nutraceutical solubility and, consequently, bioavailability and the potential for delivery to specific sites in food (Fan et al. 2011; Kim et al. 2018; Subramani and Ganapathyswamy 2020). Liposome size can be reduced substantially by increasing the energy input. When their size decreases to nanometer scale, the spherical or oval vesicles obtained are called nanoliposomes (Zarrabi et al. 2020). These conserve the chemical, physicochemical, and structural properties of liposomes, but have additional attributes due to their size and exposure area (e.g. modified release and spatial ubication, high transfer surface, enhanced diffusion potential) that may be attractive for developing nutraceutical products (Beltrán et al. 2020). Diverse food substances can be incorporated into nanoliposomes: antioxidants, minerals, nutrients, enzymes, antimicrobials, vitamins, flavors, aromas, essential fatty acids and oils, plant extracts, nutraceuticals, and additives, among others. Their inclusion can enhance several properties – protection, enrichment, preservation, modified, or controlled target release, and better sensory characteristics (taste, flavor, color, and texture) – and aid in designing intelligent packaging materials, and strengthening certain foods, nutraceuticals, and other functional products (Rehman et al. 2020). This approach is especially interesting for sensitive food actives, like nutraceuticals (Kim et al. 2018). Figure 3.3 summarizes the specific advantages of nanoliposome formulations for nutraceuticals, though several challenges for producing acceptable, nutraceutical-nanoliposome systems for food applications persist, some toxicological, technological, and economic, others related to safety (Zarrabi et al. 2020).

Selecting the ingredients is a key step in developing acceptable nutraceutical-liposomal formulations (Mathew et al. 2017). Though various natural and synthetic indigenous-body lipids and phospholipids are available for preparing lipid vesicles, phosphatidylcholine derived from natural

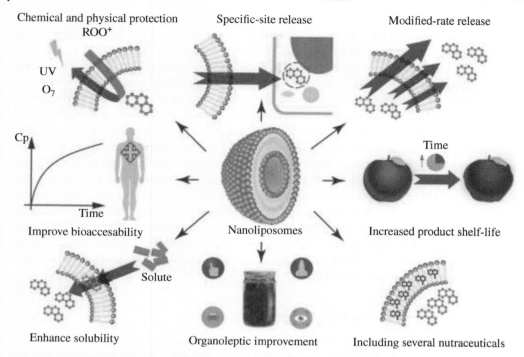

Figure 3.3 Schematic representation of some specific advantages to formulating nanoliposomes for nutraceuticals.

sources (egg, soy, milk, etc.) is omnipresent (Thompson and Singh 2006). All these molecules can be used safely in the food, feed, and nutraceutical industries, and some claim to have health benefits, but their high cost is a drawback that has not yet been resolved. It is important to understand that all the raw materials used in preparing nanoliposomes for food-grade products must be GRAS (Generally Recognized as Safe) in order to obtain regulatory approval (Rehman et al. 2020). Special attention must be paid to the content of residual organic solvents that are deemed acceptable in nutraceutical products (Tsai and Rizvi 2016) because solvent residues are potentially toxic and can affect nanoliposome stability (Mozafari 2010).

Another challenge is that nanoliposome encapsulation systems are more susceptible to chemical and physical destabilization. Consequently, the interaction among the nutraceutical, surrounding medium, and components of the nanoliposome must be assessed when designing nanoliposomes (Nayak et al. 2016). Phospholipids can be degraded by hydrolysis of the ether bonds and peroxidation of unsaturated acyl chains. Nutraceutical molecules, moreover, have poor stability, leaving them susceptible to chemical degradation, while their activity depends on such environmental conditions as pH, temperature, and ions, etc. Another important aspect is that nanoliposomes may change their size due to aggregation or fusion, and may expel the nutraceutical due to various effects, including physicochemical changes and degradation processes. These changes can also be triggered by the physical stress applied during their elaboration. Formulators must evaluate all these elements to prevent potential problems and deterioration during dispersion. Another task is to successfully incorporate the nutraceutical nanoliposome dispersion into the final food product. Here, various approaches can be adopted: solutions, solids, and dispersions in the form of emulsions, suspensions, pastas, and gels, among others, that vary in composition and structure and, hence, also in physical and chemical properties like pH, ionic strength, temperature-time profile, light, surfactant and/or polymer presence, and ionic interacting-molecules, etc., all of which can affect nanoliposome integrity (Zarrabi et al. 2020). This explains why a rigorous program of quality control of these parameters is required, based on both analytic and sensory evaluations of organoleptic and textural properties, particle size, zeta potential, colorimetry, rheology, degradation, and physical stability, among others (Kharat and McClements 2019).

As will be discussed in greater detail below, several methods for preparing nanoliposomes exist. Selecting the optimal system depends on various parameters: food safety, cost, equipment availability, the potential for scale-up, simplicity, and the potential physical and chemical stress to which the nutraceutical molecules will be subjected. As a general rule, formulators should avoid methods that require potentially toxic solvents, or large amounts of organic solvent, or that leave residues in the final product. Other methods to be avoided are those that are difficult to implement, time-consuming, nonreproducible, or expensive, or that require high temperatures, leave contaminating residues after processing, or generate oxidant-species or degradative stress, and require complicated purification steps. If it is necessary to use such systems, their potential effects must be assessed thoroughly before formulating the nutraceuticals.

Another important element is the nature of the lipid and its source, since preparation and homogenization techniques can significantly influence the structure of the nanoliposome, the number and position of the lamellae, particle size, uniformity, charge, and bilayer rigidity. Formulators must keep all these parameters in mind. In addition, the preparation process of nutraceutical nanoliposomes must guarantee production that is predictable and reproducible, with adequate particle size distribution (polydispersity), all determined by light-scattering techniques, which are the recommended control measures for these parameters. Validating preparation techniques is highly recommended to determine batch-to-batch scores (Mozafari 2010). Finally, most molecules, including nutraceuticals, are not totally encapsulated in nanoliposomes. This nonencapsulated compound can either be removed from, or allowed to remain in, the dispersion. The latter enhances the purpose and stability of the system. If separation techniques (e.g. dialysis, ultrafiltration, gel permeation, and ion exchange) are used, their selection must consider such aspects as food industry parameters, toxicity, and sustainability (Colas et al. 2007).

3.7.4 Preparation Methods

Nanoliposomes are prepared by assembling amphiphilic molecules, especially phospholipids (Hassane Hamadou et al. 2020). Two broad classifications are recognized based on the type of process: (i) chemical means (thin-film hydration, solvent injection, solvent diffusion, supercritical fluid process, reverse phase evaporation, etc.); and (ii) physical means (mechanical, microfluidization, high-pressure hot and cold homogenization, sonication, etc.). Techniques are classified by energy consumption as low-energy or high-energy. In general, the physical means coincide with high-energy techniques (Katouzian et al. 2017; Wang et al. 2017), but several preparation methods combine various approaches. Techniques that avoid the use of solvents are preferred for food applications (Tsai and Rizvi 2016). All these methods share three aspects: (i) a hydration step is required; (ii) the vesicles obtained must be homogenized; and (iii) purification is required to eliminate nonencapsulated nutraceutical molecules. The following sections describe various preparation techniques that can be used in designing nutraceutical nanoliposomes:

a) *Thin-film hydration (traditional) method and modalities.* This consists in forming a thin lipid film from an organic (chloroform, methanol, hexane, etc.) solution on a glass wall (distillation flask) that will be hydrated with an appropriate buffer solution by shaking (vortex, hand, or rotary evaporator). It requires a temperature above the phospholipid phase transition temperature. Multilamellar vesicles with broad size distributions are obtained (Hassane Hamadou et al. 2020). One interesting modality involves forming the lipid film by melting the phospholipids, thus avoiding the use of organic solvents *(heating method)*. During phospholipid humectation, an inert gas (e.g. N_2) can be bubbled into the formed dispersion to obtain multilamellar and large, unilamellar vesicles. Mozafari et al. (2008b) proposed a modality of the heating method that adds liposome ingredients to a preheated (60°C/5 min) mixture containing the material to be encapsulated and glycerol (final concentration 3% v/v) to form a film on a baffled wall glass flask by rotation (1000 rpm) on a hotplate stirrer (60°/45–60 minutes). However, the excess energy required to heat the materials can negatively affect the chemical or physicochemical properties of the nutraceuticals produced (da Silva Malheiros et al. 2012; Gülseren et al. 2007; Lagoueyte and Paquin 1998; Sant'Anna et al. 2011; Zarrabi et al. 2020). Another modality is called in situ liposome preparation, or the pro-liposome technique (Payne et al. 1986). In this case, the phospholipids are deposited as a thin film on particles of fine sodium chloride or sorbitol, and a highly concentrated dispersion is formed by hydrating. The application of mechanical energy as a secondary process can promote the transformation of multilamellar into large unilamellar, or even small unilamellar, vesicles depending on the device used and the specific working conditions (energy input). Homogenization by membrane extrusion, for example, can generate – depending on pore size – large unilamellar vesicles or nanoliposomes. In contrast, if microfluidization, colloid mill, or high-shear homogenization is used, most of the nanoliposomes obtained will have diameters as small as 100 nm (Leung et al. 2019). Sonication is another simple way to reduce liposomes to nanometric size, as it uses ultrasonic waves to break down the cavitation particles. Sonication, however, requires strict temperature control, is difficult to raise to an industrial scale, and can contaminate. Significantly, any of these homogenization systems can be used to transform liposomes into nanoliposomes by almost any method (Beltrán et al. 2020; Gulzar and Benjakul 2020).

b) *Microfluidization*. This is an attractive method for preparing food nanoliposomes because it does not use organic solvents. Industrial scale-up is possible that is both continuous and reproducible. Nanoliposome particle size is narrow, and high-efficiency encapsulation (>75%) can be obtained (Beltrán et al. 2020). The microfluidizer is a device that uses high pressure (up to 10 000 psi) to create a high-shear fluid that passes through specifically configured microchannels that generate shear, impact, and cavitation inside an interaction chamber. The process is quite simple as the components of the nanoliposomes are dispersed in the aqueous medium by mechanical stirring or a rotor/stator homogenizer. This raw pre-dispersion passes through the microfluidizer and recycled until the required size is obtained. Finally, a cooling chamber lowers the temperature generated during homogenization (Mozafari 2010).

c) *Methods based on replacing an organic with an aqueous phase*. These fairly simple methods dissolve the phospholipids in an organic solvent, which is then placed in contact with an aqueous phase and eliminated to form the liposomes. The properties of the vesicles obtained depend on the modality applied. If the organic solvent is immiscible in water, an emulsion results. Generally speaking, a phospholipid/ether or ether/methanol solution is slowly injected under agitation. After the organic solvent is removed by evaporation under reduced pressure, large unilamellar vesicles are obtained. Other structures reported modify the organic/lipid/aqueous phase ratio and stirring rate. In one common modality, the phospholipid is dissolved in an organic solvent with a low boiling point (e.g. chloroform, diethyl ether, and methanol) and an aqueous solution is added to the organic phase using either low-energy sonication or vortex shaking to form a water-in-oil emulsion (reverse system). Under controlled conditions, the solvent is removed by vacuum evaporation and the emulsion is inverted. Large unilamellar or oligolamellar liposomes called reverse-phase evaporation vesicles (REV) with a high loading capacity are obtained (Szoka et al. 1980; Szoka and Papahadjopoulos 1978; Tsai and Rizvi 2016). A 3:1 organic/aqueous phase ratio is commonly reported. If the organic content is increased, or the phospholipid concentration is above 20 µmol/ml, multilamellar REVs are formed (concentric vesicles with high hydro-loading capacity). If the entire process, including evaporation, is performed under stable sonication, plurilamellar vesicles (inter-bilayer vesicles with high lipoloading capacity) result (Demirci et al. 2017). This method can be performed using supercritical gas (e.g. carbon dioxide) instead of organic solvents, to provide significant advantages related to sustainability, toxicity, nutraceutical industry acceptability, and potential scale-up, etc. This process is called supercritical reverse-phase evaporation (Otake et al. 2006).

d) *Solvents miscible in water (solvent injection method).* This approach solubilizes lipids in a miscible aqueous solvent (e.g. ethanol) and injects them into the aqueous phase to form nanoliposomes immediately after diffusion of the solvent by lipid precipitation in bilayer fragments that quickly self-assemble in vesicles (Batzri and Korn 1973). The nanoprecipitation and solvent displacement methods are nanotechnological names that describe the interfacial turbulence formation mechanism (Quintanar-Guerrero et al. 1997). This method has several advantages: (i) simple and rapid implementation; (ii) reproducibility; (iii) solvent acceptability; (iv) size control dependent on injection speed; (v) potential industrial scale-up; and (vi) nutraceutical compatibility. Disadvantages are: (i) low phospholipid solubility; (ii) difficulty in encapsulating hydrophilic nutraceuticals; and iii) ethanol removal (Tsai and Rizvi 2016).

e) *Detergent removal methods.* Mixed micelles can be formed with phospholipids, detergents, and lipophilic nutraceuticals, among other compounds (e.g. amphipathic proteins). If the detergent is removed (by dialysis, gel filtration, or adding polymeric adsorbents), small vesicles will form. This method was first used to study the behavior of membranes in the presence of various proteins, tumor membranes, and virus envelopes (Chandler 1992; Nelson et al. 1972; Racker 1972). Important drawbacks of formulating nutraceuticals in this way are: (i) low encapsulation of hydrophilic low-molecular molecules; (ii) cost; (iii) time; and (iv) content of nonfood-grade detergent residues (Mozafari et al. 2008b).

f) *Methods based on pH adjustment.* Phosphatidic acid dispersions can form small unilamellar or large vesicles upon transient exposure to alkaline solutions. This method has had little impact due to its low efficiency, problems with size control, cost, and potential degradation (Hauser 1989).

g) *Supercritical fluid process.* This method arose to provide a continuous green process that does not require an organic solvent. So, it is more susceptible to implementation in alimentary industries. These methods use a supercritical, nontoxic incombustible gas with low critical temperature and moderate critical pressure as the solubilizer medium for phospholipids. Supercritical carbon dioxide is recommended to prepare various dispersions because it evaporates completely under ambient conditions. In rapid expansion of supercritical solution processes, the phospholipid dissolved in the supercritical carbon dioxide passes through a small orifice and is mixed with an aqueous loading solution (Cabrera et al. 2013; Castor 1994). The vesicles are formed by the desolvation of the phospholipids as they pass through a non-solvent medium. An intermediate, oil-in-water emulsion is formed during gas expansion. The type, size, and encapsulation efficiency of the liposomes obtained depend on several preparation variables: pre-expansion pressure, orifice diameter, solubility of components, and the presence of cosolvents, etc. The versatility of this method is countered by the fragility of the liposomes obtained and their low encapsulation efficiency. Several modifications of rapid expansion of supercritical solution have been proposed to encapsulate specific molecules more efficiently or improve process performance. These include using cosolvents to increase phospholipid solubility, encapsulating hydrophilic molecules, incorporating a pressure pump, utilizing a high-pressure reactor and collector (improved rapid expansion of supercritical solution), incorporating vacuum-driven cargo suction to make the process continuous, depressurizing an expanded solution in aqueous media to prepare bulk liposomal dispersions in a vessel, spraying the organic phospholipid solution onto a continuous phase of supercritical gas that functions as an antisolvent to cause phospholipid precipitation by diffusion, implementing a continuous antisolvent process for industrial applications, and depressurizing an expanded liquid solution-suspension, among others (Cabrera et al. 2013; Lesoin et al. 2011; Otake et al. 2006; Tsai and Rizvi 2016).

3.7.5 Mechanism of Formation

When an amphiphilic material is dissolved or dispersed in an aqueous medium, various chemical interactions occur among the polar head, lipophilic tails, and expressed solvent (Subramani and Ganapathyswamy 2020). Different colloidal association structures can be formed by self-assembly. When phospholipid bilayers are humected, Van der Waals and hydrophilic/hydrophobic interactions manifest the formation of spherical bilayer structures. Perhaps the best way to explain the type of association structure formed by an amphiphilic molecule is based on the molecular shape using the critical packing parameter (Israelachvili 2011; Israelachvili et al. 1980), which expresses the ratio between the surfactant parameters:

$$CPP = \frac{v}{al} \tag{3.1}$$

where v is the volume of the hydrophobic tail, a is the area of the polar head, and l is the length of the hydrophobic chain (Šegota and Težak 2006). For double-chained, "fluid state" lipids with a large head-group area that behave as a non-soluble swelling amphiphile, like phosphatidyl choline, phosphatidyl serine, phosphatidyl glycerol, phosphatidyl inositol, phosphatidic acid, sphingomyelin DGDG, and most alpha-tocopherol phosphates, a 0.5> critical packing parameter <1 will be obtained. This value suggests that the molecule has a truncated, cone-critical packing shape and will form flexible bilayer vesicles (called Lam, Lα, D, G, etc.) with the largest aggregation number (g_{max}) of 2 l/v. In this context, polar groups of phosphatides are oriented toward the interior and exterior of the aqueous phase, while hydrocarbon chains reduce unfavorable interactions (concentric packing), and bilayer sheets are formed that fold to form a closed-stable vesicle (minimum thermodynamic energy level) with an interior aqueous phase. It is important to note that generating this bilayer association requires administering minimal energy to the system, whether through physical, mechanical, thermal, or acoustic (e.g. ultrasonication) means, or a combination of these (Mozafari 2010) (Figure 3.4). If nutraceutical (hydro- or lipophilic) molecules are added during the process, they will be encapsulated – depending on their nature – in the bilayer or aqueous-core reservoir (Demirci et al. 2017). Significantly, while critical packing parameter is a highly didactic way of explaining the formation of bilayer vesicles, several conditions can modify the aggregation state and, hence, the critical packing parameter value, including pH, temperature, the inclusion of proteins and/or carbohydrates as vesicle stabilizers, contra-ion molecules (ion-pair formation), interaction and/or fusion among structures, and mixtures with other lipids or amphiphilic molecules (Cheng et al. 2019).

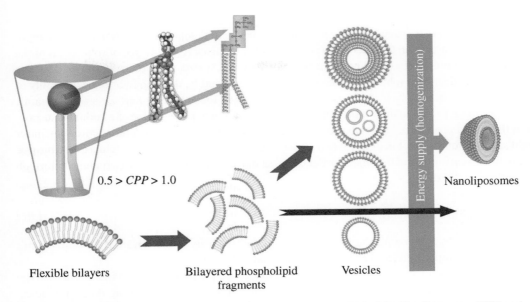

Figure 3.4 Schematic representation of liposome formation by the Critical Packing Parameter (CPP) and bilayer phospholipid fragments (BPF).

One issue that requires additional explanation is the process of vesicle formation from stacks of hydrated lipid bilayers. The *budding off theory* holds that large sheets of a bilayer bud off multilamellar (mother liposomes) to form small or large vesicles (daughter vesicles). The curvature elastic theory for an uncharged molecule suggests that this process is not spontaneous, but requires energy because the curvature energy of vesicles is higher than in the stacked form (Jesenek et al. 2013). This implies that these liposomes are in a metastable state that can subsist for months or even years. In contrast, charged phospholipids can form spontaneously under favorable conditions as uni- or oligolamellar vesicles. It is well-known that a higher curvature of the bilayer produces a smaller liposome. So, in some cases, high energy or mixtures with other amphiphilic molecules are used to obtain nanometer size (Hassane Hamadou et al. 2020).

Another widely recognized mechanism used to explain liposome formation sets out from intermediate structures called bilayer phospholipid fragments, which self-close in liposomes (Lasic 1995; Racker 1988). This model makes it possible to explain liposome formation by means of detergent removal but can be extended to any vesicle preparation procedure. Thus, liposomes can be formed from mixed micelles containing at least one phospholipid and detergents, as long as the latter is reduced (detergent depletion) to a certain concentration in the solution. The alkyl chains of phospholipids express their lipophilic nature by minimizing their interfacial area to form, first, BPFs, and then vesicles (Lesoin et al. 2011).

3.7.6 Characterization

Various process controls are applied to achieve specific, reproducible parameters when elaborating nanoliposomes (Weissing 2017). The most common controls are determining particle size, zeta potential, and morphology by electron microscopy. This strategy requires expensive equipment but is essential for verifying the key parameters of formulations.

3.7.6.1 Particle Size

Average particle size is crucial in these formulations because biological interaction and final applications depend largely on this factor. It is even possible to measure the degree of robustness of the manufacturing process by oscillations in the average particle size. In some cases, as particle size decreases, the degree of robustness also begins to decline; that is, the degree of reproducibility of the formulation diminishes. The most common technique for analyzing particle size is dynamic light-scattering. Dynamic light-scattering measures the average particle size of a colloidal suspension through a procedure in which the colloidal sample is illuminated by a monochromatic laser light scattered onto a photon detector (Xu 2008). The scattered light intensity fluctuates in time due to the Brownian motion of the small particles. These movements are related to particle size through the following equation:

$$D_h = \frac{k_B T}{3\pi\eta D_t} \tag{3.2}$$

where D_h is the hydrodynamic diameter, η is the relative viscosity of the solvent, k_B is Boltzmann's constant, T is temperature, and D_t is the translational diffusion coefficient.

In addition to average particle size, it is normal to include the polydispersion index and the type of distribution of the particle populations present in samples when describing them in studies. While one might desire only a specific population of particles with a peak in the graphs, at times, insufficient control of critical variables in the manufacturing process generates two or more populations of particle sizes that will be reflected in two or more spikes in the distribution charts.

3.7.6.2 Zeta Potential

Measuring zeta potential is a complement to particle size assessment. This parameter can usually be measured using the type of instrumentation mentioned above, but based on a different principle. Zeta potential helps predict the stability of the dispersed nanoliposomes: those with a high absolute zeta potential are electrically stable, while those with a low value tend to be less stable. Less frequent, but also useful, is using zeta potential to predict possible interactions with cells. A positive charge on the surface of nanoliposomes can increase interaction with the negative charge of the cell membrane or, where appropriate, with bacteria. Zeta potential analysis is generally performed by electrophoresis (Kathe et al. 2014). The principle involved is to measure the electrophoretic mobility of charged particles under an applied electrical potential. Henry's equation is used to calculate zeta potential (z):

$$U_e = \frac{2\varepsilon z f\left(\kappa a\right)}{3\eta} \tag{3.3}$$

where U_e is electrophoretic mobility, ε is the dielectric constant, η is the absolute zero-shear viscosity of the medium, $f(\kappa a)$ is Henry's function, and κa is a measure of the ratio of the particle radius to the Debye length (Clogston and Patri 2011).

3.7.6.3 Structure and Morphology

The structure and morphology of nanoliposomes can be determined by transmission electron microscopy (TEM). Samples placed on a copper grid are negatively stained with a 2% phosphotungstic acid solution and air-dried before observation under TEM (Figure 3.5).

Though morphology under TEM may differ from the original form that dispersed liposomes acquire, the cryo-TEM modality can be useful in maintaining the original features. The advantage

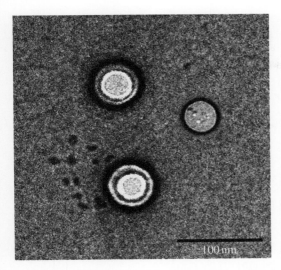

Figure 3.5 ω3 polyunsaturated fatty acids incorporated into nanoliposomes for food enrichment. *Source:* Reproduced with permission from Rasti et al. (2017) © 2017 Elsevier.

of TEM over scanning electron or atomic force microscopy is the appreciation of the inner layers of the nanoliposome. As Figure 3.5 shows, at least one bilayer of phospholipids can be distinguished compared to the images observed by AFM, though its resolution reaches 3Å (Figure 3.6). Another option for determining lamellarity is Mn^{2+} labeling, which interacts with the negative charge of the phosphate groups on the phospholipids to cause a broadening and reduction of the quantifiable signal using ^{31}P NMR.

3.7.6.4 Encapsulation Efficiency

The methods employed to determine the entrapment efficiency of nanoliposomes coincide with the traditional strategies used with nanoparticles. A sample can be centrifuged under moderate conditions to form sediments of nanoliposomes and the supernatant can then be quantified. Another procedure removes the supernatant and dissolves the nanoliposomes to release the drug. It is important to use moderate centrifugation conditions to avoid breaking the nanoliposomes and releasing more drug than is anticipated. The quantification method and type of instrumentation adapted for quantification depend on the physicochemical properties of the drug, especially stability, solubility, and the molar absorptivity coefficient (Weissing 2017).

3.7.7 Uses of Nanoliposomes in Nutraceutical Systems

The properties of nanoliposomes differ from those of liposomes larger than 1 μm as their small size increases both the surface area and the probability of interaction with various structures in the cell membrane. Most biological reactions occur at the nanometric level. So, nanoliposomes greatly improve the biological functionality of nutraceuticals, including bioactive compounds of natural origin (Khorasani et al. 2018). Nanoliposomes have been used to encapsulate essential oils combined with other micronutrients, hydrosoluble compounds like vitamin C, and plant extracts that are currently of great interest as an attractive option for developing sustainable nutraceutical systems that utilize parts of plants not normally consumed as food, and/or byproducts of food preparation, including bagasse, seeds, and remains of pulp, among others, which contain innumerable

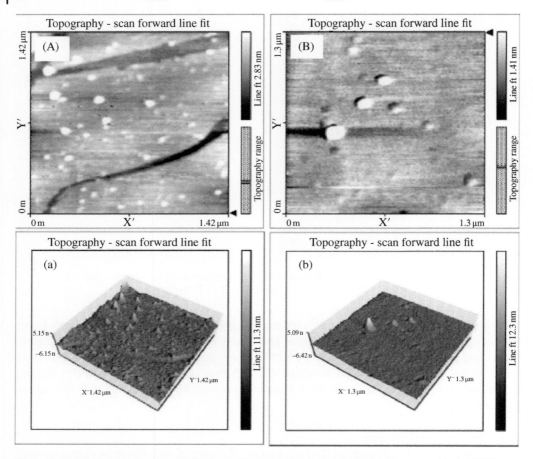

Figure 3.6 AFM images (topography) of nanoliposomes loaded with charantin extract: (A, a) 0.5E1L (0.5% extract and 1% lecithin) and (B, b) 0.5E5L (0.5% extract and 5% lecithin). *Source:* Reproduced with permission from Rezaei Erami et al. (2019) © 2017 Elsevier.

substances that can be extracted by different methods and used to form bioactive and functional compounds. Components like quercetin, thymoquinone, essential cinnamon oil, and resveratrol, for example, have been used in cancer treatments (Ballout et al. 2018; Saneja et al. 2018; Vergallo 2020). Some of these substances also have anti-inflammatory and cardiovascular protector functions; for example, phospholipids, the principal components of nanoliposomes (Lordan et al. 2017). In addition, extracts from cherries, ginger, blueberries, and similar natural products contain polyphenols with anti-inflammatory properties, while others perform the function of protecting the heart through their capacity to reduce the formation of cholesterol plaques in the venous system, as studies of endothelial cells have demonstrated (Beconcini et al. 2020; Rubió et al. 2014). In fact, numerous antioxidant substances with diverse effects on organisms are being studied for their possible beneficial health effects; for example, polyphenols, which include the essential oils of cardamom, cinnamon, rice, and Curcuma, among many others (Keivani Nahr et al. 2019; Meghani et al. 2018; Quagliariello et al. 2018; Rodriguez et al. 2019).

Because nanoliposomes are thermodynamically unstable systems, there is a high probability of aggregation that will rupture the membrane formed by the phospholipids, thereby reducing the lipophilic components' capacity to penetrate the organism and make itself bioavailable. Phenols in aqueous and lipid plant extracts have also sparked interest in recent years. Here again, nanoliposomes are a good option for increasing the penetrability of components and improving their beneficial action for health (Khorasani et al. 2018).

Nanoliposomes have the capacity to incorporate new types of amphiphilic lipids with nutraceutical properties because they function as anti-inflammatories, anti-carcinogens, or antioxidants with many health benefits. One such case involves using marine phospholipids which have advantages over phospholipids derived from soy or egg lecithin. Marine phospholipids are less susceptible to lipid oxidation because they are packed intermolecularly at the sn-2 position of glycerol, giving them greater stability (Lordan et al. 2017). Phospholipids of marine origin have been used to encapsulate carotenoids in nanoliposomes prepared by the thin film method that, compared to nanoliposomes formed with phospholipids derived from egg, show greater encapsulation capacity, zeta potential, and stability during 70 days of storage, as well as the ability to protect encapsulated β-carotene, as shown by their greater antioxidant capacity (Hassane Hamadou et al. 2020).

Some current research on the preparation of nanoliposomes uses microfluidization and ultrasonic processing to evaluate the effect of these processes on system stability and changes in particle size associated with their passage through the GIT. A study of palm oil rich in lycopene and β-carotene encapsulated in nanoliposomes prepared by the film hydration method and a microfluidization or ultrasound process found that the nanoliposomes formed with microfluidization maintained greater stability in terms of particle size as they passed through a simulated GIT system. That study established that particle size increased in the gastric medium from 141–180 to 445–481 nm for nanoliposomes prepared by microfluidization and ultrasound, respectively. Particle size decreased slightly in the intestinal phase (Beltrán et al. 2019).

Using natural polymers to coat nanoliposomes to improve their stability by limiting the oxidation of the lipid bilayer is another current topic of study. The methods employed to conduct this process are layer-by-layer deposition and crossover (Zamani Ghaleshahi and Rajabzadeh 2020). While the latter is more effective in improving the physical and chemical properties and controlled release, its utilization is limited because the substance added as the crossover agent can form toxic components; hence, it is preferable to use self-assembling methods or to select natural crossover compounds like tartaric acid, genipin, lychee procyanidins, or various other phenols obtained from byproducts of the food industry that can potentialize the nutraceutical effect of several components of food and food byproducts (Luo et al. 2020; Zamani Ghaleshahi and Rajabzadeh 2020). For layer-by-layer coating systems, it is possible to use various polymers – chitosan, sodium alginate, and whey, among others – to form multiple layers, as they permit modeling systems that allow bioactive functional-wall, and polymeric-gastrointestinal environment interactions that are capable of achieving absorption, bioaccessibility, and bioavailability of nutraceuticals with the longest possible storage stability. Table 3.3 shows some of the studies that have been conducted with nanoliposomes to prepare nutraceutical ingredients, considering the method of preparation and potential action site of nutraceutical ingredient.

3.7.8 Safety, Regulatory, and Sustainability Issues Related to Nanoliposomes

Liposomal technology has been developing over several decades. Today, some well-established products on the market contain this technology in areas, including pharmaceuticals, cosmetics, and food. However, they do not bear a statement indicating that they contain nanoscale particles, but are presented in the generic form of liposomes. In fact, there is no formal, established regulatory framework for nanoliposomes. So, products that contain nanoscale particles already available

Table 3.3 Nanoliposomes as releases systems of different nutraceutical substances.

Component encapsulated	Phospholipid and other components	Nutraceutical effect	Preparation method	Principal characteristics
Cardamom	PC, C	Anti-inflammatory and antioxidant	Layer hydration/homogenization/Ultrasonication Solvent: Methanol	Particle size < 150 nm. Stable up to 40 days which decrease at pH = 7.0. Encapsulation efficiency > 60%. Release increase with increase cardamom amount (Keivani Nahr et al. 2019).
Lycopene	Lecithin	Cardiovascular disease, cancer prevention, improve immunity, photoprotective effect	Layer hydration/Ultrasonication Solvent: Chloroform	*In vivo* nanoliposomes shows that POD, CAT and SOD were higher respect to control liver mice whit less MDA. Nanoliposomes improve water solubility of lycopene and increases its oral bioavailability (Fan et al. 2011).
High oleic palm oil; rich in carotenoids and Vitamin E	Lecithin	Antioxidant	Mozafari method	Particle size increases in the intestinal phase *in vitro* maintaining nanometric size. Microfluidization had best digestibility (Beltrán et al. 2019).
Betalains from *Basella rubra L.* leaf	Soyabean lecithin	Malignancy, aggravation, joint inflammation, neurodegenerative, and cardiovascular diseases	Thin-film hydration-sonication technique	The betalains nanoliposomes showed higher thermal stability respect to nanoliposomes unloaded. This type of encapsulation is a novel method to encapsulation of betalains (Sravan Kumar et al. 2020).
Orange seed protein	Soya lecithin C Coating: Chitosan	Immuno-modulatory, antibacterial, antithrombotic, reducing the blood pressure, hypocholestero-lemic, antioxidant, and anti-cancer activities	Thin-film hydration method	The study revealed the effect of peptide type loaded and chitosan concentration determined the particle size, polydispersity index and encapsulation efficiency The peptide protection and antioxidant effect using coated nanoliposomes was confirmed (Mazloomi et al. 2020).
Bioactive polyphenolic: Phloridzin	Soybean lecithin, 90% phosphatidylcholine (LIPOID P 100) Cationic lipid 1,2-dioleoyl-3-trimethylammoniumpropane. Coating: Pectin	Anti-diabetic activity	Organic solvent-free, heating-stirring-sonication method	Pectine-coating nanoliposomes are potential carriers for polyphenolic compounds. They showed best immobilization, encapsulation efficiencies and physical storage stability. The optimized nanoliposomes were stable during 4 months at 4 °C (Haghighi et al. 2018).

PC: phosphatidylcholine; C: cholesterol; POD: peroxidase; CAT: catalase; MDA: malondialdehyde; SOD: superoxide dismutase.

in the market emerged in the absence of such regulations. For two decades, regulatory agencies like the FDA and EMEA have made efforts to produce guidelines and recommendations for developing products that contain liposomes. In 2018, the FDA released a guide titled "Liposome Drug Products: chemistry, manufacturing, and controls; human pharmacokinetics and bioavailability; and labeling documentation" (Food and Drug Administration 2018). This document contains a series of guidelines exclusively for liposome drug products submitted as new drug applications (NDAs). Significantly, this document describes the characteristics of liposomal systems and their differences from other lipid systems but fails to differentiate in detail between liposomal and nanoliposomal systems. In 2011, the FDA published another document, "Guidance for Industry Considering Whether an FDA-Regulated Product Involves the Application of Nanotechnology" (Food and Drug Administration 2011), which described current thinking on determining whether FDA-regulated products involve the application of nanotechnology. In the specific case of nanoliposomal nutraceuticals, these could be considered in cases 1 and 2 of the guide, though they also appear in one of the categories of FDA-Regulated Products (drug or food supplements). The guide establishes the importance of evaluating the safety, effectiveness, performance, quality, and public health impact of such systems, whose physical and chemical properties and biological behavior are attributable to their reduced size. The EMEA, in a publication titled "Reflection paper on nanotechnology-based medicinal products for human use" (European Medicines Agency 2006), makes it clear that some pharmaceutical products are already on the market and have been approved even though they contain nanoparticles with no requirement for specific legislation. This report establishes that any request to place a nanomedical product on the market must be evaluated by the corresponding authority based on the established principles of risk/benefit analysis, in addition to a technology-based assessment. The EMEA urges all manufacturers of nanomedicinal products to conduct the necessary pre-marketing toxicological and ecotoxicological tests. Finally, in this context of the vacuum of specific guidelines, the EMEA urges applicants to contact it in the early stages of the development of their products through a committee called the Innovation Task Force (ITF).

In this setting, some nutraceuticals formulated with nanoliposomes may find a favorable path for acceptance by regulatory agencies because they already have, on the one hand, guidelines that clarify the criteria for the correct classification of what is "nano" and what is not, and, on the other, because some liposomal products are already available, having emerged despite the lack of specific regulations. Without doubt, nanoliposome-based nutraceutical products should demonstrate markedly greater efficiency and safety than nonencapsulated nutraceuticals to justify the advantage gained through nanoencapsulation. As well, they should demonstrate significant benefits with a low risk for patients and the environment. Manufacturing methods should reduce the environmental impact, especially by avoiding the use of potentially toxic solvents. The basic materials (phospholipids) are generally obtained from soy or egg and represent sustainable sources of production, but much remains to be done in the area of extraction and purification methods to achieve a truly green approach.

3.8 Future Trends

Nanoliposomes constitute a field that needs to implement and optimize preparation methods that limit the use of organic solvents to reduce toxicity in systems designed to administer nutraceuticals. The key factors to be addressed include the ability to escalate the methods to the industrial level, for this is currently a severe limitation of these systems. It is also necessary to evaluate the development of protein-coated nanoliposomes, as this would help increase their nutraceutical properties and biocompatibility with cells. Another area that requires research centers on targeting mechanisms to conduct nutraceuticals to specific action sites. Incorporating new ingredients with antioxidant capacity that reduces lipid oxidation of the phospholipid used as the wall is also crucial. Future considerations must also include characterizing the molecules present in different extracts obtained to elucidate their functions as nutraceuticals, studying interaction with vesicle walls, and incorporating hydrophilic and lipophilic components; this, in light of the synergic effect of the components that may potentialize their functionality and beneficial effects on human health.

As the study of different polymeric materials to enhance the stability of nanoliposomes and considerably improve their properties advances, it will become possible to develop novel systems that can be protected through the different stages of the process and passage through the GIT until they are absorbed at a specific action site. These could be designed specifically for controlled release under varying conditions of pH, ions, viscosity, and the characteristics of functional components. Another particularly important point regarding nutraceutical systems added to foods are changes in particle size and limitations on absorption due to the formation and modification of their structures, caused by interaction with other components of the foods, the effects of conditions in the GIT, the composition of microflora, and consumption habits, all of which must be considered when recommending sizes and forms of dosing.

One clear tendency in the preparation of nanoliposomes consists in optimizing new processes to obtain phospholipids from marine sources, or through biotechnological processes that will make ingredients available that are capable of forming stable systems that conserve their nutraceutical properties. Searching for new stabilization systems obtained through byproducts that reduce the use of cholesterol as the stabilizer, and that mediate other mechanisms, will help prevent oxidation of the phospholipids, thus increasing their shelf life. This has led to studies that will enable the incorporation of natural antioxidants and phase transition temperature modifiers.

3.9 Conclusion

There is growing interest in the food industry in developing products with novel, enhanced properties. Liposomal nanotechnology represents a viable alternative for facilitating the incorporation of nutraceutical components found in foods, food byproducts, and plant extracts that are susceptible to degradation. This chapter discussed our current knowledge of nutraceutical nanoliposomes to provide consolidated information that can be used by nutraceutical formulators to satisfy specific objectives in encapsulation design. As we have seen, nanoliposomes can be prepared by various methods with the only condition being that the organic solvents used cannot be toxic. Methods such as thin-film hydration have been modified using polyols in film formation. While several other methods – microfluidization, supercritical fluids, water-miscible solvents like ethanol – are important for preparing nanoliposomes, they require additional modifications to increase encapsulation efficiency and stability. Characterization is a critical step in demonstrating the particle size, surface characteristics, and encapsulation efficiency, among other key parameters for establishing compatibility, documenting their impact on the properties of systems, and studying their behavior in the GIT. It is also important to determine which characteristics of bioactives with nutraceutical properties provide the best bioavailability and targeting at the action site, as well as the stability and shelf-life of products, and the effects of transit through the GIT. Finally, the design of nutraceuticals for incorporation in foods and beverages must consider the characteristics of both the functional bioactive and the food into which it will be incorporated to ensure that it will remain stable during commercialization and perform its health-promoting action upon ingestion.

Acknowledgments

The authors acknowledge support for this work provided by PAPIIT IN 222520 and IN 222420 (DGAPA), PIAPI2060.

References

Akbari-Alavijeh, S., Shaddel, R., and Jafari, S.M. (2020). Encapsulation of food bioactives and nutraceuticals by various chitosan-based nanocarriers. *Food Hydrocolloids 105*: 105774. https://doi.org/10.1016/j.foodhyd.2020.105774.

Akbarzadeh, A., Rezaei-Sadabady, R., Davaran, S. et al. (2013). Liposome: classification, preparation, and applications. *Nanoscale Research Letters 102* (8): 1–9. https://doi.org/10.1186/1556-276X-8-102.

Akhavan, S., Assadpour, E., Katouzian, I., and Jafari, S.M. (2018). Lipid nano scale cargos for the protection and delivery of food bioactive ingredients and nutraceuticals. *Trends in Food Science and Technology 74*: 132–146. https://doi.org/10.1016/j.tifs.2018.02.001.

Ali, A., Ahmad, U., Akhtar, J. et al. (2019). Engineered nano scale formulation strategies to augment efficiency of nutraceuticals. *Journal of Functional Foods 62*: 103554. https://doi.org/10.1016/j.jff.2019.103554.

Allen, T.M. and Cullis, P.R. (2013). Liposomal drug delivery systems: from concept to clinical applications. *Advanced Drug Delivery Reviews 65* (1): 36–48. https://doi.org/10.1016/j.addr.2012.09.037.

Amidon, G.L., Lennernäs, H., Shah, V.P., and Crison, J.R. (1995). A theoretical basis for a biopharmaceutic drug clasification: the correlation of in vitro drug product dissolution and in vivo bioavailability. *Pharmaceutical Research 12* (3): 413–420.

Assadpour, E. and Mahdi Jafari, S. (2019). A systematic review on nanoencapsulation of food bioactive ingredients and nutraceuticals by various nanocarriers. *Critical Reviews in Food Science and Nutrition 59* (19): 3129–3151. https://doi.org/10.1080/10408398.2018.1484687.

Ballout, F., Habli, Z., Rahal, O.N. et al. (2018). Thymoquinone-based nanotechnology for cancer therapy: promises and challenges. *Drug Discovery Today 23* (5): 1089–1098. https://doi.org/10.1016/j.drudis.2018.01.043.

Barenholz, Y. (2012). Doxil® – the first FDA-approved nano-drug: lessons learned. *Journal of Controlled Release 160* (2): 117–134. https://doi.org/10.1016/j.jconrel.2012.03.020.

Batzri, S. and Korn, E.D. (1973). Single bilayer liposomes prepared without sonieation. *Biochemica et Biophysica Acta (BBA)-Biomembranes 298* (4): 1015–1019.

Beconcini, D., Felice, F., Fabiano, A. et al. (2020). Antioxidant and anti-inflammatory properties of cherry extract: nanosystems-based strategies to improve endothelial function and intestinal absorption. *Food 9* (2): 207. https://doi.org/10.3390/foods9020207.

Beltrán, J.D., Sandoval-Cuellar, C.E., Bauer, K., and Quintanilla-Carvajal, M.X. (2019). In-vitro digestion of high-oleic palm oil nanoliposomes prepared with unpurified soy lecithin: physical stability and nano-liposome digestibility. *Colloids and Surfaces A: Physicochemical and Engineering Aspects 578*: 123603. https://doi.org/10.1016/j.colsurfa.2019.123603.

Beltrán, J.D., Ricaurte, L., Estrada, K.B., and Quintanilla-Carvajal, M.X. (2020). Effect of homogenization methods on the physical stability of nutrition grade nanoliposomes used for encapsulating high oleic palm oil. *Lwt 118*: 108801. https://doi.org/10.1016/j.lwt.2019.108801.

Bonechi, C., Donati, A., Tamasi, G. et al. (2019). Chemical characterization of liposomes containing nutraceutical compounds: tyrosol, hydroxytyrosol and oleuropein. *Biophysical Chemistry 246*: 25–34. https://doi.org/10.1016/j.bpc.2019.01.002.

Brotons-Canto, A., Gonzalez-Navarro, C.J., Gurrea, J. et al. (2020). Zein nanoparticles improve the oral bioavailability of resveratrol in humans. *Journal of Drug Delivery Science and Technology 57*: 101704. https://doi.org/10.1016/j.jddst.2020.101704.

Cabrera, I., Elizondo, E., Esteban, O. et al. (2013). Multifunctional nanovesicle-bioactive conjugates prepared by a one-step scalable method using CO_2-expanded solvents. *Nano Letters 13* (8): 3766–3774. https://doi.org/10.1021/nl4017072.

Cassidy, A. and Minihane, A.M. (2017). The role of metabolism (and the microbiome) in defining the clinical efficacy of dietary flavonoids. *American Journal of Clinical Nutrition 105* (1): 10–22. https://doi.org/10.3945/ajcn.116.136051.

Castor, T. P. (1994). *Methods and apparatus for making liposomes using critical, supercritical or near critical fluids*. WO1994US05933 19940526.

Chandler, R. (1992). Artificial viral envelopes containing recombinant human immunodeficiency virus (HIV) gp160. *Life Science Journal 50*(7): 481–489.

Chen, W., Ju, X., Aluko, R.E. et al. (2020). Rice bran protein-based nanoemulsion carrier for improving stability and bioavailability of quercetin. *Food Hydrocolloids 108*: 106042. https://doi.org/10.1016/j.foodhyd.2020.106042.

Cheng, C., Wu, Z., McClements, D.J. et al. (2019). Improvement on stability, loading capacity and sustained release of rhamnolipids modified curcumin liposomes. *Colloids and Surfaces B: Biointerfaces 183*: 110460. https://doi.org/10.1016/j.colsurfb.2019.110460.

Chi, J., Ge, J., Yue, X. et al. (2019). Preparation of nanoliposomal carriers to improve the stability of anthocyanins. *LWT 109*: 101–107. https://doi.org/10.1016/j.lwt.2019.03.070.

Clogston, J.D. and Patri, A.K. (2011). Zeta potential measurement. In: *National Institute of Standards and TechnologyCharacterization of Nanoparticles Intended for Drug Delivery*, vol. 697 (ed. S.E. McNeil), 71–82. Humana Press https://doi.org/10.1007/978-1-60327-198-1.

Colas, J., Shi, W., Rao, V.S.N.M. et al. (2007). Microscopical investigations of nisin-loaded nanoliposomes prepared by Mozafari method and their bacterial targeting. *Micron 38*: 841–847. https://doi.org/10.1016/j.micron.2007.06.013.

Coupland, J.N. and Hayes, J.E. (2014). Physical approaches to masking bitter taste: lessons from food and pharmaceuticals. *Pharmaceutical Research 31* (11): 2921–2939. https://doi.org/10.1007/s11095-014-1480-6.

Crommelin, D.J.A., van Hoogevest, P., and Storm, G. (2020). The role of liposomes in clinical nanomedicine development. What now? Now what? *Journal of Controlled Release 318*: 256–263. https://doi.org/10.1016/j.jconrel.2019.12.023.

Dahiya, M. and Dureja, H. (2018). Recent developments in the formulation of nanoliposomal delivery systems. *Current Nanomaterials 3* (2): 62–74. https://doi.org/10.2174/2405461503666180821093033.

Deamer, D.W. (2010). From "Banghasomes" to liposomes: a memoir of Alec Bangham, 1921–2010. *The FASEB Journal 24* (5): 1308–1310. https://doi.org/10.1096/fj.10-0503.

Demirci, M., Caglar, M.Y., Cakir, B., and Gülseren, I. (2017). Encapsulation by nanoliposomes. In: *Nanoencapsulation Technologies for the Food and Nutraceutical Industries*, 1e (ed. S. Mahdi Jafari), 74–113. Elsevier https://doi.org/10.1016/B978-0-12-809436-5.00003-3.

Dima, C., Assadpour, E., Dima, S., and Jafari, S.M. (2020). Bioavailability of nutraceuticals: role of the food matrix, processing conditions, the gastrointestinal tract, and nanodelivery systems. *Comprehensive Reviews in Food Science and Food Safety 19* (3): 954–994. https://doi.org/10.1111/154 1-4337.12547.

Durazzo, A., Nazhand, A., Lucarini, M. et al. (2020). An updated overview on nanonutraceuticals: focus on nanoprebiotics and nanoprobiotics. *International Journal of Molecular Sciences 21* (7): 1–24. https://doi.org/10.3390/ijms21072285.

Dutta, S., Moses, J.A., and Anandharamakrishnan, C. (2018). Encapsulation of nutraceutical ingredients in liposomes and their potential for cancer treatment. *Nutrition and Cancer 70* (8): 1184–1198. https://doi.org/10.1080/01635581.2018.1557212.

European Medicines Agency (2006). *Reflection Paper on Nanotechnology-Based Medicinal Products for Human Use*. European Medicinees Agency.

Fan, Y., Xie, X., Zhang, B., and Zhang, Z. (2011). Absorption and antioxidant activity of lycopene nanoliposomes in vivo. *Current Topics in Nutraceutical Research 9* (4): 131–138.

Food and Drug Administration. (2011). *Guidance for industry considering whether an FDA-regulated product involves the application of nanotechnology.* https://doi.org/10.1089/blr.2011.9814

Food and Drug Administration. (2018). Liposome drug products: chemistry, manufacturing, and controls; human pharmacokinetics and bioavailability; and labeling. In *Food and Drug Administration*.

Galindo-Pérez, M.J., Quintanar-Guerrero, D., Cornejo-Villegas, M.D.L.Á., and Zambrano-Zaragoza, M.D.L.L. (2018). Optimization of the emulsification-diffusion method using ultrasound to prepare nanocapsules of different food-core oils. *LWT – Food Science and Technology* https://doi.org/10.1016/j.lwt.2017.09.008.

Gülseren, I., Güzey, D., Bruce, B.D., and Weiss, J. (2007). Structural and functional changes in ultrasonicated bovine serum albumin solutions. *Ultrasonics Sonochemistry 14* (2): 173–183. https://doi.org/10.1016/j.ultsonch.2005.07.006.

Gulzar, S. and Benjakul, S. (2020). Characteristics and storage stability of nanoliposomes loaded with shrimp oil as affected by ultrasonication and microfluidization. *Food Chemistry 310*: 125916. https://doi.org/10.1016/j.foodchem.2019.125916.

Haghighi, M., Yarmand, M.S., Emam-Djomeh, Z. et al. (2018). Design and fabrication of pectin-coated nanoliposomal delivery systems for a bioactive polyphenolic: Phloridzin. *International Journal of Biological Macromolecules 112*: 626–637. https://doi.org/10.1016/j.ijbiomac.2018.01.108.

Hassane Hamadou, A., Huang, W.C., Xue, C., and Mao, X. (2020). Comparison of β-carotene loaded marine and egg phospholipids nanoliposomes. *Journal of Food Engineering 283*: 110055. https://doi.org/10.1016/j.jfoodeng.2020.110055.

Hauser, H. (1989). Mechanism of spontaneous vesiculation. *Proceedings of the National Academy of Sciences of the United States of America 86* (14): 5351–5355. https://doi.org/10.1073/pnas.86.14.5351.

He, H., Lu, Y., Qi, J. et al. (2019). Adapting liposomes for oral drug delivery. *Acta Pharmaceutica Sinica B 9* (1): 36–48. https://doi.org/10.1016/j.apsb.2018.06.005.

Huang, Z., Li, X., Zhang, T. et al. (2014). Progress involving new techniques for liposome preparation. *Asian Journal of Pharmaceutical Sciences 9* (4): 176–182. https://doi.org/10.1016/j.ajps.2014.06.001.

Huang, M., Su, E., Zheng, F., and Tan, C. (2017). Encapsulation of flavonoids in liposomal delivery systems: the case of quercetin, kaempferol and luteolin. *Food & Function 8* (9): 3198–3208. https://doi.org/10.1039/c7fo00508c.

Israelachvili, J.N. (2011). Thermodynamic principles of self-assembly. In: *Intermolecular and Surface Forces*, 503–534. Elsevier https://doi.org/10.1016/B978-0-12-391927-4.10019-2.

Israelachvili, J.N., Marcelja, S., Horn, R.G., and Israelachvili, J.N. (1980). Physical principles of membrane organization. *Quarterly Reviews of Biophysics* 13 (2) https://doi.org/10.1017/S0033583500001645.

Jesenek, D., Perutková, Š., Góźdź, W. et al. (2013). Vesiculation of biological membrane driven by curvature induced frustrations in membrane orientational ordering. *International Journal of Nanomedicine 8*: 677–687. https://doi.org/10.2147/IJN.S38314.

Kathe, N., Henriksen, B., and Chauhan, H. (2014). Physicochemical characterization techniques for solid lipid nanoparticles: principles and limitations. *Drug Development and Industrial Pharmacy 40* (12): 1565–1575. https://doi.org/10.3109/03639045.2014.909840.

Katouzian, I., Faridi Esfanjani, A., Jafari, S.M., and Akhavan, S. (2017). Formulation and application of a new generation of lipid nano-carriers for the food bioactive ingredients. *Trends in Food Science and Technology 68*: 14–25. https://doi.org/10.1016/j.tifs.2017.07.017.

Keivani Nahr, F., Ghanbarzadeh, B., Hamishehkar, H. et al. (2019). Investigation of physicochemical properties of essential oil loaded nanoliposome for enrichment purposes. *LWT 105*: 282–289. https://doi.org/10.1016/j.lwt.2019.02.010.

Kharat, M. and McClements, D.J. (2019). Recent advances in colloidal delivery systems for nutraceuticals: a case study – delivery by design of curcumin. *Journal of Colloid and Interface Science 557*: 506–518. https://doi.org/10.1016/j.jcis.2019.09.045.

Khorasani, S., Danaei, M., and Mozafari, M.R. (2018). Nanoliposome technology for the food and nutraceutical industries. *Trends in Food Science and Technology 79*: 106–115. https://doi.org/10.1016/j.tifs.2018.07.009.

Kim, H., Lee, J.H., Kim, J.E. et al. (2018). Micro-/nano-sized delivery systems of ginsenosides for improved systemic bioavailability. *Journal of Ginseng Research 42* (3): 361–369. https://doi.org/10.1016/j.jgr.2017.12.003.

Lagoueyte, N. and Paquin, P. (1998). Effects of microfluidization on the functional properties of xanthan gum. *Food Hydrocolloids 12* (3): 365–371.

Lasic, D.D. (1995). Mechanisms of liposome formation. *Journal of Liposome Research 5* (3): 431–441. https://doi.org/10.3109/08982109509010233.

Lesoin, L., Boutin, O., Crampon, C., and Badens, E. (2011). CO2/water/surfactant ternary systems and liposome formation using supercritical CO_2: a review. *Colloids and Surfaces A: Physicochemical and Engineering Aspects 377*: 1–3), 1–14. https://doi.org/10.1016/j.colsurfa.2011.01.027.

Leung, A.W.Y., Amador, C., Wang, L.C. et al. (2019). What drives innovation: the Canadian touch on liposomal therapeutics. *Pharmaceutics 11* (3): 1–26. https://doi.org/10.3390/pharmaceutics11030124.

Liu, W., Ye, A., Han, F., and Han, J. (2019). Advances and challenges in liposome digestion: surface interaction, biological fate, and GIT modeling. *Advances in Colloid and Interface Science 263*: 52–67. https://doi.org/10.1016/j.cis.2018.11.007.

Lordan, R., Tsoupras, A., and Zabetakis, I. (2017). Phospholipids of animal and marine origin: structure, function, and anti-inflammatory properties. *Molecules 22* (11): 1–32. https://doi.org/10.3390/molecules22111964.

Luo, M., Zhang, R., Liu, L. et al. (2020). Preparation, stability and antioxidant capacity of nano liposomes loaded with procyandins from lychee pericarp. *Journal of Food Engineering 284*: 110065. https://doi.org/10.1016/j.jfoodeng.2020.110065.

Mathew, A., Marotta, F., and Sakthi Kumar, D. (2017). Nanotechnology in anti-aging: nutraceutical delivery and related applications. *RSC Drug Discovery Series* 2017 (57): 2443. https://doi.org/10.1039/9781782626602-00142.

Maurya, V.K. and Aggarwal, M. (2019). Fabrication of nano-structured lipid carrier for encapsulation of vitamin D3 for fortification of "Lassi"; A milk based beverage. *Journal of Steroid Biochemistry and Molecular Biology* 193: 105429. https://doi.org/10.1016/j.jsbmb.2019.105429.

Mazloomi, S.N., Mahoonak, A.S., Ghorbani, M., and Houshmand, G. (2020). Physicochemical properties of chitosan-coated nanoliposome loaded with orange seed protein hydrolysate. *Journal of Food Engineering 280*: 109976. https://doi.org/10.1016/j.jfoodeng.2020.109976.

McClements, D.J., Li, F., and Xiao, H. (2015). The nutraceutical bioavailability classification scheme: classifying nutraceuticals according to factors limiting their oral bioavailability. *Annual Review of Food Science and Technology 6* (1): 299–327. https://doi.org/10.1146/annurev-food-032814-014043.

Meghani, N., Patel, P., Kansara, K. et al. (2018). Formulation of vitamin D encapsulated cinnamon oil nanoemulsion: its potential anti-cancerous activity in human alveolar carcinoma cells. *Colloids and Surfaces B: Biointerfaces 166*: 349–357. https://doi.org/10.1016/j.colsurfb.2018.03.041.

Mehta, J. (2010). Practical challenges of stability testing of nutraceutical formulations. In: *Pharmaceutical Stability Testing to Support Global Markets* (ed. K. Huynh-Ba), 85–91. New York: Springer https://doi.org/10.1007/978-1-4419-0889-6_12.

Mohan, A., Rajendran, S.R.C.K., He, Q.S. et al. (2015). Encapsulation of food protein hydrolysates and peptides: a review. *RSC Advances 5* (97): 79270–79278. https://doi.org/10.1039/C5RA13419F.

Mozafari, R.M. (2010). Nanoliposomes: preparation and analysis. *Methods in Molecular Biology (Clifton, N.J.) 605*: 29–50. https://doi.org/10.1007/978-1-60327-360-2_2.

Mozafari, M.R., Johnson, C., Hatziantoniou, S., and Demetzos, C. (2008a). Nanoliposomes and their applications in food nanotechnology. *Journal of Liposome Research 18* (4): 309–327. https://doi.org/10.1080/08982100802465941.

Mozafari, R.M., Khosravi-darani, K., Borazan, G.G., and Cui, J. (2008b). Encapsulation of food ingredients using nanoliposome technology. *International Journal of Food Properties 11* (4): 833–844. https://doi.org/10.1080/10942910701648115.

Nayak, A., Mills, T., and Norton, I. (2016). Lipid based nanosystems for curcumin: past, present and future. *Current Pharmaceutical Design 22* (27): 4247–4256. https://doi.org/10.2174/1381612822666160614083412.

Nedovic, V., Kalusevic, A., Manojlovic, V. et al. (2011). An overview of encapsulation technologies for food applications. *Procedia Food Science Science 1*: 1806–1801815. https://doi.org/10.1016/j.profoo.2011.09.266.

Nelson, N., Nelson, H., and Racker, E. (1972). Partial resolution of the enzymes catalyzing photophosphorylation. XII. Purification and properties of an inhibitor isolated from chloroplast coupling factor 1. *Journal of Biological Chemistry 247* (23): 7657–7662.

Nii, T. and Ishii, F. (2005). Encapsulation efficiency of water-soluble and insoluble drugs in liposomes prepared by the microencapsulation vesicle method. *International Journal of Pharmaceutics 298* (1): 198–205. https://doi.org/10.1016/j.ijpharm.2005.04.029.

Otake, K., Shimomura, T., Goto, T. et al. (2006). Preparation of liposomes using an improved supercritical reverse phase evaporation method. *Langmuir 22* (6): 2543–2550. https://doi.org/10.1021/la051654u.

Payne, N.I., Ambrose, C.V., Timmins, P. et al. (1986). Proliposomes: a novel solution to an old problem. *Journal of Pharmaceutical Sciences 75* (4): 325–329. https://doi.org/https://doi.org/10.1002/jps.2600750402.

Quagliariello, V., Vecchione, R., Coppola, C. et al. (2018). Cardioprotective effects of nanoemulsions loaded with anti-inflammatory nutraceuticals against doxorubicin-induced cardiotoxicity. *Nutrients 10* (9) https://doi.org/10.3390/nu10091304.

Quintanar-Guerrero, D., Allémann, E., Doelker, E., and Fessi, H. (1997). A mechanistic study of the formation of polymer nanoparticles by the emulsification-diffusion technique. *Colloid and Polymer Science 275* (7): 640–647. https://doi.org/10.1007/s003960050130.

Racker, E. (1972). Reconstitution of a calcium pump with phospholipids and a purified Ca ++ - adenosine triphosphatase from sacroplasmic reticulum. *Journal of Biological Chemistry 247* (24): 8198–8200.

Racker (1988). Reconstitution of a calcium pump with phospholipids and a purified Ca ++ - adenosine triphosphatase from sacroplasmic reticulum. *The Journal of Biological Chemistry 256*: 1–11.

Raslan, M.-E. (2013). Effect of some formulation variables on the entrapment efficiency and in vitro release of ketoprofen from ketoprofen niosomes. *Journal of Medicines 1*: 15–22. https://doi.org/10.14511/jlm.2013.010201.

Rasti, B., Erfanian, A., and Selamat, J. (2017). Novel nanoliposomal encapsulated omega-3 fatty acids and their applications in food. *Food Chemistry 230*: 690–696. https://doi.org/10.1016/j.foodchem.2017.03.089.

Rehman, A., Tong, Q., Jafari, S.M. et al. (2020). Carotenoid-loaded nanocarriers: a comprehensive review. *Advances in Colloid and Interface Science 275*: 102048. https://doi.org/10.1016/j.cis.2019.102048.

Rezaei Erami, S., Raftani Amiri, Z., and Jafari, S.M. (2019). Nanoliposomal encapsulation of Bitter Gourd (Momordica charantia) fruit extract as a rich source of health-promoting bioactive compounds. *LWT 116*: 108581. https://doi.org/10.1016/j.lwt.2019.108581.

Rodriguez, E.B., Almeda, R.A., Vidallon, M.L.P., and Reyes, C.T. (2019). Enhanced bioactivity and efficient delivery of quercetin through nanoliposomal encapsulation using rice bran phospholipids. *Journal of the Science of Food and Agriculture 99* (4): 1980–1989. https://doi.org/10.1002/jsfa.9396.

Rubió, L., Maciá, A., and Motilva, M.-J. (2014). Impact of various factors on pharmacokinetics of bioactive polyphenols: an overview. *Current Drug Metabolism 15*: 62–76.

Ruiz Canizales, J., Velderrain Rodríguez, G.R., Domínguez Avila, J.A. et al. (2019). Encapsulation to protect different bioactives to be used as nutraceuticals and food ingredients. In: *Bioactive Molecules in Food. Reference Series in Phytochemistry* (eds. J. Mérillon and K. Ramawat), 2163–2182. New York: Springer https://doi.org/10.1007/978-3-319-78030-6_84.

Salminen, H., Stübler, A.S., and Weiss, J. (2020). Preparation, characterization, and physical stability of cocoa butter and tristearin nanoparticles containing β-carotene. *European Food Research and Technology 246* (3): 599–608. https://doi.org/10.1007/s00217-020-03431-0.

Saneja, A., Arora, D., Kumar, R. et al. (2018). Therapeutic applications of betulinic acid nanoformulations. *Annals of the New York Academy of Sciences 1421* (1): 5–18. https://doi.org/10.1111/nyas.13570.

Sant'Anna, V., Malheiros, P.d.S., and Brandelli, A. (2011). Liposome encapsulation protects bacteriocin-like substance P34 against inhibition by Maillard reaction products. *Food Research International 44* (1): 326–330. https://doi.org/10.1016/j.foodres.2010.10.012.

Sarabandi, K. and Jafari, S.M. (2020). Effect of chitosan coating on the properties of nanoliposomes loaded with flaxseed-peptide fractions: stability during spray-drying. *Food Chemistry 310* (December 2019): 125951. https://doi.org/10.1016/j.foodchem.2019.125951.

Schwendener, R.A. and Schott, H. (2010). Liposome formulations of hydrophobic drugs. In: *Liposomes – Methods and Protocols, Volume 1: Pharmaceutical Nanocarriers*, vol. 605 (ed. V. Weissig), 129–138. Humana Press https://doi.org/10.1007/978-1-60327-360-2_8.

Šegota, S. and Težak, D.u.i. (2006). Spontaneous formation of vesicles. *Advances in Colloid and Interface Science 121* (1–3): 51–75. https://doi.org/10.1016/j.cis.2006.01.002.

da Silva Malheiros, P., Sant'Anna, V., Utpott, M., and Brandelli, A. (2012). Antilisterial activity and stability of nanovesicle-encapsulated antimicrobial peptide P34 in milk. *Food Control 23* (1): 42–47. https://doi.org/10.1016/j.foodcont.2011.06.008.

Singh, H., Thompson, A., Liu, W., and Corredig, M. (2012). Liposomes as food ingredients and nutraceutical delivery systems. In: *Encapsulation Technologies and Delivery Systems for Food Ingredients and Nutraceuticals*, 287–318. Woodhead Publishing https://doi.org/10.1533/9780857095909.3.287.

Sravan Kumar, S., Singh Chauhan, A., and Giridhar, P. (2020). Nanoliposomal encapsulation mediated enhancement of betalain stability: characterisation, storage stability and antioxidant activity of Basella rubra L. fruits for its applications in vegan gummy candies. *Food Chemistry 333*: 127442. https://doi.org/10.1016/j.foodchem.2020.127442.

Subramani, T. and Ganapathyswamy, H. (2020). An overview of liposomal nano-encapsulation techniques and its applications in food and nutraceutical. *Journal of Food Science and Technology*: 1–11. https://doi.org/10.1007/s13197-020-04360-2.

Sun, J., Chen, J., Mei, Z. et al. (2020). Synthesis, structural characterization, and evaluation of cyanidin-3-O-glucoside-loaded chitosan nanoparticles. *Food Chemistry 330*: 127239. https://doi.org/10.1016/j.foodchem.2020.127239.

Szoka, F. and Papahadjopoulos, D. (1978). Procedure for preparation of liposomes with large internal aqueous space and high capture by reverse-phase evaporation. *Proceedings of the National Academy of Sciences 75* (9): 4194–4198. https://doi.org/10.1073/pnas.75.9.4194.

Szoka, F., Olson, F., Heath, T. et al. (1980). Preparation of unilamellar liposomes of intermediate size (0.1–0.2 μm) by a combination of reverse phase evaporation and extrusion through polycarbonate membranes. *Biochimica et Biophysica Acta (BBA) – Biomembranes 601* (C): 559–571. https://doi.org/10.1016/0005-2736(80)90558-1.

Tan, C., Xia, S., Xue, J. et al. (2013). Liposomes as vehicles for lutein: preparation, stability, liposomal membrane dynamics, and structure. *Journal of Agricultural and Food Chemistry 61* (34): 8175–8184. https://doi.org/10.1021/jf402085f.

Thompson, A.K. and Singh, H. (2006). Preparation of liposomes from milk fat globule membrane phospholipids using a microfluidizer. *Journal of Dairy Science 89* (2): 410–419. https://doi.org/10.3168/jds.S0022-0302(06)72105-1.

Torres-Giner, S., Martinez-Abad, A., Ocio, M.J., and Lagaron, J.M. (2010). Stabilization of a nutraceutical omega-3 fatty acid by encapsulation in ultrathin electrosprayed zein prolamine. *Journal of Food Science 75* (6): N69–N79. https://doi.org/10.1111/j.1750-3841.2010.01678.x.

Tsai, W.C. and Rizvi, S.S.H. (2016). Liposomal microencapsulation using the conventional methods and novel supercritical fluid processes. *Trends in Food Science and Technology 55*: 61–71. https://doi.org/10.1016/j.tifs.2016.06.012.

Vahabi, S. and Eatemadi, A. (2017). Nanoliposome encapsulated anesthetics for local anesthesia application. *Biomedicine and Pharmacotherapy 86* (2017): 1–7. https://doi.org/10.1016/j.biopha.2016.11.137.

Vergallo, C. (2020). Nutraceutical vegetable oil nanoformulations for prevention and management of diseases. *Nanomaterials 10* (6): 1–30. https://doi.org/10.3390/nano10061232.

Wagner, A. and Vorauer-Uhl, K. (2011). Liposome technology for industrial purposes. *Journal of Drug Delivery 2011*: 1–9. https://doi.org/10.1155/2011/591325.

Wang, T., Xue, J., Hu, Q. et al. (2017). Preparation of lipid nanoparticles with high loading capacity and exceptional gastrointestinal stability for potential oral delivery applications. *Journal of Colloid and Interface Science 507*: 119–130. https://doi.org/10.1016/j.jcis.2017.07.090.

Weissing, V. (2017). Liposomes. In: *Methods in Molecular Biology*, 2e, vol. 1522 (ed. G.G.M. D'Souza). New York: Springer https://doi.org/10.1007/978-1-4939-6591-5.

Xia, S., Tan, C., Zhang, Y. et al. (2015). Modulating effect of lipid bilayer-carotenoid interactions on the property of liposome encapsulation. *Colloids and Surfaces B: Biointerfaces 128*: 172–180. https://doi.org/10.1016/j.colsurfb.2015.02.004.

Xu, R. (2008). Progress in nanoparticles characterization: sizing and zeta potential measurement. *Particuology 6* (2): 112–115. https://doi.org/10.1016/j.partic.2007.12.002.

Zamani Ghaleshahi, A. and Rajabzadeh, G. (2020). The influence of sodium alginate and genipin on physico-chemical properties and stability of WPI coated liposomes. *Food Research International 130*: 108966. https://doi.org/10.1016/j.foodres.2019.108966.

Zarrabi, A., Alipoor Amro Abadi, M., Khorasani, S. et al. (2020). Nanoliposomes and tocosomes as multifunctional nanocarriers for the encapsulation of nutraceutical and dietary molecules. *Molecules 25* (3): 638. https://doi.org/10.3390/molecules25030638.

Zhang, Y., Pu, C., Tang, W. et al. (2020). Effects of four polyphenols loading on the attributes of lipid bilayers. *Journal of Food Engineering 282* (March): 110008. https://doi.org/10.1016/j.jfoodeng.2020.110008.

4

Bioavailability and Delivery of Nutraceuticals by Nanoparticles

Shalvi Sinai Kunde, Varunesh Sanjay Tambe, and Sarika Wairkar

Shobhaben Pratapbhai Patel School of Pharmacy & Technology Management, SVKM's NMIMS, Mumbai, Maharashtra, India

4.1 Introduction

In the present day, consumers across the globe are inclined toward a junk food-eating lifestyle which has increased the risk of ailments like obesity, heart disease, and several metabolic disorders due to improper nutrition (Das et al. 2012). However, as life expectancy and health awareness persist to grow, people have become more health-conscious and adopting nutritious diet habits. This evolving health paradigm has paved the path for "Nutraceuticals" as a new field healthcare system. The current trends in nutritious diet and public demand has led to the emergence of nutraceuticals as a strong market globally and encouraging researchers to work on natural products to erase the thin line between food and drugs (Mishra and Verma 2016).

The term "Nutraceutical" is a combination of "nutrition" and "pharmaceutical," coined by Dr. Stephen De Felice, founder of "Foundation for Innovation in Medicine." He has redefined nutraceuticals as "foods or parts of food offering health benefits, including the prevention and treatment of diseases." In the United States, since nutraceuticals are not regulated by Food and Drug Administration (FDA), they are considered under dietary supplements. Health Canada has also proposed a definition of nutraceuticals as products obtained from food but is delivered in the form of pills, powders, or capsules to provide physiological benefits (Wildman and Kelley 2007). Similarly in Europe, nutraceuticals are categorized as food supplements by the Food Supplements Directive which is regulated under food law itself (Giunta et al. 2010). While the regulatory body of Japan, the Ministry of Health, Labour and Welfare has categorized "health foods" under regulatory systems such as foods for specified health uses, foods for special dietary uses, foods with nutrient function claims, and foods with health claims (Umegaki 2016). Since nutraceuticals are natural food products or biotechnologically produced foods, they show less toxicities in comparison to pharmaceuticals (Shahidi 2006). They are bound to less regulatory rules and laws, thus allowing easy marketing of products by companies. The global nutraceutical market is expected to grow at a compound annual growth rate (CAGR) rate of 8.3% with market size of USD 722.49 billion by the year 2027 (Daniels et al. 2020) and market statistics with different segments is described in Figure 4.1 (Statistic n.d.).

Handbook of Nutraceuticals and Natural Products: Biological, Medicinal, and Nutritional Properties and Applications,
Volume 1, First Edition. Edited by Sreerag Gopi and Preetha Balakrishnan.
© 2022 John Wiley & Sons, Inc. Published 2022 by John Wiley & Sons, Inc.

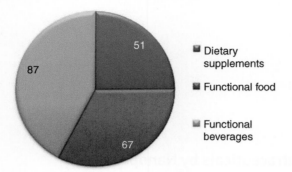

Figure 4.1 Global nutraceutical market size in billion USD in the year 2016.

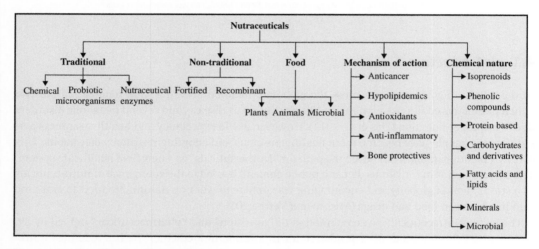

Figure 4.2 Classification of nutraceuticals.

The nutraceuticals are classified into different categories as shown in Figure 4.2. Additionally, their categories based on source, mechanism of action, and chemical nature of molecules are mentioned in Table 4.1.

4.2 Constraints in Delivery of Nutraceuticals

FDA defines bioavailability (BA) as "the rate and extent to which the drug moiety is absorbed from the drug product and becomes available to the site of action" (Yao et al. 2015). Various exogenous as well as endogenous factors affect the oral bioavailability of nutraceuticals. Exogenous factors are particularly those which are responsible before entering the gastrointestinal tract (GIT), such as their solubility, physicochemical properties, and lipophilicity. Nutraceuticals are mainly obtained from natural sources having different physicochemical properties which affect their bioavailability. They exhibit crystalline or amorphous nature and a wide range of water solubility. Three major parameters related to oral bioavailability are namely solubility, lipophilicity, and permeability which are interlinked and usually affected by the chemical structure and molecular weight of the biomolecule. There are three types of biomolecules with a combination of lipophilicity and

Table 4.1 List of nutraceuticals based on source, mechanism of action, and chemical nature.

S. No.	Category	Subcategory	Examples
1.	Source	Plant origin	β-glucans, Ascorbic acid, Quercetin, Luteolin, Lutein, Cellulose, γ-tocotrienol, Gallic acid, Pectin, Glutathione, Capsaicin, Curcumin, α-tocopherol, Geraniol, β-Ionone, β-carotene, Allicin, δ-limonene, Lignin, Daedzein
		Animal origin	Conjugated linonelic acid, Eicosapentanoic acid, Docosahexanoic acid, Sphingolipids, Choline, Lecithin
		Microbial origin	*Saccharomyces boulardii* (yeast), *Bifidobacterium bifidum, B. longum, B. infactus, Lactobacillus acidophilus, Streptococcus salvarius*
		Plant origin	β-glucans, Ascorbic acid, Quercetin, Luteolin, Lutein, Cellulose, γ-tocotrienol, Gallic acid, Pectin, Glutathione, Capsaicin, Curcumin, α-tocopherol, Geraniol, β-Ionone, β-carotene, Allicin, δ-limonene, Lignin, Daedzein
2.	Mechanism of action	Anticancer	Capsaicin, Genestein, Daidzein, α-tocotrienol, γ-tocotrienol, Sphingolipids, Limonene, Diallyl sulphide, Ajoene, α-tocopherol, Enterolactone, Glycyrrhizin, Curcumin, Quercetin, Ellagic acid, Lutein, Carnosol, L. Bulgaricus, *Lactobacillus acidophilus*
		Hypolipidemic	β-glucans, δ-tocotrienol, γ-tocotrienol, MUFA, Quercetin, ω-3PUFAs, Resveratrol, Tannins, β-sitosterol, Guar, Pectins, Saponins
		Antioxidant	Ascorbic acid, β-carotene, Polyphenolics, Tocopherols, Tocotrienols, Ellagic acid, Lycopene, Lutein, Glutathione, Luteolin, Catechins, Gingerol, Tannins, Oleuropein
		Anti-inflammatory	Linolenic acid, EPA, DHA, γ-linolenic acid (GLA), Capsaicin, Quercetin, Curcumin
		Osteogenetic (Bone protectives)	CLA, soy protein, Genestein, Daidzein, Inulin, Casein
3.	Chemical nature	Isoprenoids (Terpenoids)	Carotenoids, Saponins, tocotrienols, tocopherols, terpenes
		Phenolic compounds	Coumarins, tannins, lignin, flavones, isoflavones, flavonones, anthrocyanins
		Protein/Amino acid-based	Allyl-S-compounds, capsaicinoids, isothiocyanates, indoles, folate, choline
		Carbohydrate and derivatives	Ascorbic acid, oligosaccharides, non-starch polysaccharides
		Fatty acid and structured lipids	CLA, n-3 PUFAs, MUFA, sphingolipids, lecithin
		Minerals	Ca, Se, K, Cu, Zn
		Microbial	Prebiotics, probiotics

solubility affecting the bioavailability. First, biomolecules such as curcumin having nonpolar nature show low solubility in GI fluids and have poor bioavailability. Second, polar biomolecules show high solubility but face difficulty in passage through lipophilic endothelial bilayer (water-soluble vitamins). The third type is biomolecules like resveratrol which have nonpolar nature with low solubility but high membrane permeability through lipoidal bilayer (Dima et al. 2020). Another exogenous constraint affecting the bioavailability of nutraceuticals is their chemical instability during storage. The biomolecules undergo rapid degradation under environmental conditions such as temperature, pH, light, microbial action, oxidative stress, in turn, reducing the nutritional value (Gupta and Sen 2016).

Endogenous factors are the ones that influence bioavailability during food digestion, namely absorption, microbiota, and digestive enzymes. The absorption of nutraceuticals in the GIT is a major endogenous factor affecting bioavailability. Ingested food undergoes breakdown from high molecular weight to lower molecular weight compounds as a result of physiological processes throughout GIT aiding absorption. The human GIT possesses varied physiological conditions beginning from the oral cavity up to the intestinal part for absorption. The inherent microbial flora and digestive enzymes also affect their absorption (Acosta 2009).

4.3 Delivery Systems for Bioavailability Improvement of Nutraceuticals

Although nutraceutical or dietary supplement expands its reach in the daily lives of human beings, but the bioavailability of the majority of the nutraceuticals is the foremost limitation. In recent years, scientists have worked on various platforms to enhance the bioavailability of nutraceuticals by developing many novel delivery systems. Considering the fact that the bioactives or nutraceuticals are part of the daily diet, they can be supplemented in the form of tablets or any conventional formulation by oral route. However, the physicochemical properties of bioactives and certain drawbacks of conventional dosage forms make it difficult to be readily absorbed from GIT to be bioavailable (Ting et al. 2014). The existing delivery systems of nutraceuticals are administered mainly via three routes – oral, dermal, and ophthalmic, among which the oral route is preferred due to its noninvasive feature.

Various formulation approaches like encapsulation and solid dispersion were designed to address the issue of bioavailability of nutraceuticals (Chang et al. 2017).

In the current era of nanotechnology, various food-grade engineered nanomaterials are developed to serve the purpose of attaining maximum bioavailability. Nanotechnology encompasses a number of formulations from liposome to the latest technology of functionalized nanoparticles (NPs). Delivery of nutraceuticals by nanotechnology using lipid-based, polymer-based, carbon-based, or metal-based nanoparticulate delivery system has been studied in the last few decades. It includes delivery platforms like NPs, nanosuspension, nanospheres, nanoemulsion, self-emulsifying delivery system, nanocapsules, liposomes, phytosome, niosomes, carbon nanotubes, etc. (Oehlke et al. 2014).

4.4 Nanoparticle Delivery of Nutraceuticals

NPs have revolutionized the arena of nanotechnology and this nanocarrier has gained immense importance due to the versatility of the materials used to encapsulate or entrap actives within and successfully deliver the cargo at the target site. NPs are defined as materials ranging in nanometer scale ideally less than 100 nm in size and are made up of materials such as polymers, lipids, metals, metal oxide, or any organic matter (Wang et al. 2014). Before the emergence of the term "nanoparticle," they were known as "nanoscale structures" (Pan and Zhong 2016). The properties of NPs can be altered by varying composition, aspect ratio, their shell thickness, and polymer/lipid quantity, etc. In nutshell, their advantages are high drug loading, targeted delivery with controlled and/or sustained release pattern, reduction in effective dose, improved solubility, and bioavailability of actives (Mohanraj and Chen 2006). Thus, the nanoparticle concept was successfully used for delivering insoluble, incompatible nutraceuticals in an efficient manner. However, NPs face the challenge of stability and particle aggregation upon standing and can lead to problems such as burst release or dose dumping which may hamper its performance (Ealias and Saravanakumar 2017). To address the aforesaid issues, various types of NPs are now innovated to deliver the nutraceuticals and the classification of NPs is shown in Figure 4.3.

4.4.1 Organic Nanoparticles

Organic NPs are fabricated using natural or synthetic organic materials. These NPs constitute systems such as dendrimers, liposomes, solid lipid nanoparticles (SLNs), micellar delivery system, etc. Their unique characteristics are biocompatibility, improved physicochemical parameters like solubility and enhanced bioavailability. These are further subdivided into polymer-based, lipid-based, and protein-based according to the nature and properties of the materials.

4.4.1.1 Polymeric Nanoparticles

Polymeric nanoparticles (PNPs) are made up of polymers and counted among those nanosystems having the potential of site-specific delivery with modified drug release pattern (Kim and Martin 2006). Prior to the introduction of biodegradable polymers which are most preferred currently, the use of nonbiodegradable polymers such as poly (methyl methacrylate) (PMMA), polyacrylamides (PA), polyacrylates, polystyrene was practiced until the observations related to chronic toxicities and inflammatory reactions were reported (Banik et al. 2016). Biodegradable polymers possess good biocompatibility, reduced toxicity and noticeable biomimetic features. Their improved oral bioavailability is also credited to flexibility in designing surface modification and desired functionalization. Biodegradable polymers are obtained from natural origin, namely chitosan, alginates,

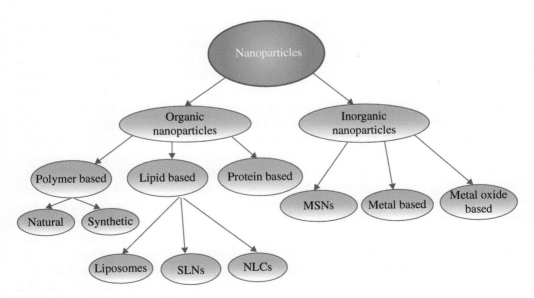

Figure 4.3 Types of nanoparticles.

gelatin, etc., as well as synthetic polymerization reactions like polylactic acid (PLA), poly (caprolactone) (PCL), poly (lactide-co-glycolic acid) (PLGA) (Kumari et al. 2010). PNPs can be obtained as nanospheres and nanocapsules wherein nanosphere is a matrix system in which biomolecule is uniformly dispersed in the polymeric matrix whereas nanocapsules are reservoir type of system which contains biomolecule encapsulated in the polymeric membrane cavity. PNPs portray certain disadvantages regarding batch-to-batch reproducibility, degradation, and antigenicity in a few cases (El-Say and El-Sawy 2017).

Among the available natural polymers, chitosan has several applications in targeted delivery, gene therapy, and tissue engineering. Chitosan is a linear biopolymer obtained as the deacetylated product from chitin (Cai et al. 2006). The presence of the amino group in chitosan molecule permits surface modification and obtaining derivatives conferring unique properties (Varlamov et al. 2020). Pedro et al. developed pH-sensitive NPs using the amphiphilic derivative of chitosan with varied concentration of hydrophobic-grafting agent to deliver quercetin, a multifunctional flavonoid to breast cancer cells. The encapsulation efficiency of quercetin was higher in a more hydrophobic sample due to more number of sites for interaction and showed higher release in an acidic medium. Quercetin nanoformulation had improved release, reduced side effects, and satisfactory biocompatibility (de Oliveira et al. 2018). Similarly, Rahimi et al. studied quercetin-loaded pH-responsive chitosan-quinoline NPs for anticancer activity. The in vitro quercetin release was faster in an acidic medium as compared to physiological pH which is beneficial in the acidic tumor microenvironment. 3-[4,5-Dimethylthiazole-2-yl]-2,5-diphenyltetrazolium bromide (MTT) cell viability assay showed that these NPs had a higher cytotoxic effect as compared to free quercetin against HeLa (Henrietta Lacks) cancer cells (Rahimi et al. 2019). In another study, derivatized chitosan was used for the delivery of curcumin to study anticancer activity. Curcumin loaded *N,O*-Carboxymethyl chitosan NPs (*N,O*-CMC NPs) showed 80% encapsulation efficiency and a pH-dependent sustained release from the polymer matrix. *in vitro* cytotoxicity studies performed by MTT assay, lactate dehydrogenase (LDH) assay, and apoptosis assay revealed concentration-dependent cytotoxic effects of curcumin-loaded *N,O*-CMC NPs as compared to free curcumin (Anitha et al. 2012).

Chitosan NPs with folate modification were studied for targeted curcumin delivery toward the overexpressed folate receptors in cancerous tissues. This nanoformulation exhibited a biphasic release pattern; specifically, a burst release in an acidic medium in the first three hours followed by 90% sustained release over a week. in vitro cytotoxicity effects on Michigan Cancer Foundation (MCF-7) cells compared for free curcumin and loaded curcumin which showed that cytotoxic effects were higher in case of later than free curcumin (Esfandiarpour-Boroujeni et al. 2017). Similarly, genistein was studied in chitosan NPs with folic acid to enhance its anticancer activity. The in vitro studies revealed that folate-targeted formulation had a greater cellular uptake and cytotoxic effect in HeLa cells for cervical cancer than the nontargeted NPs (Cai et al. 2017). In an experiment performed by Kumar et al., bioflavonoid naringenin (NAR) was loaded in chitosan NPs for antioxidant and anticancer activities. Antioxidant assays such as nitrate scavenging assay, 2,2-diphenyl-1-picrylhydrazyl (DPPH) scavenging assay, and hydroxyl radical scavenging assay were performed to study the scavenging property of free naringenin and encapsulated naringenin. This revealed that NAR nanoformulation had effective antioxidant property due to sustained release of naringenin in cells. To measure the cytotoxic effects of NAR, an MTT assay was performed that showed significant cytotoxic effects on A549 lung cancer cells as compared to blank chitosan NPs and free NAR (Kumar et al. 2015). Lin et al. developed surface-modified chitosan NPs for hepatocyte-targeted delivery of glycyrrhizin. in vitro cellular uptake study showed 4.9 times greater uptake in hepatocytes as compared to hepatic non-parenchymal cells (Lin et al. 2008).

In another study, glycyrrhizin NPs were prepared using a chitosan-gum arabic combinational polymeric matrix having particle size 140–200 nm and showed a sustained release pattern (Rani et al. 2015). The same research group has further reported the antidiabetic activity of these NPs in streptozocin-induced diabetic Wistar rats. It was observed that the nanoformulation containing 1/4th amount of glycyrrhizin showed an equivalent antidiabetic activity to that of pure glycyrrhizin (Rani et al. 2017).

Another polymer, alginate was used to prepare nanoparticle of peppermint phenolic extract by internal gelation technique. The nanoformulation had an encapsulation efficiency of 5.6% and particle size was 785 nm (Mokhtari et al. 2017). Velayudhan et al. developed catechin-loaded alginate NPs to evaluate the antioxidant and hepatoprotective activity. The in vitro release carried out in simulated intestinal fluid showed a sustained release of catechin up to 85% at the end of 96 hours. An experimental rat hepatic injury model revealed hepatocyte regeneration of damaged liver cells by oxidative stress marker assays and histopathological studies (Mullakkalparambil Velayudhan et al. 2020). In another study, catechin extract from white tea was encapsulated in a polymeric shell of PCL and alginate combinational polymers for controlled drug delivery. The in vitro release performed in simulated intestinal fluid showed a gradual release of encapsulated polyphenol up to 80% within five hours at pH 7.4. The free radical scavenging activity of catechins in the nanoformulation was greater than the free tea extract as observed by the DPPH inhibition assay (Sanna et al. 2015).

By virtue of drawbacks shown by natural polymers, biodegradable synthetic polyesters are of great interest to researchers in nano-systems. In an investigation done by Xie et al., the oral bioavailability of curcumin from PLGA NPs was carried out in Sprague Dawley rats which showed that NPs exhibited five times more relative oral bioavailability than free curcumin (Xie et al. 2011). In one more experiment, ellagic acid was loaded into a PCL carrier to improve oral bioavailability and obtain higher antitumor activity. Ellagic acid NPs presented a sustained release pattern as well as a superior cytotoxic effect on HCT-116 colon carcinoma cells in comparison to free ellagic acid (Mady and Shaker 2017). Peng et al. formulated NP using a polymeric combination of methoxy-polyethylene glycol and PCL to deliver capsaicin orally. It depicted a sustained release of capsaicin from the polymeric system. The nanoformulation exhibited improved bioavailability and reduced gastric mucosal irritation as observed by the pharmacokinetic and histopathological study respectively (Peng et al. 2015).

4.4.1.2 Lipid-based NPs

Lipid-based NPs or lipid nanocarriers are formulated mainly using the lipidic component along with the surfactants and solubilizers and very useful in the delivery of the hydrophobic bioactives to the target site. Structurally, these NPs are composed of the lipid bilayer enclosing the hydrophilic or lipophilic bioactives, arranged either in a concentric fashion or as a distinct entity (McClements 2020). Further, the types of lipid NPs delivering the bioactives of nutraceuticals that enhance the bioavailability are explained below.

4.4.1.2.1 Liposomes

Liposomes are the nanometric version of the novel system made up of amphiphilic material known as phospholipids in the year 1965 (Bangham et al. 1965). These systems are used for encapsulation of bioactives having both lipid-soluble and water-soluble nature such as nutraceuticals, enzymes, or essential oils. Tea polyphenols found in green tea were formulated into liposomes by Lu et al., which showed a cumulative release rate of 50% after six hours and 94% release within 24 hours by first-order kinetic. The formulated liposomes showed good stability in refrigerated condition (Lu et al. 2011). In addition to this, the same polyphenols were further researched by Gülseren et al. and the effects on the cytotoxicity were studied on HT-29 human carcinoma cells which proved the greater bioavailability of the polyphenol encapsulated in liposomes as compared to free polyphenols (Gülseren et al. 2012). Flavonoids, such as luteolin, kaempferol, and quercetin were loaded in a liposomal carrier and their antioxidant properties were studied with respective DPPH-free radical scavenging assays, where quercetin-loaded liposomes showed higher stability and antioxidant activity as compared to luteolin and kaempferol. The IR spectroscopy results indicated good stability of quercetin and luteolin with the lipid envelope whereas kaempferol indicated some interactions with the lipids (Huang et al. 2017). Flavonoid such as Fisetin was also explored for its antiangiogenic and anticancer activity where Mignet et al. developed stable nanoliposomes with acceptable cytotoxicity results to treat angiogenesis (Mignet et al. 2012).

Fortification of beverages can be achieved to suffice the need for Vitamin D_3 and, hence, Mohammadi et al. developed Vitamin D_3 liposomes to treat hypovitaminosis D. It showed 93% of encapsulation efficiency due to the lipid-soluble nature of vitamin D_3 and stability of one month achieved with minimal leakage from liposomes at 2–3 °C (Mohammadi et al. 2014). Fish oils, a good source of omega-3-fatty acid, showing cardioprotective activity, were encapsulated into liposomes which showed 92% of encapsulation efficiency. A constant peroxide value of 0.6 which lasted for 21 days indicated the stable nature of fish oil achieved by incorporation into liposomes (Ghorbanzade et al. 2017). Curcumin, a natural anticancer agent obtained from *Curcuma longa*, was nanosized into a stable liposomal formulation with enhanced bioavailability and an attempt of co-encapsulation with resveratrol was done to show synergism in the treatment of cancer. The in vivo studies conducted in phosphatase and tensin homolog (PTEN) knockout mice showed a five-fold increase in the rate of apoptosis (55–62%) in the case of co-encapsulated nanoformulation as compared to the single bioactive liposomal formulation. Further confirmation on the apoptotic activity of encapsulated bioactives was done by transfection assays using small interfering ribonucleic acid (si-RNA) and modulated signaling pathways for the treatment of prostate cancer (Dutta et al. 2018).

4.4.1.2.2   Solid Lipid Nanoparticles (SLNs)

SLNs are one of the prominent delivery options under a lipid-based delivery system. They are nanostructured vesicles that encapsulate the actives inside the lipid coat and now used in the field of nutraceuticals (Mehnert and Mäder 2012). Curcumin was formulated into SLNs to enhance oral bioavailability and studies performed in Wistar rats showed a 32-fold increase in the bioavailability as compared to free curcumin (Kakkar et al. 2011). Similarly, Campos et al. developed SLNs of rosmarinic acid, a natural polyphenol, having antioxidant, antimutagenic, and another nutraceutical potential. The formulation was optimized to enhance its storage ability for about 28 days in normal conditions which showed no leakage or aggregation of SLNs (Campos et al. 2015). Surface-modified SLNs using chitosan derivatives were used to load resveratrol and cell viability studies performed (20–1000 µg/ml) showed no cytotoxic response indicating the safety of SLNs. The in vitro release study showed a sustained release pattern in simulated intestinal fluid and a 3.8-fold increase in bioavailability was shown by developed SLNs as compared to unmodified nanoformulation in pharmacokinetic studies (Young and Ko 2015).

Li et al. formulated quercetin-loaded SLNs to enhance oral absorption. The in situ perfusion model in rat was adopted to study the gastrointestinal absorption of SLN and it was revealed that the intestine, mainly the ileum and colon, are major absorption sites than the stomach. The pharmacokinetic study in rats confirmed nanoformulation showed five times increase in relative bioavailability as compared to quercetin suspension (Li and Zhao 2009). In an added study for quercetin,

SLNs were prepared to enhance its brain delivery and the optimized formulation was studied in Wistar rats. The behavioral activities were assessed by utilizing behavioral models such as spatial navigation task, elevated plus maze paradigm which revealed improved memory retention than the free quercetin. The biochemical estimation done in brain tissue homogenates exhibited maintained levels of malondialdehyde and nitrites and reduced glutathione levels in the rats administered with aluminium chloride and quercetin loaded nanoformulation (Dhawan et al. 2011).

4.4.1.2.3   Nanostructured Lipid Carriers (NLCs)

Nanostructured lipid carriers (NLCs) are the second generation of lipid carrier developed to overcome the pitfalls of SLNs in terms of drug-carrying or loading capacity (Braithwaite et al. 2014). Carotenoids, which belong to the class of terpenoids, are considered to have antioxidant potential and relieve oxidative stress. Tamjidi et al., developed NLCs of astaxanthin, a carotenoid, to enhance its oral bioavailability. Characterizations showed that the particle size of NLCs is governed by the ratio of lipid components and oleic acid and Tween 80 (22.4:1.8) ratio has found to have the optimal size of NLCs (Tamjidi et al. 2014). Quercetin was also loaded into NLCs and compared with other lipid nanocarriers like SLNs. The lipid-based carriers were compared to study the bioaccessibility using simulated intestinal fluid. The results indicated that NLCs loaded with quercetin showed 52.7% of bioaccessibility while SLNs showed approximately 39.7% after two hours, concluding the potential of NLCs towards increased absorption and enhanced bioavailability (Aditya et al. 2014). The same polyphenol, quercetin was studied by Ni et al. as an NLC formulation which showed entrapment efficiency of 93.50 and 65% drug release in six hours. The antioxidant activity was studied by superoxide radical scavenging assay which showed $36.39 \pm 2.63\%$ activity as compared to free quercetin ($35.45 \pm 1.38\%$) (Ni et al. 2014). To overcome the problems of poor bioavailability and low intestinal absorption, Granja et al. formulated folic acid-functionalized epigallocatechin gallate (EGCG)-loaded NLCs to target folate receptors on the intestinal epithelial cells. The in vitro release studies showed a higher release of functionalized NLCs as compared to nonfunctionalized NLCs after 21 hours. Also, functionalized NLCs protected the bioactive from the harsh gastric environment to enhance the bioavailability (Granja et al. 2017).

Similarly, curcumin NLCs were reported for their antioxidant, antibacterial and antimicrobial properties. in vitro release study conducted on formulation showed 42.3% of curcumin release after 20 hours at pH 7. The antioxidant property confirmed by the DPPH assay showed improved results for oxidative radical scavenging of curcumin NLCs as compared to free curcumin. Microbial assays such as agar-dilution assay and macro-broth-dilution assay were performed to check the antimicrobial activity. The minimum inhibitory concentration (MIC) and minimum bactericidal concentration (MBC) of curcumin-loaded NLCs were found to be higher than free curcumin extract confirming the antibacterial activity against gram-negative bacteria (Karimi et al. 2018).

4.4.1.3   Protein-based Nanoparticles

The protein-based nanocarriers, generally recognized as safe (GRAS), are being developed with improved nutritional value. They also exhibit biodegradable, biocompatible, nontoxic and nonantigenic characteristics along with the presence of numerous binding sites for surface modifications (Chen et al. 2006). Protein-based NPs are synthesized using natural proteins from abundantly available renewable sources from either animal or plant origin. Proteins obtained from the animal source have good absorbing ability as well as low toxicity such as gelatin, collagen, albumin, elastin, and milk proteins. They are hydrophilic in nature, thus limiting the incorporation of highly hydrophobic molecules. Due to its water-loving nature, the addition of crosslinking agents is necessary to attain a hard and strong core of NPs (Elzoghby et al. 2012). The plant-originated proteins such as zein, soy protein, gliadin, lectins are comparably less expensive than animal proteins. They are hydrophobic in nature; thus, the use of crosslinkers or any physical and chemical treatments can be avoided to encapsulate fat-soluble molecules. Usage of plant proteins also reduces the risk of acquiring any animal protein-related disease like mad cow's disease (Lohcharoenkal et al. 2014).

Albumin is considered an attractive water-soluble protein carrier by virtue of its biodegradable, nontoxic nature as well as high ligand-binding capacity (Elzoghby et al. 2012). In an experiment performed by Saha et al., BAB triblock copolymer and albumin complex was developed to prepare quercetin NP for anti-inflammatory action. Cytotoxicity assay against Madin-Darby Canine Kidney (MDCK) cells in presence of oxalates confirmed the nontoxic and biocompatible nature of quercetin NPs. Anti-inflammatory activity studied in mouse bone marrow-derived dendritic cells and interleukin (IL-β) pathway revealed the anti-inflammatory potential of quercetin by downregulation of various inflammatory mediators (Saha et al. 2020). Li et al. formulated conjugate NPs incorporating ovalbumin and dextran by Maillard reaction to promote enhanced absorption of EGCG that displayed greater permeability in cancel coli-2 (Caco-2) cells as compared to free EGCG (Li et al. 2014). In another experiment, capsaicin-loaded albumin NPs were formulated for antioxidant, anti-inflammatory action. The antioxidant activity demonstrated concentration as well as time-dependent activity and in vivo study of nanoencapsulated capsaicin revealed reduced levels of tumor necrosis factor α (TNF-α) suggesting capsaicin as a potential anti-inflammatory agent (De Freitas et al. 2018).

Zein is a highly hydrophobic, alcohol soluble protein obtained from corn kernels, approved by FDA for human consumption (Lohcharoenkal et al. 2014). Penalva et al. developed quercetin-loaded zein NPs complexed with hydroxypropyl-β-cyclodextrin to improve its oral bioavailability. The anti-inflammatory efficacy involving endotoxic mouse model showed reduced endotoxic symptoms in presence of quercetin-loaded NPs than free quercetin (Penalva et al. 2017). In another study, curcumin and piperine were loaded into core-shell NPs of zein protein and carrageenan polysaccharide to produce a synergistic effect aiding bioavailability and activity of curcumin. The stability study and antioxidant assay suggested good photostability and thermal stability along with remarkable DPPH radical scavenging ability (71%) after encapsulation of curcumin, confirming the ability of carrier for co-delivery of biomolecules (Chen et al. 2020). Zein NPs were adopted to deliver polyphenol resveratrol with enhanced oral bioavailability. The pharmacokinetics was studied in sixteen healthy volunteers by administering resveratrol-loaded zein NPs. The sample analysis by mass spectrometry confirmed the presence of resveratrol and with t_{max} as 2.84 hours and C_{max} values as 21.85 ng/ml (Brotons-Canto et al. 2020).

Soyprotein is a plant-derived protein obtained from an inexpensive, renewable source having surface-active proteins such as β-conglycinin and glycinin (Elzoghby et al. 2012). In an experiment conducted by Teng et al., curcumin-loaded soy protein NPs were synthesized with a high encapsulation efficiency of 97.2% as well as biphasic release kinetics in phosphate buffer recommending soy protein as a promising carrier for delivery of nutraceuticals (Teng et al. 2012). β-conglycinin, a type of soy protein was used as a carrier to encapsulate vitamin D_3. Simulated shelf life study of NPs done for simulated gastric digestion revealed a high amount (70 and 90%) retainment of vitamin D_3 in pH 6.8 and 2.5, respectively as a result of vitamin and peptide interaction (Levinson et al. 2014). Apart from soyprotein and other plant proteins, pea protein is another upcoming protein obtained from dry peas. Fan et al. used pea protein as a biomaterial crosslinked with calcium ions to deliver hydrophobic resveratrol. Antioxidant assays, namely DPPH, 2,2'-azino-bis(3-ethylbenzothiazoline-6-sulfonic acid) (ABTS), and oxygen radical absorbance capacity (ORAC) confirmed the effective antioxidant activity of resveratrol loaded in pea protein NPs (Fan et al. 2020).

Milk proteins are animal-based food-grade proteins used as natural vehicles for the delivery of bioactives. On the basis of structure, milk proteins are categorized as caseins (flexible) and whey proteins (globular) such as β-lactoglobulin. Casein has high emulsifying property while whey proteins exhibit gelling property (Kimpel and Schmitt 2015). Penalva et al. used sodium caseinate to prepare oral NPs of folic acid that showed biphasic release of vitamin in simulated intestinal fluid up to 90%. The higher oral bioavailability of folic acid was observed after encapsulation in casein nanocarriers as compared to plain vitamin in a pharmacokinetic study using Wistar rats (Penalva et al. 2015). Similarly, casein NPs were used as carriers for the oral delivery of resveratrol. The in vitro drug release study performed in simulated GI fluids suggested pH-independent sustained release of the polyphenol. The in vivo pharmacokinetic study in Wistar rats revealed that oral bioavailability of encapsulated resveratrol increased 10 times than the conventional oral resveratrol. in vitro-in vivo correlation data was reviewed by plotting the percentage amount of resveratrol release versus the fraction of resveratrol absorbed until eight hours showed a linear correlation (R^2 = 0.996) (Peñalva et al. 2018).

Teng et al. formulated and evaluated grafted cationic β-lactoglobulin as a nutraceutical carrier. Curcumin-loaded cationic β-lactoglobulin NPs showed remarkable permeability across Caco-2 cells along with sustained-release kinetics as well as high cellular uptake (Teng et al. 2016). Additionally, Ron et al. synthesized a β-lactoglobulin-pectin nanocomplex to enhance the electrostatic stability for delivery of hydrophobic nutraceuticals such as vitamin D_2. The stability study conducted on polysaccharide-free sample and protein-polysaccharide complex demonstrated that vitamin D_2 was highly protected and stable in the case of the latter (Ron et al. 2010).

Gliadin is another plant-originated protein obtained from wheat gluten having aqueous solubility (Joye et al. 2015). Wu et al. formulated gliadin NPs loaded with resveratrol using gum Arabic and chitosan polymers to enhance the stability. The nanoformulation with polymer showed high encapsulation efficiency of resveratrol (68.2%) as well as higher release in simulated gastric fluid (84.4%) as compared to polymer-free resveratrol gliadin NPs. in vivo antioxidant activity study, namely DPPH radical scavenging activity and Fe^{3+} reducing power suggested these NPs showed improved antioxidant activity as well as chemical stability (Wu et al. 2020).

Organic NPs have a wide range of applications in the field of nutraceuticals. They can be fabricated to achieve the desired release pattern as well as better targeting, thereby increasing the bioavailability of nutraceuticals. The safe and effective nature of synthetic materials in organic NPs has promoted them as a choice of nanocarrier for nutraceuticals.

4.4.2 Inorganic Nanoparticles

An inorganic nanoparticle is a new class of NPs made up of non-carbon materials. They are subdivided into mesoporous silica NPs, metal, and metal-oxide-based NPs. These inorganic systems are also receiving a considerable response from the field of research which can be evidenced below.

4.4.2.1 Mesoporous Silica Nanoparticles (MSNs)

Mesoporous silica nanoparticles unlike organic or lipid-based systems have a proper and definite honeycomb-like structure having a solid framework with a large surface area, providing an option for fabrication with materials that can be used for targeting the organs (Bharti et al. 2015). Amongst all the mesoporous materials of silica, MCM-41 (Mobil Crystalline Materials of silica or Mobil Composition of Matter Grade 41) has been explored widely due to its size range (2–50 nm) (Narayan et al. 2018). Nutraceuticals were not an exception to these emerging systems of inorganic NPs and polyphenols, essential oils, antioxidants are loaded into MSNs.

Quercetin, a well-known polyphenol, was studied by Sarkar et al. in which folic acid was conjugated with quercetin to increase its targeting due to overexpression of folate cancer cells. in vitro drug release studies show a pH-dependent pattern whereas the in vitro cellular uptake studies using rhodamine isothiocyanate (RITC), a fluorescent dye revealed that folic acid tagged MSNs with quercetin (RITC-tagged-MSN-FA) showed more uptake with proportional folate receptors placed on the cell lines promoting internalization (Sarkar et al. 2016). Grape extracts-based polyphenols were loaded into MCM-41 silica-based MSNs and were subjected to DPPH assay which showed enhanced antioxidant ability. in vitro cytocompatibility evaluation which triggered proliferation showed satisfactory results obtained by grape extract-loaded MSNs (Brezoiu et al. 2019). Resveratrol, due to its multifunctional activity, was loaded into MSNs for the treatment of inflammation and cancer. in vitro cytotoxicity studies by using various cell lines and nuclear factor kappa-light-chain-enhancer of activated B cells (NF-kB)-responsive endothelial leukocyte adhesion molecule 1 (ELAM 1) promotor set-up-infected Ralph and William's (RAW) 264.7 macrophage cells were experimented to show anti-inflammatory response which revealed dose-dependent activity of MSNs which was significant than free resveratrol. Moreover, oral permeability using Caco-2 cell lines confirmed the transfer of resveratrol MSNs via the tight junctions revealing oral bioavailability improvement with this innovative technology (Juère et al. 2017).

Also, curcumin was encapsulated by Elbialy et al. into the MSN framework to enhance the bioavailability for cancer treatment. The anticancer activity confirmed by in vitro cell lines such as hepatoma G2 (HepG2) and HeLa cells showed promising results in terms of cytotoxicity with a pH-dependent and acidic-environment-triggered release of bioactive (Elbialy et al. 2020). On a similar note, essential oil bioactive-like thymoquinone-loaded MSNs were fabricated to release in favorable acidic pH ranging from 5.5 to 6.8 to treat glioma cells. in vitro tests of MSNs as compared to the free form of thymoquinone confirmed by enhanced anti-proliferative action of MSNs with improved targeting (Shahein et al. 2019).

4.4.2.2 Metal-based NPs

Metallic NPs are obtained from elemental metals. They are produced by either chemical treatments or biosynthesized using microbial enzymatic process, also known as green synthesis. The use of the former method faces limitations such as high cost of production, noxious waste products while the latter technique is easy, economical, and environment-friendly (Kulkarni and Muddapur 2014; Li et al. 2011). The nanometric-sized particles obtained from green synthesis provide a large surface area and passive accumulation in tumor cells due to their small particle size, high catalytic reactivity, and photothermal and surface plasmonic resonance properties allowing their use in theranostics (Sardoiwala et al. 2018). Elemental metals such as Gold (Au), Silver (Ag), Platinum (Pt), Selenium (Se), Palladium (Pd), Lead (Pb), Cobalt (Co), and their alloys are used to produce metal-based nanocarriers (Li et al. 2011).

Gold nanoparticles (AuNPs) are used in biomedical applications due to their biocompatible nature, high zeta potential, electro-magnetic properties (Jain et al. 2012). In an experiment performed by Muddineti et al., curcumin-loaded AuNPs were formulated by using ascorbic acid as a reducing agent and polyethylene glycol-xanthan gum (PEG/XG) as a stabilizing agent. The in vitro cellular uptake and cytotoxicity study of curcumin in Murine melanoma (B16F10) cells indicated that these AuNPs showed increased cell internalization of curcumin and improved cytotoxic activity in comparison to free curcumin (Muddineti et al. 2016). In another study, AuNPs were synthesized to deliver resveratrol radiolabeled with Technetium-99m for effective cancer targeting. The radiolabeled complex was found to be stable with 90% radiolabeled efficiency up to six hours at room temperature. The in vitro cytotoxicity and cellular uptake performed on HT29 colon cancer cells revealed that radiolabeled resveratrol-loaded AuNPs showed low toxicity and increased cellular uptake as compared to plain AuNPs and resveratrol (Kamal et al. 2018).

Silver nanoparticles (AgNPs) are one of those metallic NPs exhibiting antimicrobial activity against bacteria, fungi, virus, etc. (Thakkar et al. 2010). In an experiment performed by Duraipandy et al., AgNPs were used to deliver Plumbagin, an anticancer nutraceutical. The in vitro cytotoxicity and apoptosis study were performed on HaCaT normal cells and A431 cancer cells that indicated no toxicity in HaCaT cells with 95% cell viability. The nanoformulation showed selective apoptosis by adopting the caspase-3-dependent apoptotic pathway at the same concentration as observed by the mitochondria-mediated apoptosis study (Duraipandy et al. 2014). In another study by Park et al., AuNPs and AgNPs were used as a nanocarrier for resveratrol. Resveratrol was used as a reducing/capping agent in the biosynthesis of both NPs. The metallic NPs and resveratrol produced a synergistic effect and enhanced the antibacterial activity of the polyphenol. in vitro antibacterial activity of AuNPs and AgNPs was measured in twenty-two strains of gram-positive bacteria and gram-negative bacteria, among which Streptococcus pneumonia being most susceptible showed a twofold increase in antibacterial activity of resveratrol AuNPs as compared to free resveratrol (Park et al. 2016).

Yu et al. developed platinum NPs by conjugation of curcumin. Antimicrobial assay performed for these NPs against both gram-positive bacteria and gram-negative bacteria showed excellent antimicrobial activity with MIC of 32-64 nM. The anti-fibrotic activity conducted using NIH/3 T3 cells revealed that curcumin-platinum NPs exhibited considerable anti-fibrotic activity as compared to free curcumin (Yu et al. 2019).

4.4.2.3 Metal Oxide-based Nanoparticles

Metal oxides, another subcategory of inorganically synthesized NPs have gained importance which is attributed to their physiochemical, optical, electronic properties, and chemical stability. This nanocarrier has widespread use, initially in the field of biosensors and later in drug delivery supported by green synthesis (Khalil et al. 2017). Recently, metal oxides such as iron oxides, copper oxides, titanium oxide, and zinc oxide are widely explored for loading of bioactives and fabrication of nutraceutical delivery systems.

Due to its superparamagnetic nature, iron oxide NPs are majorly used to enhance the bioavailability of nutraceuticals. Quercetin was loaded into iron oxide NPs which were detected in plasma and brain during in vivo evaluation in rats, but no significant amount of iron accumulation was observed in the brain (Enteshari Najafabadi et al. 2018). A nerve regeneration study was conducted by Katebi et al. with quercetin and nerve growth factor loaded in superparamagnetic iron oxide NPs. There was significant improvement observed in neurite outgrowth promotion and neuronal branching trees studied in pheochromocytoma (PC12) cells and, thus, this nanocarrier may be useful for improving neuronal growth (Katebi et al. 2019).

Formulations developed using copper oxide (CuO) NPs were essentially based on loading curcumin as a bioactive for its anticancer, antibacterial, and miscellaneous properties. Sriram et al. formulated curcumin-conjugated CuO NPs aiming at the enhancement in the bioavailability of curcumin. Anticancer activity was confirmed by using cell lines such as M19-MEL (skin cancer), HeLa (ovarian cancer), and MCF-7 (breast cancer), where the IC_{50} results of curcumin-conjugated CuO NPs showed inhibition in a range of 12–19 μg/ml for experimented cell lines (Sriram et al. 2017). Similarly, antibacterial properties of curcumin using CuO NPs were studied with the findings promising toward increased bioavailability of nutraceutical (Varaprasad et al. 2019). Further, bovine serum albumin (BSA)-based curcumin CuO NPs showed a sustained release for 24 hours with 85% cumulative release in contrast with plain curcumin. Significant ($p < 0.05$) decrease in reactive oxygen species (ROS) generation was observed indicating beneficial effects of these NPs to suppress ROS production (Zhang et al. 2016).

Sawant et al. developed pH-sensitive curcumin-loaded titanium dioxide NPs to check anticancer potential. The results on MCF-7 breast cell lines showed 47.61% of suppression of cancer cells at 10 µg/ml concentration (Sawant et al. 2016). Sherin et al. developed curcumin-loaded titanium dioxide NPs and biodistribution studies using Sprague Dawley rats showed the first-hour distribution of curcumin in highly perfused organs such as the liver, spleen, and heart (Sherin et al. 2017).

Zinc oxide (ZnO) NPs are majorly used in the field of electronics and biomedical fields. A lot of researchers focus on the anticancer properties of zinc oxide. Majorly curcumin and quercetin are the choice of bioactives loaded into ZnO NPs. Sawant et al. synthesized PEG-fabricated zinc oxide NPs loaded with curcumin under the rationale of pH-sensitive delivery and the inherent property of zinc oxide of cellular imaging. This study showed sustained release of curcumin at pH 4.8 and sustained release for 50 hours with 83% bioactive release. Anticancer activity of curcumin was characterized by MTT assay using MCF-7 cells in which 85.5% of apoptosis was observed at 21.25 µg/ml concentration of curcumin-loaded zinc oxide NPs (Sawant and Bamane 2017).

Inorganic NPs made up of different inorganic elements are also considered a carrier for nutraceuticals. However, they are not preferred over organic NPs due to the nonbiodegradable nature and threat of bioaccumulation of inorganic elements in the biological system.

4.5 Conclusion

Nutraceuticals are gaining importance in the commercial market due to their beneficial effects over synthetic products. Poor solubility, limited absorption, and susceptibility to degradations affect the oral bioavailability of nutraceuticals. In order to overcome these constraints, novel formulations are designed and developed by considering advanced nanotechnological systems. A nanoparticulate system is a preferred approach for the delivery of several nutraceuticals to improve the bioavailability as well as aiding its targeted delivery. However, limited clinical data on the delivery system of nutraceuticals hinders commercial translation. Therefore, extensive development and clinical studies should be done to bridge the gap of knowledge and promote the development of effective formulations.

References

Acosta, E. (2009). Bioavailability of nanoparticles in nutrient and nutraceutical delivery. *Curr. Opin. Colloid Interface Sci.* 14 (1): 3–15.

Aditya, N.P., Macedo, A.S., Doktorovova, S. et al. (2014). Development and evaluation of lipid nanocarriers for quercetin delivery: a comparative study of solid lipid nanoparticles (SLN), nanostructured lipid carriers (NLC), and lipid nanoemulsions (LNE). *LWT Food Sci. Technol.* 59 (1): 115–121.

Anitha, A., Maya, S., Deepa, N. et al. (2012). Curcumin-loaded N, O-carboxymethyl chitosan nanoparticles for cancer drug delivery. *J. Biomater. Sci. Polym. Ed.* 23 (11): 1381–1400.

Bangham, A.D., Standish, M.M., and Watkins, J.C. (1965). Diffusion of Univalent Ions across the Lamellae of Swollen Phospholipids. *J. Mol. Biol.* 13 (1): 238–252. IN26–7.

Banik, B.L., Fattahi, P., and Brown, J.L. (2016). Polymeric nanoparticles: the future of nanomedicine. *Wiley Interdiscip. Rev. Nanomed. Nanobiotechnol.* 8 (2): 271–299.

Bharti, C., Gulati, N., Nagaich, U., and Pal, A. (2015). Mesoporous silica nanoparticles in target drug delivery system: a review. *Int. J. Pharm. Investig.* 5 (3): 124.

Braithwaite, M.C., Tyagi, C., Tomar, L.K. et al. (2014). Nutraceutical-based therapeutics and formulation strategies augmenting their efficiency to complement modern medicine: an overview. *J. Funct. Foods* 6: 82–99.

Brezoiu, A.M., Matei, C., Deaconu, M. et al. (2019). Polyphenols extract from grape pomace. Characterization and valorisation through encapsulation into mesoporous silica-type matrices. *Food Chem. Toxicol.* 133 (June): 110787.

Brotons-Canto, A., Gonzalez-Navarro, C.J., Gurrea, J. et al. (2020). Zein nanoparticles improve the oral bioavailability of resveratrol in humans. *J. Drug Delivery Sci. Technol.* 57 (March): 101704.

Cai, J., Yang, J., Du, Y. et al. (2006). Enzymatic preparation of chitosan from the waste Aspergillus niger mycelium of citric acid production plant. *Carbohydr. Polym.* 64 (2): 151–157.

Cai, L., Yu, R., Hao, X., and Ding, X. (2017). Folate receptor-targeted bioflavonoid genistein-loaded chitosan nanoparticles for enhanced anticancer effect in cervical cancers. *Nanoscale Res. Lett.* 12: 1–8.

Campos, A., Fonte, P., Nunes, S. et al. (2015). RSC advances characterization of solid lipid nanoparticles produced with carnauba wax for rosmarinic acid oral delivery. *RSC Adv.* 5: 22665–22673.

Chang, C.W., Wong, C.Y., Wu, Y.T., and Hsu, M.C. (2017). Development of a solid dispersion system for improving the oral bioavailability of resveratrol in rats. *Eur. J. Drug Metab. Pharmacokinet.* 42 (2): 239–249.

Chen, L., Remondetto, G.E., and Subirade, M. (2006). Food protein-based materials as nutraceutical delivery systems. *Trends Food Sci. Technol.* 17 (5): 272–283.

Chen, S., Li, Q., McClements, D.J. et al. (2020). Co-delivery of curcumin and piperine in zein-carrageenan core-shell nanoparticles: formation, structure, stability and in vitro gastrointestinal digestion. *Food Hydrocoll.* 99 (August 2019): 105334.

Daniels, A., Company, M., Mills, G. et al. (2020). https://www.grandviewresearch.com/press-release/global-nutraceuticals-market 1/5. 2027:5–9.

Das, L., Bhaumik, E., Raychaudhuri, U., and Chakraborty, R. (2012). Role of nutraceuticals in human health. *J. Food Sci. Technol.* 49 (2): 173–183.

De Freitas, G.B.L., De Almeida, D.J., Carraro, E. et al. (2018). Formulation, characterization, and in vitro/in vivo studies of capsaicin-loaded albumin nanoparticles. *Mater. Sci. Eng. C* 93 (October 2017): 70–79.

Dhawan, S., Kapil, R., and Singh, B. (2011). Formulation development and systematic optimization of solid lipid nanoparticles of quercetin for improved brain delivery. *J. Pharm. Pharmacol.* 63 (3): 342–351.

Dima, C., Assadpour, E., Dima, S., and Jafari, S.M. (2020). Bioavailability of nutraceuticals: role of the food matrix, processing conditions, the gastrointestinal tract, and nanodelivery systems. *Compr. Rev. Food Sci. Food Saf.* 19 (3): 1–41.

Duraipandy, N., Lakra, R., Vinjimur, S.K. et al. (2014). Caging of plumbagin on silver nanoparticles imparts selectivity and sensitivity to plumbagin for targeted cancer cell apoptosis. *Metallomics* 6 (11): 2025–2033.

Dutta, S., Moses, J.A., and Anandharamakrishnan, C. (2018). Encapsulation of nutraceutical ingredients in liposomes and their potential for cancer treatment. *Nutr. Cancer* 70 (8): 1184–1198.

Ealias, A.M. and Saravanakumar, M.P. (2017). A review on the classification, characterisation, synthesis of nanoparticles and their application. *IOP Conf. Ser. Mater. Sci. Eng.* 263 (3).

Elbialy, N.S., Aboushoushah, S.F., Sofi, B.F., and Noorwali, A. (2020). Multifunctional curcumin-loaded mesoporous silica nanoparticles for cancer chemoprevention and therapy. *Microporous Mesoporous Mater.* 291: 109540.

El-Say, K.M. and El-Sawy, H.S. (2017). Polymeric nanoparticles: promising platform for drug delivery. *Int. J. Pharm.* 528 (1–2): 675–691.

Elzoghby, A.O., Samy, W.M., and Elgindy, N.A. (2012). Protein-based nanocarriers as promising drug and gene delivery systems. *J. Control. Release* 161 (1): 38–49.

Elzoghby, A.O., Samy, W.M., and Elgindy, N.A. (2012). Albumin-based nanoparticles as potential controlled release drug delivery systems. *J. Control. Release* 157 (2): 168–182.

Enteshari Najafabadi, R., Kazemipour, N., Esmaeili, A. et al. (2018). Using superparamagnetic iron oxide nanoparticles to enhance bioavailability of quercetin in the intact rat brain. *BMC Pharmacol. Toxicol.* 19 (1): 1–12.

Esfandiarpour-Boroujeni, S., Bagheri-Khoulenjani, S., Mirzadeh, H., and Amanpour, S. (2017). Fabrication and study of curcumin loaded nanoparticles based on folate-chitosan for breast cancer therapy application. *Carbohydr. Polym.* 168: 14–21.

Fan, Y., Zeng, X., Yi, J., and Zhang, Y. (2020). Fabrication of pea protein nanoparticles with calcium-induced cross-linking for the stabilization and delivery of antioxidative resveratrol. *Int. J. Biol. Macromol.* 152: 189–198.

Ghorbanzade, T., Jafari, S.M., Akhavan, S., and Hadavi, R. (2017). Nano-encapsulation of fish oil in nano-liposomes and its application in fortification of yogurt. *Food Chem.* 216: 146–152.

Giunta, R., Basile, G., and Tibuzzi, A. (2010). Legislation on nutraceuticals and food supplements: a comparison between regulations in USA and EU. In: *Bio-Farms for Nutraceuticals*, 322–328. Boston, MA: Springer.

Granja, A., Vieira, A.C.C., Chaves, L.L. et al. (2017). Folate-targeted nanostructured lipid carriers for enhanced oral delivery of Epigallocatechin-3-gallate. *Food Chem.* 237: 803–810.

Gülseren, İ., Guri, A., and Corredig, M. (2012). Encapsulation of tea polyphenols in nanoliposomes prepared with milk phospholipids and their effect on the viability of HT-29 human carcinoma cells. *Food Digestion* 3: 36–45.

Gupta, S. and Sen, G.M. (2016). Formulations and challenges: A special emphasis on stability and safety evaluations. In: *Developing New Functional Food and Nutraceutical Products*, 149–159. Elsevier Inc.

Huang, M., Su, E., Zheng, F., and Tan, C. (2017). Encapsulation of flavonoids in liposomal delivery systems: the case of quercetin, kaempferol and luteolin. *Food Funct.* 8 (9): 3198–4208.

Jain, S., Hirst, D.G., and O'Sullivan, J.M. (2012). Gold nanoparticles as novel agents for cancer therapy. *Br. J. Radiol.* 85 (1010): 101–113.

Joye, I.J., Nelis, V.A., and McClements, D.J. (2015). Gliadin-based nanoparticles: fabrication and stability of food-grade colloidal delivery systems. *Food Hydrocoll.* 44: 86–93.

Juère, E., Florek, J., Bouchoucha, M. et al. (2017). in vitro dissolution, cellular membrane permeability, and anti-inflammatory response of resveratrol-encapsulated mesoporous silica nanoparticles. *Mol. Pharm.* 14 (12): 4431–4441.

Kakkar, V., Singh, S., Singla, D., and Kaur, I.P. (2011). Exploring solid lipid nanoparticles to enhance the oral bioavailability of curcumin. *Mol. Nutr. Food Res.* 55 (3): 495–503.

Kamal, R., Chadha, V.D., and Dhawan, D.K. (2018). Physiological uptake and retention of radiolabeled resveratrol loaded gold nanoparticles (99mTc-Res-AuNP) in colon cancer tissue. *Nanomed. Nanotechnol. Biol. Med.* 14 (3): 1059–1071.

Karimi, N., Ghanbarzadeh, B., Hamishehkar, H., and Mehramuz, B. (2018). Antioxidant, antimicrobial and physicochemical properties of turmeric extract-loaded nanostructured lipid carrier (NLC). *Colloid Interface Sci. Commu.* 22 (November 2017): 18–24.

Katebi, S., Esmaeili, A., Ghaedi, K., and Zarrabi, A. (2019). Superparamagnetic iron oxide nanoparticles combined with NGF and quercetin promote neuronal branching morphogenesis of PC12 cells. *Int. J. Nanomedicine* 14: 2157–2169.

Khalil, A.T., Ovais, M., Ullah, I. et al. (2017). Sageretia thea (Osbeck.) modulated biosynthesis of NiO nanoparticles and their in vitro pharmacognostic, antioxidant and cytotoxic potential. *Artif Cells Nanomed. Nanotechnol.* 0 (0): 1–15.

Kim, D.H. and Martin, D.C. (2006). Sustained release of dexamethasone from hydrophilic matrices using PLGA nanoparticles for neural drug delivery. *Biomaterials* 27 (15): 3031–3037.

Kimpel, F. and Schmitt, J.J. (2015). Review: milk proteins as nanocarrier systems for hydrophobic nutraceuticals. *J. Food Sci.* 80 (11): R2361–R2366.

Kulkarni, N. and Muddapur, U. (2014). Biosynthesis of metal nanoparticles: a review. *J Nanotechnol.* 2014: 1–8.

Kumar, S.P., Birundha, K., Kaveri, K., and Devi, K.T.R. (2015). Antioxidant studies of chitosan nanoparticles containing naringenin and their cytotoxicity effects in lung cancer cells. *Int. J. Biol. Macromol.* 78: 87–95.

Kumari, A., Yadav, S.K., and Yadav, S.C. (2010). Biodegradable polymeric nanoparticles based drug delivery systems. *Colloids Surf. B: Biointerfaces* 75 (1): 1–18.

Levinson, Y., Israeli-Lev, G., and Livney, Y.D. (2014). Soybean β-Conglycinin nanoparticles for delivery of hydrophobic nutraceuticals. *Food Biophys.* 9 (4): 332–340.

Li, H.L. and Zhao, X. (2009). Bin, Ma YK, Zhai GX, Li LB, Lou HX. Enhancement of gastrointestinal absorption of quercetin by solid lipid nanoparticles. *J. Control. Release* 133 (3): 238–244.

Li, X., Xu, H., Chen, Z.S., and Chen, G. (2011). Biosynthesis of nanoparticles by microorganisms and their applications. *J. Nanomater.* 2011: 1–16.

Li, Z., Ha, J., Zou, T., and Gu, L. (2014). Fabrication of coated bovine serum albumin (BSA)-epigallocatechin gallate (EGCG) nanoparticles and their transport across monolayers of human intestinal epithelial Caco-2 cells. *Food Funct.* 5 (6): 1278–1285.

Lin, A., Liu, Y., Huang, Y. et al. (2008). Glycyrrhizin surface-modified chitosan nanoparticles for hepatocyte-targeted delivery. *Int. J. Pharm.* 359 (1–2): 247–253.

Lohcharoenkal, W., Wang, L., Chen, Y.C., and Rojanasakul, Y. (2014). Protein nanoparticles as drug delivery carriers for cancer therapy. *Biomed. Res. Int.* 2014.

Lu, Q., Li, D., and Jiang, J. (2011). Preparation of a tea polyphenol nanoliposome system and its physicochemical properties. *J. Agric. Food Chem.* 59: 13004–13011.

Mady, F.M. and Shaker, M.A. (2017). Enhanced anticancer activity and oral bioavailability of ellagic acid through encapsulation in biodegradable polymeric nanoparticles. *Int. J. Nanomedicine* 12: 7405–7417.

McClements, D.J. (2020). Advances in nanoparticle and microparticle delivery systems for increasing the dispersibility, stability, and bioactivity of phytochemicals. *Biotechnol. Adv.* 38: 107287.

Mehnert, W. and Mäder, K. (2012). Solid lipid nanoparticles production, characterization and applications. *Adv. Drug Deliv. Rev.* 64: 83–101.

Mignet, N., Seguin, J., Romano, M.R. et al. (2012). Development of a liposomal formulation of the natural flavonoid fisetin. *Int. J. Pharm.* 423 (1): 69–76.

Mishra, M. and Verma, G. (2016). A review on nutraceuticals: classification and its role in various disease. *Int J Pharm Ter.* 7 (4): 152–160.

Mohammadi, M., Ghanbarzadeh, B., and Hamishehkar, H. (2014). Formulation of nanoliposomal vitamin D3 for potential application in beverage fortification. *Adv Pharm Bull.* 4 (Suppl 2): 569–575.

Mohanraj, V.J. and Chen, Y. (2006). Nanoparticles – a review. *Trop. J. Pharm. Res.* 5 (June): 561–573.

Mokhtari, S., Jafari, S.M., and Assadpour, E. (2017). Development of a nutraceutical nano-delivery system through emulsification/internal gelation of alginate. *Food Chem.* 229: 286–295.

Muddineti, O.S., Kumari, P., Ajjarapu, S. et al. (2016). Xanthan gum stabilized PEGylated gold nanoparticles for improved delivery of curcumin in cancer. *Nanotechnology* 27 (32): 1–13.

Mullakkalparambil Velayudhan, J., Mondal, D., Raja, R. et al. (2020). Hepatoprotectant potential of sodium alginate coated catechin nanoparticles (SACC-NPs) in rat model. *Inorg. Nano-Metal Chem.* 50: 1–9.

Narayan, R., Nayak, U.Y., Raichur, A.M., and Garg, S. (2018). Mesoporous silica nanoparticles: a comprehensive review on synthesis and recent advances. *Pharmaceutics.* 10 (3): 1–49.

Ni, S., Sun, R.U.I., Zhao, G. et al. (2014). Quercetin loaded nanostructured lipid carrier for food fortification: preparation, characterization and in vitro study. *J. Food Process Eng.* 38 (1): 93–106.

Oehlke, K., Adamiuk, M., Behsnilian, D. et al. (2014). Potential bioavailability enhancement of bioactive compounds using food-grade engineered nanomaterials: a review of the existing evidence. *Food Funct.* 5 (7): 1341–1359.

de Oliveira, P.R., Hoffmann, S., Pereira, S. et al. (2018). Self-assembled amphiphilic chitosan nanoparticles for quercetin delivery to breast cancer cells. *Eur. J. Pharm. Biopharm.* 131: 203–210.

Pan, K. and Zhong, Q. (2016). Organic nanoparticles in foods: fabrication, characterization, and utilization. *Annu. Rev. Food Sci. Technol.* 7 (1): 245–266.

Park, S., Cha, S.H., Cho, I. et al. (2016). Antibacterial nanocarriers of resveratrol with gold and silver nanoparticles. *Mater. Sci. Eng. C* 58: 1160–1169.

Penalva, R., Esparza, I., Agüeros, M. et al. (2015). Casein nanoparticles as carriers for the oral delivery of folic acid. *Food Hydrocoll.* 44: 399–406.

Penalva, R., Gonzalez-Navarro, C.J., Gamazo, C. et al. (2017). Zein nanoparticles for oral delivery of quercetin: pharmacokinetic studies and preventive anti-inflammatory effects in a mouse model of endotoxemia. *Nanomedicine* 13 (1): 103–110.

Peñalva, R., Morales, J., González-Navarro, C.J. et al. (2018). Increased oral bioavailability of resveratrol by its encapsulation in casein nanoparticles. *Int. J. Mol. Sci.* 19 (9): 2816.

Peng, W., Jiang, X.Y., Zhu, Y. et al. (2015). Oral delivery of capsaicin using MPEG-PCL nanoparticles. *Acta Pharmacol. Sin.* 36 (1): 139–148.

Rahimi, S., Khoee, S., and Ghandi, M. (2019). Preparation and characterization of rod-like chitosan–quinoline nanoparticles as pH-responsive nanocarriers for quercetin delivery. *Int. J. Biol. Macromol.* 128: 279–289.

Rani, R., Dilbaghi, N., Dhingra, D., and Kumar, S. (2015). Optimization and evaluation of bioactive drug-loaded polymeric nanoparticles for drug delivery. *Int. J. Biol. Macromol.* 78: 173–179.

Rani, R., Dahiya, S., Dhingra, D. et al. (2017). Evaluation of anti-diabetic activity of glycyrrhizin-loaded nanoparticles in nicotinamide-streptozotocin-induced diabetic rats. *Eur. J. Pharm. Sci.* 106 (May): 220–230.

Ron, N., Zimet, P., Bargarum, J., and Livney, Y.D. (2010). Beta-lactoglobulin e polysaccharide complexes as nanovehicles for hydrophobic nutraceuticals in non-fat foods and clear beverages. *Int. Dairy J.* 20 (10): 686–693.

Saha, S., Kundu, J., Verma, R.J., and Chowdhury, P.K. (2020). Albumin coated polymer nanoparticles loaded with plant extract derived quercetin for modulation of inflammation. *Materialia* 9: 100605.

Sanna, V., Lubinu, G., Madau, P. et al. (2015). Polymeric nanoparticles encapsulating white tea extract for nutraceutical application. *J. Agric. Food Chem.* 63 (7): 2026–2032.

Sardoiwala, M.N., Kaundal, B., and Choudhury, S.R. (2018). Development of engineered nanoparticles expediting diagnostic and therapeutic applications across blood-brain barrier. In: *Handbook of Nanomaterials for Industrial Applications* (ed. C.M. Hussain), 696–709. Elsevier Inc.

Sarkar, A., Ghosh, S., Chowdhury, S. et al. (2016). Targeted delivery of quercetin loaded mesoporous silica nanoparticles to the breast cancer cells. *Biochim. Biophys. Acta, Gen. Subj.* 1860 (10): 2065–2075.

Sawant, V.J. and Bamane, S.R. (2017). PEG-beta-cyclodextrin functionalized zinc oxide nanoparticles show cell imaging with high drug payload and sustained pH responsive delivery of curcumin in to MCF-7 cells. *J. Drug Delivery Sci. Technol.* 43: 397–408.

Sawant, V.J., Bamane, S.R., Kanase, D.G. et al. (2016). Encapsulation of curcumin over carbon dot coated TiO 2 nanoparticles for pH sensitive enhancement of anticancer and anti-psoriatic potential. *RSC Adv.* 6: 66745–66755.

Shahein, S.A., Aboul-Enein, A.M., Higazy, I.M. et al. (2019). Targeted anticancer potential against glioma cells of thymoquinone delivered by mesoporous silica core-shell nanoformulations with pH-dependent release. *Int. J. Nanomedicine* 14: 5503–5526.

Shahidi, F. (2006). Functional foods: their role in health promotion and disease prevention. *J. Food Sci.* 69 (5): R146–R149.

Sherin, S., Sheeja, S., Devi, R.S. et al. (2017). in vitro and in vivo pharmacokinetics and toxicity evaluation of curcumin incorporated titanium dioxide nanoparticles for biomedical applications. *Chem. Biol. Interact.* 275: 35–46.

Sriram, K., Maheswari, P.U., and Ezhilarasu, A. (2017). CuO-loaded hydrophobically modified chitosan as hybrid carrier for curcumin delivery and anticancer activity. *Asia Pacific Journal of Chemical Engineering* 12 (6): 858–871.

Statistic (n.d.). statistic_id591536_global-market-size-of-nutraceuticals-2016-by-category.pdf.

Tamjidi, F., Shahedi, M., Varshosaz, J., and Nasirpour, A. (2014). Design and characterization of astaxanthin-loaded nanostructured lipid carriers. *Innov. Food Sci. Emerg. Technol.* 26: 366–374.

Teng, Z., Luo, Y., and Wang, Q. (2012). Nanoparticles synthesized from soy protein: preparation, characterization, and application for nutraceutical encapsulation. *J. Agric. Food Chem.* 60 (10): 2712–2720.

Teng, Z., Luo, Y., Li, Y., and Wang, Q. (2016). Cationic beta-lactoglobulin nanoparticles as a bioavailability enhancer: effect of surface properties and size on the transport and delivery in vitro. *Food Chem.* 204: 391–399.

Thakkar, K.N., Mhatre, S.S., and Parikh, R.Y. (2010). Biological synthesis of metallic nanoparticles. *Nanomed. Nanotechnol. Biol. Med.* 6 (2): 257–262.

Ting, Y., Jiang, Y., Ho, C.T., and Huang, Q. (2014). Common delivery systems for enhancing in vivo bioavailability and biological efficacy of nutraceuticals. *J. Funct. Foods* 7 (1): 112–128.

Umegaki, K. (2016). *Regulatory Aspects of Nutraceuticals: Japanese Perspective. Nutraceuticals: Efficacy, Safety and Toxicity*, 933–940. Elsevier Inc.

Varaprasad, K., López, M., Núñez, D. et al. (2019). Antibiotic copper oxide-curcumin nanomaterials for antibacterial applications. *J. Mol. Liq.* 300: 112353.

Varlamov, V.P., Il, A.V., Shagdarova, B.T. et al. (2020). Chitin/chitosan and its derivatives: fundamental problems and practical approaches. *Biochemistry* 85: 154–176.

Wang, S., Su, R., Nie, S. et al. (2014). Application of nanotechnology in improving bioavailability and bioactivity of diet-derived phytochemicals. *J. Nutr. Biochem.* 25 (4): 363–376.

Wildman, R.E.C. and Kelley, M. (2007). *Nutraceuticals Functional Foods*, 1–21. New York: Taylor & Francis.

Wu, W., Kong, X., Zhang, C. et al. (2020). Fabrication and characterization of resveratrol-loaded gliadin nanoparticles stabilized by gum Arabic and chitosan hydrochloride. *Lwt.* 129 (March): 109532.

Xie, X., Tao, Q., Zou, Y. et al. (2011). PLGA nanoparticles improve the oral bioavailability of curcumin in rats: characterizations and mechanisms. *J. Agric. Food Chem.* 59 (17): 9280–9289.

Yao, M., McClements, D.J., and Xiao, H. (2015). Improving oral bioavailability of nutraceuticals by engineered nanoparticle-based delivery systems. *Curr. Opin. Food Sci.* 2 (April): 14–19.

Young, P. and Ko, T. (2015). Improved oral delivery of resveratrol from N -trimethyl chitosan- g – palmitic acid surface-modified solid lipid nanoparticles. *Mass Spectrometry Reviews* 139: 52–61.

Yu, X., Yuan, L., Zhu, N. et al. (2019). Fabrication of antimicrobial curcumin stabilized platinum nanoparticles and their anti-liver fibrosis activity for potential use in nursing care. *J. Photochem. Photobiol. B Biol.* 195 (March): 27–32.

Zhang, W., Jiang, P., Chen, Y. et al. (2016). Suppressing the cytotoxicity of CuO nanoparticles by uptake of curcumin/BSA particles. *Nanoscale* 8 (18): 9572–9582.

5

Prebiotics and Probiotics

Concept and Advances

Hammad Ullah[1], Maria Daglia[1], and Haroon Khan[2]

[1] Department of Pharmacy, School of Medicine and Surgery, University of Naples Federico II, Naples, Italy
[2] Department of Pharmacy, Faculty of Chemical & Life Sciences, Abdul Wali Khan University, Mardan, Pakistan

5.1 Introduction

The human body is colonized with a vast number of microorganisms such as bacteria, viruses, fungi, and protozoans living in coexistence with their host and is known as microbiota or normal flora (Sekirov et al. 2010). Joshua Lederberg introduced the concept of human microbiota for the first time and defined it as "the ecological community of symbiotic and pathogenic microorganisms that literally share our body space and have been all but ignored as determinants of health and disease" (Lederberg and McCray 2001). Bacteria are most extensively studied for their beneficial effects on human health and disease, while viruses, fungi, and protozoans are less known for favorable effects. The microbiota is known to colonize every part of the human body, exposed to the external environment including skin, genitourinary, respiratory, and GI tracts. The human body has been estimated to contain about 10^{14} bacterial cells, where the gastrointestinal (GI) tract alone is colonized with about 70% of all microbes present in the body (Sekirov et al. 2010; Sommer and Bäckhed 2013; Jandhyala et al., 2015).

The gut microbiota is dominated by species of Bacteroidetes and Firmicutes phyla, representing 90% of gut microbiota. Other phyla include Actinobacteria, Proteobacteria, Fusobacteria, and Verrucomicrobia (Table 5.1) (Rinninella et al. 2019). The number of gut microbiota shows continuum, with 10^1 to 10^3 bacteria per gram of contents in the stomach and duodenum, progresses to 10^4 to 10^7 bacteria per gram in the jejunum and ileum, and 10^{11} to 10^{12} bacteria per gram in the colon (O'Hara and Shanahan 2006). Studies have demonstrated that colonization of gut microbiota begins at birth, as newborns exposed to a complex microbial population of the birth canal during delivery. Moreover, the composition of intestinal microbial composition depends upon the mode of delivery, vaginally delivered infants show a high abundance of *Lactobacilli* during the early stage of life while C-section-delivered babies show depleted and delayed colonization of the *Bacteroides* species, though they are colonized with facultative anaerobes like *Clostridium* species (Thursby and Juge 2017).

Gut microbiota possesses complex interaction with their host and they can help their host with digestion, production of vitamins (vitamins B12 and K), modulating the body's immune system and restricting the growth and/or activity of harmful pathogens (Ho et al. 2015). Several factors

Table 5.1 A detailed list of gut microbiota composition (Rinninella et al. 2019).

Phylum	Class	Order	Family	Genus	Species
Actinobacteria	Actinobacteria	Actinomycetales	Corynebacteriacea	*Corynebacterium*	*C. accolens*
		Bifidobacteriales	Bifidobacteriaceae	*Bifidobacterium*	*B. longum*, *B. bifidum*
	Coriobacteriia	Coriobacteriales	Coriobacteriaceae	*Atopobium*	*A. parvulum*
Firmicutes[a]	Clostridia	Clostridiales	Clostridiaceae	*Faecalibacterium*	*F. prausnitzii*
				Clostridium	*Clostridium* spp.
			Lachnospiraceae	*Roseburia*	*R. intestinalis*
			Ruminococcaceae	*Ruminococcus*	*R. faecis*
	Negativicutes	Veillonellales	Veillonellaceae	*Dialister*	*D. invisus*
	Bacilli	Lactobacillus	Lactobacillaceae	*Lactobacillus*	*L. reuteri*
			Enterococcaceae	*Enterococcus*	*E. faecium*
		Bacillales	Staphylococcaceae	*Staphylococcus*	*S. lei*
Bacteroidetes[a]	Sphingobacteria	Sphingobacteriales	Sphingobacteriaceae	*Sphingobacterium*	*Sphingobacterium* spp.
	Bacteroidia	Bacteroidales	Bacteroidaceae	*Bacteroides*	*B. fragilis*, *B. vulgatus*
			Tannerellaceae	*Tannerella*	*T. forsythia*
				Parabacteroides	*P. distasonis*
			Rikenellaceae	*Alistipes*	*A. finegoldii*
			Prevotellaceae	*Prevotella*	*Prevotella* spp.
Proteobacteria	Gamma proteobacteria	Enterobacterales	Enterobacteriaceae	*Escherichia*	*E. coli*
				Shigella	*S. flexneri*
	Delta proteobacteria	Desulfovibrionales	Desulfovibrionaceae	*Desulfovibrio*	*D. intestinalis*
				Bilophila	*B. wadsworthia*
	Epsilon proteobacteria	Campylobacterales	Helicobacteraceae	*Helicobacter*	*H. pylori*
Fusobacteria	Fusobacteria	Fusobacteriales	Fusobacteriaceae	*Fusobacterium*	*F. nucleatum*
Verrucomicrobia	Verrucomicrobiae	Verrucomicrobiales	Akkermansiaceae	*Akkermansia*	*A. muciniphila*

[a] Firmicutes and Bacteroidetes represent about 90% of gut microbiota.

can be associated with the imbalance of the gut microbiota composition and integrity of the intestinal epithelial layer (Cani et al. 2008). Dysregulated gut microbiota may result in the pathogenesis of several intestinal and extraintestinal disorders including inflammatory disorders of the GI tract, hepatitis, cholelithiasis, obesity, diabetes, allergy, autism spectrum disorder (ASD), and infections (Sekirov et al. 2010).

Numerous strategies have been proposed to regulate imbalances in the gut microbiota composition such as consumption of probiotics and prebiotics (Bagarolli et al. 2017).

5.2 Probiotics

Lilly and Stillwell used the term "probiotics" in 1965 for the first time to describe the substances secreted by one microorganism stimulating the growth of another (Lilly and Stillwell 1965). In 1974, Parker proposed probiotics as organisms and substances contributing to intestinal microbial balance (Parker 1974). The most practical definition of probiotics is microbial food supplements that offer health benefits beyond nutrition when consumed in enough amount, usually by modulating gut flora (Mack 2005). They should be nontoxic, nonpathogenic, being able to adhere to gut epithelial tissues and produce short-chain fatty acids (SCFAs) on interaction with dietary fibers and prebiotics. Lactic acid bacteria (LAB) such as *Lactobacillus* and *Bifidobacterium*, genus *Saccharomyces*, some strains of *Escherichia coli*, and some gram-positive cocci are some commonly used probiotics (Suvarna and Boby 2005; Chugh and Kamal-Eldin 2020; Delgado et al. 2020).

The genus *Lactobacillus* has 56 species widely distributed throughout GI and genital tracts constitute an important part of the microflora of human and higher animals. The genus *Bifidobacterium* has 30 species, 10 of which are from human sources including feces, vagina, and dental caries. The remaining 17 species are from animal intestinal tracts, 2 from wastewater and 1 from fermented milk (Soccol et al. 2010). The probiotic supplements contain either a single or multiple strain(s), where a probiotic species may exert different therapeutic benefits or efficacy when used as a single strain or in combination with other strains (Pandey et al. 2015). The commercially available probiotic products should contain the optimal number of colony-forming units (CFUs) for each bacterial strain above the critical threshold (10^6 CFU). Moreover, the recommended daily dose of probiotic species for their beneficial effects is about 10^6 to 10^9, though the optimal number of CFUs for each strain delivered remains unknown (Sreeja and Prajapati 2013; Jesus et al. 2016).

5.2.1 Therapeutic Benefits

Probiotic supplementation offers health benefits to the host in a number of ways such as enhancing intestinal integrity, regulating immune pathways, inhibiting the growth and/or activity of pathogenic microbes and protecting against gut barrier disruption (De Filippis et al. 2020). Because of their multiple targets, they can be used in preventing and treating a number of chronic pathologies (Aureli et al. 2011). Figure 5.1 represents the commonly used probiotic species. Figure 5.2 illustrates the proposed mechanisms of probiotic actions relating to the health benefits of the host. Some of the elite properties of probiotics in relation to their antioxidant effects, immune-modulating activities, vitamins production, metabolic disorders, psychiatric diseases, neurodegenerative diseases, GI diseases and anti-infective activities as depicted in Figure 5.3 are discussed below.

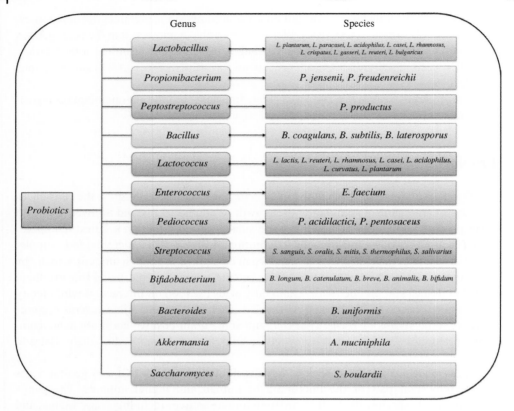

Figure 5.1 Commonly used probiotic species.

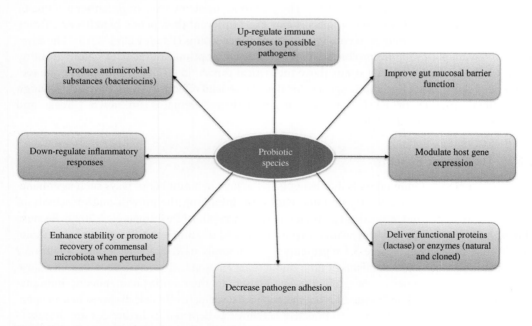

Figure 5.2 Proposed mechanisms of probiotic actions.

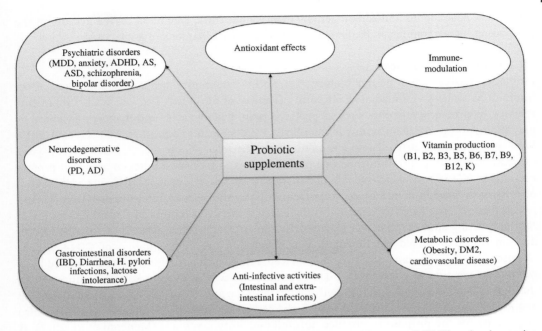

Figure 5.3 Health benefits of probiotic supplementation. Diabetes mellitus type 2 (DM2), major depressive disorder (MDD), attention deficit hyperactivity disorder (ADHD), Asperger syndrome (AS), ASD, Parkinson's disorder (PD), Alzheimer's disorder (AD), and inflammatory bowel disorder (IBD).

5.2.1.1 Antioxidant Effects

As indicated by in vitro and in vivo studies, specific strains of probiotics alone or in foods exert antioxidant effects by increasing free radical scavenging rate and upregulating the expression of antioxidant enzymes (Mishra et al. 2015). Some species of LAB such as *Lactobacillus*, *Lactococcus*, *Streptococcus*, and *Leuconostoc* genera showed greater antioxidant effects, more probably through resisting reactive oxygen species (ROS) including superoxide anions, peroxide, and hydroxyl radicals (Wang et al. 2017; Fardet and Rock 2018; Gholamhosseinpour and Hashemi 2019). Rats showed higher antioxidant ability when supplemented with *Lactobacillus plantarum* P-8, as reflected by reducing the accumulation of hepatic lipids and protecting the liver against oxidative damage (Bao et al. 2012). *Lactobacillus rhamnosus* exerted strong antioxidant activity in case of elevated physical stress and thus athletes can be benefited from *L. rhamnosus* supplementation to neutralize the ROS effects (Martarelli et al. 2011).

Bifidobacterium species (*B. longum* and *B. animalis* 01) are reported to exert their antioxidant effects through increased ROS scavenging, enhanced production and expression of antioxidant enzymes, decreased lipid peroxidation and reduced oxidative DNA damage (Nowak et al. 2019). Lim et al. reported that the antioxidant activity of probiotics is strain-specific, as he observed higher antioxidant activity with yoghurt obtained with *Lactobacillus acidophilus* strain PC16 than yoghurt produced with *Lactobacillus casei* strain PC05 (Lim 2013). Yoghurt and fermented milk possess higher antioxidant activity as compared to milk because of the presence of fermenting microorganisms (Melini et al. 2019). Moreover, milk origin may also affect the antioxidant potential of fermented milk and yoghurt. Yoghurt produced through fermentation of goat milk with *Pediococcus pentosaceus* has more radical scavenging properties than yoghurt from cow, camel, and goat milk. Similarly, yoghurt fermented with *Lactobacillus rhamnosus* strain PTCC 1637 from camel milk have higher antioxidant activity than yoghurt from cow milk, maybe because of the presence of higher contents of proline in camel milk caseins (Fardet and Rock 2018).

5.2.1.2 Immune Modulation

Probiotics possess immune-modulatory and anti-inflammatory properties, and they affect humoral as well as cell-mediated immunity (Pandey et al. 2015). The cell wall components released by probiotic microbes such as peptidoglycan, teichoic acid, and lipoteichoic acid may play an important role in immunity homeostasis (Weidenmaier and Peschel 2008; Xia et al. 2010; Wolf and Underhill 2018). Factors secreting from *Lactobacillus reuteri* decrease NF-kB gene expression, resulting in diminished cell proliferation and increased mitogen-activated protein kinase (MAPK) activity, which may induce apoptosis (Delcenserie et al. 2008). A down-regulation of mRNA expression of tumor necrosis factor-alpha (TNF-α) and interleukin-1 beta (IL-1β), released by macrophages in intestinal inflammation has been reported in probiotic strains of *Bifidobacterium* species (Okada et al. 2009). Moreover, *Enterococcus faecalis* triggers IL-12 production from stimulated macrophages, which helps in the differentiation of CD4+ T cells (Menconi et al. 2014). Yan and coresearchers were reported that a soluble protein released by *L. rhamnosus* was found effective in treating colitis induced by dextran sulfate sodium (DSS), through activation of epidermal growth factor receptor and reduction of intestinal epithelial apoptosis (Yan et al. 2011). More interestingly, genetically modified probiotic species are also engineered for the purpose to produce anti-inflammatory cytokines (Menconi et al. 2014). A strain of genetically modified *Lactococcus lactis* minimized the effects of DSS-induced colitis through secretion of anti-inflammatory IL-10 (Steidler et al. 2000). in vitro models using dendritic cell cultures showed an increased release of IL-10 by the mixture of probiotic strains known as VSL VSL#3, comprising *L. acidophilus*, *L. casei*, *L. plantarum*, *Lactobacillus delbrueckii* subsp. *bulgaricus*, *B. longum*, *B. breve*, *B. infantis*, and *Streptococcus salivarius* subsp. *thermophilus* (Drakes et al. 2004; Hart et al. 2004). An in vivo experiment with mice by Pagnini et al. showed the stimulation of epithelial innate immunity (Pagnini et al. 2010).

5.2.1.3 Vitamins' Production

Several microbial groups have been evaluated for their potential to produce essential vitamins that are neither synthesized by the body nor consumed through diet. The vitamins that are produced by the gut microbiota in humans include vitamins B1, B2, B3, B5, B6, B7, B9, B12, and vitamin K (LeBlanc et al. 2013). As these vitamins are produced by intestinal flora, their nutritional requirements for individuals with a low intake of these vitamins depends on gut microbial production (Hugenholtz and Smid 2002; Crittenden et al. 2003). LAB species are reportedly using in the food industry for the production of riboflavin and folate (Hugenholtz et al. 2002; Kehagias et al. 2008). Among 179 LAB strains isolated from a variety of foods, *L. plantarum* CRL 725 was shown to two-fold increase in the concentration of riboflavin in soy milk (Juarez del Valle et al. 2014). Colonic microbes such as *B. longum* and *B. bifidum* have been reported to synthesize folate (Lee et al. 2018). in vivo study showed an increased production of folate by intake of folate-producing *Bifidobacteria* strains such as *B. adolescentis* MB 239, *B. adolescentis* MB 227, and *B. pseudocatenulatum* MB 116 (Pompei et al. 2007). Though it remains controversial, fortification of foods with probiotics may also improve the vitamin status of the individual's body by increasing their availability in the gut (Pompei et al. 2007). Previously, fermentation of soymilk with *B. longum* resulted in moderately increased production of thiamine (Hou et al. 2000). More recently, soy beverages fermented with *Lactobacillus helveticus* R0052 and *Streptococcus thermophilus* ST5 did not affect the concentrations of thiamine and pyridoxine (Champagne et al. 2010).

5.2.1.4 Metabolic Disorders

It has been evidenced that gut microbiota plays a role in energy homeostasis from the diet and they could suppress the metabolic stresses through regulation of G-protein-coupled receptors (GPR41 and GPRF43) via SCFAs production and suppression of hepatic and skeletal muscle 5' AMP-activated protein kinase (AMPK)-dependent fatty acid oxidation (Cani and Delzenne 2009). Gut dysbiosis may provide a way for the pathogenesis of metabolic disorders such as obesity, diabetes mellitus type 2 (DM2), and cardiovascular diseases (Jin et al. 2019; Vallianou et al. 2019; Sikalidis and Maykish 2020). Dysbiosis of intestinal flora may result in β-cell dysfunction, increased adiposity, oxidative stress, systemic inflammation, and metabolic endotoxemia (Yoo and Kim 2016). Probiotics are considered an effective alternative treatment for metabolic diseases as they modulate gut microbial modulation resulting in insulin signaling stimulation (Delzenne et al. 2011; Yoo and Kim 2016). SCFAs, the end-products of carbohydrate metabolism help in improving glucose tolerance, decreasing glucagon levels in a dose-dependent manner and activating glucagon-like peptide (GLP), which, in turn, stimulates insulin production and enhances insulin sensitivity (Everard et al. 2011; Parnell and Reimer 2012).

Lactobacillus species (*L. acidophilus, L. curvatus* HY7601, *L. Plantarum* KY1034, *L. salivarius* UCC118, *L. casei* NCDC 19, *L. brevis* OK56, *L. rhamnosus* NCDC17) and *Bifidobacterium* species (*B. longum, B. lactis*) have proven anti-obesity effects, more possibly through decreasing fat storage, altering serum lipid profiles, inducing fatty acid oxidation genes, interacting with host TLRs, reducing inflammatory cascade and stimulating the production of satiety-inducing peptides (Dahiya et al. 2017). An oral probiotic supplementation comprising of viable strains of *L. acidophilus, L. rhamnosus, L. bulgaricus, L. casei, B. longum, B. breve* and *S. thermophilus* for eight weeks in randomized, placebo-controlled, and parallel designed study significantly lowers fasting plasma glucose levels (Asemi et al. 2013). Probiotics could also decrease oxidative stress and prevent against oxidative damage in pancreatic tissues, as evidenced by the administration of *L. acidophilus* and *L. casei* with yoghurt, which inhibits lipid peroxidation and nitric oxide formation (Yadav et al. 2008). However, studies explained that probiotics could fail in maintaining normal cholesterol levels in diabetic patients, as no significant changes in the levels of total cholesterol (TC), low-density lipoprotein (LDL), high-density lipoprotein (HDL), and triglycerides (TG) were noted (Lewis and Burmeister 2005; Andreasen et al. 2010; Mahboobi et al. 2014).

5.2.1.5 Psychiatric Disorders

Literature has linked the gut-brain axis and dysbiosis of intestinal flora with psychiatric disorders, and the gut microbiome is a potential therapeutic target using probiotics and prebiotics, though the research is still very limited to make any directions of clinical use of probiotics in psychiatric diseases (Barbosa and Vieira-Coelho 2020). Patients with MDD normally have increased oxidative and inflammatory stresses, altered GI function with lower micronutrient, and omega-3 fatty acid status. Overgrowth of small intestinal bacteria is likely to contribute to limited nutrient absorption. MDD-associated stress may alter intestinal flora by reducing *Lactobacilli* and *Bifidobacterium* levels. Probiotics can be used as adjuvant therapy in MDD as they have the potential to lower oxidative stress and systemic inflammatory cytokines, improve nutritional status, and correct small intestinal bacterial overgrowth. The positive regulation of oxidative stress and inflammatory mediators may result in increasing brain-derived neurotrophic factor (BDNF) concentration (Logan and Katzman 2005).

A randomized trial revealed a reduced risk of the development of neuropsychiatric disorders such as ADHD and AS, later in life in subjects supplemented with *L. rhamnosus* GG early in life. *L. rhamnosus* GG was shown to stabilize the gut permeability barrier and regulate the central

GABAergic system (Pärtty et al. 2015). A prospective, open-label study demonstrated the improvement in the severity of ASD and GI symptoms in autistic children when treated with probiotic nutritional supplement formula comprising *L. acidophilus*, *L. rhamnosus*, and *B. longum* (Shaaban et al. 2018). Quite differences in gut microbiome quantification have been reported in chronic psychiatric disorders such as schizophrenia and bipolar disorder, and studies have linked these differences with the symptom's severity. Probiotic supplementation of these patients with probiotics including *L. acidophilus* W22, *L. casei* W56, *L. plantarum* W62, *L. rhamnosus* GG, *L. paracasei* W20, *B. bifidum* W23, *B. breve* A,1 *B. animalis* subs. *Lactis* BB-12, and *L. lactis* W19 has shown to reduce the symptoms' severity and rehospitalization rates with the improvement of cognitive function (Genedi et al. 2019).

5.2.1.6 Neurodegenerative Disorders

Gut microbiota, when in a state of dysbiosis, may influence the neurological disease progression and even initiates the onset of the disorder (Catanzaro et al. 2014). Reduced diversity may be one of the contributing factors in the development of the neurodegenerative disorder in aging where neuroinflammation is the possible mechanism linking gut microbiota to age-related diseases (Jyothi et al. 2015; A Kohler et al. 2016; Dinan and Cryan 2017). This relationship could also explain the high rate of GI comorbid pathologies in patients with neurodegenerative diseases such as gut dysbiosis, diarrhea, constipation, vitamin deficiency, and metabolic dysregulations (Westfall et al. 2017). Manipulation of the gut microbiome with SCFAs producing bacteria can modulate neuroimmune activation and thus may halt the progression of neurodegeneration (Dinan and Cryan 2017; Vickers 2017).

Probiotic species may reduce pro-inflammatory cytokines while upregulating anti-inflammatory mediators, which ultimately results in downstream regulation of neuroinflammation in the enteric nervous system (ENS) (Heiss and Olofsson 2019). The first clinical study conducted in 2011, with the aim of investigating the role of probiotics on defecation habits in patients with Parkinson's disease (PD), concluded the improvement of stool consistency and defecation habits in patients treated with *L. casei* Shirota (Cassani et al. 2011). in vitro study suggests the production of L-dopa from L-tyrosine by *Bacillus* species, which can then be converted to dopamine through dopa decarboxylase enzyme (Surwase and Jadhav 2011). More recently, probiotics alleviate the progressive deterioration of motor functions in a mouse model of Parkinson's disease, as the motor impairments in gait pattern, balance function, and motor coordination were found to be significantly reduced (Hsieh et al. 2020).

Probiotic supplementation of patients with Alzheimer's disease in randomized, double-blind, and controlled clinical trial comprising *L. acidophilus*, *L. fermentum*, *L. casei*, and *B. bifidum* for 12 weeks positively affects cognitive function, insulin secretion and sensitivity, serum TG, and malondialdehyde (MDA) levels (Akbari et al. 2016). BDNF signaling is critical for neuronal protection, survival and plasticity, and *B. breve* 6330 enhances the BDNF levels in the dentate gyrus of the hippocampus in rats (O'Sullivan et al. 2011).

5.2.1.7 Gastrointestinal Disorders

Growing evidence suggests that gut dysbiosis is closely linked with the pathogenesis of intestinal disorders (De Filippis et al. 2020). Selected probiotic strains can be used in the treatment of some common GI disorders by regulating immunity of GI mucosa, decreasing gut barrier disruption, inhibiting pathogenic microbial growth and activity, improving functional GI symptoms, reducing *Helicobacter pylori* infection and improving lactose tolerance (Almeida et al. 2012; Srinarong et al. 2014; Kang and Im 2015; Bron et al. 2017; Xue et al. 2017). Supplementation of probiotic species like *Saccharomyces boulardii*, *L. casei B. bifidum*, *L. rhamnosus*, and VSL#3 showed promising results in preventing inflammatory bowel diseases (IBD) including ulcerative colitis and Crohn's disease (Kelesidis and Pothoulakis 2012; Jonkers et al. 2012). Fermented milk containing *L. acidophilus*, *B. breve*, and *B. bifidum* was found affective in inducing mild-degree remission of IBD as revealed by a pilot study (Sheil et al. 2007). Probiotic strains may also be efficacious in the management of IBD due to their potential of restoring the integrity of the protective intestinal mucosa (Peña 2007).

Evidence from animal and human studies depicted that selected probiotic strains can be useful in the management of *Clostridium difficile*-associated colitis (*S. boulardii*), antibiotic-associated diarrhea (*L. acidophilus*, *L. fermentum*, *L. rhamnosus* GG, *L. delbruckii*, and *S. boulardii*) and traveler's diarrhea (*Lactobacilli*, *Bifidobacteria*, *Enterococci*, and *Streptococci*) (McFarland 2006). The possible antidiarrheal mechanisms of probiotics include stimulation of immune system, competing for binding sites on intestinal epithelial cells or secretion of bacteriocins (Pandey et al. 2015). Lactose intolerance is the most common type of carbohydrate intolerance and can be treated either with commercially available lactase or with probiotics such as *L. bulgaricus* and *S. thermophiles*. It has also been evident that milk consumption containing *L. acidophilus* and *B. longum* significantly decreases hydrogen production and flatulence (Vonk et al. 2012; Pandey et al. 2015).

5.2.1.8 Anti-infective Activities

Unlike antibiotics, probiotics may inhibit the disturbance or alteration in the complex population of gut microbiota, and, thus, anti-infective activities are regarded as one of the most beneficial effects of probiotics (Kerry et al. 2018). As available literature suggests, supplementation of probiotics can be useful in intestinal (gastroenteritis, *C. difficile*-associated diarrhea, *H. pylori* infections, and food-borne pathogens) as well as extraintestinal (hepatic, respiratory, and vaginal) infections (Britton and Versalovic 2008; Kim and Park 2017; El-Khadragy et al. 2019; Shinde et al. 2020). The influence of probiotics on the survival of *Salmonella enterica*, *C. difficile*, and *Serovar typhimurium* have been investigated by Tejero-Sarinena and colleagues, using in vitro model of study and it was concluded that probiotics inhibited the growth of these pathogens by the production of SCFAs (Tejero-Sariñena et al. 2013).

Regulation of immune cell function, induction of microphage differentiation, reduction of the mammalian target of rapamycin (mTOR) kinase activity, and production of antimicrobial peptides in the absence of increased inflammatory cytokine response are some of the basic mechanisms responsible for the anti-pathogenic activities of SCFAs (Corrêa-Oliveira et al. 2016; Schulthess et al. 2019). Probiotics also produced some other substances like bacteriocins, ethanol, organic acids, and hydrogen peroxide (H_2O_2) which may aid in their anti-pathogenic properties (Kerry et al. 2018). Bacteriocins possess antimicrobial potential by increasing membrane permeability of the target cells, resulting in the depolarization of the membrane potential and, ultimately, cell death (Simova et al. 2009). H_2O_2 is known to cause oxidation of sulfhydryl groups which may denature several enzymes, which leads to peroxidation of membrane lipids, thus increasing membrane permeability of the pathogenic microbes (Ammor et al. 2006). Organic acids like acetic and lactic acids may act by lowering pH (Kareem et al. 2014). Direct mechanisms exerted by probiotics include the production of defensins (Figueroa-González et al. 2011) or competitive inhibition of pathogen-binding and receptor sites (Kerry et al. 2018).

5.2.2 Safety Concerns

A growing number of evidence has suggested the probiotic species safe and well-tolerated for use in clinical settings, though the number of studies about safety profiles of these species are not sufficient and it needs further evaluation in preclinical and clinical trials (Agostoni et al. 2004). As concluded by a report published by Agency for Healthcare Research and Quality in 2011, however, no evidence exists regarding the increased risk of toxicity with the existing clinical trials of probiotics, the current literature is not well equipped to answer questions on the safety of probiotics with confidence (Doron and Snydman 2015). Unlike other food or drug ingredients, probiotics or live microorganisms and the possibility for infectivity or in situ toxin production will always exist (Sanders et al. 2010). Four types of adverse effects may be considered with the use of probiotics, including the risk of systemic infections, adjuvant side effects and immunomodulation, deleterious metabolic activities, and risk of gene transfer (Zielińska et al. 2018).

The most common systemic infection reported is fungemia associated with *Saccharomyces cerevisiae* or *S. boulardii* (Cassone et al. 2003). Some cases of bacteremia have also been reported with *Lactobacilli* strains including *L. acidophilus*, *L. casei*, and *Lactobacillus GG* (Russo et al. 2010; Lee et al. 2015; Haghighat and Crum-Cianflone 2016). Events of endocarditis with *Lactobacillus* and *Streptococcus* probiotics, and abscess with *L. rhamnosus* have been reported (Vankerckhoven et al. 2007; Conrads et al. 2018). A double-blind, randomized clinical trial showed a higher mortality rate in patients supplemented with probiotics, which was attributed to bowel ischemia in critically ill patients. The authors postulated that probiotics may increase oxygen demand in gut mucosa in the setting of already reduced blood supply (Besselink et al. 2008). Literature also supported the increased risk of antibiotic resistance, as LAB possess plasmid-containing resistance promoting genes to tetracycline, macrolide, erythromycin, streptomycin, streptogramin, chloramphenicol, and lincosamide (Doron and Snydman 2015). GI side effects include nausea, abdominal cramping, flatulence, taste disturbances, and stool softening. However, patients receiving probiotics for *C. difficile* associated diarrhea are 18–20% less likely to experience GI adverse events than controls (Johnston et al. 2012; Goldenberg et al. 2017).

5.3 Prebiotics

A subclass of dietary fibers, prebiotics can be defined as food supplements selectively enhancing the growth and/or activity of favorable indigenous probiotic bacteria (Zheng et al. 2019). They are basically resistant to gastric juices and enzymes (Patel and Goyal 2012). There is a long list of prebiotics with diverse dietary sources and chemical properties, but the most commonly used are fructans (fructo-oligosaccharides (FOS) and inulin) and galacto-oligosaccharides (GOS) (Roberfroid et al. 2010). Raw oats, soybeans, yacon, nondigestible carbohydrates, and unrefined wheat and barley are the richest dietary sources of prebiotics (Rovinaru and Pasarin 2019). Chemically, fructans contain a linear chain of fructose with β $(2 \rightarrow 1)$ linkage, where the degree of polymerization (DOP) of FOS is less than 10 and that of inulin is about 60 (Gibson et al. 2010).

Fructans were thought to selectively stimulate LAB, but recent literature shows that chain length of fructans is an important determinant to select bacterial species for their fermentation and, thus, they may also directly or indirectly influence other bacterial species (Scott et al. 2014). GOS is the product of lactose extension and is divided into two subgroups: one group contains excess galactose at C_3, C_4, and C_6 positions and the second group also known as trans-galacto-oligosaccharides (TOS), manufactured by enzymatic trans-glycosylation from lactose (Macfarlane et al. 2008; Gibson et al. 2010; Johnson et al. 2013; Whelan 2013). GOS can stimulate LAB (*Lactobacilli* and *bifidobacteria*) up to a greater extent but they may also affect other species of Firmicutes and Bacteroidetes up to a lesser degree (Maathuis et al. 2012). Nonresistant starches have been supported for their high selectivity toward Firmicutes and are known to produce high level of butyrate (Fuentes-Zaragoza et al. 2011; Walker et al. 2011; Davani-Davari et al. 2019). Some noncarbohydrate entities such as flavonoids are also including in prebiotics as numerous in vitro and in vivo studies showed the stimulation of LAB with flavanols (Tzounis et al. 2011).

5.3.1 Health Impact

SCFAs are the byproducts of the degradation of prebiotics by gut microbial species, which gain attention due to their critical role in maintaining health and wellness. SCFAs can reduce luminal pH, increase the absorption of several nutrients, improve the composition of gut flora, inhibit the growth of pathogenic microbes like food-borne pathogens and serve as a source of energy to colonocytes (Feng et al. 2018). SCFAs are small molecules enough to enter blood circulation through gut enterocytes, which make prebiotics being able to exert beneficial effects not only on GI tract but also on extra GI sites (Den Besten et al. 2013).

Prebiotics may improve intestinal functions such as stool bulking, stool regularity, and stool consistency. Supplementation of infants with GOS/inulin softens stools, enhances stool frequency, and acidifies stool pH (Gibson et al. 2010; Roberfroid et al. 2010; Tabbers et al. 2011). On the other hand, inulin possesses no effects on stool weight in adults (Slavin 2013). The differential effect on stool bulking between infants and adults may be because of differences in fermentation intensity. The stool-bulking capability in infants is attributed to an increase in stool water content by osmolarity, as the prebiotics are likely to be incompletely fermented (Moro et al. 2005). Low-dose intake of prebiotics may downregulate mucosal inflammatory cascade and may reverse the pathogenesis of inflammatory bowel syndrome (IBS). However, the majority of studies showed no clinical benefits (Wilson and Whelan 2017; Davani-Davari et al. 2019).

Fructans showed an improvement in the homeostasis of glucose and lipid metabolism. An in vivo study depicted a decrease in levels of TC, LDL, and triglyceride levels (Vulevic et al. 2013). As revealed by clinical trial, an improvement of blood glucose level was seen with prebiotics in healthy adults but not in diabetic patients (Cani et al. 2009; Roberfroid et al. 2010). Prebiotics affect the immune system through direct (increase in the population of beneficial microbes) and indirect (through SCFAs production) mechanisms (Roberfroid et al. 2010; Macfarlane et al. 2008). SCFAs alter immune responses through GPR41 and GPR43, which are expressed on leukocytes, as well as on enterocytes and enteroendocrine cells in the human colon (Roberfroid et al. 2010). One of the most widely studied SCFAs, butyrate alters the expression of chemokines in intestinal epithelial cells, and the production of anti-inflammatory (IL-10) and proinflammatory (IL-2 and IF-γ) cytokines (Macfarlane et al. 2008; Roberfroid et al. 2010). Acetate enhances NF-kB activity and peripheral blood antibody production (Macfarlane et al. 2008).

5.4 Synbiotics

Progress in microbial research leads to the development of synbiotics which are the products formulated by the fusion of probiotics and prebiotics, intended for synergistic activities (Tufarelli and Laudadio 2016). The synbiotics are designed to affect their host in improving the survival and implantation of live species of beneficial microorganisms in the GI tract (Pandey et al. 2015). The word "synbiotics" alludes to synergism, suggesting that the term should be reserved only for products in which prebiotic substances selectively enhance the growth and/or activity of probiotic microbes (Cecic and Chingwaru 2010). Live microbial species used as probiotics are generally sensible to stomach acidity and length of exposure to acid and bile salts. Prebiotics produce specific substrates which support the survival of live microbial species during their passage in the upper intestinal tract in a sufficient number, with little or no stimulation of other microorganisms (Peña 2007). Table 5.2 enlisted synbiotic compositions of probiotics and prebiotics.

Some of the most common benefits to the human population attributed to the intake of synbiotics include an enhanced level of *Lactobacilli* and *Bifidobacteria*, balanced gut microbiota, improved immune-modulation, improved hepatic function in patients with cirrhosis, and reduced incidences of nosocomial infections in surgical patients (Zhang et al. 2010). There is growing scientific evidence that the fusion of probiotics and prebiotics in a single formulation contributes appreciably to health (Kearney and Gibbons 2018). Preclinical and clinical trials revealed that supplementation of synbiotics gives a better therapeutic response, comparatively to probiotics or prebiotics when consumed alone (Ringel-Kulka et al. 2015; Krumbeck et al. 2016; Shinde et al. 2019). The commercial market showed an increased interest in functional foods containing synbiotics, which may be due to the awareness of the benefits of gut microbiota, contributing toward disease prevention and treatment (Kerry et al. 2018).

5.5 Microencapsulation

Probiotics have been incorporated into a range of dairy products because of their health benefits such as yoghurt, cheese, milk powder, ice cream, and frozen dairy desserts. But still, there are issues with the low viability of the probiotic species in dairy products (Menezes et al. 2013). They lose viability during GI transit due to an unfavorable intestinal environment while the minimum most important criterion for preserving consumer acceptance is maintaining the minimum viability and activity of probiotics through the end of shelf-life. Several techniques have been designed to enhance the viability of probiotic bacteria including selection acid and bile resistance strains, stress adaptation, use of oxygen impermeable packaging materials, the inclusion of micronutrients, two-step fermentation, and sonication of bacteria but microencapsulation offers the best

Table 5.2 Common synbiotic compositions of probiotics and prebiotics (Kerry et al. 2018).

Probiotics	Prebiotics
Bifidobacteria, Bacteroides fragilis, Peptostreptococcaceae, Klebsiellae	Fructo-oligosaccharides
Bifidobacterium animalis, Lactobacillus acidophilus, Lactobacillus paracasei	Inulin
Bifidobacteria, Bacteroides fragilis group	Isomalto-oligosaccharides
Bifidobacteria lactis, Lactobacillus bulgaricus, Lactobacillus acidophilus, Lactobacillus rhamnosus	Lactulose
Zymomonas mobilis	Lactosucrose
Bifidobacterium adolescentis, Lactobacillus plantarum	Xylo-oligosaccharides
Bifidobacterium longum, Bifidobacterium catenulatum	Galacto-oligosaccharides
Bifidobacterium bifidum, Bifidobacterium lactis	Fructo-oligosaccharides
Bifidobacterium spp.	Arabinoxylan and Arabinoxylan oligosaccharides
Bacteroides, Eubacterium rectal	Resistant starch-1,2,3,4

solution that can increase the viability of probiotic bacteria during processing and in the GI environment (Sarkar 2010). It is a technique used for packaging particles of finely grounded solids, droplets of liquids or gaseous materials in small capsules with the help of protective membranes, releasing their contents at controlled rates over a prolonged period of time under the influence of specific conditions (Anal and Singh 2007).

Different techniques have been employed for encapsulating probiotic microbes including (i) spray drying using water-soluble polymers for coating, (ii) spray congealing using waxes, fatty acids, water-soluble and water-insoluble polymers, and monomers, (iii) fluidized bed coating using water-soluble and water-insoluble polymers, lipids, and waxes, (iv) extrusion using water-soluble and insoluble polymers, (v) coacervation/phase separation technique using water-soluble polymers, and (vi) electrostatic method using oppositely charged polymers or compounds (Anal and Singh 2007). Alginate is a natural polymer extracted from algae containing β-D-mannuronic and α-L-guluronic acids and can be applied as a successful pH-sensitive material for the microencapsulation of probiotics (Allan-Wojtas et al. 2008; Burgain et al. 2013). Alginate microencapsulation was established for the protection of the viability of probiotic strains in the GI tract (Hansen et al. 2002). Ca-alginate has been generally used for the encapsulation of LAB in the concentration of 0.5–4%. Alginate polymers easily form gel matrices around bacterial cells, are biocompatible, cheap, and easily prepared (Mortazavian et al. 2007). *L. lactis* microencapsulated in alginate showed improved resistance to environmental stresses (Yeung et al. 2016) while *Bifidobacterium* BB-12 microencapsulated with alginate showed improved viability in storage and simulated GI conditions with controlled release of probiotics (Holkem et al. 2016; Holkem et al. 2017). Some disadvantages associated with the use of these types of polymers include their susceptibility to the acidic environment, loss of integrity when subjected to chelating agents or monovalent ions such as phosphates, citrates, or lactates (Mortazavian et al. 2007).

Chitosan is a cationic polymer that can form gels with sodium alginate by ionic cross-linking (Lucinda-Silva et al. 2010). The coating of alginate microcapsules with chitosan can increase the stability of alginate beads and, thus, can enhance the survival rate of encapsulated probiotics (Krasaekoopt et al. 2003). Alginate complex with chitosan may decrease the porosity of alginate beads, decreases the leak of encapsulated probiotics, and shows stability at low pH (Chávarri et al. 2010). Kanmani and colleagues reported that *Enterococcus faecium* MC13 cells encapsulated into the alginate-chitosan complex were not released for 144 hours in simulated gastric fluid (Kanmani et al. 2011). Another study demonstrated the increased survival rate of *L. gasseri* and *B. bifidum* (10^7 CFU/ml) in simulated gastric conditions after two hours when compared to free cells (10 CFU/ml) (Chávarri et al. 2010).

Plant-based materials can also be used for the encapsulation of probiotics, which may play a role in food applications (Shori 2017). As reported, pea protein-alginate microspheres with FOS improved the viability of *B. adolescentis* (10^8 CFU/ml) as compared to free cells (10 CFU/ml) after two hours in simulated gastric fluid (Klemmer et al. 2011). Milk proteins, especially whey proteins, have good chelation properties and pH-responsive gel-swelling behavior and can be used to encapsulate LAB, as an encapsulation of *Lactobacillus bulgaricus* in skim milk-alginatemicrospheres gave yield about 100% (Livney 2010; Pan et al. 2013). *B. lactis* and *L. paracasei* encapsulated in milk proteins showed increased survival rate at pH 2.5 in comparison to free cells (Heidebach et al. 2009). However, *L. paracasei* was found more pH-sensitive than *B. lactis*, suggesting that the survival rate of probiotics in low pH is strain-dependent and that microencapsulation cannot fully recover the pH-responsive mechanisms of each strain to tolerate low pH (Muthukumarasamy et al. 2006; Heidebach et al. 2009).

5.6 Conclusion

Probiotics, prebiotics, and synbiotics are designated as health-promoting agents owing to their potential of preventing local and systemic diseases. Probiotics are essential to balance gut dysbiosis and thus can regulate immune pathways, enhance intestinal integrity, and prevent the gut barrier disruption. Prebiotics utilization by probiotics is a prerequisite for symbiotic selection that could maximize their beneficial effects. As probiotic microbes are sensitive to the GI environment such as stomach acidity and the length of exposure to acid and bile salts, which may affect the viability of live microorganisms. Microencapsulation is a technique that is most widely accepted to protect the viability of probiotics from the beginning of production to the end of shelf-life, and, thus, it could preserve consumer acceptance. By knowing the underlying mechanisms and safety aspects of probiotic species and prebiotics, scientists would be able to design functional foods that could improve host health.

Conflicts of Interest: The authors declare no conflict of interest.

References

Köhler, C.A., Maes, M., Slyepchenko, A. et al. (2016). The gut-brain axis, including the microbiome, leaky gut and bacterial translocation: mechanisms and pathophysiological role in Alzheimer's disease. *Current Pharmaceutical Design* 22: 6152–6166.

Agostoni, C., Axelsson, I., Braegger, C. et al. (2004). Probiotic bacteria in dietetic products for infants: a commentary by the ESPGHAN Committee on Nutrition. *Journal of Pediatric Gastroenterology and Nutrition* 38: 365–374.

Akbari, E., Asemi, Z., Daneshvar Kakhaki, R. et al. (2016). Effect of probiotic supplementation on cognitive function and metabolic status in Alzheimer's disease: a randomized, double-blind and controlled trial. *Frontiers in Aging Neuroscience* 8: 256.

Allan-Wojtas, P., Hansen, L.T., and Paulson, A.T. (2008). Microstructural studies of probiotic bacteria-loaded alginate microcapsules using standard electron microscopy techniques and anhydrous fixation. *LWT- Food Science and Technology* 41: 101–108.

Almeida, C.C., Lorena, S.L.S., Pavan, C.R. et al. (2012). Beneficial effects of long-term consumption of a probiotic combination of Lactobacillus casei Shirota and Bifidobacterium breve Yakult may persist after suspension of therapy in lactose-intolerant patients. *Nutrition in Clinical Practice* 27: 247–251.

Ammor, S., Tauveron, G., Dufour, E., and Chevallier, I. (2006). Antibacterial activity of lactic acid bacteria against spoilage and pathogenic bacteria isolated from the same meat small-scale facility: 1 – screening and characterization of the antibacterial compounds. *Food Control* 17: 454–461.

Anal, A.K. and Singh, H. (2007). Recent advances in microencapsulation of probiotics for industrial applications and targeted delivery. *Trends in Food Science & Technology* 18: 240–251.

Andreasen, A.S., Larsen, N., Pedersen-Skovsgaard, T. et al. (2010). Effects of Lactobacillus acidophilus NCFM on insulin sensitivity and the systemic inflammatory response in human subjects. *British Journal of Nutrition* 104: 1831–1838.

Asemi, Z., Zare, Z., Shakeri, H. et al. (2013). Effect of multispecies probiotic supplements on metabolic profiles, hs-CRP, and oxidative stress in patients with type 2 diabetes. *Annals of Nutrition and Metabolism* 63: 1–9.

Aureli, P., Capurso, L., Castellazzi, A.M. et al. (2011). Probiotics and health: an evidence-based review. *Pharmacological Research* 63: 366–376.

Bagarolli, R.A., Tobar, N., Oliveira, A.G. et al. (2017). Probiotics modulate gut microbiota and improve insulin sensitivity in DIO mice. *The Journal of Nutritional Biochemistry* 50: 16–25.

Bao, Y., Wang, Z., Zhang, Y. et al. (2012). Effect of Lactobacillus plantarum P-8 on lipid metabolism in hyperlipidemic rat model. *European Journal of Lipid Science and Technology* 114: 1230–1236.

Barbosa, R.S. and Vieira-Coelho, M.A. (2020). Probiotics and prebiotics: focus on psychiatric disorders–a systematic review. *Nutrition Reviews* 78: 437–450.

Besselink, M.G., Van Santvoort, H.C., Buskens, E. et al. (2008). Probiotic prophylaxis in predicted severe acute pancreatitis: a randomised, double-blind, placebo-controlled trial. *The Lancet* 371: 651–659.

Britton, R.A. and Versalovic, J. (2008). Probiotics and gastrointestinal infections. *Interdisciplinary Perspectives on Infectious Diseases* 2008: 1–10.

Bron, P.A., Kleerebezem, M., Brummer, R.-J. et al. (2017). Can probiotics modulate human disease by impacting intestinal barrier function? *British Journal of Nutrition* 117: 93–107.

Burgain, J., Gaiani, C., Francius, G. et al. (2013). in vitro interactions between probiotic bacteria and milk proteins probed by atomic force microscopy. *Colloids and Surfaces B: Biointerfaces* 104: 153–162.

Cani, P.D., Bibiloni, R., Knauf, C. et al. (2008). Changes in gut microbiota control metabolic endotoxemia-induced inflammation in high-fat diet–induced obesity and diabetes in mice. *Diabetes* 57: 1470–1481.

Cani, P.D. and Delzenne, N.M. (2009). Interplay between obesity and associated metabolic disorders: new insights into the gut microbiota. *Current Opinion in Pharmacology* 9: 737–743.

Cani, P.D., Possemiers, S., Van De Wiele, T. et al. (2009). Changes in gut microbiota control inflammation in obese mice through a mechanism involving GLP-2-driven improvement of gut permeability. *Gut* 58: 1091–1103.

Cassani, E., Privitera, G., Pezzoli, G. et al. (2011). Use of probiotics for the treatment of constipation in Parkinson's disease patients. *Minerva Gastroenterologica e Dietologica* 57: 117–121.

Cassone, M., Serra, P., Mondello, F. et al. (2003). Outbreak of Saccharomyces cerevisiae subtype boulardii fungemia in patients neighboring those treated with a probiotic preparation of the organism. *Journal of Clinical Microbiology* 41: 5340–5343.

Catanzaro, R., Anzalone, M., Calabrese, F. et al. (2014). The gut microbiota and its correlations with the central nervous system disorders. *Panminerva Medica* 57: 127–143.

Cecic, A. and Chingwaru, W. (2010). The role of functional foods. *Nutraceuticals, and food supplements in intestinal health. Nutrients* 2: 611–625.

Champagne, C.P., Tompkins, T.A., Buckley, N.D., and Green-Johnson, J.M. (2010). Effect of fermentation by pure and mixed cultures of Streptococcus thermophilus and Lactobacillus helveticus on isoflavone and B-vitamin content of a fermented soy beverage. *Food Microbiology* 27: 968–972.

Chávarri, M., Marañón, I., Ares, R. et al. (2010). Microencapsulation of a probiotic and prebiotic in alginate-chitosan capsules improves survival in simulated gastro-intestinal conditions. *International Journal of Food Microbiology* 142: 185–189.

Chugh, B. and Kamal-Eldin, A. (2020). Bioactive compounds produced by probiotics in food products. *Current Opinion in Food Science* 32: 76–82.

Conrads, G., Bockwoldt, J.A., Kniebs, C., and Abdelbary, M.M. (2018). Commentary: health-associated niche inhabitants as oral probiotics: the case of Streptococcus dentisani. *Frontiers in Microbiology* 9: 340.

Corrêa-Oliveira, R., Fachi, J.L., Vieira, A. et al. (2016). Regulation of immune cell function by short-chain fatty acids. *Clinical & Translational Immunology* 5: e73.

Crittenden, R., Martinez, N., and Playne, M. (2003). Synthesis and utilisation of folate by yoghurt starter cultures and probiotic bacteria. *International Journal of Food Microbiology* 80: 217–222.

Dahiya, D.K., Puniya, M., Shandilya, U.K. et al. (2017). Gut microbiota modulation and its relationship with obesity using prebiotic fibers and probiotics: a review. *Frontiers in Microbiology* 8: 563.

Davani-Davari, D., Negahdaripour, M., Karimzadeh, I. et al. (2019). Prebiotics: definition, types, sources, mechanisms, and clinical applications. *Food* 8: 92.

De Filippis, A., Ullah, H., Baldi, A. et al. (2020). Gastrointestinal disorders and metabolic syndrome: Dysbiosis as a key link and common bioactive dietary components useful for their treatment. *International Journal of Molecular Sciences* 21: 4929.

Delcenserie, V., Martel, D., Lamoureux, M. et al. (2008). Immunomodulatory effects of probiotics in the intestinal tract. *Current Issues in Molecular Biology* 10: 37.

Delgado, S., Sánchez, B., Margolles, A. et al. (2020). Molecules produced by probiotics and intestinal microorganisms with immunomodulatory activity. *Nutrients* 12: 391.

Delzenne, N.M., Neyrinck, A.M., Bäckhed, F., and Cani, P.D. (2011). Targeting gut microbiota in obesity: effects of prebiotics and probiotics. *Nature Reviews Endocrinology* 7: 639.

Den Besten, G., Van Eunen, K., Groen, A.K. et al. (2013). The role of short-chain fatty acids in the interplay between diet, gut microbiota, and host energy metabolism. *Journal of Lipid Research* 54: 2325–2340.

Dinan, T.G. and Cryan, J.F. (2017). Gut instincts: microbiota as a key regulator of brain development, ageing and neurodegeneration. *The Journal of Physiology* 595: 489–503.

Doron, S. and Snydman, D.R. (2015). Risk and safety of probiotics. *Clinical Infectious Diseases* 60: S129–S134.

Drakes, M., Blanchard, T., and Czinn, S. (2004). Bacterial probiotic modulation of dendritic cells. *Infection and Immunity* 72: 3299–3309.

El-Khadragy, M.F., Al-Olayan, E.M., Elmallah, M.I. et al. (2019). Probiotics and yogurt modulate oxidative stress and fibrosis in livers of Schistosoma mansoni-infected mice. *BMC Complementary and Alternative Medicine* 19: 3.

Everard, A., Lazarevic, V., Derrien, M. et al. (2011). Responses of gut microbiota and glucose and lipid metabolism to prebiotics in genetic obese and diet-induced leptin-resistant mice. *Diabetes* 60: 2775–2786.

Fardet, A. and Rock, E. (2018). in vitro and in vivo antioxidant potential of milks, yoghurts, fermented milks and cheeses: a narrative review of evidence. *Nutrition Research Reviews* 31: 52–70.

Feng, W., Ao, H., and Peng, C. (2018). Gut microbiota, short-chain fatty acids, and herbal medicines. *Frontiers in Pharmacology* 9: 1354.

Figueroa-González, I., Cruz-Guerrero, A., and Quijano, G. (2011). The benefits of probiotics on human health. *Journal of Microbial and Biochemical Technology* 1: 1948–5948.

Fuentes-Zaragoza, E., Sánchez-Zapata, E., Sendra, E. et al. (2011). Resistant starch as prebiotic: a review. *Starch-Stärke* 63: 406–415.

Genedi, M., Janmaat, I.E., Haarman, B.B.C., and Sommer, I.E. (2019). Dysregulation of the gut–brain axis in schizophrenia and bipolar disorder: probiotic supplementation as a supportive treatment in psychiatric disorders. *Current Opinion in Psychiatry* 32: 185–195.

Gholamhosseinpour, A. and Hashemi, S.M.B. (2019). Ultrasound pretreatment of fermented milk containing probiotic Lactobacillus plantarum AF1: Carbohydrate metabolism and antioxidant activity. *Journal of Food Process Engineering* 42: e12930.

Gibson, G.R., Scott, K.P., Rastall, R.A. et al. (2010). Dietary prebiotics: current status and new definition. *Food Science and Technology Bulletin Functional Foods* 7: 1–19.

Goldenberg, J.Z., Yap, C., Lytvyn, L. et al. (2017). Probiotics for the prevention of Clostridium difficile-associated diarrhea in adults and children. *Cochrane Database of Systematic Reviews* 12: CD006095.

Haghighat, L. and Crum-Cianflone, N.F. (2016). The potential risks of probiotics among HIV-infected persons: Bacteraemia due to Lactobacillus acidophilus and review of the literature. *International Journal of STD & AIDS* 27: 1223–1230.

Hansen, L.T., Allan-Wojtas, P.M., Jin, Y.L., and Paulson, A.T. (2002). Survival of Ca-alginate microencapsulated Bifidobacterium spp. in milk and simulated gastrointestinal conditions. *Food Microbiology* 19: 35–45.

Hart, A., Lammers, K., Brigidi, P. et al. (2004). Modulation of human dendritic cell phenotype and function by probiotic bacteria. *Gut* 53: 1602–1609.

Heidebach, T., Först, P., and Kulozik, U. (2009). Microencapsulation of probiotic cells by means of rennet-gelation of milk proteins. *Food Hydrocolloids* 23: 1670–1677.

Heiss, C.N. and Olofsson, L.E. (2019). The role of the gut microbiota in development, function and disorders of the central nervous system and the enteric nervous system. *Journal of Neuroendocrinology* 31: e12684.

Ho, J.T., Chan, G.C., and Li, J.C. (2015). Systemic effects of gut microbiota and its relationship with disease and modulation. *BMC Immunology* 16: 1–6.

Holkem, A.T., Raddatz, G.C., Barin, J.S. et al. (2017). Production of microcapsules containing Bifidobacterium BB-12 by emulsification/internal gelation. *LWT- Food Science and Technology* 76: 216–221.

Holkem, A.T., Raddatz, G.C., Nunes, G.L. et al. (2016). Development and characterization of alginate microcapsules containing Bifidobacterium BB-12 produced by emulsification/internal gelation followed by freeze drying. *LWT- Food Science and Technology* 71: 302–308.

Hou, J.-W., Yu, R.-C., and Chou, C.-C. (2000). Changes in some components of soymilk during fermentation with bifidobacteria. *Food Research International* 33: 393–397.

Hsieh, T.H., Kuo, C.W., Hsieh, K.H. et al. (2020). Probiotics alleviate the progressive deterioration of motor functions in a mouse model of Parkinson's disease. *Brain Sciences* 10: 206.

Hugenholtz, J. and Smid, E.J. (2002). Nutraceutical production with food-grade microorganisms. *Current Opinion in Biotechnology* 13: 497–507.

Hugenholtz, J., Sybesma, W., Groot, M. N., Wisselink, W., Ladero, V., Burgess, K., VAN Sinderen, D., Piard, J.-C., Eggink, G. & Smid, E. J. 2002. Metabolic Engineering of Lactic Acid Bacteria for the Production of Nutraceuticals. *Lactic Acid Bacteria: Genetics, Metabolism and Applications*. Springer.

Jandhyala, S.M., Talukdar, R., Subramanyam, C. et al. (2015). Role of the normal gut microbiota. *World Journal of Gastroenterology* 21: 8787.

Jesus, A.L.T., Fernandes, M.S., Kamimura, B.A. et al. (2016). Growth potential of Listeria monocytogenes in probiotic cottage cheese formulations with reduced sodium content. *Food Research International* 81: 180–187.

Jin, M., Qian, Z., Yin, J. et al. (2019). The role of intestinal microbiota in cardiovascular disease. *Journal of Cellular and Molecular Medicine* 23: 2343–2350.

Johnson, C.R., Combs, J.R.,.G.F., and Thavarajah, P. (2013). Lentil (Lens culinaris L.): a prebiotic-rich whole food legume. *Food Research International* 51: 107–113.

Johnston, B.C., Ma, S.S., Goldenberg, J.Z. et al. (2012). Probiotics for the prevention of Clostridium difficile–associated diarrhea: a systematic review and meta-analysis. *Annals of Internal Medicine* 157: 878–888.

Jonkers, D., Penders, J., Masclee, A., and Pierik, M. (2012). Probiotics in the management of inflammatory bowel disease. *Drugs* 72: 803–823.

Juarez Del Valle, M., Laiño, J.E., Savoy, G., and Leblanc, J.G.J. (2014). Riboflavin producing lactic acid bacteria as a biotechnological strategy to obtain bio-enriched soymilk. *Food Research International* 62: 1015–1019.

Jyothi, H.J., Vidyadhara, D.J., Mahadevan, A. et al. (2015). Aging causes morphological alterations in astrocytes and microglia in human substantia nigra pars compacta. *Neurobiology of Aging* 36: 3321–3333.

Kang, H.-J. and Im, S.-H. (2015). Probiotics as an immune modulator. *Journal of Nutritional Science and Vitaminology* 61: S103–S105.

Kanmani, P., Kumar, R.S., Yuvaraj, N. et al. (2011). Effect of cryopreservation and microencapsulation of lactic acid bacterium Enterococcus faecium MC13 for long-term storage. *Biochemical Engineering Journal* 58: 140–147.

Kareem, K.Y., Ling, F.H., Chwen, L.T. et al. (2014). Inhibitory activity of postbiotic produced by strains of Lactobacillus plantarum using reconstituted media supplemented with inulin. *Gut Pathogens* 6: 23.

Kearney, S.M. and Gibbons, S.M. (2018). Designing synbiotics for improved human health. *Microbial Biotechnology* 11: 141–144.

Kehagias, C., Csapó, J., Konteles, S. et al. (2008). Support of growth and formation of d-amino acids by Bifidobacterium longum in cows', ewes', goats' milk and modified whey powder products. *International Dairy Journal* 18: 396–402.

Kelesidis, T. and Pothoulakis, C. (2012). Efficacy and safety of the probiotic Saccharomyces boulardii for the prevention and therapy of gastrointestinal disorders. *Therapeutic Advances in Gastroenterology* 5: 111–125.

Kerry, R.G., Patra, J.K., Gouda, S. et al. (2018). Benefaction of probiotics for human health: a review. *Journal of Food and Drug Analysis* 26: 927–939.

Kim, J.-M. and Park, Y.J. (2017). Probiotics in the prevention and treatment of postmenopausal vaginal infections. *Journal of Menopausal Medicine* 23: 139–145.

Klemmer, K.J., Korber, D.R., Low, N.H., and Nickerson, M.T. (2011). Pea protein-based capsules for probiotic and prebiotic delivery. *International Journal of Food Science & Technology* 46: 2248–2256.

Krasaekoopt, W., Bhandari, B., and Deeth, H. (2003). Evaluation of encapsulation techniques of probiotics for yoghurt. *International Dairy Journal* 13: 3–13.

Krumbeck, J.A., Maldonado-Gomez, M.X., Ramer-Tait, A.E., and Hutkins, R.W. (2016). Prebiotics and synbiotics: dietary strategies for improving gut health. *Current Opinion in Gastroenterology* 32: 110–119.

Leblanc, J.G., Milani, C., De Giori, G.S. et al. (2013). Bacteria as vitamin suppliers to their host: a gut microbiota perspective. *Current Opinion in Biotechnology* 24: 160–168.

Lederberg, J. and Mccray, A.T. (2001). Ome SweetOmics – a genealogical treasury of words. *The scientist* 15: 8.

Lee, E.-S., Song, E.-J., Nam, Y.-D., and Lee, S.-Y. (2018). Probiotics in human health and disease: from nutribiotics to pharmabiotics. *Journal of Microbiology* 56: 773–782.

Lee, M.-R., Tsai, C.-J., Liang, S.-K. et al. (2015). Clinical characteristics of bacteraemia caused by Lactobacillus spp. and antimicrobial susceptibilities of the isolates at a medical centre in Taiwan, 2000–2014. *International Journal of Antimicrobial Agents* 46: 439–445.

Lewis, S. and Burmeister, S. (2005). A double-blind placebo-controlled study of the effects of Lactobacillus acidophilus on plasma lipids. *European Journal of Clinical Nutrition* 59: 776–780.

Lilly, D.M. and Stillwell, R.H. (1965). Probiotics: growth-promoting factors produced by microorganisms. *Science* 147: 747–748.

Lim, S.-M. (2013). Microbiological, physicochemical, and antioxidant properties of plain yogurt and soy yogurt. *Korean Journal of Microbiology* 49: 403–414.

Livney, Y.D. (2010). Milk proteins as vehicles for bioactives. *Current Opinion in Colloid & Interface Science* 15: 73–83.

Logan, A.C. and Katzman, M. (2005). Major depressive disorder: probiotics may be an adjuvant therapy. *Medical Hypotheses* 64: 533–538.

Lucinda-Silva, R.M., Salgado, H.R.N., and Evangelista, R.C. (2010). Alginate-chitosan systems: in vitro controlled release of triamcinolone and in vivo gastrointestinal transit. *Carbohydrate Polymers* 81: 260–268.

Maathuis, A.J., Van Den Heuvel, E.G., Schoterman, M.H., and Venema, K. (2012). Galacto-oligosaccharides have prebiotic activity in a dynamic in vitro colon model using a 13C-labeling technique. *The Journal of Nutrition* 142: 1205–1212.

Macfarlane, G., Steed, H., and Macfarlane, S. (2008). Bacterial metabolism and health-related effects of galacto-oligosaccharides and other prebiotics. *Journal of Applied Microbiology* 104: 305–344.

Mack, D.R. (2005). Probiotics: mixed messages. *Canadian Family Physician* 51: 1455.

Mahboobi, S., Iraj, B., Maghsoudi, Z. et al. (2014). The effects of probiotic supplementation on markers of blood lipids, and blood pressure in patients with prediabetes: a randomized clinical trial. *International Journal of Preventive Medicine* 5: 1239.

Martarelli, D., Verdenelli, M.C., Scuri, S. et al. (2011). Effect of a probiotic intake on oxidant and antioxidant parameters in plasma of athletes during intense exercise training. *Current Microbiology* 62: 1689–1696.

Mcfarland, L.V. (2006). Meta-analysis of probiotics for the prevention of antibiotic associated diarrhea and the treatment of Clostridium difficile disease. *American Journal of Gastroenterology* 101: 812–822.

Melini, F., Melini, V., Luziatelli, F. et al. (2019). Health-promoting components in fermented foods: an up-to-date systematic review. *Nutrients* 11: 1189.

Menconi, A., Bielke, L.R., Hargis, B.M., and Tellez, G. (2014). Immuno-modulation and anti-inflammatory effects of antibiotic growth promoters versus probiotics in the intestinal tract. *Journal of Microbiology Research and Reviews* 2: 62–67.

Menezes, C.R.D., Barin, J.S., Chicoski, A.J. et al. (2013). Microencapsulation of probiotics: progress and prospects. *Ciência Rural* 43: 1309–1316.

Mishra, V., Shah, C., Mokashe, N. et al. (2015). Probiotics as potential antioxidants: a systematic review. *Journal of Agricultural and Food Chemistry* 63: 3615–3626.

Moro, G.E., Stahl, B., Fanaro, S. et al. (2005). Dietary prebiotic oligosaccharides are detectable in the faeces of formula-fed infants. *Acta Paediatrica* 94: 27–30.

Mortazavian, A., Razavi, S.H., Ehsani, M.R., and Sohrabvandi, S. (2007). Principles and methods of microencapsulation of probiotic microorganisms. *Iranian Journal of Biotechnology* 5: 1–18.

Muthukumarasamy, P., Allan-Wojtas, P., and Holley, R.A. (2006). Stability of Lactobacillus reuteri in different types of microcapsules. *Journal of Food Science* 71: M20–M24.

Nowak, A., Paliwoda, A., and Błasiak, J. (2019). Anti-proliferative, pro-apoptotic and anti-oxidative activity of Lactobacillus and Bifidobacterium strains: a review of mechanisms and therapeutic perspectives. *Critical Reviews in Food Science and Nutrition* 59: 3456–3467.

O'hara, A.M. and Shanahan, F. (2006). The gut flora as a forgotten organ. *EMBO Reports* 7: 688–693.

O'sullivan, E., Barrett, E., Grenham, S. et al. (2011). BDNF expression in the hippocampus of maternally separated rats: does Bifidobacterium breve 6330 alter BDNF levels? *Beneficial Microbes* 2: 199–207.

Okada, Y., Tsuzuki, Y., Hokari, R. et al. (2009). Anti-inflammatory effects of the genus Bifidobacterium on macrophages by modification of phospho-IκB and SOCS gene expression. *International Journal of Experimental Pathology* 90: 131–140.

Pagnini, C., Saeed, R., Bamias, G. et al. (2010). Probiotics promote gut health through stimulation of epithelial innate immunity. *Proceedings of the National Academy of Sciences* 107: 454–459.

Pan, L.X., Fang, X.J., Yu, Z. et al. (2013). Encapsulation in alginate–skim milk microspheres improves viability of Lactobacillus bulgaricus in stimulated gastrointestinal conditions. *International Journal of Food Sciences and Nutrition* 64: 380–384.

Pandey, K.R., Naik, S.R., and Vakil, B.V. (2015). Probiotics, prebiotics and synbiotics-a review. *Journal of Food Science and Technology* 52: 7577–7587.

Parker, R. (1974). Probiotics, the other half of the antibiotic story. *Animal Nutrition and Health* 29: 4–8.

Parnell, J.A. and Reimer, R.A. (2012). Prebiotic fibres dose-dependently increase satiety hormones and alter Bacteroidetes and Firmicutes in lean and obese JCR: LA-cp rats. *British Journal of Nutrition* 107: 601–613.

Pärtty, A., Kalliomäki, M., Wacklin, P. et al. (2015). A possible link between early probiotic intervention and the risk of neuropsychiatric disorders later in childhood: a randomized trial. *Pediatric Research* 77: 823–828.

Patel, S. and Goyal, A. (2012). The current trends and future perspectives of prebiotics research: a review. *3 Biotech* 2: 115–125.

Peña, A. (2007). Intestinal flora, probiotics, prebiotics, synbiotics and novel foods. *Revista Española de Enfermedades Digestivas* 99: 653.

Pompei, A., Cordisco, L., Amaretti, A. et al. (2007). Administration of folate-producing bifidobacteria enhances folate status in Wistar rats. *The Journal of Nutrition* 137: 2742–2746.

Ringel-Kulka, T., Kotch, J.B., Jensen, E.T. et al. (2015). Randomized, double-blind, placebo-controlled study of synbiotic yogurt effect on the health of children. *The Journal of Pediatrics* 166: 1475–1481.

Rinninella, E., Raoul, P., Cintoni, M. et al. (2019). What is the healthy gut microbiota composition? A changing ecosystem across age, environment, diet, and diseases. *Microorganisms* 7: 14.

Roberfroid, M., Gibson, G.R., Hoyles, L. et al. (2010). Prebiotic effects: metabolic and health benefits. *British Journal of Nutrition* 104: S1–S63.

Rovinaru, C. and Pasarin, D. (2019). Application of microencapsulated synbiotics in fruit-based beverages. *Probiotics and Antimicrobial Proteins* 12: 1–10.

Russo, A., Angeletti, S., Lorino, G. et al. (2010). A case of Lactobacillus casei bacteraemia associated with aortic dissection: is there a link? *The New Microbiologica* 33: 175.

Sanders, M.E., Akkermans, L.M., Haller, D. et al. (2010). Safety assessment of probiotics for human use. *Gut Microbes* 1: 164–185.

Sarkar, S. (2010). Approaches for enhancing the viability of probiotics: a review. *British Food Journal* 112: 329–349.

Schulthess, J., Pandey, S., Capitani, M. et al. (2019). The short chain fatty acid butyrate imprints an antimicrobial program in macrophages. *Immunity* 50: 432–445.

Scott, K.P., Martin, J.C., Duncan, S.H., and Flint, H.J. (2014). Prebiotic stimulation of human colonic butyrate-producing bacteria and bifidobacteria, in vitro. *FEMS Microbiology Ecology* 87: 30–40.

Sekirov, I., Russell, S.L., Antunes, L.C.M., and Finlay, B.B. (2010). Gut microbiota in health and disease. *Physiological Reviews* 90: 859–904.

Shaaban, S.Y., El Gendy, Y.G., Mehanna, N.S. et al. (2018). The role of probiotics in children with autism spectrum disorder: a prospective, open-label study. *Nutritional Neuroscience* 21: 676–681.

Sheil, B., Shanahan, F., and O'mahony, L. (2007). Probiotic effects on inflammatory bowel disease. *The Journal of Nutrition* 137: 819S–824S.

Shinde, T., Hansbro, P.M., Sohal, S.S. et al. (2020). Microbiota modulating nutritional approaches to countering the effects of viral respiratory infections including SARS-CoV-2 through promoting metabolic and immune fitness with probiotics and plant bioactives. *Microorganisms* 8: 921.

Shinde, T., Perera, A.P., Vemuri, R. et al. (2019). Synbiotic supplementation containing whole plant sugar cane fibre and probiotic spores potentiates protective synergistic effects in mouse model of IBD. *Nutrients* 11: 818.

Shori, A.B. (2017). Microencapsulation improved probiotics survival during gastric transit. *HAYATI Journal of Biosciences* 24: 1–5.

Sikalidis, A.K. and Maykish, A. (2020). The gut microbiome and type 2 diabetes mellitus: discussing a complex relationship. *Biomedicine* 8: 8.

Simova, E., Beshkova, D., and Dimitrov, Z.P. (2009). Characterization and antimicrobial spectrum of bacteriocins produced by lactic acid bacteria isolated from traditional Bulgarian dairy products. *Journal of Applied Microbiology* 106: 692–701.

Slavin, J. (2013). Fiber and prebiotics: mechanisms and health benefits. *Nutrients* 5: 1417–1435.

Soccol, C.R., Vandenberghe, L.P.D.S., Spier, M.R. et al. (2010). The potential of probiotics: a review. *Food Technology and Biotechnology* 48: 413–434.

Sommer, F. and Bäckhed, F. (2013). The gut microbiota – masters of host development and physiology. *Nature Reviews Microbiology* 11: 227–238.

Sreeja, V. and Prajapati, J.B. (2013). Probiotic formulations: application and status as pharmaceuticals – a review. *Probiotics and Antimicrobial Proteins* 5: 81–91.

Srinarong, C., Siramolpiwat, S., Wongcha-Um, A. et al. (2014). Improved eradication rate of standard triple therapy by adding bismuth and probiotic supplement for Helicobacter pylori treatment in Thailand. *Asian Pacific Journal of Cancer Prevention* 15: 9909–9913.

Steidler, L., Hans, W., Schotte, L. et al. (2000). Treatment of murine colitis by Lactococcus lactis secreting interleukin-10. *Science* 289: 1352–1355.

Surwase, S.N. and Jadhav, J.P. (2011). Bioconversion of L-tyrosine to L-DOPA by a novel bacterium Bacillus sp. JPJ. *Amino Acids* 41: 495–506.

Suvarna, V. and Boby, V. (2005). Probiotics in human health: a current assessment. *Current Science* 88: 1744–1748.

Tabbers, M.M., Boluyt, N., Berger, M.Y., and Benninga, M.A. (2011). Nonpharmacologic treatments for childhood constipation: systematic review. *Pediatrics* 128: 753–761.

Tejero-Sariñena, S., Barlow, J., Costabile, A. et al. (2013). Antipathogenic activity of probiotics against Salmonella Typhimurium and Clostridium difficile in anaerobic batch culture systems: is it due to synergies in probiotic mixtures or the specificity of single strains? *Anaerobe* 24: 60–65.

Thursby, E. and Juge, N. (2017). Introduction to the human gut microbiota. *Biochemical Journal* 474: 1823–1836.

Tufarelli, V. and Laudadio, V. (2016). An overview on the functional food concept: prospectives and applied researches in probiotics, prebiotics and synbiotics. *Journal of Experimental Biology and Agricultural Sciences* 4: 273–278.

Tzounis, X., Rodriguez-Mateos, A., Vulevic, J. et al. (2011). Prebiotic evaluation of cocoa-derived flavanols in healthy humans by using a randomized, controlled, double-blind, crossover intervention study. *The American Journal of Clinical Nutrition* 93: 62–72.

Vallianou, N., Stratigou, T., Christodoulatos, G.S., and Dalamaga, M. (2019). Understanding the role of the gut microbiome and microbial metabolites in obesity and obesity-associated metabolic disorders: current evidence and perspectives. *Current Obesity Reports* 8: 317–332.

Vankerckhoven, V., Moreillon, P., Piu, S. et al. (2007). Infectivity of Lactobacillus rhamnosus and Lactobacillus paracasei isolates in a rat model of experimental endocarditis. *Journal of Medical Microbiology* 56: 1017–1024.

Vickers, N.J. (2017). Animal communication: when i'm calling you, will you answer too? *Current Biology* 27: R713–R715.

Vonk, R.J., Reckman, G.A., Harmsen, H.J., and Priebe, M.G. (2012). Probiotics and lactose intolerance. *INTECH* 7: 149–160.

Vulevic, J., Juric, A., Tzortzis, G., and Gibson, G.R. (2013). A mixture of trans-galactooligosaccharides reduces markers of metabolic syndrome and modulates the fecal microbiota and immune function of overweight adults. *The Journal of Nutrition* 143: 324–331.

Walker, A.W., Ince, J., Duncan, S.H. et al. (2011). Dominant and diet-responsive groups of bacteria within the human colonic microbiota. *The ISME Journal* 5: 220–230.

Wang, Y., Wu, Y., Wang, Y. et al. (2017). Antioxidant properties of probiotic bacteria. *Nutrients* 9: 521.

Weidenmaier, C. and Peschel, A. (2008). Teichoic acids and related cell-wall glycopolymers in Gram-positive physiology and host interactions. *Nature Reviews Microbiology* 6: 276–287.

Westfall, S., Lomis, N., Kahouli, I. et al. (2017). Microbiome, probiotics and neurodegenerative diseases: deciphering the gut brain axis. *Cellular and Molecular Life Sciences* 74: 3769–3787.

Whelan, K. (2013). Mechanisms and effectiveness of prebiotics in modifying the gastrointestinal microbiota for the management of digestive disorders. *Proceedings of the Nutrition Society* 72: 288–298.

Wilson, B. and Whelan, K. (2017). Prebiotic inulin-type fructans and galacto-oligosaccharides: definition, specificity, function, and application in gastrointestinal disorders. *Journal of Gastroenterology and Hepatology* 32: 64–68.

Wolf, A.J. and Underhill, D.M. (2018). Peptidoglycan recognition by the innate immune system. *Nature Reviews Immunology* 18: 243.

Xia, G., Kohler, T., and Peschel, A. (2010). The wall teichoic acid and lipoteichoic acid polymers of Staphylococcus aureus. *International Journal of Medical Microbiology* 300: 148–154.

Xue, L., He, J., Gao, N. et al. (2017). Probiotics may delay the progression of nonalcoholic fatty liver disease by restoring the gut microbiota structure and improving intestinal endotoxemia. *Scientific Reports* 7: 45176.

Yadav, H., Jain, S., and Sinha, P.R. (2008). Oral administration of dahi containing probiotic Lactobacillus acidophilus and Lactobacillus casei delayed the progression of streptozotocin-induced diabetes in rats. *The Journal of Dairy Research* 75: 189.

Yan, F., Cao, H., Cover, T.L. et al. (2011). Colon-specific delivery of a probiotic-derived soluble protein ameliorates intestinal inflammation in mice through an EGFR-dependent mechanism. *The Journal of Clinical Investigation* 121: 2242–2253.

Yeung, T.W., Arroyo-Maya, I.J., Mcclements, D.J., and Sela, D.A. (2016). Microencapsulation of probiotics in hydrogel particles: enhancing Lactococcus lactis subsp. cremoris LM0230 viability using calcium alginate beads. *Food & Function* 7: 2909–2909.

Yoo, J.Y. and Kim, S.S. (2016). Probiotics and prebiotics: present status and future perspectives on metabolic disorders. *Nutrients* 8: 173.

Zhang, M.-M., Cheng, J.-Q., Lu, Y.-R. et al. (2010). Use of pre-, pro-and synbiotics in patients with acute pancreatitis: a meta-analysis. *World Journal of Gastroenterology* 16: 3970.

Zheng, H.J., Guo, J., Jia, Q. et al. (2019). The effect of probiotic and synbiotic supplementation on biomarkers of inflammation and oxidative stress in diabetic patients: a systematic review and meta-analysis of randomized controlled trials. *Pharmacological Research* 142: 303–313.

Zielińska, D., Sionek, B., and KołoŻyn-Krajewska, D. (2018). Safety of probiotics. In: *Diet, Microbiome and Health* (eds. A.M. Holban and A.M. Grumezescu), 131–161. Cambridge, Massachusetts, United States: Elsevier.

6

Marine Nutraceuticals

Giuseppe Derosa[1,2] and Pamela Maffioli[1]

[1] Department of Internal Medicine and Therapeutics, University of Pavia, Pavia, Italy
[2] Laboratory of Molecular Medicine, University of Pavia, Pavia, Italy

6.1   Introduction

In the latest years, the science of nutraceuticals is constantly evolving, different substances have shown a favorable effect in controlling lipid profile, glycemia, hypertension, insulin resistance, and metabolic parameters (Derosa et al. 2014; Derosa and Maffioli 2015). The ocean contains numerous marine organisms, including algae, animals, and plants, from which diverse marine polysaccharides with useful physicochemical and biological properties can be extracted. The enormous amounts of biodiversity marine water contains make it a source of huge amounts and wide varieties of novel bioactive compounds. Most of the bioactive compounds have several biological activities which are found to act as nutraceuticals for humans and animals. The potential of marine nutraceuticals in human health had already been established and their use in animal health is also found to be successful (Ande et al. 2017). In particular, fucoidan, carrageenan, alginate, and chitosan have been extensively investigated in pharmaceutical and biomedical fields owing to their desirable characteristics, such as biocompatibility, biodegradability, and bioactivity.

In the next pages, we will describe how marine organisms can be helpful in treating many human diseases.

6.2   Marine Bacteria and Fungi

Bacteria and fungi are widely distributed in marine environments (from shallow water to deep sea, even down to the polar ice covers) and synthesize a high number of structurally and functionally diverse bioactive molecules.

Marine microbes have received growing attention as the sources of bioactive metabolites and have great potential to increase the number of marine natural products in clinical trials. Marine microbes play a great role in the expansion of the drug development pipeline. Actinobacteria from the genus Streptomyces, represent a rich source of biologically active molecules (Zhao et al. 2016; Hassan et al. 2017; Jose and Jha 2017; Kamjam et al. 2017; Blunt et al. 2018; Jakubiec-Krzesniak et al. 2018; Yang et al. 2019). Actinobacteria have made a substantial positive contribution to

Handbook of Nutraceuticals and Natural Products: Biological, Medicinal, and Nutritional Properties and Applications,
Volume 1, First Edition. Edited by Sreerag Gopi and Preetha Balakrishnan.

human health; they are the producers of many compounds that are used as important drugs, including most antibiotics (Hopwood 2007).

Regarding fungi, marine fungi are a rich source of terpenoids which can be divided into six groups based on their chemical structures and biogenetic pathways: monoterpenes, sesquiterpenes, diterpenes, sesterterpenes, triterpenes, and meroterpenes. Among them, sesquiterpenes (188, 40%), meroterpenes (165, 35%), and diterpenes (75, 16%) comprise the largest proportion of terpenes, while Penicillium (108, 23%), Aspergillus (99, 21%), and Trichoderma (49, 10%) are the dominant producers of terpenoids. The majority of the fungi producing these novel terpenes were isolated from live marine matter, marine animals (27%), and aquatic plants (including mangrove plants) (38%), while the remaining fungi were obtained from marine environments (i.e. deep-sea sediments (15%), other marine sediments from the shallow sea or coast (11%), and hydrothermal vents (3%)) (Minghua et al. 2020).

Terpenes are created by plants to protect against herbivores, insects, and other environmental dangers. They are also responsible for a plant's regeneration and oxygenation. In light of these functions, it makes sense that some serve as potential immunity boosters in humans. It appears that terpenes are providing immunity defenses in both the people who consume these aromatic compounds and the plants that produce them.

6.3 Marine Algae

Marine algae provide various types of bioactive compounds. The most important and striking feature of marine algae is their natural pigments. The natural pigments of the marine algae provide food by photosynthesis and also provide pigmentation. In addition to these, natural pigments are also found to exhibit health benefits which make them one of the important marine nutraceuticals.

Marine algae produce a huge number of metabolites with biological activity (Mimouni et al. 2012) including anticancer (Lauritano et al. 2016; Martinez Andrade et al. 2018), antimicrobial (Martinez et al. 2019), immunomodulatory (Riccio and Lauritano 2020), anti-diabetes (Lauritano and Ianora 2016), antituberculosis (Lauritano et al. 2018), anti-epilepsy (Brillatz et al. 2018), antihypertensive, anti-atherosclerosis, anti-osteoporosis (Giordano et al. 2018), and anti-inflammatory (Lauritano et al. 2020) activities.

Microalgae, the most primary and simply organized members of marine plant life, are rich sources of food ingredients, such as β-carotene, Vitamins C, A, E, H, B1, B2, B6, and B12, astaxanthin, polysaccharides, and polyunsaturated fatty acids (Yap and Chen 2001; Luiten et al. 2003; Grobbelaar 2004). As such, bioactive molecules from microalgae are commercially produced, used as food additives and also incorporated into infant milk formulations and dietary supplements (Alves et al. 2018).

Among the marine organisms, algae have revealed to be one of the major sources of new compounds of marine origin, including those exhibiting antitumor and cytotoxic potential. These compounds demonstrated the ability to mediate specific inhibitory activities on a number of key cellular processes, including apoptosis pathways, angiogenesis, migration, and invasion, in both in vitro and in vivo models, revealing their potential to be used as anticancer drugs (Grobbelaar 2004).

Among algae, Ascophyllum nodosum and Fucus vesiculosus have been mainly studied for their hypoglycemic effects. Ascophyllum nodosum and Fucus vesiculosus belong to a brown seaweed species harvested off the coast of Sea Nord that is commercially available as a nutritional supplement and feed additive. The polyphenolic composition is represented by phlorotannins, able to inhibit α-amylase and α-glucosidase with an important hypoglycemic action in vivo (Paradis et al. 2011; Roy et al. 2011), and, in particular, post-prandial glucose (PPG). Phlorotannins slow carbohydrate absorption with a not competitive (not focalized on catalytic site in competition with the substrate) and reversible mechanism of inhibition of the enzymes involved in carbohydrates degrading (Paradis et al. 2011). The inhibiting action toward the activity of these enzymes results in animal models (rats), in a reduction of glycemia and insulinemia after administration of acids and glucose.

In literature, a study by Paradise et al. showed that Ascophyllum nodosum and Fucus vesiculosus improve insulin homeostasis in response to carbohydrate ingestion in not diabetic men and women (Paradis et al. 2011). This was confirmed in a randomized, placebo-controlled study conducted by Derosa et al. Authors conducted a study about the effects of a hypoglycemic nutraceutical containing Ascophyllum nodosum and Fucus vesiculosus in a ratio of 95/5 and Chromium picolinate in dysglycemic patients (Derosa et al. 2019). Ascophyllum nodosum and Fucus vesiculosus act in a mechanism acarbose-like, and also in this case, we recorded a similar reduction of glycated hemoglobin, fasting plasma glucose, PPG, and HOMA-IR compared to placebo, suggesting that reducing glucose absorption can be a valid option to prevent diabetes. The combination of Ascophyllum nodosum and Fucus vesiculosus also reduced high-sensitivity C-reactive protein, and tumor necrosis factor-α compared to baseline, and to the placebo group.

The same group studied the specific polyphenolic composition (extracted from Ascophyllum nodosum and Fucus vesiculosus in ratio 95/5) and chromium picolinate also in type 2 diabetic patients (Derosa et al. 2019). The trial showed a reduction of glycemia with the nutraceutical combination compared to placebo. This action can be due to the inhibiting action of the polyphenolic composition toward enzymatic activities, in an acarbose-like mechanism. The ability of a phytocomplex obtained from these algae to inhibit both enzymes has already been reported by Roy et al. (2011) and lately by Gabbia et al. (2017). Gabbia showed that the administration of this extract in mice fed with a diet rich in fat is associated not only with a delay in carbohydrate digestion, but also with a decrease in its assimilation. Furthermore, Ascophyllum nodosum and Fucus vesiculosus contain polyunsaturated fatty acids (PUFAs) and the quantity is abundant, ranging from near 44 to 48% for the Ascophyllum nodosum and Fucus vesiculosus, respectively (Lorenzo et al. 2017).

6.4 Marine Plants

Marine plants have been studied because they can play a role in treating infectious diseases which are the world's leading cause of premature deaths. Various hard works have been made to discover new antimicrobial compounds from many kinds of natural sources such as plants, animals, fungi, bacteria, and other microorganisms. Among marine plants, the most studied are seagrasses and mangroves. Seagrasses are angiosperms (flowering plants), evolved from terrestrial plants, which have adapted to live in marine environments, and that live fully submerged in the sea. Seagrasses contain several compounds in their secondary metabolism in which they differ from terrestrial plants. They produce novel chemicals to withstand extreme variations in pressure, salinity, temperature, and so forth, prevailing in their environment, and the chemicals produced are unique in diversity, structural, and functional. The phytochemicals present in seagrasses exhibit antibacterial, antioxidant, and antitumor activities (Bharathi et al. 2016). These entities could be the source of new lead form treatment of many diseases such as cancer, AIDS, inflammatory condition, arthritis, malaria, and a large variety of viral, bacterial, and fungal diseases (Bharathi et al. 2016). Yuvaraj et al. (2012) evaluated the antibacterial activity of crude methanol extract of seagrass

Halophila ovalis R. Br. Hooke (Hydrocharitaceae) against marine and human pathogens, antioxidant potential, and anti-inflammatory effect on peripheral blood mononuclear cells (PBMCs). The study showed that the methanol extract of seagrass H. ovalis collected from Chunnambar estuary, Pondicherry coastal line, exhibited antibacterial activity against Gram-positive Bacillus cereus and Gram-negative pathogens such as Vibrio parahaemolyticus, *Vibrio fischeri*, *Vibrio anguillarum*, *Vibrio vulnificus*, and *Acinetobacter baumannii*. Similar results were reported by some preceding studies of seagrass antibacterial activity conducted by Rengasamy et al. (2008).

On the other hand, mangroves are woody trees or shrubs and the salt marsh halophytes are herbs and sledges. The mangrove plants are distributed in 121 countries and the Pichavaram forest is one of the coastal ecosystems of Tamil Nadu, India with rich vegetation. Mangroves are used in traditional medicine for the treatment of many diseases (Kirtikar and Basu 2009). Several species of mangroves produce bioactive compounds that may control microbial growth (Miki et al. 1994). Moreover, preliminary studies have demonstrated that the mangrove plant extracts have antibacterial activity against pathogenic bacterial strains: *Staphylococcus* sp., *Escherichia coli*, and *Pseudomonas* sp. and resistant bacterial strains: *Staphylococcus* sp. and Proteus sp. (Ishibashi et al. 1993). Mangrove extracts can also be the research of the possible sources of mosquito larvicides, antifungal, antiviral, anticancer, and antidiabetic compounds (Wu et al. 1997).

Mangrove and mangrove associates contain biologically active antiviral, antibacterial, and antifungal compounds. The effects of mangrove extracts on some microorganisms including *Shigella* sp., *Staphylococcus* sp., and *Pseudomonas* sp. have been reported in some studies in the area of pharmacology (Abeysinghe and Pathirana 2006).

6.5 Marine Animals

A marine organism can be divided into invertebrates and vertebrates. Organisms belonging to marine invertebrates are composed of different taxonomic groups, which can be classified into several major phyla, namely Porifera (sponges), Cnidaria (corals, sea anemones, hydrozoans, and jellyfish), Annelida (polychaetes and marine worms), Bryozoa (moss animals or sea mats), Mollusca (oysters, abalone, clams, mussels, squid, cuttlefish, and octopuses), Arthropoda (lobsters, crabs, shrimps, prawns, and crayfish), and Echinodermata (sea stars, sea cucumbers, and sea urchins).

Several antiviral agents have been described from marine invertebrates, but, despite the numbers of antivirals found, only a few of them are on clinical trials or have been approved for drug marketing. The most promising organisms are represented by marine sponges, sessile animals that look like plants. They attached themselves to a rock, shell, or seafloor when they are young and live for the rest of their lives. They filter water through their porous body for the food they eat. They eat bacteria and other particles floating in the water as they move through their bodies. Some sponges have been found living on ocean floors that are up to 8800 meters deep. The potentiating effects of sponge extracts on antibiotics have been investigated by Beesoo et al. (2017). These authors showed that extracts from Neopetrosia exigua, rich in beta-sitosterol and cholesterol, displayed the widest activity spectrum against the nine tested bacterial isolates whilst the best antibacterial profile was observed by its ethyl acetate form, particularly against Staphylococcus aureus and Bacillus cereus. These findings suggest that the antibacterial properties of the tested marine sponge extracts may provide an alternative and complementary strategy to manage bacterial infections.

Fish are also a good source of taurine, an essential aminoacid for the human body. This aminoacid is found in cod, mackerel, salmon, albacore tuna, ray, shark, etc. (Kadam and Prabhasankar 2010).

Taurine has various potential applications including the reduction of blood pressure, the improvement of cardiac performances and the reduction of the cholesterol level (FAO 2021). Fish bones, on the other hand, are an excellent source of calcium, but the problem is the need for transformation of fish bones into an edible form. Grinded into powder, it can be inserted in products such as surimi (Gormley 2006). The intake of a healthy amount of calcium helps prevent or treat diseases such as osteoporosis, hypoparathyroidism, high blood pressure, premenstrual syndrome, obesity, weight loss, high cholesterol, and rickets (Shungan 1996). Shrimp and crab are good sources of chitin and chitosan (UMMS 2021). These molecules support the acceleration of wound healing (Rinaudo 2006), are involved in immune-enhancement, disease recovery and are used as dietary fibers. Chitin and chitosan are present in the scale of these animals, and need to be extracted in order to implement these molecules in other food sources. Marine-based fish is also rich of n-3 polyunsaturated fatty acids (n-3 PUFAs), which can have beneficial effects on arrhythmia (Tavazzi et al. 2008), on high levels of triglycerides (Patterson et al. 2012), on the atherosclerotic plaque (Thies et al. 2003), on the impaired endothelial function (Derosa et al. 2009), and on platelet aggregation and inflammation (Derosa et al. 2009, 2011, 2012; Cicero et al. 2010; Patterson et al. 2012). Supplementation with n-3 PUFAs reduced the levels of metalloproteinases two and nine in patients with mixed dyslipidemia (Derosa et al. 2009), with a further positive effect on blood pressure levels in subjects with and without high cardiovascular risk (Kim and Reaven 2004; Cicero et al. 2010). It has also been shown that patients with type 2 diabetes mellitus, impaired fasting glucose (IFG), or impaired glucose tolerance (IGT) have an increased risk for cardiovascular events (Gerstein 2010), while several epidemiological studies have shown a reduced risk of cardiovascular events among people who regularly consume fish or n-3 PUFAs (Hu et al. 2002, 2003; Calder 2004; Saravanan et al. 2010). In this regard, the ORIGIN study (Outcome Reduction with an Initial Glargine Intervention) (ORIGIN Trial Investigators et al. 2012) suggested that the use of n-3 PUFAs in the long-term may reduce the risk of cardiovascular events in subjects with IFG, IGT, or diabetes. The results of this study, however, have shown that supplementation with 1 g of omega-3 does not appear to reduce the risk of cardiovascular events, while reducing triglyceride levels compared to placebo. Different results were observed in a substudy of the study JELIS (Japan EPA Lipid Intervention Study) which showed that patients with impaired glucose metabolism have a higher cardiovascular risk than those with normal blood sugar and that the intake of n-3 PUFAs reduces the incidence of cardiovascular events (Oikawa et al. 2009). n-3 PUFAs, at the dose of 3 g/day, also showed to be effective in reducing glycemia in patients affected by IFG or IGT and seem to be helpful to slow the development of type 2 diabetes mellitus (Derosa et al. 2016).

6.6 Conclusion

Data reported above suggest that marine microorganisms can be helpful for treating several human diseases. Obviously, all these substances cannot replace conventional treatments, but can be useful in addition to conventional therapies.

References

Abeysinghe, P.D. and Pathirana, R.N. (2006). Evaluation of antibacterial activity of different mangrove plant extracts. *Ruhuna J. Sci.* 1: 104–112.

Alves, C., Silva, J., Pinteus, S. et al. (2018). From marine origin to therapeutics: the antitumor potential of marine algae-derived compounds. *Front. Pharmacol.* 9: 777.

Ande, M.P., Syamala, K., SrinivasaRao, P. et al. (2017). Marine Nutraceuticals. *Aquaculture Times* 3 (2): 06.

Beesoo, R., Bhagooli, R., Neergheen-Bhujun, V.S. et al. (2017). Antibacterial and antibiotic potentiating activities of tropical marine sponge extracts. *Comp. Biochem. Physiol. Part C: Toxicol. Pharmacol.* 196: 81–90.

Bharathi, N.P., Amudha, P., and Vanitha, V. (2016). Sea grasses – novel marine nutraceuticals. *Int. J. Pharm. Bio. Sci* 7 (4): 567–573.

Blunt, J.W., Carroll, A.R., Copp, B.R. et al. (2018). Marine natural products. *Nat. Prod. Rep.* 35: 8–53.

Brillatz, T., Lauritano, C., Jacmin, M. et al. (2018). Zebrafish-based identification of the antiseizure nucleoside inosine from the marine diatom Skeletonema marinoi. *PLoS One* 13: e0196195.

Calder, P.C. (2004). n-3 Fatty acids and cardiovascular disease: evidence explained and mechanisms explored. *Clin. Sci. (Lond.)* 107 (1): 1–11.

Cicero, A.F., Derosa, G., Di Gregori, V. et al. (2010). Omega 3 polyunsaturated fatty acids supplementation and blood pressure levels in hypertriglyceridemic patients with untreated normal-high blood pressure and with or without metabolic syndrome: a retrospective study. *Clin. Exp. Hypertens.* 32 (2): 137–144.

Derosa, G. and Maffioli, P. (2015). Nutraceuticals for the treatment of metabolic diseases: evidence from clinical practice. *Expert. Rev. Endocrinol. Metab.* 10 (3): 297–304.

Derosa, G., Maffioli, P., D'Angelo, A. et al. (2009). Effects of long chain omega-3 fatty acids on metalloproteinases and their inhibitors in combined dyslipidemia patients. *Expert. Opin. Pharmacother.* 10 (8): 1239–1247.

Derosa, G., Cicero, A.F., Fogari, E. et al. (2011). Effects of n-3 PUFAs on insulin resistance after an oral fat load. *Eur. J. Lipid Sci. Technol.* 113 (8): 950–960.

Derosa, G., Cicero, A.F., Fogari, E. et al. (2012). n-3 PUFAs effects on post-prandial variation of metalloproteinases, inflammatory and insulin resistance parameters in dyslipidemic patients: evaluation with euglycemic clamp and oral fat load. *J. Clin. Lipidol.* 6 (6): 553–564.

Derosa, G., Limas, C.P., Macías, P.C. et al. (2014). Dietary and nutraceutical approach to type 2 diabetes. *Arch. Med. Sci.* 10: 336–344.

Derosa, G., Cicero, A.F., D'Angelo, A. et al. (2016). Effects of n-3 PUFAs on fasting plasma glucose and insulin resistance in patients with impaired fasting glucose or impaired glucose tolerance. *Biofactors* 42 (3): 316–322.

Derosa, G., Cicero, A.F.G., D'Angelo, A., and Maffioli, P. (2019). Ascophyllum nodosum and Fucus vesiculosus on glycemic status and on endothelial damage markers in dysglicemic patients. *Phytother. Res.* 33 (3): 791–797.

Derosa, G., Pascuzzo, M.D., D'Angelo, A., and Ascophyllum Nodosum, M.P. (2019). Fucus Vesiculosus and chromium picolinate nutraceutical composition can help to treat type 2 diabetic patients. *Diabetes Metab. Syndr. Obes.* 12: 1861–1865.

FAO (2021). http://www.fao.org/fishery/aquaculture/en (accessed July 2021).

Gabbia, D., Dall'Acqua, S., Di Gangi, I.M. et al. (2017). The phytocomplex from fucus vesiculosus and ascophyllum nodosum controls postprandial plasma glucose levels: an in vitro and in vivo study in a mouse model of NASH. *Mar. Drugs* 15: 41.

Gerstein, H.C. (2010). More insights on the dysglycaemia-cardiovascular connection. *Lancet* 375 (9733): 2195–2196.

Giordano, D., Costantini, M., Coppola, D. et al. (2018). Biotechnological applications of bioactive peptides from marine sources. *Adv. Microb. Physiol.* 73: 171–220.

Gormley, R. (2006). Fish as a functional food. *Proceedings of the Functional Food Network Conference*, Turku, Finland, March 8–10.

Grobbelaar, J.U. (2004). Algal biotechnology: real opportunities for Africa. *S. Afr. J. Bot.* 70: 140–144.

Hassan, S.S., Anjum, K., Abbas, S.Q. et al. (2017). Emerging biopharmaceuticals from marine actinobacteria. *Environ. Toxicol. Pharmacol.* 49: 34–47.

Hopwood, D.A. (2007). *Nature and Medicine: The Antibiotic Makers*. New York: Oxford University Press Streptomyces.

Hu, F.B., Bronner, L., Willett, W.C. et al. (2002). Fish and omega-3 fatty acid intake and risk of coronary heart disease in women. *JAMA* 287 (14): 1815–1821.

Hu, F.B., Cho, E., Rexrode, K.M. et al. (2003). Fish and long-chain omega-3 fatty acid intake and risk of coronary heart disease and total mortality in diabetic women. *Circulation* 107 (14): 1852–1857.

Ishibashi, S.N., Isman, M.B., and Neil Towers, N.H. (1993). Insecticidal 1H – Cyclopentatetrahydro Benzofurans from Aglaia odorata. *Phytochemistry* 32: 307–310.

Jakubiec-Krzesniak, K., Rajnisz-Mateusiak, A., Guspiel, A. et al. (2018). Secondary metabolites of actinomycetes and their antibacterial, antifungal and antiviral properties. *Pol. J. Microbiol.* 67: 259–272.

Jose, P.A. and Jha, B. (2017). Intertidal marine sediment harbours Actinobacteria with promising bioactive and biosynthetic potential. *Sci. Rep.* 7: 10041.

Kadam, S.U. and Prabhasankar, P. (2010). Marine foods as functional ingredients in bakery and pasta products. *Food Res. Int.* 43: 1975–1980.

Kamjam, M., Sivalingam, P., Deng, Z., and Hong, K. (2017). Deep sea actinomycetes and their secondary metabolites. *Front. Microbiol.* 8: 760.

Kim, S.H. and Reaven, G.M. (2004). The metabolic syndrome: one step forward, two steps back. *Diab. Vasc. Dis. Res.* 1 (2): 68–75.

Kirtikar, K.R. and Basu, B.D. (2009). *Indian Medicinal Plants*, 1–2793. Allahabad, India: Lalit Mohan Basu Publishers I-IV.

Lauritano, C. and Ianora, A. (2016). Marine organisms with anti-diabetes properties. *Mar. Drugs* 14: 220.

Lauritano, C., Andersen, J.H., Hansen, E. et al. (2016). Bioactivity screening of microalgae for antioxidant, anti-inflammatory, anticancer, anti-diabetes, and antibacterial activities. *Front. Mar. Sci.* 3: 68.

Lauritano, C., Martín, J., De La Cruz, M. et al. (2018). First identification of marine diatoms with anti-tuberculosis activity. *Sci. Rep.* 8: 2284.

Lauritano, C., Helland, K., Riccio, G. et al. (2020). Lysophosphatidylcholines and chlorophyll-derived molecules from the diatom Cylindrotheca closterium with anti-inflammatory activity. *Mar. Drugs* 18: 166.

Lorenzo, J.M., Agregán, R., Munekata, P.E.S. et al. (2017). Proximate composition and nutritional value of three macroalgae: Ascophyllum nodosum, Fucus vesiculosus and Bifurcaria bifurcata. *Mar. Drugs* 15: 360.

Luiten, E.E., Akkerman, I., Koulman, A. et al. (2003). Realizing the promises of marine biotechnology. *Biomol. Eng.* 20: 429–439.

Martinez Andrade, K.A., Lauritano, C., Romano, G., and Ianora, A. (2018). Marine microalgae with anti-cancer properties. *Mar. Drugs* 16: 165.

Martinez, K.A., Lauritano, C., Druka, D. et al. (2019). Amphidinol 22, a new cytotoxic and antifungal amphidinol from the dinoflagellate amphidinium carterae. *Mar. Drugs* 17: 385.

Miki, T., Sakaki, T., Shibata, M. et al. (1994). Soxhlet extraction of mangrove and biological activities of extracts. *Kyushu Kogyo Gijutsu Kenkyusho Hokoku* 1004 (53): 3347–3352.

Mimouni, V., Ulmann, L., Pasquet, V. et al. (2012). The potential of microalgae for the production of bioactive molecules of pharmaceutical interest. *Curr. Pharm. Biotechnol.* 13: 2733–2750.

Minghua, J., Zhenger, W., Heng, G. et al. (2020). A review of terpenes from marine-derived fungi: 2015-2019. *Mar Drugs* 18 (6): 321.

Oikawa, S., Yokoyama, M., Origasa, H. et al. (2009). Suppressive effect of EPA on the incidence of coronary events in hypercholesterolemia with impaired glucose metabolism: sub-analysis of the Japan EPA Lipid Intervention Study (JELIS). *Atherosclerosis* 206 (2): 535–539.

ORIGIN Trial Investigators, Bosch, J., Gerstein, H.C. et al. (2012). n-3 fatty acids and cardiovascular outcomes in patients with dysglycemia. *N. Engl. J. Med.* 367 (4): 309–318.

Paradis, M.E., Couture, P., and Lamarche, B. (2011). A randomised crossover placebo-controlled trial investigating the effect of brown seaweed (Ascophyllum nodosum e Fucus vesiculosus) on postchallenge plasma glucose and insulin levels in men and women. *Appl. Physiol. Nutr. Metab.* 36: 913–919.

Patterson, E., Wall, R., Fitzgerald, G.F. et al. (2012). Health implications of high dietary omega-6 polyunsaturated Fatty acids. *J. Nutr. Metab.* 539426.

Rengasamy, R., Kumar, C.S., Sarada, D.V.L., and Gideon, T.P. (2008). Antibacterial activity of three South Indian seagrasses, Cymodocea serrulata, Halophila ovalis and Zostera capensis. *World J. Microbiol. Biotechnol.* 24: 1989–1992.

Riccio, G. and Lauritano, C. (2020). Microalgae with immunomodulatory activities. *Mar. Drugs* 18: 2.

Rinaudo, M. (2006). Chitin and chitosan: properties and applications. *Prog. Polym. Sci.* 31: 603–632.

Roy, M.C., Anguenot, R., Fillion, C. et al. (2011). Effect of a commercially-available algal phlorotannins extract on digestive enzymes and carbohydrate absorption in vivo. *Food Res. Int.* 44: 3026–3029.

Saravanan, P., Davidson, N.C., Schmidt, E.B., and Calder, P.C. (2010). Cardiovascular effects of marine omega-3 fatty acids. *Lancet* 376 (9740): 540–550.

Shungan, X. (1996). Calcium powder of freshwater fish bone. *J. Shanghai Fish. Univ.* 5: 246.

Tavazzi, L., Maggioni, A.P., Marchioli, R. et al. (2008). Gissi-HF Investigators. Effect of n-3 polyunsaturated fatty acids in patients with chronic heart failure (the GISSI-HF trial): a randomised, double-blind, placebo-controlled trial. *Lancet* 372 (9645): 1223–1230.

Thies, F., Garry, J.M., Yaqoob, P. et al. (2003). Association of n-3 polyunsaturated fatty acids with stability of atherosclerotic plaques: a randomised controlled trial. *Lancet* 361 (9356): 477–485.

UMMS (2021). https://www.umms.org/ummc/ (accessed July 2021).

Wu, T.S., Liou, M.J., Kuon, C.S. et al. (1997). Cytotoxic and antiplatelet aggregation principles from Aglaia elliptifolia. *J. Nat. Prod.* 60: 606–608.

Yang, C., Qian, R., Xu, Y. et al. (2019). Marine Actinomycetes-derived. Natural Products. *Curr. Top. Med. Chem.* 19: 2868–2918.

Yap, C.Y. and Chen, F. (2001). Polyunsaturated fatty acids: biological significance, biosynthesis, and production by microalgae and microalgae-like organisms. In: *Algae and Their Biotechnological Potential* (eds. F. Chen and Y. Jiang), 1–32. Dordrecht, The Netherlands: Kluwer Academic Publishers.

Yuvaraj, N., Kanmani, P., Satishkumar, R. et al. (2012). Seagrass as a potential source of natural antioxidant and anti-inflammatory agents. *Pharm. Biol.* 50 (4): 458–467.

Zhao F, Qin YH, Zheng X, Zhao HW, Chai DY, Li W, Pu MX, Zuo XS, Qian W, Ni P et al. Biogeography and adaptive evolution of Streptomyces Strains from saline environments. *Sci. Rep.* 2016; 6: 32718.34.

7

Nutraceuticals as Therapeutic Agents

O.J. Onaolapo[1] and A.Y. Onaolapo[2]

[1] *Behavioural Neuroscience Unit, Neuropharmacology Subdivision, Department of Pharmacology, Ladoke Akintola University of Technology, Ogbomosho, Oyo State, Nigeria*
[2] *Behavioural Neuroscience Unit, Neurobiology Subdivision, Department of Anatomy, Ladoke Akintola University of Technology, Ogbomosho, Oyo State, Nigeria*

7.1 Introduction

"Nutraceuticals" is a term coined more than three decades ago to emphasize the relationship that exists between nutrition and pharmaceutical agents in the maintenance of health and well-being. Although it has no universally accepted definition (Aronson 2017; Andrew and Izzo 2017), a nutraceutical has been defined as food or parts of food that have health benefits such as the prevention and/or treatment of disease (Brower 1998; Kalra 2003; Chauhan et al. 2013; Onaolapo and Onaolapo 2019). Hence, the broad term "nutraceutical" generally includes a wide category of products (functional foods, fortified foods, dietary supplements, and herbal products) that have been used to improve health, prevent chronic diseases, delay the aging process, and increase life expectancy (Nasri et al. 2014; Andrew and Izzo 2017; Drake et al. 2017). The knowledge regarding the importance of good food and adequate nutrition on the maintenance of human health and the prevention of disease dates back centuries (Deb and Gupta 2015). More recently, there is increasing awareness of the beneficial effects of consuming diets rich in natural plant foods; therefore, the use of nutraceuticals in the maintenance of health, as well as the prevention and treatment of disease (Raskin et al. 2002; Zhao 2007; Trottier et al. 2010; Nasri et al. 2014) is becoming popular worldwide (Melina et al. 2016).

The results of a large number of studies and reviews (Onaolapo and Onaolapo 2018a,bc, 2019, 2020; Onaolapo et al. 2019a) have demonstrated the potential benefits of diet, dietary supplements, herbs/herbal products, and bioactive compounds (Table 7.1) in the prevention and management of a number of diseases including diabetes, metabolic syndrome (Onaolapo et al. 2011, 2012; Onaolapo and Onaolapo 2012; Akbari et al. 2013; Cicero et al. 2014; Mollica et al. 2017a,b, 2018), atherosclerosis, cardiovascular diseases (Khosravi-Boroujeni et al. 2012, 2013), cancers (Clark and Lee 2016; Nabavi et al. 2018), infections (Karimi et al. 2013), infertility (Onaolapo et al. 2018), central nervous system, and mental health disorders (Onaolapo et al. 2017a,b,c,d,e, 2019b, 2020a,b; Olofinnade et al. 2020).

The science of distinguishing between foods and drugs is gradually becoming imprecise as a number of foods are now known to contain substances or chemicals that act in the body to maintain

Handbook of Nutraceuticals and Natural Products: Biological, Medicinal, and Nutritional Properties and Applications, Volume 1, First Edition. Edited by Sreerag Gopi and Preetha Balakrishnan.
© 2022 John Wiley & Sons, Inc. Published 2022 by John Wiley & Sons, Inc.

Table 7.1 Beneficial effects of nutraceuticals.

Nutraceutical/ functional food/ dietary supplement	Species	Effects	References
Potato and white rice consumption	Humans	Decreases cardiovascular risk factors	Khosravi-Boroujeni et al. (2012, 2013)
Curcumin, Capsaicin	Humans	Ameliorative effects in cancers such as melanomas	Clark and Lee (2016), Nabavi et al. (2018)
Tulip	Rats	Antidiabetic activity	Akbari et al. (2013)
Quercus persica		Antiviral activity	Karimi et al. (2013)
Melatonin	Mice	modulates the response of adolescent mice to stress, and attenuates behavioral deficits and brain oxidative stress in a rodent model of schizophrenia	Onaolapo et al. (2017a,b)
Melatonin	Mice	behavioral, metabolic, oxidative, and organ morphological changes in mice that are fed high-fat	Onaolapo et al. (2020a)
Methionine and silymarin	Rats	Ameliorates acetaminophen-induced injuries of the liver, kidney, and cerebral cortex	Onaolapo et al. (2017c)
Silymarin	Mice	Ameliorates aspartame-induced variation in mouse behavior, oxidative stress, and cerebral cortex morphology	Onaolapo et al. (2017d)
Co-enzyme Q10 as mono and adjunct	Mice	Ameliorates changes due to drug-induced Parkinsonism	Onaolapo et al. (2019b)
Pyridoxal phosphate	Mice	Ameliorates changes due to drug-induced Parkinsonism	Olofinnade et al. (2020)
Ocimum grattisimum	Rats	Ameliorates streptozotocin-induced changes in rats	Onaolapo et al. (2011, 2012), Onaolapo and Onaolapo (2012)
Lepideium meyeni	Mice	Ameliorated cyclophosphamide-induced subfertility	Onaolapo et al. (2018)
Zinc as mono- or adjunct therapy	Mice	Ameliorated Ketamine-induced behavioral and brain oxidative changes in mice	Onaolapo et al. (2017e)
Dietary zinc	Mice	Militates against ketamine-induced changes	Onaolapo et al. (2020b)
Capparis spinosa	Rats	Ameliorates streptozotocin-induced changes	Mollica et al. (2017a)
Juglans regia	Rats	Ameliorates streptozotocin-induced changes	Mollica et al. (2017b)
Corylus avellana	Mice	Ameliorates high-fat diet-induced changes	Mollica et al. (2018)

normal physiology and prevent pathological processes leading to disease. In an era when a number of human diseases have origins that are traceable to nutrition, a number of foods that combat human diseases are also being identified, investigated and, in some cases, recommended. However, the question here is that can we improve our knowledge of nutraceuticals up to the point where a number of them become a direct substitute for known pharmaceutical agents? Or will they occupy a special class of "therapeutic agents" that are not necessarily direct replacements? In this chapter, we explore nutraceuticals as therapeutic agents, as well as their role in the future of medical treatment and disease management.

7.1.1 Definitions and Regulation of Nutraceuticals

The terms "nutraceutical," "functional foods," and "dietary supplements" have been used interchangeably, having different meanings in various countries (Spagnuolo 2020). In Canada, nutraceuticals are referred to as natural health products. Natural health products are defined as naturally occurring substances used for the restoration and maintenance of health and well-being, which are usually made from plants, but can also originate from animals, microorganisms, and marine sources (Health Products and Food Branch 2020). In the United States of America, they are referred to as dietary supplements (Spagnuolo 2020). The US Food and Drug Administration defines a dietary ingredient as an amino acid, mineral, vitamin, herb, or any other botanical or dietary substance for use in humans to supplement the diet by increasing the total dietary intake; or a concentrate, metabolite, constituent, extract, or combination of the preceding substances (CFSAN 2020a,b). In Europe, products with nutraceutical potential are considered food supplements, which are defined as concentrated sources of nutrients including minerals, proteins, vitamins, and other compounds with a beneficial nutritional effect. Stephen De Felice, who coined the terminology "nutraceuticals" meaning food (or a part of food) that provides medical or health benefits, including the prevention and/or treatment of a disease (Brower 1998; Maddi et al. 2007; Das et al., 2012). However, suggestions that the absence of a universal definition impeded the regulation of nutraceuticals globally resulted in a proposal of a working- definition that considered nutraceuticals as diet supplements used to enhance health by virtue of their ability to deliver concentrated forms of biologically active food components in a nonfood matrix (Zeisel 1999; Varzakas et al. 2016). Overall, it is generally accepted that foods that have nutraceutical value have the ability to impart physiological changes in the body in addition to their nutritional benefits (Spagnuolo 2020).

Globally, the regulation of nutraceuticals, like its definition, is not supported by a unified act or law. In the US, the Dietary Supplement Health and Education Act (1994) is the framework with which the Food and Drug Administration regulates dietary supplements. The act prohibits the sale of dietary supplements that are adulterated or misbranded, although the manufacturers and distributors of these products are responsible for evaluating the safety and labeling of their products to ensure that they meet DSHEA requirements and FDA regulation (CFSAN 2020a,b). In Canada, nutraceuticals are regulated under the Natural and Non-Prescription Health Products Directorate as subsets of drugs. They are also recognized as self-care products, allowing them to be marketed over-the-counter without the need for a prescription. In Europe, the European Food and Safety Authority regulates food supplements, the main European Union legislation and regulatory framework relating to food supplements is the Food Supplements Directive 2002/46/EC (Directive 2002/46/EC, 2002; Meštrović 2018; Santini et al. 2018).

There have been suggestions that the ambiguities created by the lack of a unified definition and gaps in the regulatory framework possess a substantial potential risk to public health, considering reports of adverse effects that have arisen from the use of nutraceuticals. There have been proposals that dietary supplements or food supplements such as vitamins and minerals should be separated from other food or botanical supplements which would then be known as nutraceuticals if they need to be consumed at doses exceeding normal human exposure in foods (Zeisel 1999; Varzakas et al. 2016). Also, regulations need to be strengthened such that the claimed benefits are properly substantiated by reproducible safety and efficacy information or in vitro and in vivo studies so as to reduce false expectations and targeted misinformation (Santini et al. 2018).

Table 7.2 Classification of nutraceuticals.

Categories	Classes
Based on the food source	Animal, plant, microbes
Mechanism of action/ specific therapeutic properties	antioxidants, anticancer, immunomodulators, anti-inflammatory and antilipemic agents, antimicrobial agents, antihyperglycemic, cytoprotective, antiparasitic, antifungal
Novelty	Traditional (herbal minerals, nutrients, phytochemicals, probiotic microorganisms, and enzymes) and nontraditional (fortified and recombinant)
Based on chemical nature/ constituent	Carotenoids, dietary fibers, collagen hydroxylates, flavonoids, tannins, lignans, phytoestrogens and phenols, fatty acids, amino acid carbohydrates, and isoprenoid derivatives

7.1.2 Classification of Nutraceuticals

There are different ways by which nutraceuticals can be classified. Nutraceuticals can be classified (Table 7.2) based on a food source (plants, animals, and microbes), mechanism of action (antioxidants, anticancer, immunomodulators, anti-inflammatory, and antilipemic agents) or chemical nature (carotenoids, dietary fibers, collagen hydroxylate, flavonoids, tannins, lignans, phytoestrogens, and phenols) (Chanda et al. 2019). Nutraceuticals have also been classified based on their novelty into traditional (herbal minerals, nutrients, phytochemicals, probiotic microorganisms, and enzymes) and nontraditional (fortified and recombinant) nutraceuticals (Swaroopa and Srinath 2017; Rajasekaran 2017).

7.1.3 Pharmacology of Nutraceuticals and Functional Foods

7.1.3.1 Bioavailability of Nutraceuticals

In therapeutics, the efficiency of any given drug is determined by its bioavailability at the target site (Aqil et al. 2013). In predicting the bioavailability of conventional drugs, Lipinski et al. (2001) suggested the bioavailability of a compound was closely linked to the number of hydrogen bonds' donors and acceptors it contained, its molecular mass, and partition coefficient log value (Lipinski et al. 2001). There have also been suggestions that the bioavailability of nutraceuticals is modulated by physicochemical characteristics, including physical state, chemical structure, solubility, and lipophilicity (Dima et al. 2020). Other factors that determine the bioavailability of nutraceuticals include the ease with which it is liberated from food matrices, chemical degradation, or metabolism, interaction with gastrointestinal components, transformation, and epithelial cell permeability (McClements et al. 2015).

However, a number of bioactive compounds, including curcumin and green tea polyphenols, do not meet all the bioavailability criteria as they exhibit low bioavailability (Gao and Hu 2010). While compounds like genistein and biochanin A meet the chemical and structural criteria, but their bioavailability is limited by the rate of excretion in the gut by efflux mechanisms (Gao and Hu 2010; Upadhyay and Dixit 2015). Also, the bioavailability of epigallocatechin gallate is limited by poor absorption and rapid first-pass metabolism. There have also been reports suggesting that the rapid conjugation of phytochemicals in the intestine and liver are responsible for poor bioavailability (Manach et al. 2004; Upadhyay and Dixit 2015).

The poor oral bioavailability of a number of the important phytochemical compounds lowers their efficacy as health-promoting agents; therefore, there have been suggestions from a number of studies that the bioavailability of these nutraceuticals can be improved through the use of biomedically engineered delivery systems (McClements et al. 2015; Yao et al. 2015; Yang et al. 2019). These delivery systems improve bioavailability by increasing the stability of nutraceuticals in foods and the gastrointestinal tract, enhancing their solubility in the intestine, facilitating absorption, and decreasing conjugation and first-pass metabolism in the intestine and liver (Yao et al. 2015).

7.1.3.2 Nutraceuticals: Active Principle

The active compounds in functional foods are chemical constituents that are present in small quantities and provide health benefits including physiological, antioxidant, immunomodulatory, anti-inflammatory, behavioral, anticarcinogenic, antimicrobial properties, and immunological effects beyond the basic nutritional value of the food (Liu 2013). The majority of these bioactive compounds are concentrated and made into different forms including capsules, tablets, and powders and marketed as nutraceuticals. The importance of bioactive compounds in the maintenance of health is behind the extensive research to discover and characterize old and new bioactive compounds to better understand their mechanism of action as it relates to health maintenance and disease prevention. Plant phytochemicals vary widely in structure and function, and they include flavonoids, carotenoids, carnitine, phytosterols, phytoestrogens, dithiolthiones, polyphenols, glucosinolates, lignans, and taurine. There have also been suggestions that because minerals and vitamins also elicit a pharmacological response, they should be classified as bioactive compounds (Liu 2013). Animals are also rich sources of bioactive compounds. In the last few decades, a growing number of natural compounds have been extracted from animal sources including polyunsaturated fatty acids, L-carnitine, L-carnosine, choline, α-lipoic acid, conjugated linoleic acid, Glutathione, Taurine, and bioactive peptides extracted from milk, bovine blood, eggs, collagen, gelatin, or fish species such as salmon, tuna, and herring (Kulczyński et al. 2019).

7.1.3.3 Nutraceuticals: Mechanism of Action

Bioactive compounds are important sources of molecules with numerous therapeutic applications. There have been reports that these natural compounds are regulators of important pathological processes, such as cancer, metabolic syndrome, diabetes mellitus, cardiovascular disease, and central nervous system disorders.

In cancers, there have been suggestions that phytochemicals, such as epigallocatechin gallate, caffeic acid phenethyl ester, genistein, kaempferol, and morin, are able to modulate the expression of coding and noncoding gene transcripts (Budisan et al. 2017). Also, the health benefits and/or the antitumor effects of bioactive compounds have been attributed to their ability to function as antioxidants, inhibit the generation of reactive oxygen and nitrogen species, mitigate lipid peroxidation, combat deoxyribonucleic acid and protein damage, and regulate the cell cycle, cell proliferation, and immune response (Budisan et al. 2017; Gan et al. 2018). Phytochemicals like epigallocathechin gallate induce apoptosis by activating mitogen-activated protein kinases, through the phosphorylation of ERK1/2 (Song et al. 2014; Cerezo-Guisado et al. 2015; Budisan et al. 2017). Compounds like curcumin have also been shown to exert their anti-inflammatory effects by inhibiting cycloxygenase 2 (a key player in the inflammatory process), and downregulating nuclear factor kappa-light-chain-enhancer of activated B cells (NF-κB) (Jurenka 2009; Cojocneanu Petric et al. 2015). A number of these natural compounds also influence the expression of several microRNAs resulting in the modulation of critical cellular processes, including inhibiting cell growth, the reduction of inflammation, and stimulation of cell differentiation and cell cycle arrest

(Budisan et al. 2017). There have also been reports associating phytochemicals with the activation of transcription factors. Studies have shown that phenethyl isothiocyanate, a glucosinolate precursor in cruciferous vegetable (watercress), has the ability to activate transcription factor nuclear factor erythroid 2 p45-related factor 2 (NRF2), transcription factor heat shock factor 1 (HSF1), and induce the expression of epigenetic regulators. NRF2 mediates the transcription of numerous detoxification and antioxidant genes, while HSF1 induces the heat shock response which is cytoprotective in normal cells and ensures adaptation and survival during stressful conditions (Ramirez et al. 2017; Dayalan Naidu et al. 2018).

In cardiovascular diseases, there are reports that phytochemicals have the ability to modulate oxidative stress response to ischemic injury, and reduce apoptosis, necrosis, and fibrosis in cardiac myocytes. Also, the antioxidant potential of a number of these bioactive compounds is dependent on their ability to upregulate antioxidant defences, scavenge, and interact with reactive oxygen species (ROS), and inhibit enzymes involved in the generation of ROS. Bioactive compounds like resveratrol are able to increase levels of intracellular Ca^{2+} and enhance endothelial nitric oxide synthase activity, resulting in the attenuation of nitric oxide release (Martin et al. 2002). Taxifolin has also been suggested to mitigate diabetic cardiomyopathy, by reducing diastolic dysfunction through the inhibition of NADPH oxidase activity, the reduction of angiotensin II levels, and induction of JAK-STAT3 signaling pathway (Sánchez et al. 2006; Sun et al. 2014).

In metabolic diseases like diabetes mellitus, the hypoglycemic/antihyperglycemic effects of phytochemicals have been ascribed to their ability to reduce intestinal uptake of carbohydrates, modulation of the activities of enzymes involved in glucose metabolism, improving β-cell function and insulin action, increasing insulin secretion/release, as well as their antioxidant and anti-inflammatory properties (Cabrera et al. 2006; Iwai et al. 2006; Sayem et al. 2018). Several phytochemicals also maintain glucose homeostasis by regulating the expression of genes and signaling pathways involved in the occurrence of type 2 diabetes mellitus (Sayem et al. 2018). Bioactive compounds like resveratrol induce protein kinase B (Akt) and vascular endothelial growth factor (VEGF), and also increase the expression of insulin-regulated glucose transporter (GLUT4) through the activation of phosphatidylinositol 3-kinase/protein kinase B (PI3K/AKT) signaling pathways (Sayem et al. 2018).

In the brain, the nootropic benefits of a number of phytochemicals including flavonoids, anthocyanins, phenols, and carotenoids have been attributed to their ability to inhibit acetylcholinesterase activity, upregulate the levels of acetylcholine as well as other neurotransmitters, and regulate intracellular signaling (Ali Hassan et al. 2013; Venkatesan et al. 2015). Also, the neuroprotective potential of bioactive compounds such as epigallocatechin-3-galate (ECCG) have been linked to their ability to prevent neuronal cell death via the inhibition of transcription factors or signaling molecules such as nuclear factor kappa-light-chain-enhancer of activated B cells (NF-κβ) and extracellular-signal-regulated kinase (ERK), respectively. This then results in a decrease in the levels of β- and γ-secretases. The upregulation of α-secretase levels by ECCG has also been associated with a reduction in the concentration of amyloid plaques due to the cleavage of amyloid precursor proteins (Smith et al. 2010; Liu et al. 2014; Velmurugan et al. 2018). The neuroprotective effect of phytochemicals like berberine have also been ascribed to the ability to scavenge-free radicals via the activation of the PI3K/Akt/Nrf2 pathway and also prevent apoptosis by decreasing the expression of Bax, caspase 1 and 3, and upregulating the expression of Bcl-2 (Asai et al. 2006; Velmurugan et al. 2018).

7.1.3.4 Nutraceuticals: Adverse Effects and Drug Interactions

Paracelsus, who is credited as the father of toxicology, is quoted as saying that *ola dosis facit venenum* – "Only the dose makes the poison." The intake of nutraceuticals is considered to be generally safe; however, regardless of this presumed safety, more recent reports show that the use of nutraceuticals is not totally without risk (Ronis et al. 2018). There have been suggestions that a number of nutraceuticals display cytotoxic effects and/or drug interactions (when used in combination with conventional pharmaceuticals), which could be due to unsuitable combinations, the use of inappropriately high doses, or improper use (Cojocneanu Petric et al. 2015; Ronis et al. 2018).

Toxicities associated with the consumption of micronutrients and vitamin supplements have been reported to increase with dose. Although toxicity is rare with water-soluble vitamins, consumption of vitamin B6 (Pyridoxine) at doses higher than 500 mg/day especially in the elderly has been associated with the development of photosensitivity, neurotoxicity, and pyridoxine-associated chronic sensory polyneuropathy (de Kruijk and Notermans 2005). Also, there have been reports of bleeding (due to platelet abnormalities), diarrhoea, blurred vision, and gonadal dysfunction following the consumption of high doses of vitamin E; while the use of vitamin E post-irradiation for head and neck cancers has been associated with high rates of cancer recurrence (Ziegler and Filer 1996; Ronis et al. 2018).

There have also been reports of toxicities associated with the use of phytochemicals. These toxicities include the hemolytic effects of fava beans (in genetically susceptible populations), the goitrogenic effects of the *Brassica* plant, and the agglutination caused by lectins (Cojocneanu Petric et al. 2015). The metabolites of epigalocatechin gallate have also been shown to induce/enhance oxidative stress and hepatic injury (Mazzanti et al. 2009; Ronis et al. 2018). Co-ingestion of nutraceuticals with conventional pharmaceuticals has also been associated with the development of adverse reactions due to drug interactions. Russo et al. (2016) reported the case of an elderly woman who developed rhabdomyolysis following the use of a dietary supplement that contained monacolin K in addition to regular drugs like sertraline and rosuvastatin. The authors deduced (from the drug interaction probability scale) that the rhabdomyolysis could have resulted from drug interactions between the dietary supplements, and the antidepressant or statin she was also using. Discontinuation of the treatments was associated with remission (Russo et al. 2016).

7.2 Therapeutic Potential of Nutraceuticals

The therapeutic potential of nutraceuticals is a globally recognized phenomenon. The prospect of deriving what goes beyond basic nourishments from foods is fascinating, and this is not only applicable to parts of the world where access to orthodox medicine is limited but it is also applicable to advanced nations and economies. Along this line, how nutraceuticals can be used alongside orthodox medications in the delivery of a total health and wellness package is currently receiving worldwide attention.

7.2.1 Nutraceuticals as Alternative or Add-on Therapies

In recent times, it will not be out of place to say that nutraceuticals are now being considered as viable options in the prevention and management of human diseases and disorders. In a number of human disorders, nutraceuticals are now being used as an add-on to conventional therapy. However, beyond this, nutraceuticals are also being considered as alternative therapies, especially in dealing with limitations occasioned by cost, availability, and possibly side effects.

Nutraceuticals that had been used and scientifically documented (by way of studies) in the management of human disorders include Lertal® which contains quercetin, perilla extract, and vitamin D_3 (agents that are known to exert antiallergic and anti-inflammatory activities), and was used in both adult and paediatric patients as an add-on for conventional antihistamines in the management of allergic rhinoconjunctivitis (Marseglia et al. 2020). The clinical study showed that Lertal® prevented clinical worsening and clinical exacerbations (Marseglia et al. 2020).

Also, in the management of atherosclerosis, a pathological condition that is rather challenging to manage despite advances in the development of pharmacotherapeutic agents, several nutraceuticals containing distinct classes of biomolecules such as polyunsaturated fatty acids, flavonoids, and other polyphenols had been shown to be of benefit in both clinical and experimental scenarios (Moss et al. 2018). Others include phytosterols (stigmasterol, beta-sitosterol, and campesterol), anthocyanins, stilbenes, tannins, octacosanol, serotonin, melatonin, and hesperidin which have been shown to prevent and alleviate vascular heart diseases including myocardial infarction, by modulating endothelial function in many instances (Golla 2018).

In neurodegenerative disorders such as Parkinson's disease (PD), Alzheimer's disease (AD), and Huntington's disease (HD), clinical trials have shown the profound neuroprotective effect of curcumin, resveratrol, Epigallocatechin-3-gallate (EGCG), Coenzyme Q10, and a number of ω-3 fatty acids; an effect that is attributable to mechanisms like antioxidation, anti-inflammation, maintenance of mitochondrial homeostasis, autophagy regulation, and promotion of neurogenesis (Chiu et al. 2020). This brings to light the potential benefits of using such nutraceuticals as add-on therapy to known neuroprotective agents in the management of such disorders, while also providing an essential solution in an aspect of therapy in which many pharmaceuticals have proven to be inadequate.

Diabetes mellitus is an endocrine disorder with systemic effects, and for which prevention and therapy have continued to be challenging despite advances in pharmacotherapy. Diabetes mellitus also happens to be one of the human disorders in which the benefits of several nutraceuticals continue to be demonstrated. A number of such nutraceuticals have been shown to target distinct aspects of the pathogenetic pathways of diabetes mellitus. Omega-3 fatty acids, phytoestrogens (isoflavones), cinnamon tea, green tea, antioxidant vitamins (vitamins C and E), vitamin D, flavonoids, conjugated linoleic acid, minerals (chromium and magnesium), and dietary fibers are among the list (Golla 2018). Mitigation of oxidative stress which is a crucial factor in the development of diabetes complications, reduction in the rate of absorption of dietary carbohydrates, improved glucose tolerance, and better body weight control are among the mechanisms of action of these nutraceuticals.

7.2.2 Nutraceuticals as Therapeutic Agents – Future Perspectives

The future holds a lot for the use of nutraceuticals as therapeutic agents. However, a lot of work needs to be done before we can get to the level where nutraceuticals can stand side by side with pharmaceuticals as options for disease prevention and management. One of the obstacles that must be overcome is to determine how much of an active constituent is found per unit mass of a nutraceutical. While this has been achieved with many packaged supplements, it is not easy to determine with food-based nutraceuticals. Also, it is believed that orthodox medical practice will continue to accept the use of nutraceuticals as long as research continues to make available data regarding safety and efficacy. Finally, we foresee that in the near future, our drugs and our foods will be contained in the same entity that is capable of bringing both sustenance and total wellness to the human body and mind.

References

Akbari, F., Ansari-Samani, R., Karimi, A. et al. (2013). Effect of turnip on glucose and lipid profiles of alloxan-induced diabetic rats. *Iran J. Endocrinol. Metab.* 14: 1–7.

Ali Hassan, S.H., Fry, J.R., and Abu Bakar, M.F. (2013). Phytochemicals content, antioxidant activity and acetylcholinesterase inhibition properties of indigenous Garcinia parvifolia fruit. *Biomed. Res. Int.* 2013: 138950. https://doi.org/10.1155/2013/138950.

Andrew, R. and Izzo, A.A. (2017). Principles of pharmacological research of nutraceuticals. *Br. J. Pharmacol.* 174 (11): 1177–1194. https://doi.org/10.1111/bph.13779.

Aqil, F., Munagala, R., Jeyabalan, J., and Vadhanam, M.V. (2013). Bioavailability of phytochemicals and its enhancement by drug delivery systems. *Cancer Lett.* 334 (1): 133–141. https://doi.org/10.1016/j.canlet.2013.02.032.

Aronson, J.K. (2017). Defining 'nutraceuticals': neither nutritious nor pharmaceutical. *Br. J. Clin. Pharmacol.* 83 (1): 8–19. https://doi.org/10.1111/bcp.12935.

Asai, M., Iwata, N., Yoshikawa, A. et al. (2006). Berberine alters the processing of Alzheimer's amyloid precursor protein to decrease Abeta secretion. *Biochem. Biophys. Res. Commun.* 352 (2): 498–502. https://doi.org/10.1016/j.bbrc.2006.11.043.

Brower, V. (1998). Nutraceuticals: poised for a healthy slice of the healthcare market? *Nat. Biotechnol.* 16 (8): 728–731.

Budisan, L., Gulei, D., Zanoaga, O.M. et al. (2017). Dietary intervention by phytochemicals and their role in modulating coding and non-coding genes in cancer. *Int. J. Mol. Sci.* 18 (6): 1178. https://doi.org/10.3390/ijms18061178.

Cabrera, C., Artacho, R., and Giménez, R. (2006). Beneficial effects of green tea – a review. *J. Am. Coll. Nutr.* 25: 79–99.

Cerezo-Guisado, M.I., Zur, R., Lorenzo, M.J. et al. (2015). Implication of Akt, ERK1/2 and alternative p38MAPK signalling pathways in human colon cancer cell apoptosis induced by green tea EGCG. *Food Chem. Toxicol.* 84: 125–132. https://doi.org/10.1016/j.fct.2015.08.017.

CFSAN: Center for Food Safety and Applied Nutrition (2020a). Dietary Supplement Products & Ingredients. U.S Food and Drug Administration Retrieved 2 July 2020.

CFSAN: Center for Food Safety and Applied Nutrition (2020b). Dietary Supplements. U.S Food and Drug Administration Retrieved 2 April 2020.

Chanda, S., Tiwari, R.K., Kumar, A., and Singh, K. (2019). Nutraceuticals Inspiring the current therapy for lifestyle diseases. *Adv. Pharmacol. Sci.* 2019 (1-5): 6908716. https://doi.org/10.1155/2019/6908716.

Chauhan, B., Kumar, G., Kalam, N., and Ansari, S.H. (2013). Current concepts and prospects of herbal nutraceutical: a review. *J. Adv. Pharm. Technol. Res.* 4 (1): 4–8.

Chiu, H.-F., Venkatakrishnan, K., and Wang, C.-K. (2020). The role of nutraceuticals as a complementary therapy against various neurodegenerative diseases: a mini-review. *J. Tradit. Complement. Med.* https://doi.org/10.1016/j.jtcme.2020.03.008.

Cicero, A.F., Tartagni, E., and Ertek, S. (2014). Nutraceuticals for metabolic syndrome management: from laboratory to benchside. *Curr. Vasc. Pharmacol.* 12 (4): 565–571. https://doi.org/10.2174/15701611113119990120.

Clark, R. and Lee, S.H. (2016). Anticancer properties of capsaicin against human cancer. *Anticancer Res.* 36 (3): 837–843.

Cojocneanu Petric, R., Braicu, C., Raduly, L. et al. (2015). Phytochemicals modulate carcinogenic signalling pathways in breast and hormone-related cancers. *Onco Targets Ther.* 8: 2053–2066. https://doi.org/10.2147/OTT.S83597.

Das, L., Bhaumik, E., Raychaudhuri, U., and Chakraborty, R. (2012). Role of nutraceuticals in human health. *J. Food Sci. Technol.* 49 (2): 173–183. https://doi.org/10.1007/s13197-011-0269-4.

Dayalan Naidu, S., Suzuki, T., Yamamoto, M. et al. (2018). Phenethyl Isothiocyanate, a dual activator of transcription factors NRF2 and HSF1. *Mol. Nutr. Food Res.* 62 (18): e1700908. https://doi.org/10.1002/mnfr.201700908.

de Kruijk, J.R. and Notermans, N.C. (2005). Gevoelsstoornissen veroorzaakt door multivitaminepreparaten [Sensory disturbances caused by multivitamin preparations]. *Ned. Tijdschr. Geneeskd.* 149 (46): 2541–2544.

Deb, G. and Gupta, S. (2015). Natural phytochemicals as epigenetic modulators. In: *Genomics, Proteomics and Metabolomics in Nutraceuticals and Functional Foods* (eds. D. Bagchi, A. Swaroop and M. Bagchi), 424–439. Hoboken, NJ: Wiley https://doi.org/10.1002/9781118930458.ch34.

Dima, C., Assadpour, E., and Dima, S. (2020). Bioavailability of nutraceuticals: role of the food matrix, processing conditions, the gastrointestinal tract, and nanodelivery systems. *Compr. Rev. Food Sci. Food Saf.* https://doi.org/10.1111/1541-4337.12547.

Directive 2002/46/EC (2002). Directive 2002/46/EC of the European Parliament and of the Council of 10 June 2002 on the approximation of the laws of the Member States relating to food supplements. Official Journal of the European Union: L136/85, 12 July 2002.

Drake, P.M., Szeto, T.H., Paul, M.J. et al. (2017). Recombinant biologic products versus nutraceuticals from plants – a regulatory choice? *Br. J. Clin. Pharmacol.* 83 (1): 82–87. https://doi.org/10.1111/bcp.13041.

Gan, R.Y., Li, H.B., Sui, Z.Q. et al. (2018). Absorption, metabolism, anti-cancer effect and molecular targets of epigallocatechin gallate (EGCG): an updated review. *Crit. Rev. Food Sci. Nutr.* 58: 924–941. https://doi.org/10.1080/10408398.2016.1231168.

Gao, S. and Hu, M. (2010). Bioavailability challenges associated with development of anti-cancer phenolics. *Mini-Rev. Med. Chem.* 10 (6): 550–567.

Golla, U. (2018). Emergence of nutraceuticals as the alternative medications for pharmaceuticals. *Int. J. Complement. Altern. Med.* 11 (3): 155–158. https://doi.org/10.15406/ijcam.2018.11.00388.

Liu, R.H. (2013). Dietary bioactive compounds and their health implications. *J. Food Sci.* 78 (Suppl 1): A18–A25. https://doi.org/10.1111/1750-3841.12101. PMID: 23789932.

Health Products and Food Branch (2020). The Natural and Non-prescription Health Products Directorate Health Canada. https://www.canada.ca/en/health-canada/ (Retrieved 2 July 2020).

Iwai, K., Kim, M.Y., Onodera, A. et al. (2006). α-Glucosidase inhibitory and antihyperglycemic effects of polyphenols in the fruit of *Viburnum dilatatum* Thunb. *Agric. Food Chem.* 54: 4588–4592.

Jurenka, J.S. (2009). Anti-inflammatory properties of curcumin, a major constituent of Curcuma longa: a review of preclinical and clinical research. *Altern. Med. Rev.* 14 (2): 141–153.

Kalra, E.K. (2003). Nutraceutical – definition and introduction. *AAPS PharmSci.* 5: E25.

Karimi, A., Moradi, M.T., Saeedi, M. et al. (2013). Antiviral activity of Quercus persica L.: high efficacy and low toxicity. *Adv. Biomed. Res.* 2: 36. https://doi.org/10.4103/2277-9175.109722.

Khosravi-Boroujeni, H., Mohammadifard, N., Sarrafzadegan, N. et al. (2012). Potato consumption and cardiovascular disease risk factors among Iraanian population. *Int. J. Food Sci. Nutr.* 63 (8): 913–920. https://doi.org/10.3109/09637486.2012.690024.

Khosravi-Boroujeni, H., Sarrafzadegan, N., Mohammadifard, N. et al. (2013). White rice consumption and CVD risk factors among Iranian population. *J. Health Popul. Nutr.* 31 (2): 252–261. https://doi.org/10.3329/jhpn.v31i2.16390.

Kulczyński, B., Sidor, A., and Gramza-Michałowska, A. (2019). Characteristics of selected Antioxidative and Bioactive compounds in meat and animal origin products. *Antioxidants (Basel)* 8 (9): 335.

Lipinski, C.A., Lombardo, F., Dominy, B.W. et al. (2001). Experimental and computational approaches to estimate solubility and permeability in drug discovery and development settings. *Adv. Drug Deliv. Rev.* 46 (1-3): 3–26. https://doi.org/10.1016/s0169-409x(00)00129-0.

Liu, M., Chen, F., Sha, L. et al. (2014). (-)-Epigallocatechin-3-gallate ameliorates learning and memory deficits by adjusting the balance of TrkA/p75NTR signaling in APP/PS1 transgenic mice. *Mol. Neurobiol.* 49 (3): 1350–1363. https://doi.org/10.1007/s12035-013-8608-2.

Maddi, V.S., Aragade, P.D., Digge, V.G., and Nitaliker, M.N. (2007). Importance of nutraceuticals in health management. *Pharmacol. Rev.* 1: 377–379.

Manach, C., Scalbert, A., Morand, C. et al. (2004). Polyphenols: food sources and bioavailability. *Am. J. Clin. Nutr.* 79 (5): 727–747.

Marseglia, G., Licari, A., and Ciprandi, G. (2020). Complementary treatment of allergic rhinoconjunctivitis: the role of the nutraceutical Lertal® Acta Biomedica. *Acta Biomed.* https://doi.org/10.23750/abm.v91i1.9275.

Martin, S., Andriambeloson, E., Takeda, K., and Andriantsitohaina, R. (2002). Red wine polyphenols increase calcium in bovine aortic endothelial cells: a basis to elucidate signalling pathways leading to nitric oxide production. *Br. J. Pharmacol.* 135 (6): 1579–1587. https://doi.org/10.1038/sj.bjp.0704603.

Mazzanti, G., Menniti-Ippolito, F., Moro, P.A. et al. (2009). Hepatotoxicity from green tea: a review of the literature and two unpublished cases. *Eur. J. Clin. Pharmacol.* 65 (4): 331–341. https://doi.org/10.1007/s00228-008-0610-7.

McClements, D.J., Li, F., and Xiao, H. (2015). The nutraceutical bioavailability classification scheme: classifying nutraceuticals according to factors limiting their oral bioavailability. *Annu. Rev. Food Sci. Technol.* 6: 299–327. https://doi.org/10.1146/annurev-food-032814-014043.

Melina, V., Craig, W., and Levin, S. (2016). Position of the academy of nutrition and dietetics: vegetarian diets. *J. Acad. Nutr. Diet.* 116 (12): 1970–1980. https://doi.org/10.1016/j.jand.2016.09.025.

Meštrović, T. (2018). Nutraceutical Regulation. News-Medical. https://www.news-medical.net/health/Nutraceutical-Regulation.aspx (Retrieved 8 July 2020).

Mollica, A., Zengin, G., Locatelli, M. et al. (2017b). Anti-diabetic and anti-hyperlipidemic properties of Capparis spinosa L.: in vivo and in vitro evaluation of its nutraceutical potential. *J. Funct. Foods* 35: 32. https://doi.org/10.1016/j.jff.2017.05.001.

Mollica, A., Zengin, G., Locatelli, M. et al. (2017a). An assessment of the nutraceutical potential of Juglans regia L. leaf powder in diabetic rats. *Food Chem. Toxicol.* 107: 554–564. https://doi.org/10.1016/j.fct.2017.03.056.

Mollica, A., Zengin, G., Stefanucci, A. et al. (2018). Nutraceutical potential of Corylus avellana daily supplements for obesity and related dysmetabolism. *J. Funct. Foods* 47: 562–574.

Moss, J.W.E., Williams, J.O., and Ramji, D.P. (2018). Nutraceuticals as therapeutic agents for atherosclerosis. *Biochim. Biophys. Acta (BBA) - Mol. Basis Dis.* 1864 (5): 1562–1572.

Nabavi, S.M., Russo, G.L., Tedesco, I. et al. (2018). Curcumin and Melanoma: from chemistry to medicine. *Nutr. Cancer* 70 (2): 164–175. https://doi.org/10.1080/01635581.2018.1412485.

Nasri, H., Baradaran, A., Shirzad, H., and Rafieian-Kopaei, M. (2014). New concepts in nutraceuticals as alternative for pharmaceuticals. *Int. J. Prev. Med.* 5 (12): 1487–1499.

Olofinnade, A.T., Onaolapo, T.M., Oladimeji, S. et al. (2020). An evaluation of the effects of Pyridoxal Phosphate in Chlorpromazine induced Parkinsonism using Mice. *Cent. Nerv. Syst. Agents Med. Chem.* 20 (1): 13–25. https://doi.org/10.2174/1871524920666200120142508.

Onaolapo, A.Y. and Onaolapo, O.J. (2012). Ocimum Gratissimum Linn causes dose dependent hepatotoxicity in streptozotocin-induced diabetic Wistar rats. *Macedonian J. Med. Sci.* 5: 17–25.

Onaolapo, A.Y. and Onaolapo, O.J. (2019). Nutraceuticals and diet-based phytochemicals in type 2 diabetes mellitus: from whole food to components with defined roles and mechanisms. *Curr. Diabetes Rev.* 216 (1): 12–25. https://doi.org/10.2174/1573399814666181031103930.

Onaolapo, A.Y., Abdusalam, S.Z., and Onaolapo, O.J. (2017d). Silymarin attenuates aspartame-induced variation in mouse behaviour, cerebrocortical morphology and oxidative stress markers. *Pathophysiology* 24 (2): 51–62. https://doi.org/10.1016/j.pathophys.2017.01.002.

Onaolapo, A.Y., Adebayo, A.N., and Onaolapo, O.J. (2017a). Exogenous daytime melatonin modulates response of adolescent mice in a repeated unpredictable stress paradigm. *Naunyn Schmiedeberg's Arch. Pharmacol.* 390 (2): 149–161. https://doi.org/10.1007/s00210-016-1314-7.

Onaolapo, A.Y., Adebisi, E.O., Adeleye, A.E. et al. (2020a). Dietary melatonin protects against behavioural, metabolic, oxidative, and organ morphological changes in Mice that are fed high-fat, high- sugar diet. *Endocr. Metab. Immune Disord. Drug Targets* 20 (4): 570–583. https://doi.org/10.217 4/1871530319666191009161228.

Onaolapo, A.Y., Aina, O.A., and Onaolapo, O.J. (2017b). Melatonin attenuates behavioural deficits and reduces brain oxidative stress in a rodent model of schizophrenia. *Biomed. Pharmacother.* 92: 373–383. https://doi.org/10.1016/j.biopha.2017.05.094.

Onaolapo, A.Y. and Onaolapo, O.J. (2020). African plants with antidiabetic potentials: beyond Glycaemic control to central nervous system benefits. *Curr. Diabetes Rev.* 16 (5): 419–437. https://doi.org/10.2174/1573399815666191106104941.

Onaolapo, A.Y., Obelawo, A.Y., and Onaolapo, O.J. (2019a). Brain ageing, cognition and diet: a review of the emerging roles of food-based nootropics in mitigating age-related memory decline. *Curr. Aging Sci.* 12 (1): 2–14. https://doi.org/10.2174/1874609812666190311160754.

Onaolapo, A.Y., Oladipo, B.P., and Onaolapo, O.J. (2018). Cyclophosphamide-induced male subfertility in mice: an assessment of the potential benefits of Maca supplement. *Andrologia* 50 (3) https://doi.org/10.1111/and.12911.

Onaolapo, A.Y. and Onaolapo, O.J. (2018c). Circadian dysrhythmia-linked diabetes mellitus: Examining melatonin's roles in prophylaxis and management. *World J. Diabetes* 9 (7): 99–114. https://doi.org/10.4239/wjd.v9.i7.99.

Onaolapo, A.Y., Onaolapo, O.J., and Adewole, S.O. (2012). Ocimum gratissimum linn worsens streptozotocin-induced nephrotoxicity in diabetic Wistar rats. *Macedonian J. Med. Sci.* 5: 382–388.

Onaolapo, A.Y., Onaolapo, O.J., and Adewole, S.O. (2011). Ethanolic extract of Ocimum grattissimum leaves (Linn.) rapidly lowers blood glucose levels in diabetic Wistar rats. *Macedonian J. Med. Sci.* 4: 351–357.

Onaolapo, O.J., Adekola, M.A., Azeez, T.O. et al. (2017c). l-Methionine and silymarin: a comparison of prophylactic protective capabilities in acetaminophen-induced injuries of the liver, kidney and cerebral cortex. *Biomed. Pharmacother.* 85: 323–333. https://doi.org/10.1016/j.biopha.2016.11.033.

Onaolapo, O.J., Ademakinwa, O.Q., Olalekan, T.O., and Onaolapo, A.Y. (2017e). Ketamine-induced behavioural and brain oxidative changes in mice: an assessment of possible beneficial effects of zinc as mono- or adjunct therapy. *Psychopharmacology* 234 (18): 2707–2725. https://doi.org/10.1007/s00213-017-4666-x.

Onaolapo, O.J., Jegede, O.R., Adegoke, O. et al. (2020b). Dietary zinc supplement militates against ketamine-induced behaviours by age-dependent modulation of oxidative stress and acetylcholinesterase activity in mice. *Pharmacol. Rep.* 72: 55–66. https://doi.org/10.1007/s43440-019-00003-2.

Onaolapo, O.J., Odeniyi, A.O., Jonathan, S.O. et al. (2019b). An investigation of the anti-Parkinsonism potential of co-enzyme Q10 and co-enzyme Q10 /levodopa-carbidopa combination in mice. *Curr. Aging Sci.* https://doi.org/10.2174/1874609812666191023153724.

Onaolapo, O.J. and Onaolapo, A.Y. (2018a). Melatonin in drug addiction and addiction management: exploring an evolving multidimensional relationship. *World J. Psychiatry* 8 (2): 64–74. https://doi.org/10.5498/wjp.v8.i2.64.

Rajasekaran, A. (2017). 1.05 Nutraceuticals. In: *Comprehensive Medicinal Chemistry III* (eds. S. Chackalamannil, D. Rotella and S.E. Ward), 107–134. Amsterdam: Elsevier, ISBN 9780128032015, doi: https://doi.org/10.1016/B978-0-12-409547-2.12287-5.

Ramirez, C.N., Li, W., Zhang, C. et al. (2017). in vitro-in vivo dose response of Ursolic Acid, Sulforaphane, PEITC, and curcumin in cancer prevention. *AAPS J.* 20 (1): 19. https://doi.org/10.1208/s12248-017-0177-2.

Raskin, I., Ribnicky, D.M., and Komarnytsky, S.a. (2002). Plants and human health in the twenty-first century. *Trends Biotechnol.* 20 (12): 522–531. https://doi.org/10.1016/s0167-7799(02)02080-2.

Ronis, M.J.J., Pedersen, K.B., and Watt, J. (2018). Adverse effects of nutraceuticals and dietary supplements. *Annu. Rev. Pharmacol. Toxicol.* 58: 583–601. https://doi.org/10.1146/annurev-pharmtox-010617-052844.

Russo, R., Gallelli, L., Cannataro, R. et al. (2016). When nutraceuticals reinforce drugs side effects: a case report. *Curr. Drug Saf.* 11 (3): 264–266. https://doi.org/10.2174/1574886311666160201152047.

Sánchez, M., Galisteo, M., Vera, R. et al. (2006). Quercetin downregulates NADPH oxidase, increases eNOS activity and prevents endothelial dysfunction in spontaneously hypertensive rats. *J. Hypertens.* 24 (1): 75–84. https://doi.org/10.1097/01.hjh.0000198029.22472.d9.

Santini, A., Cammarata, S.M., Capone, G. et al. (2018). Nutraceuticals: opening the debate for a regulatory framework. *Br. J. Clin. Pharmacol.* 84 (4): 659–672. https://doi.org/10.1111/bcp.13496.

Sayem, A.S.M., Arya, A., Karimian, H. et al. (2018). Action of phytochemicals on insulin signaling pathways accelerating glucose transporter (GLUT4) protein translocation. *Molecules* 23 (2): 258. https://doi.org/10.3390/molecules23020258.

Smith, A., Giunta, B., Bickford, P.C. et al. (2010). Nanolipidic particles improve the bioavailability and alpha-secretase inducing ability of epigallocatechin-3-gallate (EGCG) for the treatment of Alzheimer's disease. *Int. J. Pharm.* 389 (1-2): 207–212. https://doi.org/10.1016/j.ijpharm.2010.01.012.

Song, S., Huang, Y.W., Tian, Y. et al. (2014). Mechanism of action of (-)-epigallocatechin-3-gallate: auto-oxidation-dependent activation of extracellular signal-regulated kinase 1/2 in Jurkat cells. *Chin. J. Nat. Med.* 12 (9): 654–662. https://doi.org/10.1016/S1875-5364(14)60100-X.

Spagnuolo, P.A. (ed.) (2020). Nutraceuticals. In: *Nutraceuticals and Human Health: The Food-to-supplement Paradigm*, Food Chemistry, Function and Analysis, 1–6. Royal Society of Chemistry https://doi.org/10.1039/9781839160578-00001.

Sun, X., Chen, R.C., Yang, Z.H. et al. (2014). Taxifolin prevents diabetic cardiomyopathy in vivo and in vitro by inhibition of oxidative stress and cell apoptosis. *Food Chem. Toxicol.* 63: 221–232. https://doi.org/10.1016/j.fct.2013.11.013.

Swaroopa, G. and Srinath, D. (2017). Nutraceuticals and their health benefits. *Int. J. Pure Appl. Biosci.* 5 (4): 1151–1155.

Trottier, G., Boström, P.J., Lawrentschuk, N., and Fleshner, N.E. (2010). Nutraceuticals and prostate cancer prevention: a current review. *Nat. Rev. Urol.* 7 (1): 21–30.

Upadhyay, S. and Dixit, M. (2015). Role of polyphenols and other phytochemicals on molecular signaling. *Oxidative Med. Cell. Longev.* 2015: 504253. https://doi.org/10.1155/2015/504253.

Varzakas, T., Zakynthinos, G., and Verpoort, F. (2016). Plant food residues as a source of nutraceuticals and functional foods. *Foods.* 5 (4): 88. https://doi.org/10.3390/foods5040088.

Velmurugan, B.K., Rathinasamy, B., Lohanathan, B.P. et al. (2018). Neuroprotective role of phytochemicals. *Molecules* 23 (10): 2485. https://doi.org/10.3390/molecules23102485.

Venkatesan, R., Ji, E., and Kim, S.Y. (2015). Phytochemicals that regulate neurodegenerative disease by targeting neurotrophins: a comprehensive review. *Biomed. Res. Int.* 2015: 814068. https://doi.org/10.1155/2015/814068.

Yang, W., Guo, L., Li, F. et al. (2019). Hydrophobically modified Glucan as an Amphiphilic Carbohydrate polymer for micellar delivery of Myricetin. *Molecules* 24 (20): 3747. https://doi.org/10.3390/molecules24203747.

Yao, M., McClements, D.J., and Xiao, H. (2015). Improving oral bioavailability of nutraceuticals by engineered nanoparticle-based delivery systems. *Curr. Opin. Food Sci.* 2: 14–19.

Zeisel, S.H. (1999). Regulation of nutraceuticals. *Science* 285: 185–186.

Zhao, J. (2007). Nutraceuticals, nutritional therapy, phytonutrients, and phytotherapy for improvement of human health: a perspective on plant biotechnology application. *Recent Pat. Biotechnol.* 1 (1): 75–97. https://doi.org/10.2174/187220807779813893.

Ziegler, E.E. and Filer, L.J. Jr. (1996). *Present Knowledge in Nutrition*, 7e. International Life Sciences Institute-Nutrition Foundation.

8

Antioxidant Nutraceuticals as Novel Neuroprotective Agents

Parul Katiyar[1], Souvik Ghosh[1,2], Saakshi Saini[1], Chandrachur Ghosh[1], Himanshu Agrawal[1], Debabrata Sircar[2], and Partha Roy[1]

[1] Molecular Endocrinology Laboratory, Department of Biotechnology, Indian Institute of Technology Roorkee, Roorkee, Uttarakhand, India
[2] Plant Molecular Biology Laboratory, Department of Biotechnology, Indian Institute of Technology Roorkee, Roorkee, Uttarakhand, India

8.1 Introduction

Neurodegenerative disorders (NDDs) are one of the major health concerns which are growing aggressively on a global scale. These adverse conditions appear when the brain and the peripheral nervous system are affected by some abnormal physiological conditions of the body, leading to the loss of functionality and eventually death. Although the presently used therapeutics can minimize the associated symptoms, but there are no certain cures to prevent or even slow down the progression of these NDDs (NIEHS reports 2019).

Out of many possible causes, ROS generation lays the foundation for these neurological disorders to occur. It has been shown that the oxidative status of these disorders is significantly higher than the threshold level (Singh et al. 2019). This disruption in the balance between cellular oxidants and antioxidants is effective enough for the nervous system to bring about neuronal lethality, as the neurons and other neuronal regions are extremely sensitive to the factors like oxidative status, inflammation, and glucose homeostasis (Ritter 2017; Salim 2017).

Antioxidants are the molecules, natural or artificial, which reduce the production of free radicals caused by oxidative stress. Oxidation of various biomolecules can lead to severe damage of the normal physiological condition and eventually death. Thus, maintaining the concentration of antioxidants within the physiological system is mandatory as oxygen can act as both friend and foe. The shift of this balance toward free radical production results in "oxidative stress," which is one of the main gateways of different pathophysiological conditions like cancer, atherosclerosis, neurological disorder, and diabetes (Birben et al. 2012). The endogenous oxidants, also called ROS, can be classified into two groups – free radicals and nonradicals. Free radicals are the molecules that possess one or more unpaired electrons and thus are always unstable in nature, while the nonradical form of the ROS is produced when such two free radicals share their electrons (Phaniendra et al. 2015). Among the different types, endogenous ROS, hydrogen peroxide (H_2O_2), superoxide anion (O_2^-), and hydroxyl radical ($\bullet OH$) are of special significance.

Nevertheless, the antioxidants, also known as free radical scavengers, counterbalance the deleterious effects of the oxidants or quench the formation of free radicals. The biological antioxidants are of two categories, one of them is enzymatic antioxidants which include superoxide dismutase (SOD), catalase, glutathione (GSH), thioredoxin (TRX), glutathione transferase (GST). The other one is nonenzymatic antioxidants which include the examples like uric acid, ascorbic acid, vitamin A, lipoic acid, and coenzyme Q (Poljsak et al. 2013).

As mentioned earlier, oxygen has both positive and negative roles in organismal survival. Being a beneficial agent, it oxidizes the reduced substrates by accepting electrons from them which results in the reduction of the diatomic oxygen into the water. In contrast, the negative impact of the oxygen renders in its outer orbitals. The uniformity in the spin states of both the outer orbital electrons keeps this diatomic molecule stable, except for in the presence of some transition metals like manganese, iron, nickel, copper, etc., which disorganize the electron spin states and lead to the production of partially reduced form of oxygen or ROS (Turrens 2003; Poyton et al. 2009).

In the biological systems, the mitochondrial respiratory chain is one of the main sources of intracellular ROS generation. Among the four complexes of this respiratory chain, complexes I and III are mainly responsible for the generation of O_2^-. In complex III, the auto-oxidation of ubisemiquinone (QH), a quinone-radical intermediate of the Q cycle, results in the formation of O_2^-. Coenzyme III releases O_2^- in the intermembrane space as well as in the matrix, while O_2^- produced from the coenzyme I is released only into the matrix (Han et al. 2003). The O_2^-, produced in this way, can also be converted into H_2O_2 by the action of Copper-Zinc-Superoxide Dismutase (CuZnSOD) (also called SOD1) and Manganese-Superoxide Dismutase (MnSOD) (also called SOD2), present in the intermembrane space and matrix of the mitochondria, respectively. In the cytosol, H_2O_2 can produce the hydroxyl radicals ($\cdot$OH) and hydroxyl anions (OH^-) by the involvement of some transition metals, through a reaction called "Fenton reaction" (Munro and Treberg 2017).

Neurodegenerative diseases are the abnormal condition that involves substantial damage of certain parts of the brain including neurons. In these conditions, some major regulating proteins undergo aberrant glycosylation resulting in the formation of dysfunctional proteins. The deposition of these abnormal proteins shows alteration in the physiochemical properties of the brain and peripheral nervous systems (Gitler et al. 2017). According to the World Health Organization's (WHO) report, due to neurological disorders, almost 6.8 million people die every year and across the world, more than one billion people are affected (WHO report 2016).

In a broader view, neurological disorders indicate multiple pathophysiological conditions, each of them having a different etiology. These disorders include Alzheimer's disease (AD), Parkinson's disease (PD), Huntington's disease (HD), Amyotrophic lateral sclerosis (ALS), and Spinocerebellar ataxia (SA). Among these, AD and PD are the most common neurological disorders worldwide. AD is characterized by the deposition of extracellular β-amyloid as the neuritic plaques. The patients with AD have been shown to have a distinct neuropathological profile consisting of hyperphosphorylated Tau proteins and neurofibrillary tangles (NFTs) (Polanco et al. 2018; Long and Holtzman 2019). After AD, PD is the second most common neurological disorder which affects almost 60% of adults globally. It involves bradykinesia (slow movement), tremor (involuntary twitching movements of body parts), and rigidity. The main pathological condition includes the deposition of abnormal α-synuclein proteins (often called Lewis body) in the midbrain and the dopaminergic neurons of the substantia nigra pars compacta (SNc) (Poewe et al. 2017; McGregor and Nelson 2019). Conversely, being an inherited autosomal disorder, HD has a rare prevalence status with an average age of 40 years for the onset of the disease. The etiological reason for this neurological disorder is an aberrant addition of a flexible poly-Gln (polyglutamine) chain in the N-terminal end of the huntingtin (HTT) protein which causes the protein to adopt a different shape and, ultimately, leads to aggregation (Saudou and Humbert 2016).

Though all the aforementioned disorders have different etiological reasons, they all share a common remarkable cellular condition, that is, they manifest a high level of oxidation state as their main pathogenic factor (Díaz-Hung and Fraguela 2014). The central nervous system (CNS), especially neurons and the glia, is more susceptible to oxidative stress due to some factors like an abundance of polyunsaturated fatty acids (which can be rapidly oxidized by the oxygen derivatives), lack of antioxidant mechanism, and limitation of the vitamin E (a well-known antioxidant) to cross the blood–brain barrier. Besides, the lack of the histones and the poor repair system leave the mtDNA of the CNS unprotected from the mutation and aid the oxidative stress to take place (Shukla et al. 2011). Therefore, the CNS is highly sensitive to its oxidation state and a small shift of the balance between the oxidants and antioxidants can lead to the onset of different neurological disorders.

Nutraceuticals (nutrition + pharmaceuticals) are the products that are obtained from any food sources and have additional medicinal values other than basal nutritional values which demonstrate protective roles against different chronic diseases. The nutraceutical theory is actually built upon the concept of the Greek physician Hippocrates – "Let food be your medicine" (Chauhan et al. 2013; Nasri et al. 2014). These nutraceutical products include three broad segments – natural products, dietary supplements, and functional foods which generally have several categories like alkaloids, carotenoids, flavonoids, phenolics, vitamins, probiotics, prebiotics, and melatonin. There are reports which have shown that these nutraceuticals are beneficial for health and keep diseases at bay (Cui et al. 2004; Jain and Ramawat 2013). Among various phytochemicals, epicatechin-3-gallate, quercetin and myricetin (known flavonoids) are reported to inhibit β-amyloid and tau aggregation and xanthone, another flavonoid, is known to scavenge the ROS (Ansari et al. 2009; Ayaz et al. 2019). Among phenolics, gastrodin B, and gastrol B are shown to have significant protective efficacy against the ROS-induced damage in PC12 cells (Kumar et al. 2013; Zhang et al. 2013). As a result, currently, nutraceuticals have gained considerable interest due to their therapeutic potentials, minimum side effects, and abundance in nature.

Therefore, preventing the generation of oxidative stress is one of the best possible ways to combat the onset of neurological disorders. In the following section, we will discuss the pathophysiology of neurodegenerative diseases, the role of the antioxidants in preventing these disorders, and the applications of various nutraceuticals (as the alternative of the presently used therapeutics) for regulating the progression of these diseases.

8.2 Pathophysiological Effects of Oxidative Stress on Neurodegenerative Diseases

Oxidative stress is caused by an escalated production of ROS in cells. Reactive forms of oxygen are required in the body to a certain extent, beyond which it may cause significant damage to cells. Oxidative stress may lead to damage of cellular lipids, proteins as well as DNA. In the following section, we enumerate the patterns of synthesis of ROS, the effect of oxidative stress in the brain and associated NDDs, which, ultimately, disrupts normal brain functions.

8.2.1 Synthesis of Reactive Oxygen Species (ROS)

Oxygen is one of the most important factors of life. It is a prerequisite for eukaryotic organisms for their normal functioning. The fact that it is a potential oxidizing agent with high redox potential and able to accept electrons exquisitely from reduced substances makes it highly significant for the survival of organisms. Oxygen demands for different tissues and organs depend upon their metabolic functions and requirements. Oxidative stress is a significant factor concerning cellular functions. Oxidative stress refers to the mismatch in the ratio of production of free radicals and the defense of cells against it (Halliwell 2006). The free radicals are produced if the production of free radicals increases or if scavenging of free radicals decreases or if both take place simultaneously. The consequence of this imbalance lies in a higher number of oxidatively modified molecules which might cause several dysfunctions in normal cellular pathways like postmitotic neuronal cell deaths (Coyle and Puttfarcken 1993). ROS – the term collectively involves all reactive forms of oxygen. It includes all the species – both radical and nonradical forms – that take part in initiation and/or extension of radical chain reactions. ROS are responsible for oxidative stress in cells as they possess the ability to damage lipids, proteins as well as DNA (Droge 2002). Oxygen having two unpaired electrons in the outermost shell (Held 2015) is, thereby, prone to radical formation. ROS are transient but extremely reactive due to unpaired electrons in the valence shell (Patten et al. 2010). ROS includes radicals O_2^-, $\cdot OH$, and nonradicals like H_2O_2 (Gandhi and Abramov 2012; Bolisetty and Jaimes 2013). ROS are formed by the consecutive addition of electrons in the electron transport chain while molecular oxygen gets reduced into water. The chemical reactions involved in it are as explained in Table 8.1.

O_2^- plays a pivotal role in the formation of ROS. It may be converted to a more stable form, i.e. H_2O_2 by SOD, or it may be transformed into HO_2^- by protonation. H_2O_2 might have the ability to produce highly active hydroxyl radicals, i.e. $\cdot OH$ (Bolisetty and Jaimes 2013), and broken down further into H_2O and O_2 by glutathione peroxidase, catalase, or other peroxidases (Song and Zou 2015). Hydroxyl radicals confer maximum cytotoxic effects among ROS as it is one of the most reactive classes of chemicals (Bolisetty and Jaimes 2013). It may be produced from H_2O_2 and O_2^- through Haber–Weiss reaction and catalyzed by ferrous ions (Fe^{3+}) through the Fenton reaction, i.e. Fe^{2+}-mediated decomposition of H_2O_2 (Zorov et al. 2014) (Table 8.1).

8.2.2 Impacts of ROS at the Cellular Level

ROS have a significant role in cellular functioning, but if these are produced beyond a threshold, these may turn into a toxic product and disrupt the normal functioning of cells. Excess ROS in brain cells can cause oxidative stress and, thereby, may lead to neurodegenerative complications. The human brain is vulnerable to ROS stress to a great extent, causing several brain-related problems.

Table 8.1 Formation of ROS by reduction of molecular oxygen in the electron transport chain.

S. No.	Reactions	Products
1.	$O_2 + e^- + H^+$	Hydroperoxyl radical (HO_2)
2.	HO_2	Superoxide radical ($H^+ + O_2^-$)
3.	$2H^+ + O_2^- + e^-$	Hydrogen peroxide (H_2O_2)
4.	$H_2O_2 + e^-$	Hydroxyl radical ($\cdot OH$)
5.	$OH + e^- + H^+$	Water (H_2O)
6.	$O_2^- + H_2O_2$	$OH^- + OH + O_2$ (Haber–Weiss reaction)
7.	$Fe^{2+} + H_2O_2$	$OH^- + OH + Fe^{3+}$ (Fenton reaction)

8.2.2.1 ROS and Oxidative Stress

As a consequence of high reactivity, ROS level, if increased in the cells beyond normal cellular requirements, causes structural and functional disintegration of the latter. In spite of the fact that cells possess multiple and a variety of coping mechanisms against the mighty ROSs, they may still run out of ways to defend against the ROS, leading to oxidative stress, if they surpass the antioxidant defense. There are implications of both chronic and acute oxidative stresses in multiple diseases, mostly degenerative in nature, where these ROSs affect the normal physiological functioning of the cells. Such diseases are – atherosclerosis, inflammatory diseases (e.g. rheumatoid arthritis, pancreatitis, and inflammatory bowel disease), neurological diseases, ischemia/reperfusion (I/R) injury, cancer, diabetes, hypertension, pulmonary diseases, ocular diseases like cataract, retrolental fibroplasia, and hematological diseases (Robles 2013; Patel 2016; Asmat et al. 2016; Yang et al. 2017; Dogru et al. 2018; Boukhenouna et al. 2018; Rubattu et al. 2019; Soares et al. 2019; Dasari et al. 2020; Touyz et al. 2020).

8.2.2.2 Vulnerability of the Brain to Oxidative Stress

The human brain is a complex structure made of nerve cells, nerve fibers, and a bulky lipid portion. It weighs only ~1400 g and consumes ~20% of the basal O_2 ravenously to meet the needs of ~86 billion neurons that it possesses and also the intricately complicated interconnections, i.e. trillions of synapses (Mink et al. 1981; Goyal et al. 2014; Magistretti and Allaman 2015) along with ~250–300 billions of glial cells (Araque et al. 1999; Nedergaard et al. 2003). The effect of oxidative stress upon neurodegeneration still has ambiguities because a number of reasons concerning its susceptibility to oxidative stress are still unknown. There are several findings that suggest that our brain might be distinctly vulnerable to oxidative stress (Halliwell 2001; Murphy et al. 2011). Some of these are as explained below.

i) The brain is only 2% of the body weight, but it consumes 1/5th of the total oxygen inspired to produce a substantial amount of adenosine triphosphate (ATP) at an elevated rate. About 5% of the total oxygen that is consumed by the brain reduces to ROS. This actually confers that copious amounts of ROS might be generated in the brain contrary to tissues with lesser oxygen demands, relatively.

ii) The presence of high concentrations of PUFAs in the brain, having an explicit inclination toward ROS-induced injury.

iii) In cerebrospinal fluid, the presence of small molecular weight Cu and Fe complexes catalyzes ROS synthesis.

iv) A slightly overlooked explanation of the brain's susceptibility toward oxidative stress is that these ROSs play significant roles in biological functioning, e.g. reduced nicotinamide adenine dinucleotide phosphate (NADPH) oxidase-derived H_2O_2 which is involved in normal brain and retinal neuron development.

v) In presynaptic terminals, action potential generates a substantial Ca^{2+} flux, which triggers exocytosis of neuronal vesicles (Zucker 1999). It also controls bidirectional synaptic plasticity (Wheeler et al. 1993) which is a fundamental function of the brain and is concerned with learning and memory (Kim and Linden 2007; Ganguly and Poo 2013). Excessive reliance of the brain over the Ca^{2+} signaling (Carafoli and Krebs 2016) may lead to oxidative stress, thus negatively affecting the brain.

vi) The release of excitatory neurotransmitters, e.g. glutamate, causes the initiation of a cascade of reactions in the post-synaptic neuron which, ultimately, leads to the production of ROS. Glutamate excitotoxicity causes Ca^{2+} overload and mitochondrial release of O_2^-/H_2O_2 which is associated with cell death, typically via necrosis and apoptosis (Halliwell 1992; Coyle and Puttfarcken 1993; Reynolds and Hastings 1995).

vii) Endogenous amine-related neurotransmitter, e.g. dopamine metabolism produces mitochondrial H_2O_2 by monoamine oxidases (MOA). MOA-A and MOA-B catalyze deamination: Amine $+ O_2 + H_2O \rightarrow$ Aldehyde $+ H_2O_2 + NH_3$.

viii) The intercommunication of nitric oxide (NO) and superoxide radical concerns not only with normal development of neurons, but also with degeneration. NO is an endothelium-derived relaxing factor generated in cells of endothelium and nerve by virtue of nitric oxide synthase (NOS) enzyme. This enzyme, which is triggered by calmodulin, is substantially present all over the brain.

ix) The brain does not contain glutathione reductase, catalase, and vitamin E, as extensively as the liver.

x) ROS is liberated during the oxidation of dopamine with the help of MOA which might lead to increased oxidative stress in the brain. This occurs in dopaminergic neuronal terminals.

xi) Pineal gland-secreted melatonin is a potent ROS scavenger. However, its production is eventually decreased as a person grows old.

8.2.3 Oxidative Stress and Neurodegenerative Disorders

Oxidative stress and neurodegeneration are intricately connected. Oxidative stress confers a large number of neurodegenerative diseases which cause severe disruption of cognition, motor function, and normal brain function. Here we discussed some of the major neurodegenerative diseases that are triggered by oxidative stress.

8.2.3.1 Oxidative Stress and Alzheimer's Disease (AD)

AD is one of the most prevailing forms of neurodegeneration which are designated by escalated loss of normal behavior, cognition as well as normal brain function (Zuo et al. 2015b). Pathophysiology of this very disease concerns amyloid-beta (Aβ) plaques accumulation in extracellular region and progressive storage of intracellular NFT (Butterfield 2014; Querfurth and Laferla 2018). Aβ plaques possess the ability to deplete calcium ion storage in the endoplasmic reticulum as a consequence of which cytosolic overload of calcium occurs. Due to this increase in cytosolic Ca^{2+}, endogenous glutathione levels get reduced and ROS gets accumulated inside cells (Ferreiro et al. 2008). Oxidative stress induced by ROS is found to be a significant factor controlling AD pathogenesis because of overproduction of ROS, which is conceived to be a crucial factor regarding the deposition of Aβ protein in AD (Bonda et al. 2010) (Figure 8.1).

Dysfunction of mitochondria can lead to disruption in the regulation of ROS and decreased yield of ATP, defective calcium homeostasis, thereby leading to excitotoxicity. The aforementioned

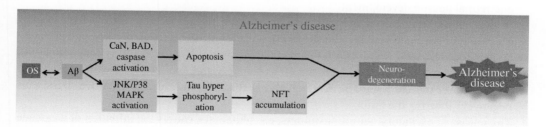

Figure 8.1 Schematic diagram representing the major roles of OS in the development of Alzheimer's disease. OS, oxidative stress; Aβ, amyloid-beta; CaN, calcineurin; BAD, Bcl-2-associated death promoter; JNK, c-Jun N-terminal kinase; MAPK, mitogen-activated protein kinase; NFT: neurofibrillary tangle.

variations may be related to the progression of AD (Moreira et al. 2007). Severe oxidative stress, recorded in AD patients, can be considered as a consequence of overactivating N-methyl-D-aspartate-type glutamate receptors (NMDARs). This NMDAR activation is observed to cause substantial Ca^{2+} influx by inducing permeability as well as ROS/reactive nitrogen species (RNS) production at neurotoxic levels (Nakamura and Lipton 2010; Nakamura and Lipton 2011). ROS is conceived to play a significant part in the activation of JNK/protein pathways mediated by stress and activation of this cascade is found to be involved in tau proteins hyperphosphorylation along with cell death induced by Aβ-protein (Patten et al. 2010). Furthermore, Aβ-proteins induce the formation of free radicals directly by NADPH oxidase activation (Shelat et al. 2008). Overproduction of ROS, induced by Aβ-plaques, alters cell signaling pathways. It also activates mitogen-activated protein kinase (MAPK) induced by p38 and, thereby, begins hyperphosphorylation of tau protein. When hyperphosphorylated tau protein aggregation reaches beyond a certain limit, it causes NFT formation (Bulat and Widmann 2009; Giraldo et al. 2014) (Figure 8.1). Moreover, Aβ proteins play a significant role concerning the regulation of apoptosis (Agostinho et al. 2008). Aβ protein may cause enhanced calcineurin action, which consequently sets off Bcl-2-associated death promoter, thus finally bringing about the release of mitochondrial cytochrome C (Awasthi et al. 2005). Also, direct association of Aβ with caspases triggers neuronal apoptosis (Awasthi et al. 2005) (Figure 8.1). Various factors such as, environmental stress, aging, inflammation, and selective nutritional factors like metals that are redox-active promote supplemental production of ROS causing the enhanced formation of Aβ-plaques (Block 2008; Smith et al. 2010; Hamilton and Holscher 2012; Aseervatham et al. 2013). Aged people have increased proneness to oxidative stress; precisely that is the reason why they are more prone to AD (Hamilton and Holscher 2012).

8.2.3.2 Oxidative Stress and Huntington's Disease (HD)

HD is a type of neurodegeneration concerning the increase of cytosine, adenine, guanine (CAG) repeats within the HTT gene, thus making it unstable (Labbadia and Morimoto 2013; Gil-Mohapel et al. 2014). The aggregation of mutated HTT in the entire brain of diseased individual causes interruption in the process of protein quality control and transcription. These modifications account for the cognitive and aberrant motor problems in HD patients (Labbadia and Morimoto 2013). Exploring how HD affects the energy levels of the brain is a broad field of research. While initial research found HD to lower energy levels due to a decrease in utilization of glucose as well as an enhanced level of lactate (Mochel et al. 2011; Covarrubias-Pinto et al. 2015) but the recent studies showed that oxidative damage leads to reduced glucose transporter (GLUT-3) expression, which further hinders uptake of glucose, thereby causing lactate accumulation (Reagan et al. 2000; Covarrubias-Pinto et al. 2015) (Figure 8.2). ATP synthesis is mostly driven by a proton motive force in the electron transport chain (Bonora et al. 2015). Mutated HTT plays a pivotal role regarding mitochondrial abnormalities. Using electron microscopy, it was shown by Panov et al. that N-terminal end of mutated HTT showed a cross-talk with mitochondrial membranes, thus leading to Ca^{2+}-related complications of mitochondria. Mutated HTT directly inhibits respiratory complex II (Panov et al. 2002; Bossy-Wetzel et al. 2008). Hindrances in mitochondrial ETC leads to a higher amount of ROS production along with reduced production of ATP (Lin and Beal 2006; Bossy-Wetzel et al. 2008). A novel mechanism of mitochondrial impairment suggested that oxidative stress might inactivate glyceraldehyde-3- phosphate dehydrogenase (GAPDH) catalytic activity. Inactive GAPDH concerns with impaired mitochondria along with acting like a signaling molecule to trigger the dysfunctional mitochondria for engulfment by lysosome and selective degradation. In HD, inactive GAPDH interacts at the outer membrane of mitochondria, with extended polyglutamine of mutated HTT and hinders the inactive GAPDH

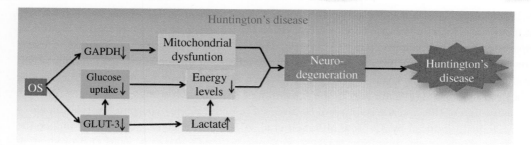

Figure 8.2 Schematic diagram representing the major roles of OS in the development of Huntington's disease. OS, oxidative stress; GAPDH, glyceraldehyde-3-phosphate dehydrogenase; GLUT-3, Glucose transporter 3.

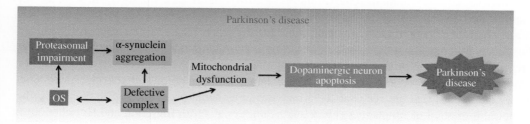

Figure 8.3 Schematic diagram representing the major roles of OS in the development of Parkinson's disease. OS, oxidative stress.

signaling. As a consequence, impaired mitochondria fail to undergo lysosomal breakdown and deposits in cells expressing mutated HTT, which eventually causes cellular death (Liot et al. 2017) (Figure 8.2). Mitochondrial alterations along with ROS induce positive feedback loops, thus leading to more oxidative stress along with loss of neuronal cells in the cortex and striatum (Gil-Mohapel et al. 2014).

8.2.3.3 Oxidative Stress and Parkinson's Disease (PD)

PD is one of the most prevalent diseases concerning neurodegeneration which is designated by loss of neurons in substantia nigra pars compacta in the brain (McCormack et al. 2002; Qin et al. 2017; Deng et al. 2018). The pathophysiology of degenerating dopaminergic neurons is correlated to overaccumulation of ROS. In the brain, ROS-generating sites are primarily mitochondria of glia and neurons (Dias et al. 2013). This free-radical generation is amplified in this very disease because of neuroinflammation, mitochondrial dysfunction, GSH depletion, dopamine degradation, aging along with high Ca^{2+} levels (Dias et al. 2013; Meiser et al. 2013). ROS has been observed to significantly increase dopaminergic neuronal loss (Dias et al. 2013; Meiser et al. 2013) (Figure 8.3). Certain other studies showed that dopaminergic neuron loss might also be concerned with neuromelanin presence as neurons that are heavily pigmented are more prone to impairment (Perfeito et al. 2012). Neuromelanin generation corresponds to dopamine auto-oxidation, which is promoted by the overproduction of ROS (Perfeito et al. 2012). Dysfunction of mitochondria leads to increased synthesis of free radicals in the electron transport chain (Dias et al. 2013). Especially, respiratory complex I inadequacy is mainly involved in PD. This corresponds to PTEN-induced putative kinase 1 (PINK1) mutations as well. This protein which is globally expressed in all human tissues plays a significant role to defend oxidative stress along with the maintenance of membrane potential of mitochondria (Zuo and Motherwell 2013; Valente et al. 2016). PINK1 mutation is associated with the onset of PD (Zuo and Motherwell 2013). Along with PINK1, additional mutations also confer toward the development of PD like DJ-1, parkin, leucine-rich repeat kinase 2 (LRRK2), and α-synuclein. The aforementioned alterations disrupt stable mitochondrial functions, thus leading to excessive generation of ROS and increased oxidative stress susceptibility. The accumulation of α-synuclein interferes in the activity of the respiratory complex, thus leading to compromised ATP synthesis along with mitochondrial abnormal functioning (Ganguly et al. 2017). There are several mechanisms accounting for the deposition of α-synuclein including reduced protein degradation efficiency due to abnormalities in proteasomes along with translation and post-translation-related protein overexpression (Ganguly et al. 2017). Proteasomal deterioration has been reported to be caused by dopamine-derived ROS, which acts as a key effector in neurodegeneration in PD (Ganguly et al. 2017) (Figure 8.3).

8.2.3.4 Oxidative Stress and Amyotrophic Lateral Sclerosis (ALS)

ALS is designated by progressive loss of motor neurons in the anterior horn of the spinal cord (Kiernan et al. 2011; Taylor et al. 2016). The disease is characterized as either sporadic or familial with respect to the presence of a specific genetic element with Sporadic ALS (sALS) specifically emerging between 50 and 60 years of age (Ingre et al. 2015). The factor that influences the initiation of this disease is still unknown since the responsible environmental cues and recognition of causative genes still remain elusive. According to some earlier report, ~20% of the familial ALS cases emerge due to SOD1 mutations (Gamez et al. 2006). SOD1 mutations have divergent functions including scavenging extensive O_2^-, regulating metabolism, cellular respiration, and post-translational modifications (Saccon et al. 2013). Though dysfunction of SOD leads to reduced antioxidant ability, there is evidence that neurodegeneration is not caused by genetic ablation (Hensley et al. 2006; Zuo et al. 2015a). An observation by Bastow et al. in the yeast model showed that the SOD1 mutants can disrupt amino acid biosynthesis of cells and cause disruption of cell function, thus leading to neurodegeneration in ALS (Bastow et al. 2016) (Figure 8.4). SOD1 mutant confers to familial ALS propagation by deregulating signal transduction cascade in motor neurons as well as in glial cell function (Li et al. 2011; Lee et al. 2016). SOD1 expresses in cells besides motor neurons as well (Lee et al. 2016). Mutant SOD1 modifies microglia and astrocyte activities, thus resulting in degeneration of motor neuron and this is designated as the non-cell-autonomous pathway (Lee et al. 2016).

This intercommunication between motor neurons and astrocytes can be scrutinized by using co-culture models, thereby culturing embryonic stem cell-derived or primary neurons in the presence of mutant SOD1 expressing astrocytes. According to an earlier report, a co-culture of normal motor neurons and motor neurons earlier treated with specific cell culture media from

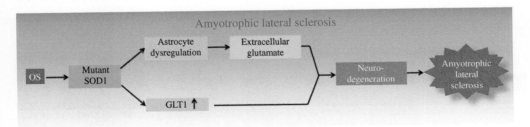

Figure 8.4 Schematic diagram representing the major roles of OS in the development of Amyotrophic lateral sclerosis. OS, oxidative stress; GLT1, Glutamate transporter-1.

mutant SOD1 expressing astrocytes, both the former and latter motor neurons were found to be experiencing increased cell damage (Nagai et al. 2007). Moreover, in motor neurons, the mutant SOD1 expressing astrocytes decreases glutamate receptor (GLT1) expression which eventually results in an enhanced concentration of glutamate in extracellular space as well as glutamate toxicity (Foran et al. 2011; Li et al. 2015) (Figure 8.4).

8.2.3.5 Oxidative Stress and Spinocerebellar Ataxia (SCA)

SCA, identified by escalated neurodegeneration, is autosomal dominant in nature. Symptoms regarding this very disease are commonly ataxic gait, dysarthria, oculomotor disorders, and cognitive impairment which ultimately may lead to death. Over 20 types of SCAs have already been characterized depending upon genetic make-up (Manto 2005; Rossi et al. 2013; Sun et al. 2016). In SCA, expanded CAG trinucleotides confer to the preliminary mutation that is responsible for pathogenesis (Manto 2005), resulting in overexpressing ataxin1 (ATXN1) mutant protein which contains an expanded polyglutamine tract. Stabilization of RAR-related orphan receptor alpha (RORα) that is conceived to play a pivotal role in Purkinje cell functioning is influenced by ATXN 1 mutant. Reduced RORα expression concerns cerebellar hypoplasia and ataxia (Zoghbi and Orr 2009; Stucki et al. 2016). As noticed by Hakonen et al. deficiency of respiratory complex I and depleting mitochondrial DNA are observed in infantile-onset SCA patients' brain (Hakonen et al. 2008). Despite reduced ROS concentration, interfering in cell signaling, ROS overaccumulation, can cause neurodegeneration because of its neurotoxic essence (Zuo et al. 2015a).

Elevated oxidative stress and salient modulations in mitochondria of Purkinje cells were observed in SCA1 by Stucki et al. (2016). They reckoned a potential interconnection between SCA progression and impairments of mitochondria which, oxidative stress brings about (Stucki et al. 2016) (Figure 8.5). The study also screened the effects of MitoQ which is an antioxidant residing in mitochondria by the virtue of an SCA mouse model. Administration of MitoQ for long-term consequently re-establishes the morphology of mitochondria and functions in Purkinje cells along with mitigating features related to SCA1, e.g. incoordination of motor activity (Stucki et al. 2016).

8.3 Classification of Nutraceuticals

On the basis of their food sources, nutraceuticals can be divided into two categories, viz. phytochemicals and non-phytochemicals, which, in turn, are subcategorized into distinct groups (Figure 8.6). Phytochemicals are nutraceuticals which are mainly derived from plant sources, whereas non-phytochemicals are derived from sources other than plants, like microbes, seafood

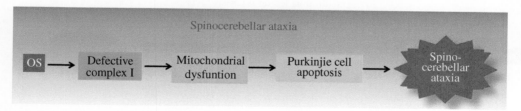

Figure 8.5 Schematic diagram representing the major roles of OS in the development of Spinocerebellar ataxia. OS, oxidative stress.

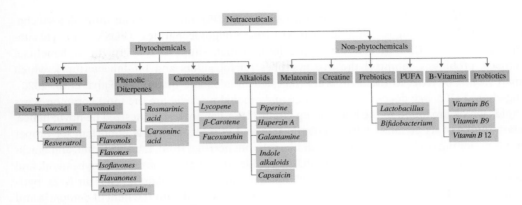

Figure 8.6 Classification of nutraceuticals.

and livestock (Aruoma et al. 2003; Al-Alawi and Laleye 2008; Kim and Dewapriya 2012; Ashraf et al. 2020). The phytochemicals have been divided into several groups on the basis of their chemical structures like alkaloids, flavonoid polyphenols, non-flavonoid polyphenols, carotenoids, diterpenes, phenolic acids, and others. Alkaloid forms a wide class of phytochemicals whose structures contain carbon (C), oxygen (O), hydrogen (H), and nitrogen (N). Alkaloids are especially derived from flowering plants belonging to Solanaceae, Papaveraceae, Ranunculaceae, and Amaryllidaceae families (Hussain et al. 2018).

Compounds belonging to the carotenoid family are generally fat-soluble pigments that possess strong antioxidant properties. Oxygenated carotenoids such as lutein, β-cryptoxanthin, and zeaxanthin comprise 66–77% of the total carotenoids in the human brain and assist in cognitive functioning. Green leafy vegetables like kale and spinach, corn, zucchini, red and orange peppers, and oranges are the major sources of natural carotenoids. It is envisaged that AD patients might have lower levels of xanthophylls (oxygenated carotenoids) in their dietary intakes (Wang et al. 2008). The flavonoid polyphenols consist of six subgroups that share a common structure. Each flavonoid polyphenol contains two aromatic rings, designated as A and B, which are connected to each other through a heterocyclic ring, designated as C. Flavonols are widely present flavonoids, which are mainly present in onions, leeks, curly kale, blueberries, red wine, tea, and broccoli. Important sources of flavones are celery and parsley. The highest concentrations of flavanones are found in citrus fruits, followed by mint and tomato. Isoflavones are structurally similar to estrogen, which gives them pseudo-hormonal properties. Leguminous plants are the exclusive sources of isoflavones and soya products form an important source of isoflavones in the human diet. Flavanols like catechins are found in green tea and fruits like apricots. Anthocyanidins are the naturally occurring pigments that are mostly found in berries (Manach et al. 2004). Phenolic diterpenes are another important class of phytochemical nutraceuticals. The most common forms of phenolic diterpenes are carnosic acid and rosmarinic acid, which are extracted from rosemary plants (Kelsey et al. 2010). The antioxidant properties of these compounds are imparted by two catechol structures ($-C_6H_6O_2$) conjugated with a carboxylic acid group (–RCOOH) (Del Bano et al. 2003).

In addition to phytochemicals, non-phytochemicals like prebiotics, probiotics, polyunsaturated fatty acid (PUFA), Vitamin B complex, melatonin, and creatine also form an important class of nutraceuticals. Prebiotics are nondigestible carbohydrates or selectively fermented compounds that promote the growth of friendly bacteria like lactobacillus and bifidobacteria in our gut and exert anti-inflammatory and anxiolytic properties (Paiva et al. 2020). Prebiotics are mostly carbohydrates, like mannan-oligosaccharides (MOS), inulin, human milk oligosaccharides (HMO), xylo-oligosaccharides (XOS), fructo-oligosaccharides (FOS), and galacto-oligosaccharides (GOS). In contrast to prebiotics which supports the growth of beneficial microbes, probiotics comprise the live microbes (lactobacillus and bifidobacterium), which impart health benefits to the host, when ingested in adequate quantities (Paiva et al. 2020). Long-chain PUFA like docosahexaenoic acid and arachidonic acid are the most common types of lipids which are found in the brain. Long-chain PUFA cannot be synthesized de novo; hence, dietary intake of its precursors like linolenic acid and α-linolenic acid is important for proper brain functioning (Eckert et al. 2013). Fish like salmon, herring, trout, albacore tuna, and mackerel are important sources of long-chain PUFA. Besides fish, walnut, flex seeds, soybean oil, and sunflower seeds are also rich sources of PUFA. Vitamins like cobalamin (vitamin B12), pyridoxin (vitamin B6), and folate (vitamin B9) are mostly associated with the field of dementia and cognitive decline (Sun et al. 2007). Cobalamin deficiency leads to digestive disorders which, in turn, result in neurological disorders in adults. Vitamin B6 consists of three distinct chemical groups, namely pyridoxal, pyridoxine, and pyridoxamine, which are important in the regulation of the mood and mental functioning of an individual. Vitamin B6 is mainly obtained through the dietary intake of meats, pork, whole grains, legumes, cereals, and green leafy vegetables. Folate is recommended especially for pregnant females to reduce the chances of neural defects in the fetus (Bellows and Moore 2012). Dietary sources of folate include dark green leafy vegetables, fish, meat, some whole grains, legumes, cereals, and citrus fruits. Vitamin B12 is important for neural system maintenance and is mainly obtained from non-vegan diet like liver, kidney, meats, fish, oysters, eggs, shellfish, milk, and milk products (Bellows and Moore 2012). Creatine is an organic acid consisting of nitrogen and is produced de novo in all vertebrates. Red meat is a major source of creatine, which is also produced by the pancreas, liver, and kidney (Toler 1997). Melatonin or *N*-acetyl-5-methoxy tryptamine occurs naturally in the pineal glands of humans and was first extracted from the bovine pineal gland. Fish and eggs are the rich sources of melatonin found in animals. Besides animals, melatonin is found in cereals (rice and corn), fruits (grapes, strawberries, and cherries), nuts (pistachio and others), yeast (*Saccharomyces cerevisiae*), medicinal herbs, juices, and legumes (Meng et al. 2017).

8.4 Potential Antioxidant Activity of Nutraceuticals in Neuroprotection

"Nutraceutical" is a combined term of pharmaceuticals associated with the food from the natural reservoirs with potent therapeutic properties. The most studied categories of nutraceuticals are dietary components from various sources that possess high nutritional value with antioxidant properties. The antioxidant properties of these dietary components are attributed to their micronutrient composition. Mitochondria, the primary site for the energy production in a cell, is also a site prone to the generation of various free radicals, HO_2, $O_2 + e^- + H^+$, H_2O_2, and the development of oxidative stress. In neuronal cells, the repetitive generation of oxidative stress leads to the accumulation of ROS, which causes inflammatory damage to the vital cellular organelles and leads to NDDs (Fiedor and Burda 2014; Guo et al. 2018). The diverse components of dietary items act in a synergistic manner to execute the neuroprotective effects. In this section, we have elaborated the previously classified nutraceuticals of Table 8.2 for their role in the amelioration of oxidative stress in the neurons, which have drawn an impact on the clinical methodology for neurological diseases.

Table 8.2 List of some nutraceuticals and their mechanism of action.

S. No.	Compound	Source	Target pathways/activities	References
1.	**Creatine**	Fish and Red meat	Activation of PI3K/Akt/GSK3β.	Toler (1997), Cunha et al. (2014)
2.	***Flavonoid polyphenols***			
	EGCG	Green tea	Improves the Nrf2/HO-1 (antioxidant pathway) and suppresses NF-κB/JNK/MAPK signaling pathway and reduces cell death.	Kelsey et al. (2010), Chiu et al. (2020)
	Quercetin	Capers and apples	Enhances memory and motor function.	Kelsey et al. (2010)
	Kaempferol	Broccoli, vegetables	Activation of Nrf2/HO1 signaling pathway.	Velagapudi et al. (2019)
3.	***Non-flavonoid polyphenols***			
	Resveratrol	Berries, red grapes, peanut, red cherries and pomegranate.	Improves the Nrf2/HO-1 and PI3K/Akt signaling pathway and NF-κB, increases SIRT-1 activity and suppresses JNK/MAPK signaling pathway.	Kelsey (2010), Chiu et al. (2020), Dey et al. (2020)
	Curcumin	*Curcumin longa*	Inhibits NF-κB, TLR4/RAGE, JNK, ERK, and MAPK (p38) signaling pathway.	Kelsey (2010), Chiu et al. (2020)
	Phenolic acids	Sea-weeds, cereals, fruits.	Enhances Nrf2/ARE pathway.	Schepers et al. (2020)
	Diterpenes	Rosemary.	Enhances Nrf-2 pathway.	Dey et al. (2020)
4.	Coenzyme Q 10 (A ubiquinone)	Organ meat, fatty fish, broccoli, and cauliflower	Improves the Nrf2/HO-1 (ARE) signaling pathway; suppresses NF-κB signaling pathway.	Chiu et al. (2020)
5.	PUFA	Sardines, salmon, (fatty fishes), flaxseed, walnuts, and algae.	Inactivates microglia/astrocytes via JNK and PPAR-γ signaling pathway.	Eckert et al. (2013), Cotas et al. (2020)
6.	Lycopene (Carotenoid)	Red fruits and vegetables.	Enhances Nrf2/HO-1 signaling pathway.	Lei et al. (2016), Lama et al. (2020)
7.	Vitamin B12 (Coumarin class)	Fish, meat, eggs, and milk.	Inhibits endoplasmic reticulum stress signaling pathway.	Wu et al. (2019)
8.	Melatonin	Eggs and meat	Antioxidant property through activation of Nrf2/ARE pathway; restore the functioning of mitochondria by activating SIRT1 signaling pathway.	Meng et al. (2017)
9.	**Alkaloids**			
	Capsaicin	Capsicum sp. (chilli)	Suppresses convulsions and inhibits tau hyperphosphorylation; enhances memory.	Dey et al. (2020)
	Piperine	Long pepper (*Piper longum* L.) and Black pepper (*Piper nigrum* L.	Increases BDNF and displays antioxidant property; decreases lipid peroxidation.	Dey et al. (2020)

8.4.1 Alkaloids

Alkaloids are well-studied plant phytochemicals that contain amino acid with a nitrogen group exerting neuroprotective effects. Alkaloids act as congenital disease modifiers or modulators of numerous molecular markers that regulate complex neurological disorders (Dey and Mukherjee 2018). In the ancient era, alkaloids were used extensively for various therapeutic purposes as has been reported in many pharmacopeias depending on the isolation method of bioactive components. Galantamine, an alkaloid-based pharmaceutical, is commercially available for the treatment of mild-to-moderate AD.

8.4.1.1 Indole Alkaloids

Indole alkaloids are extracted massively from fungi especially from *Ascomycota*. Indole alkaloids consist of nitrogen lone pair in its indole ring. As the study reveals, the indole alkaloids group acts as a prominent inhibitor of acetylcholinesterase. The indole alkaloid interacts with the positively charged nitrogen atom present in the active catalytic site of the cholinesterase enzyme leading to its inhibition. It has been reported that the progression of AD in patients is slowed down by indole alkaloids *Psychotrialaciniata* (augustine, lactone) by blocking the active site of esterase enzyme of acetylcholine receptor (Fadaeinasab et al. 2015). Several types of alkaloids exist in natural products and have been reported to exert neuroprotective activities.

Uncaria hook is one of the medicinal plants used in Chinese herbal medicine and contains majorly isorhynchophylline alkaloid. Isorhynchophylline obstructs the intracellular calcium release, thereby protecting the brain from glutamate-induced cytotoxicity. Isorhynchophylline also exhibits protective effects against ischemia-induced neuronal cell death. In addition, this phytochemical has also been reported to display an inhibitory role against inflammatory molecules like TNF-α, NO, and IL-1β. Thus, it is implied that isorhynchophylline is a potent neuroprotectant (Wu et al. 2020).

8.4.1.2 Huperzine A

Huperzine A, extracted from *Huperzia serrate*, is extensively used in Chinese medicine for the treatment of patients suffering from AD. Several studies suggested that Huperzine A acts as a neuroprotective alkaloid by inhibiting the activity of acetylcholinesterase in a similar mode of action like donepezil and galantamine (Hussain et al. 2018). It regulates apoptosis in AD patients by inhibiting the alpha subunit of the acetylcholine receptor. The bioavailability of Huperzine is more potent in the form of oral dosing and can easily cross the blood–brain barrier. According to a recent study, Huperzine A inhibits the Aβ accumulation by cleaving amyloid precursor protein via the Wnt/β-catenin signaling pathway in the transgenic mice (Dey and Mukherjee 2018).

8.4.1.3 Aloperine

Aloperine is a quinolizidine alkaloid with a neuroprotective property. The neuroprotective effects of aloperine have been established in an AD's cellular model and in primary cultured rat neurons from the hippocampal region against oxygen–glucose deficiency (Zhao et al. 2018). It has been observed that aloperine restores the cellular level of enzyme cofactor GSH and antioxidant enzyme glutathione peroxidase, simultaneously reducing the level of free radicals to maintain mitochondrial membrane potential. Additionally, aloperine protects the rat brain from lipid peroxidation-led ischemic injury and improves cerebral blood flow (Ma et al. 2015).

8.4.1.4 Alstonine

Alstonine, a key antipsychotic indoloquinolizidine alkaloid extracted from *Picralima nitida*, is known to control the psychotic behavior in adult albino mice (Linck et al. 2011). Alstonine is an anxiolytic compound affecting the response to the light/dark cycle in mice by modulating 5-hydroxytryptamine (5-HT) receptors. Alstonine protects the hippocampal neurons from glutamate toxicity by reducing the uptake of glutamate via boosting glutathione peroxidase activity (Herrmann et al. 2012). Alstonine also helps in the uptake of dopamine through dopamine receptor to employ the antipsychotic activity in two-month-old albino mice (Linck et al. 2011) and also regulate schizophrenia (de Moura Linck et al. 2008).

8.4.1.5 Berberine

Berberine is a member of the isoquinoline class and used frequently in Indian traditional medicine for the treatment of various ailments. In a study, berberine has been established as an efficient compound for protecting the neurons from neurodegenerative and neuropsychiatric disorders (Kulkarni and Dhir 2008). According to several studies, it has been found that berberine has a significant role in hippocampal neuron protection by reducing the activity of β-secretase activity. Moreover, in combination with other extracts from *C. rhizome*, the uptake and bioavailability of berberine to neurons have been found to be enhanced, which increased its efficacy (Wang et al. 2005b; Lu et al. 2015). In a study based on the AD transgenic TgCRND8 mouse model, berberine exerted neuroprotective activity against Aβ toxicity-induced oxidative stress by regulating the level of glycogen synthase kinase-3 (GSK-3). Additionally, it reduces the amyloid precursor protein (APP) aggregation and its hyperphosphorylation via activation of AKT/GSK-3 pathway (Durairajan et al. 2012). Berberine also protects the dopaminergic neurons from damage generated due to oxidative stress in PD (Hussain et al. 2018). It also enhances motor activity and short-term memory formation by regulating the apoptosis process against 1-methyl-4-phenyl-1,2 ,3,6-tetrahydropyridine (MPTP) toxicity in PD mice (Kim et al. 2014). The progression of HD involves the disruption of the autophagy process due to the generation of increased oxidative stress and neuroinflammation leading to neurodegeneration. Berberine helps in the clearance of misfolded protein by restoring the autophagy process and further improving the motor and cognition function of neurons (Jiang et al. 2015). Further, berberine has also been confirmed to rejuvenate the rat neurons from inflammation, which has occurred due to excessive free radical generation. The free radical generation involves the nuclear factor E2-related factor 2 (NRF-2) which activates the PI3K/AKT pathway by upregulation of heme oxygenase-1 (HO-1). In a clinical study, involving the 60–70 years' age population, it has been established that berberine delayed the onset of ALS, a familial inherited disorder that involves loss of scavenging property due to over 100 different mutations in SOD1 enzyme. According to an earlier report, berberine protects primary neuron culture from energy loss through the AMP-activated protein kinase (AMPK) pathway, recovering the mitochondria and endoplasmic reticulum from dysfunction and stress (Liu et al. 2015).

8.4.1.6 Capsaicin

Capsaicin is a plant alkaloid present in the chilli pepper plants belonging to the *Capsicum* genus (Family Solanaceae). Capsaicin regulates hippocampal plasticity through anxiolytic activity. It alleviates the rat brain from long-term potentiation in the dentate gyrus, spatial memory loss, and increased synapsin-I activity caused by cold water stress, and protects the neurons from tau hyperphosphorylation. This is achieved by hindering the suppressive activity of phosphatase 2A protein (Jiang et al. 2013). Furthermore, capsaicin prevents apoptosis in the primary rat neurons in the hippocampal region by reducing oxidative stress concerning PI3K/AKT signaling pathway (Guo et al. 2008), and also protects from acute ischemic stroke (Turner and Vink 2014).

8.4.1.7 Galantamine

Galantamine is a potential antioxidant compound isolated from various plants. It is a class of tertiary alkaloid phytochemical that belongs to the class of cholinesterase inhibitors and is naturally found in *Galanthusnivalis* (snowdrop), *Leucojumaestivum* (snowflake), and *Narcissus tazetta* (daffodil). This phytochemical has the potential to stimulate nicotinic receptors that enhance memory and cognition (Pearson 2001). Galantine modulates the acetylcholine receptor activity by regulating the allosteric-binding site of the receptor. Galantamine also inhibits the esterase activity of acetylcholine in the pathogenesis of AD and protects the neurons from glutamate toxicity by monitoring the *N*-Methyl-D-aspartate (NMDA) receptor. Furthermore, galantamine protects cultured rat neurons from Aβ aggregation which is caused due to oxidative stress in the cortical region of the brain (Melo et al. 2009). It also improves memory and cognition from the dopaminergic neurons and provides protection from damage against Aβ by enhancing the circulatory dopamine level (Wang et al. 2007). It has been reported that even a low dose of galantamine protects neurons from DNA damage and slows down the progression of hypoxia-ischemia condition in newborn rats via regulating the microglia movement and inflammation (Furukawa et al. 2014). Galantamine also protects the rat hippocampal neurons from ROS and promotes neurogenesis (Egea et al. 2012).

8.4.1.8 Piperine

Piperine is a principal constituent isolated from black pepper and exerts a diverse role in phytochemical-based therapies as an antitumor, anti-inflammatory, and anti-anxiolytic molecule. Piperine prevents the neurons from oxidative stress and also acts as an antidepressant. This alkaloid is extracted from *Piper longum* L. (long pepper) and *Piper nigrum* L. (black pepper), and has been observed to increase brain-derived neurotropic factor (BDNF) and antioxidant levels as well as decreased lipid peroxidation and acetylcholinesterase levels in the brain (Chonpathompikunlert et al. 2010; Mao et al. 2012). Numerous studies have suggested that even low doses of piperine could form the memory in the hippocampal region by improving neuronal thickness and progressing neurogenesis. Furthermore, a combination of piperine with quercetin improves neuroprotection and reduces the effect of oxidative stress and prevents memory loss in patients suffering from AD (Hussain et al. 2018). In another study involving the PD rat model, the level of proinflammatory cytokine level was downregulated in the presence of piperine, confirming its antioxidant property. It has also been reported in vitro study based on PC12 cells that piperine successfully enhances the mRNA expression of brain-derived neurotrophic factor (BDNF) (Mao et al. 2012). The brain-derived BDNF-mRNA expression was enhanced by using piperine against oxidative stress-induced neurotoxicity in PC12 cells (Mao et al. 2012). Moreover, in another in vivo study, it has been established that piperine, as a promising neuroprotective and antioxidant phytochemical, protects the young albino mice from autism and also regulates the Na^+ channel in case of epilepsy (Mishra et al. 2015).

8.4.2 Carotenoids

Carotenoids are predominantly present in algae, fungi, and plants as yellow, orange, or red-colored fat-soluble pigments with a C40 linear carbon chain. It is massively utilized as food products and plays an important role in maintaining the antioxidant machinery in animals and plants. Carotenoids are distributed into two major groups based on their polar and nonpolar nature: polar xanthophyll (lutein, zeaxanthin, and β-cryptoxanthin) and nonpolar carotene (lycopene, α-carotene, and β-carotene). Since animals are unable to synthesize carotenoids, they consume various dietary items such as fruits, vegetables, and seafood to accomplish the requirement of carotenoids (Cho et al. 2018). It has been reported that 16 different forms of carotenoids in *cis* and *trans* forms are present in the human brain which protect it from oxidative stress and prevent the onset of neurological disorders. Another study revealed that lycopene protects the AD mouse model from oxidative stress-led mitochondrial damage and regulates the inflammatory response expression. Several studies have suggested that lycopene improves the cognitive performance against the tau transgenic AD mouse model. Even a low level of lycopene can protect the brain from dopamine-related degeneration in the neurons in the case of a PD mouse model. Due to the potential antioxidant activity of lycopene, a combined treatment with epigallocatechin gallate (EGCG) and also with quercetin successfully downregulated the oxidative stress generated by 3-nitropropionic acid in the HD mouse model. The lycopene protects DNA fragmentation in human neurons and β-cryptoxanthin prevents external damage due to H_2O_2-persuaded injury (Wang et al. 2012). The addition of carotenoids in the supplementary diets of the patients suffering from ALS also resulted in the delay in the progression of ALS (Nieves et al. 2016). Carotenoids have also been reported to prevent neuro-inflammation in the rat brain by downregulating the nuclear factor kappa B (NF-κB) signaling pathway preventing the development of oxidative stress (Liu et al. 2017).

8.4.3 Flavonoid Polyphenols

Flavonoid polyphenols possess diverse therapeutic property toward neuroprotection. Flavonoids exist in various plants as glycoside derivatives. Various studies suggested that flavonoid-rich diets enrich the human brain and protected it from oxidative stress and other disorders like diabetes mellitus, cancer, and cardiovascular diseases. The antioxidant property of flavonoids is accredited to their low redox potential due to which they successfully form the stable radicals with ROS-generating free radicles (Gutierrez-Merino et al. 2011; Chung et al. 2016). EGCG, present in green tea, cocoa, and many other dietary items, is a widely studied flavonoid with neuroprotective activity against various neurological disorders. The glyoxalase pathway has been recognized as a vital pathway for the maintenance of neuroprotection. A detailed description of the neuroprotective role of various flavonoids is given in the following section.

8.4.3.1 Flavanols

Flavanol-rich fruits are efficient for relieving the neurons from oxidative stress, facilitating spatial memory formation, and improving cognitive behavior in mice with mental discrepancy. Lipopolysaccharides (LPS)-induced JAK/STAT3 pathway in glial cells generates the neuronal injury in the brain, which is effectively recovered by using citrus flavanol (Naringenin). Naringenin successfully reduces the production of NO and other inflammatory signals (Lau et al. 2007). Moreover, cocoa is a common flavanol-rich dietary item. Cocoa contains various amino acid-like tyrosine, and phenylalanine, which synergistically reduces the oxidative stress, promotes neurogenesis, and generates changes in the neurons belonging to the region involved in learning and memory. In human and rat brains, epicatechin and catechin are potent antioxidants that cross the blood–brain barrier. Epicatechin is more prominently present in the brain and improves the different facets of cognition in animals and humans (Nehlig 2013). EGCG has been suggested as a potent therapeutic active compound for the treatment of different neurological disorders.

8.4.3.2 Flavonols

Flavonols are a class of flavonoids having –OH in the different positions in the building block, the phytochemicals representing their structural diversity in the group found in fruits, vegetables, fruits, tea, and coffee. The well-studied flavonols are quercetin, myricetin, and kaempferol predominantly found in fruits and vegetables and tea-persisting antioxidative property, and also quercetin and myricetin can block the aggregation of tau tangles and Aβ (Ansari et al. 2009). Myricetin predominantly extracted from berries, tea, nuts, and wine possessing medicinal values as an antidiabetic, anticancer, anti-inflammatory, and potent antioxidant.

8.4.3.2.1 Quercetin Quercetin flavonoid is copiously found in dietary supplements like green veggies, fruits, tea, and beverages. It is observed that it forms a complex with other moieties such as sugar alcohol, and phenolic acid and used enormously in in vitro, in vivo, and clinical studies. Quercetin acts as a free radical scavenger and prevents the toxicity caused by hydrogen peroxide as established in the in vitro study based on glioma cells C6 cell line and adrenal gland PC12 cell line (Chen et al. 2006). In the case of the PD human model, SH-SY5Y neuroblastoma cell line, quercetin recovered the cell's encounter to 6-ODHA toxicity and also improved memory and cognition. Quercetin regulates the memory formation in the hippocampal region and maintains the plasticity of neurons against chronic ischemic trauma in vivo mice model (Kelsey et al. 2010). According to the study, quercetin reduced oxidative stress via nuclear factor erythroid 2–related factor 2 (NRF-2)-associated c-Jun N-terminal kinase (JNK) and extracellular-signal-regulated kinase (ERK) signaling pathways.

8.4.3.2.2 Kaempferol Kaempferol is a dietary phytochemical abundantly present in beverages, and vegetables such as broccoli, apple, and berries. It possesses medicinal property for curing various ailments. In various studies, it is observed that kaempferol enhances the memory and cognition activities in response to H_2O_2-induced oxidative stress (Hong et al. 2009). Kaempferol has been suggested to reduce the aggregation of Aβ by strongly inhibiting the β-subunit activity of β-secretase 1 (BACE1) enzyme in AD condition. The activity of the acetylcholinesterase enzyme in AD is downregulated by kaempferol through competitively binding to the enzyme. The analogue of kaempferol has been reported to inhibit neuroinflammation via activation of 5′ AMP-activated protein kinase (AMPK) and NRF2/HO1 signaling pathway (Velagapudi et al. 2019).

8.4.3.3 Flavones

The main flavone compounds are luteolin and apigenin, predominantly available in wheatgrass, rose merry, and various small herbs. It has been widely reported that flavones prevent the DNA damage generated in response to oxidative stress and inflammation. The copper-mediated toxicity generated in neuronal cells causes Aβ aggregation, leading to AD. Apigenin prevents this toxicity by balancing the mitochondrial potential and preventing the generation of free radicals. Apigenin also modulates the GABAnergic and glutamate receptor toxicity as observed in cultured rat cortical brain (Losi et al. 2004; Mecocci et al. 2014).

8.4.3.4 Isoflavones

Isoflavones are abundantly present in various dietary supplements like soybeans and nuts. Genistein, soy isoflavone, and folic acid together have been reported to generate the neuroprotective effect on learning and memory in the AD rat model (Ma et al. 2014). β-Estrogen is essential for long-term memory formation, which is agonized by isoflavones of estrogen in the brain (Lee et al. 2004). Due to the catalytic property of the enzyme, several derivatives of isoflavones are synthesized that perform as potent antioxidant agents (Wang et al. 2005a).

8.4.3.5 Anthocyanidin

Anthocyanidin is a coloring flavonoid group present in a rare cationic form abundantly found in berries like raspberry, blueberry, cranberry, and strawberry. Berries are useful in maintaining DNA integrity, enhancing the brain's memory and cognitive behavior. The antioxidant, anti-inflammatory property of berries is due to the presence of a high amount of anthocyanidin (Harnly et al. 2006). Anthocyanidin promotes neurogenesis in the cerebral, hippocampal, and cortex regions of the brain and supports progression in memory. In the AD animal model associated with Aβ toxicity, the diseased state is reduced in presence of berries. Anthocyanidin has been reported to regulate the expression of the BDNF/CREB-linked JNK pathway showing significant effect in memory and neuronal plasticity. Furthermore, studies suggest that the intake of berries is a potential dietary item that can be promoted with nutraceutical values for preventing neurodegeneration (Mecocci et al. 2014).

8.4.3.6 Flavanones

Flavanones are 15-carbon backbone of flavonoid-possessing ROS-scavenging property due to the functional phenyl ring that can easily cross the blood–brain barrier. SH-SY5Y cells are an efficient model to evaluate the neuroprotective efficacy of flavanones against NRF2/HO1 toxicity (Hwang et al. 2008). Citrus fruits, oranges, lemon, and grapefruit are rich in flavanone and the metabolically active constituents are hesperidin and neohesperidin that play an essential role in reducing oxidative stress in neurons. In a recent study, biologically active flavanones recovered the mitochondrial damage in AD disease models (Habtemariam 2019). Moreover, 6-hydroxydopamine (6-ODHA) toxicity in the cultured rat neurons in the PD model was also protected by naringenin flavanones.

8.4.4 Non-Flavonoid Polyphenols

Curcumin and resveratrol are widely used in Indian medicines from ancient time to treat individuals with various neurological disorders like neuroinflammation and depression. On the basis of studies separately reported by Kelsey and Mecocci, in the below section, we have elaborated the role of nonflavonoid polyphenols in neuroprotection (Kelsey et al. 2010; Mecocci et al. 2014).

8.4.4.1 Resveratrol

Resveratrol is predominantly found in dietary supplements like grapes, berries, peanuts, and cherries, which are a polyphenol shared with the phytoalexin family. It has been observed that resveratrol is an efficient antioxidant agent to persuade the neurons to dopamine synthesis by reducing the oxidative stress caused by 6-ODHA-induced toxicity in the PD rat model (Kelsey et al. 2010). Resveratrol efficiently enhances the serotonin in the hippocampal region of rat by blocking 5-HT uptake and inhibits noradrenalin activity (Xu et al. 2010). It has been established that resveratrol plays an important role in protecting the brain from H_2O_2-induced toxicity, inflammation, and oxidative stress. According to the studies, resveratrol protects the embryonic rat brain from oxygen deprivation and matrix-metalloprotease activity (Chiu et al. 2020). Furthermore, it maintains the blood–brain barrier integrity and ameliorates the inflammation due to antioxidative property via regulating MAPK/JNK pathway (Moussa et al. 2017). It has been reported that Sirtuin 1 (SIRT1) is restrained by resveratrol through the process of autophagy in order to reduce ER and mitochondrial stress and endorse neurogenesis. Additionally, the antioxidant property of resveratrol helps in protecting the neurons from the aggregation of tau tangles, Aβ protein, and amyloidogenesis, and further enhancing cognition (Gomes et al. 2018).

8.4.4.2 Curcumin

Curcumin is extensively used in Indian medicines from ancient times for its medicinal values against various diseases. Curcumin is a robust therapeutic compound as an anti-inflammatory, anticancer, antimicrobial, and extraordinary neuroprotective agent. However, the high metabolic activity and a lower rate of absorption of curcumin limits its potency for neuroprotection. It has been reported that curcumin protects neurons from damage via regulating the MAPK/ERK/JNK pathway by inhibiting NF-κB in order to suppress the microglial cells and astrocyte activation (Limanaqi et al. 2019). Additionally, curcumin restores the macrophage's autophagy process via regulating SIRT1/mTOR pathway resulting in delaying the onset of AD and neuro-inflammation (Tiwari et al. 2014). It has been established that curcumin is the most prominent compound for the antioxidant activity in mouse Neuro2A cells against Japanese encephalitis virus that results in the reduction of ROS generation, inhibition of pro-apoptosis and, ultimately, leading to cell survival (Dutta et al. 2009). Furthermore, recently a clinical trial was performed in AD patients by administrating curcumin and it was found to reduce the disease's progression rate and enhance cognitive function (Chiu et al. 2020).

8.4.5 Phenolic Acid and Diterpenes

Rosmarinic acid and carnosic acid are two biologically proficient antioxidant nutraceutical agents belonging to the category of phenolic acid and diterpenes, which are present abundantly in rosemary herbs. These two phytochemicals act as reactive nitrogen scavengers and also inhibit ROS production in the neurons (Del Bano et al. 2003). in vitro study based on SH-SY5Y cells has reported that rosmarinic acid prevents the H_2O_2-induced toxicity, which basically occurs due to the generation of oxidative-free radicals (Kelsey et al. 2010). It has also been reported that rosmarinic acid and carnosic acid efficiently inhibit Aβ aggregation in the AD mouse models. Numerous in vivo studies have proposed that rosmarinic acid considerably slows the disease progression rate in the AD and ALS mouse models, and also in SOD1-induced mouse, which generally leads to Aβ aggregation and memory loss. Additionally, carnosic acid protects the neurons from mitochondrial damage and oxidative stress by activating the NRF2 pathway (Satoh et al. 2008; Taram et al. 2018). It has been established that both rosmarinic acid and carnosic acid can easily cross the blood–brain barrier, and protect the brain from cerebral ischemia injury generated due to oxidative stress. These phytochemicals also restore the reduced glutathione level as studied in in vivo mouse model (Kelsey et al. 2010).

8.4.6 Probiotics

Probiotics are a group of microorganisms that are claimed to be healthy and are used as bacteria-based dietary supplements applicable as medicinal constituents. It has been reported that the relationship between gut microbes and the brain is a bidirectional process, thus concerning both the gut and central nervous system, it solely depends on the diet of an individual. The dietary habit of a person can alter the gut microbiota, ultimately leading to the permeable gut, which generates inflammatory cytokines. The bacterial participants of the gut microbiota and the produced proinflammatory cytokines may release into the blood circulation, and lead to the progression of PD. The whole process results in the loss of dopaminergic neuron and generation of the symptoms, such as depression, motor defect, tremor, and rigidity. A clinical study has established that the transplantation of microbiota and stem cells slows down the PD progression and also reduces the ROS generation. Recently, the most advanced probiotic formulation, SLAB51, was examined in the AD mouse model. The studies confirmed a decline in Aβ clump and protected the brain from ROS-induced toxicity through activation of the SIRT1 pathway. Furthermore, in another study, the administration of SLAB51 reportedly resulted in an improvement in the neuroprotection by upregulation of neuroprotective markers like BDNF, cAMP-response element-binding protein (CREB), and also improved the neuronal plasticity (Castelli et al. 2020). SLAB51 also exhibited neuroprotective effects in dopaminergic neurons, which is mediated through activation of the NRF2/HO1 pathway. Thus, SLAB51 acts as a potent antioxidant as it also suppresses the NF-κB signaling cascade.

8.4.7 Prebiotics

Prebiotics are members of nondigestible carbohydrates, which endorse the growth of gut microbiota, persisting trillions of favorable microbes like lactobacillus, bifidobacillus, and other various bacterial species. A superior gut microbiota will lead to a healthy human life, and its composition is crucial for nutritional value. It has been suggested that the intestinal microbes give rise to carbohydrates, ethanol, other gases, and short fatty acids, resulting in the generation of inflammation (Bu et al. 2007; Rios-Covian et al. 2016). Several studies revealed that LPS-induced disturbance in gut microbes causes permeability of cytokines in the circulation, which ultimately leads to development of chronic inflammation (Cario and Podolsky 2005, Schachter et al. 2018). The proinflammatory cytokines cross the blood–brain barrier, and affect the sensory neurons in the medulla, forebrain, and hypothalamus. In a study, researchers have used prebiotics from the food, mainly from saccharides like mannanosaccharides, fructosaccharides, and galactosaccharides extracted from banana, garlic, and onion, which has been reported to be anti-inflammatory and antioxidative agents (Pandey et al. 2015). Prebiotic components on supplementation to AD and PD patients reduced oxidative stress and also inhibited the release of proinflammatory cytokines, such as TNF-α and IL-6 (Paiva et al. 2020). Another study has reported that the Aβ aggregation in AD mouse is reduced by chitosan derivative treatment (Paiva et al. 2020). Furthermore, fructosaccharide has also been reported to promote the secretion of neurotransmitter, enhance the signal transduction at the synapse, and improve the cognition in the hippocampal region of mice brain (Sun et al. 2019).

8.4.8 Polyunsaturated Fatty Acid (PUFA)

PUFA are short and long carbon fatty acid chains that are present in the essential fatty acids like omega 3 fatty acid (ω-3 FA). PUFA deactivates the astrocyte/microglia via the JNK pathway to reduce the inflammation of neurons and expand memory formation. It has been reported that PUFA shows an inhibitory effect against Aβ aggregation and tau clump formation by enhancing phagocytosis. Furthermore, it efficiently blocks the β/γ secretase enzyme to promote neurogenesis and the production of neurotransmitters, growth factors, which confirms its neuroprotective effect. The long-chain PUFA such as docosahexaenoic acid (DHA) is important for the normal central nervous system development. Its deficiency might lead to cerebral function impairment, as it is an important part of neuronal cell membranes. Our brain is unable to produce long-chain PUFA de novo. Hence, its requirement is fulfilled by dietary intake, mainly fish, sunflower seeds, and soybean oil. Several neurodegenerative disorders like PD, AD, ischemic stroke, and HD exhibit mitochondrial impairment. Enhanced intake of DHA following the oxidative damage has been reported to improve mitochondrial and motor functions of neurons in various animal models (Eckert et al. 2013).

8.4.9 Vitamin B

Vitamin B6 (pyridoxine), B9 (folate), and B12 (cobalamin) are extensively studied vitamins in the field of neurodegeneration. It has been reported that deficiency of vitamin B9 results in homocysteine accumulation in the brain, which leads to the generation of neuropsychological symptoms. Furthermore, vitamin B12 plays a vital role in the generation of methyl acceptor methionine, which is important for the synthesis of neurotransmitters, membrane lipids, and myelination of neurons. Vitamin B6 plays an important role in the improvement of cognition and efficiency of the brain toward thinking. Both vitamin B6 and B12 administration slows the progression of Aβ aggregation in AD patients (Sun et al. 2007). It has also been reported that various neurological disorders like AD, PD, and vascular dementia are directly related to the lower levels of vitamin B12 (Sun et al. 2007). Vitamin B12 produces methionine after methylation of homocysteine, which, if remains unmethylated, induces neurotoxicity in the brain. Like vitamin B12, vitamin B6 also methylates homocysteine and thus reduces the chances of neurotoxicity. Vitamin B9 deficiency leads to peripheral neuropathy. Hence, it is important to obtain vitamin B9 through dietary sources (Mecocci et al. 2014).

8.4.10 Creatine

Creatine is known to play an important role as the buffering agent to utilize ATP from the storehouse and provide energy to the brain and muscles, and also reverses the ADP to ATP synthesis by adding phosphate moiety. Creatine is an organic compound present abundantly in the pancreas, liver, and kidney and is absorbed mainly from red meat. Being an organic compound, creatine is rigorously consumed by a sportsperson. Studies have shown that creatine has antidepressant and antiapoptotic properties and, at the same time, reduces oxidative stress and also activates the PI3K/Akt cell survival pathway (Sestili et al. 2011; Bender and Klopstock 2016). Additionally, for an elderly person to reduce the risk of PD and oxidative stress, creatine-rich fish and meat as a dietary supplement can be beneficial. It has been reported that dopaminergic neurons are rescued from MPTP-induced toxicity by creatine administration in mice. Furthermore, oral dosing of creatine in the rats recovered them from the mitochondrial oxidative stress-led dysfunction, and excitotoxicity through enhancing the ATP level in the brain (Bender and Klopstock 2016). Creatine has a potent antidepressant property which is attributed to its ability to scavenge free radicals (Bakian et al. 2020).

8.4.11 Melatonin

The premium synthesis site of melatonin is the penial gland located behind the third cerebral ventricle of the brain. Melatonin is synthesized by *N*-acetyltransferase enzyme by converting serotonin moieties to melatonin. Melatonin's natural resources are dietary supplements, such as nuts, seeds, fruits, and vegetables. It has been reported that in the rat ischemia model, the injury caused by oxidative stress in the brain is protected by melatonin (Alghamdi 2018). In addition, melatonin also reduces glutamate toxicity in the ischemic rat model by maintaining Ca^+ homeostasis in the hippocampal and cerebral cortex regions of the brain. Various studies have suggested that melatonin improves blood–brain barrier integrity by reducing the generation of ROS, inflammatory cytokines, and also by downregulating the apoptotic markers through the Nrf2 pathway (Paredes et al. 2015). Furthermore, melatonin decreases the soluble amyloid precursor protein synthesis in PC12 cells that may further inhibit the Aβ aggregation in the case of AD, acting as a prominent antioxidant. Additionally, in 6-ODHA-induced PD mouse, melatonin reduces oxidative stress to protect mitochondria from damage and prevent the loss of dopaminergic neurons by lipid peroxidation (Alghamdi 2018) (Figure 8.7).

8.5 Clinical Approach

Recently, biomedical research is more focused on the use of nutraceuticals from natural resources for the therapeutic target of various neurodegenerative diseases. According to various clinical studies, alkaloids, berberine, galantamine, capsaicin, and piperine are the major members of the class that shows effectiveness in neuroprotection (Ogle et al. 2013). Furthermore, capsaicin is used for pain and stress relief and galantamine is applied in multiple patient-age groups suffering from AD and PD at different times resulting in improved cognition and recovery from glutamate excitotoxicity (Prins et al. 2014; Blautzik et al. 2016). Among the mostly studied phytochemicals, lycopene and β-cryptoxanthin are thriving in clinical trials against H_2O_2-induced neuronal injury (Castelli et al. 2020b). Moderate and severe AD patients have also been reported to show progress in cognitive performance after consumption of lycopene and β-cryptoxanthin (Wang et al. 2016). Moreover, among all well-studied flavonoid polyphenol groups, the two most essential flavonoids, quercetin and kaempferol have been included in the daily diet of patients suffering from neurological disorders (Spencer et al. 2008; Mao et al. 2018). In a clinical trial, both quercetin and kaempferol have improved the condition of AD and PD patients, enhancing memory formation

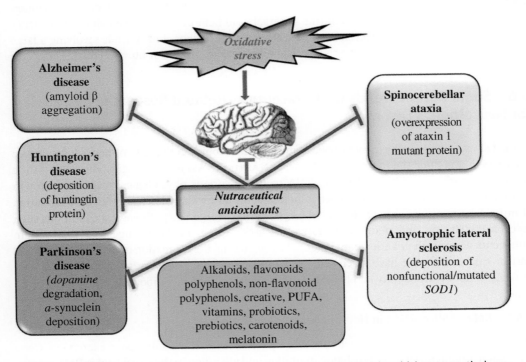

Figure 8.7 The schematic illustration depicting various mechanistic ways by which nutraceuticals can impart neuroprotection. Various nutraceutical antioxidants obtained from natural resources are potent therapeutic targets for neurological disorders.

and cognition in different age groups (Mecocci et al. 2014). In recent clinical trials, other flavonoids were also examined as neuroprotective nutraceuticals, like *Ginkgo biloba* extract was used in animal models and in clinical trials involving AD patients (Brown et al. 2009). In another study, curcumin was used prominently to conduct a clinical trial in terms of the management of AD, PD, and other neurological diseases. The study was based on the fact that a diet rich in curcumin can reduce the risk of AD by inhibiting the Aβ aggregation and ROS generation (Ganguli et al. 2000). However, to the best of our knowledge, nutraceutical-based neuroprotective compounds like rosmarinic acid and carnosic acid have not been investigated so well till date.

Furthermore, recently, probiotic and prebiotic constituents were selected for antioxidant activity. Based on in vitro and in vivo studies, SLAB51 has been reported as a potent formulation for further clinical investigation involving various neurological diseases (Castelli et al. 2020a). Recently, a clinical trial was conducted to examine the efficiency of dietary PUFA in AD patients' treatment (Chiu et al. 2020). It has been observed that PUFA reduced the risk of progression of AD via supplementary ω-fatty acid. Various studies have been conducted in a clinical trial by using oligofructose, lactulose, beta-glycan, and fructosaccharide, where significant improvement of cognitive functioning and reduced stress have been reported. According to previous studies, a combination of vitamins B6, B9, and B12 was supplemented to AD patients but it failed to attain the expected result in cognitive terms (Sun et al. 2007). A clinical trial reported that melatonin treatment results in the reversal of AD and PD since melatonin falls in the category of neuroimmunoendocrine regulator family that is responsible for its antiapoptotic and anti-inflammatory properties (Meng et al. 2017). It has been reported that melatonin imparts antioxidant property via activation of Nrf2-ARE pathway and protects mitochondrial functioning by activating SIRT-1 signaling pathway. Melatonin was also found to alleviate the levels of proinflammatory cytokines, thereby reducing edema during subarachnoid hemorrhage in vivo (Meng et al. 2017). Based on these data, it is conceived that there is a need for further clinical trials involving a large number of patients in order to better appreciate these nutraceuticals for human health.

8.6 Some Recent Trends in Nutraceutical-Related Research for Neurological Disorders

In the below section, we have mentioned some advanced topics in the field of neurodegenerative disorders that include the functioning of microRNAs (miRNAs) in neurological disorders with a special emphasis on oxidative stress. miRNA regulates various physiological responses through modulating the expression of several genes including the antioxidant defense system. Deregulation of miRNA homeostasis participates in the progression of numerous pathological conditions such as cancer, diabetes, and neurodegenerative diseases. Recent evidence suggested that certain nutraceuticals exert their antioxidant potential by regulating the expression of miRNAs. In the last part of this section, we have discussed the nanoparticle-based delivery of nutraceuticals that provides better bioavailability and potential future neuroprotective compounds.

8.6.1 Role of MicroRNAs in Neurodegenerative Diseases

MiRNAs belong to small regulatory noncoding RNA molecules that control gene expression. Gene expression is regulated due to translation inhibition and alteration in the stability of mRNA targets. MiRNAs are synthesized in the form of a hairpin structure by the RNA polymerase II and then processed by ribonuclease-protein complex Drosha in the nucleus to form pre-miRNA. Pre-miRNA is then cleaved by RNAase III enzyme Dicer in the cytoplasm, resulting in to double standard RNA duplex. Next, a guide strand of mature miRNA is loaded into Argonaute family protein Ago2 of RNA-induced silencing complex (RISC complex). Interaction of seed region of miRNA and 3′ untranslated region (UTR) of mRNA causes the degradation of target mRNA (Bartel 2004).

A critical role of miRNAs has been established during the developmental process and functioning of the adult brain. Knockout studies provide an insight into the significance of miRNA where genetic deletion of Ago2 and Dicer resulted in embryonic lethality (Bernstein et al. 2003). Likewise, Neuronal development during embryogenesis is severely hampered in the animal knocked out for Dicer. The dopamine neurons form neuronal networks in the ventral midbrain and play a major role in the regulation of emotion and voluntary motion. Dicer deletion in these neurons resulted in progressive degeneration and loss of their function (Cuellar et al. 2008). Similarly, Dicer deficiency in adult mice forebrain caused the development of neurodegenerative type phenotype that confirms the essential role of miRNA in neuronal development. However, Ago2 loss did not obstruct neuronal survival but found crucial for the normal functioning of neurons and behavior. Simultaneously, miRNAs are also associated with normal neuronal signaling. miRNAs play a vital role in the regulation of the release of neurotransmitter, dendritogenesis, and excitability of neurons (Schratt 2009). Alteration in miRNA expression due to inhibition of dicer activity is accompanied by several neurodegenerative and age-related diseases. Disturbance in the miRNA biogenesis creates oxidative stress in cells and conversely, the presence of oxidative stress adversely affects the expression of various miRNA molecules. The progression of this cycle in the cells ultimately resulted in cell death (Emde and Hornstein 2014; Engedal et al. 2018). In the following section, we have discussed the role of miRNAs in relation to specific neurodegenerative diseases.

8.6.1.1 Alzheimer's Disease

The most characteristic pathological features of AD are neuronal inflammation that causes the formation of intracellular Hirano bodies and NFT along with Aβ plaques inside the cells. All these abnormal structures resulted in excessive neuronal degeneration. Recent studies have demonstrated the significant role of miRNA in the excessive Aβ peptide accumulation and hyperphosphorylation of Tau (Liu et al. 2014; Konovalova et al. 2019). Oxidative stress also plays a crucial role in AD development particularly at the initial stage of neural degeneration. Oxidative stress caused damage to nucleic acid, lipid, and protein structure and alters gene expression. These entire factors contribute significantly to the development of AD development. Oxidative stress has been found to affect the expression of several miRNAs both positively and negatively. Similarly, various miRNAs also participate in the regulation of oxidative stress by affecting the associated gene expression (Prasad 2016; Amakiri et al. 2019).

BACE1 is the enzyme that produces the Aβ peptide by cleaving amyloid precursor protein (APP). Different miRNAs have been identified to regulate the Aβ deposition and their altered expressions have been recognized in different AD model systems like the human brain, mouse model and cell lines. miR-107, miR-298, miR-101, miR-9, and miR29a/b-1 negatively regulates the synthesis of BACE1 and APP (Wang et al. 2008). In human patients and mouse model decreased expression of these miRNAs contributes to the development of AD by increasing the Aβ production (Zhao et al. 2017; Chopra et al. 2020). In another study, researchers analyzed the role of miR-138 in the phosphorylation of tau using AD model cell lines and found that higher levels of miR-138 augmented the tau phosphorylation by targeting retinoic acid receptor alpha (Wang et al. 2008). Excessive formation of soluble Aβ peptides (sAβ) peptide leads to the formation of ROS that in turn specifically stimulate the level of miR-134, miR-145, and miR-210, whereas decreased the expression of miR-107 (Li et al. 2014; Wang et al. 2019). Persons with ε4 allele of the apolipoprotein

E (*APOE4*) genotype are at higher risk for the progression of AD. In AD patient with APOE4 genotype, accumulation of Aβ peptide is co-related with a decreased level of miR-107 (Verghese et al. 2011).

Curcumin participates in protection against AD through regulating the Aβ metabolism (Goozee et al. 2016). Curcumin is also known to regulate the expression of several miRNAs in various disease conditions (Ma et al. 2014; Toden et al. 2015; Ye et al. 2015). However, participation of miRNA in the protective effect of curcumin in AD is not studied in detail and information is scanty. Liu et al. (2019) investigated the association of curcumin and miRNA using a swAPP695-HEK293 cell line as a model. A negative connection between the miR-15b-5p and amyloid precursor protein and amyloid-β was established. Curcumin was found to enhance the expression of miR-15b-5p that in turn suppressed the level of amyloid precursor protein and Aβ in the AD model cell line. Recently, Gong and Sun (2020) conducted a clinical study, in this they examined the level of mir-146a in the cerebrospinal fluid and peripheral blood of AD patient and age-matched healthy person. A significantly higher level of mir-146a was observed in the AD patients' cerebrospinal fluid as compared to the control group. The authors also conducted animal studies to establish an association among curcumin, mir-146a and AD. Curcumin at la ow dose remarkably reduces the level of proinflammatory miR-146a in APP/PS1 mice temporal lobe compared to the control group and concurrently help in the clearance of Aβ by modulating the phagocytosis. In a previous study, Hong et al. (2017) examined the expression of certain circulatory miRNA, miR-125b, miR9 and miR-191-5p in the AD mouse model (APP/PS1 model). A decreased level of miR-125b, miR9 and miR-191-5- was observed in APP/PS1 mice as compared to control mice. Supplementation of EGCG remarkably improved the disease condition of AD mice and reverses the level of the above-mentioned miRNA. EGCG supplementation also enhanced the level of miR-125b in the SH-SY5Y cells compared to the control group.

8.6.1.2 Parkinson's Disease

In PD pathogenesis, oxidative stress contributes significantly to driving neuronal degeneration. The factors responsible for oxidative stress generation are impairment in dopamine metabolism, mitochondrial functioning, and the antioxidant system (Konovalova et al. 2019). Dopamine uptake is mediated by the dopamine transporter (DAT). A direct association between the miRNA dysregulation, oxidative stress, and dopamine transporter was established by Kim et al. (2007). In PD patient midbrain, downregulation of miR-133b caused the elevated level of dopamine transporter that contributes to oxidative stress-mediated neuronal degeneration. Increased activity of dopamine transporter resulted in an enhanced level of dopamine in the cytoplasm that oxidizes rapidly and leads to oxidative stress generation and finally neuronal degeneration (Masoud et al. 2015). MiR-137 and miR491 were also found to suppress the dopamine transporter level in in vitro condition, this might be associated with PD-induced oxidative stress (Jia et al. 2016). Nrf2 ARE pathway plays an important role in different neurodegenerative diseases. Nrf-2 translocates to the nucleus and enhances the expression of antioxidant responsive genes like SOD and GSH. Keap1 protein degrades Nrf-2 and regulates its level. miR-7 participates in the activation of the Nrf-2 pathway by repressing the Keap1 level (Kabaria et al. 2015; Xie and Chen 2016).

Downregulation of miR-7 was observed in the substantia nigra pars compacta (SNpc) of PD patients that impaired the Nrf-2 pathway and eventually led to dopamine neuron degeneration (Mcmillan et al. 2017). Conversely, Narasimhan et al. (2012) identified miR-27a, miR-142-5p, and miR-144 as a negative regulator of Nrf-2 expression, thus these miRNAs could be potential molecules responsible for impaired oxidative stress. Few miRNAs are also reported to play a role in neuroinflammation. miR-155 functions as a proinflammatory molecule and its upregulation mediate α-synuclein induced inflammation in the PD animal model, whereas miR-146a shows anti-inflammatory activities (Caggiu et al. 2018). MALAT1 participate in PD pathogenesis by increasing and inhibiting the expression of α-synuclein and f miR-129 respectively. Xia et al. (2019) established a relationship between the resveratrol, miR-129, SNCA and MALT1 expression. They identified that resveratrol regulates the level of MALAT1 by increasing the level of miR-129 that acts as a negative regulator of MALT1 and SNCA by suppressing their expressions. In another study, Wang et al. (2015) examined the expression of miR-214 and α-synuclein in the midbrain of PD mice model and PD-induced SH-SY5Y cells. They identified a lower expression of miR-214 of increased expression of α-synuclein in both cell line and animal PD models, respectively. Interestingly, treatment with resveratrol protects against PD progression by reversing the level of miR-214 and α-synuclein.

8.6.1.3 Amyotrophic Lateral Sclerosis and Huntington's Disease

In ALS patients, the differential expression of miRNAs contributes to the regulation of oxidative stress genes. Similar to PD, miR27a, miR-142-5p, and miR34a suppressed the Nrf-2 level that resulted in impaired Nrf-2 ARE pathway in ALS as well. Conversely, miR-107 affects Nrf-2 in a positive manner by downregulating the Keap1 expression. miR-155 and miR338-3p were found to be upregulated in both sporadic and familial ALS and their higher expression is correlated with mitochondrial dysfunction (Paladino et al. 2018). In HD pathogenesis, a close interaction between miRNA expression and oxidative stress is not fully investigated. However, it is evident that mutant Huntingtin protein interacts with Repressor Element 1 Silencing Transcription Factor (REST) and alters the expression of REST-regulated miRNA. Mutant Huntingtin protein is also found to inhibit Ago2 and RISC complex activity. In HD patients, at different stages, downregulation of miR-9, miR29b, and miR-124a and upregulation of miR-132 was observed. In the mice HD model, dicer and drosha mRNA level were found to be decreased as compared to normal control mice (Konovalova et al. 2019).

8.6.2 Nano-Formulation-Based Delivery of Natural Products

Oral delivery of drugs is highly accepted due to certain associated advantages like better patient acquiescence and self-administration. This is in spite of the fact that the efficacy is significantly affected by chemical and enzymatic barriers present in the gastrointestinal (GI) tract. Poor aqueous solubility and permeability across the epithelial membrane also decrease the bioavailability of such drugs. Therefore, the use of an efficient drug delivery system can ameliorate these difficulties. Currently, nanocarrier systems are being investigated for the oral delivery of several drugs and phytochemicals. Active ingredients or drugs are either encapsulated or linked to the nanoparticle surface. Various types of biodegradable and biocompatible polymer-based nanostructures have been designed for efficient delivery. Most studied nanostructures are nanospheres (NSs), nanocapsule (NCs), solid nanoparticles (SLNs), and liposomes. These nanostructures are designed to protect the bioactive compound from the gastrointestinal tract barrier, enhance the absorption and bioavailability and proper targeting to a defined organ (Squillaro et al. 2018). Curcumin, ginsenosides, piperine, and various other natural plant products have been incorporated into different types of nanoformulations. These nanoformulations have been comprehensively examined for their role as a therapeutic reagent for various diseases such as diabetes, cardiovascular disease, and cancer, though information about the application of nanoformulation for neurodegenerative disease treatment is quite scanty.

Curcumin has shown neuroprotective property against different neurological disorders including AD, PD, HD, and multiple sclerosis. However, poor brain bioavailability limits its efficacy as a neuroprotective agent. Tiwari et al. (2014) encapsulated curcumin using poly lactic-co-glycolic acid (PLGA) nanoparticles (Cur-PLGA-NPs) and evaluated its potential on the neuronal stem cells for their proliferation and differentiation under in vitro condition and in the hippocampus and subventricular zone of adult rats in vivo. The study reported that Cur-PLGA-NPs increased neuronal stem cell proliferation and differentiation in both in vitro and in vivo conditions. The study further showed that the said nanoparticle exerted its effect by modulating Wnt/β-catenin pathway and increasing the expression of genes related to neuronal proliferation and differentiation. Results of this further study suggested that Cur-PLGA-NPs could be a potential therapeutic approach for the treatment of neurological disorders via modifying the brain's self-repair machinery. Previously, Sandhir et al. (2014) encapsulated curcumin in solid lipid nanoparticles (C-SLN) and evaluated their effectiveness against mitochondrial impairments in the HD rat model. The obtained results demonstrated a remarkable decrease in lipid peroxidation and reactive oxygen species in solid lipid nanoparticles-treated animals compared to nontreated animals. A decrease in oxidative stress was found to be mediated by improving the SOD activity and activation of the Nrf-2 pathway. Furthermore, the said nanoparticles-treated animals demonstrated better neuromotor coordination. Based on these data, the authors claimed that the solid lipid nanoparticles could be used as a potential therapeutic option against HD mitochondrial impairment.

Recently, Kundu et al. (2016) examined the potency of curcumin and piperine co-loaded glycerylmonooleate (GMO) nanoparticles to cross the blood–brain barrier using a mouse PD model. The data showed that the dual-loaded nanoparticles inhibited the oligomerization of α-synuclein protein and fibril formation. Administration of dual nanoparticles also suppressed rotenone-mediated oxidative stress and apoptosis in comparison to free counterpart as evident from in vitro study. Remarkably, dual nanoparticles were also helpful in protecting against the rotenone-mediated motor coordination injury and repair the dopaminergic neuronal degeneration in the PD mouse model. Mathew et al. (2011) formulated PGLA-encapsulated curcumin nanoparticles and incubated them with amyloid proteins using an in vitro model. The authors demonstrated the binding of curcumin nanoparticles with amyloid aggregates that prevented their aggregation, rather induced their dissociation. Further, Taylor et al. (2011) developed different types of nanoliposome for encapsulation of curcumin and examined their efficacy against (Aβ1–42) peptide aggregation. All types of curcumin nanoparticles prevented Aβ aggregation and fibril formation but the nanoliposome formed by click chemistry showed more promising results as compared to free curcumin. As a whole, the nutraceutical-loaded/encapsulated nanoparticles showed higher efficacy in terms of their neuroprotective activities as compared to their natural forms. Some of them were even found to be efficient in crossing the blood–brain barrier. All these indicate that these advanced formulations of nutraceuticals have tremendous therapeutic potential. But in spite of these advantages, there still remains a gap in relation to the toxicity profile of these nanoformulations. Once this aspect is addressed with proper preclinical in vitro and in vivo experimental models followed by their clinical trials in large populations, these formulations will really provide a solid base for the cure and management of neurological disorders.

8.6.3 Future Neuroprotective Compounds

Marine sponges (Porifera) are found in different types of marine environments and considered ancient multicellular animals. Marine sponges are a very rich source of marine drugs and approximately 30% of natural products are derived from marine sponges (Mehbub et al. 2014). The compounds isolated from sponges have shown diverse biological activities including antimalarial, antiviral anti-inflammatory, and antibacterial (Mayer et al. 2011). Ninety marine sponges' derived compounds have been isolated from 18 different countries and evaluated for their neuroprotective competencies. These compounds belong to different categories like alkaloid, amino acid, a quaternary amine, betaine, and diterpenes. These natural products inhibit the activity of BACE1, enhance the serotonin level, and protect the neuronal cells against oxidative stress. They also modulate the activity of GSK-3β and cell cycle-related kinases (Alghazwi et al. 2016). However, these compounds have not been investigated thoroughly and utilized effectively as a therapeutic reagent for different neurodegenerative diseases. Therefore, these marine natural products could be accepted and appreciated as the future neuroprotective molecules/compounds, though continuous in-depth research is required to validate their therapeutic potential.

8.7 Present Research Gap and Future Prospective

Strong scientific evidence suggests nutraceutical antioxidants as novel therapeutic molecules against various neurodegenerative diseases. Different neuronal cell types participate in the development of individual neurodegenerative disease; oxidative stress generation followed by the formation of dysfunctional proteins, impairment in mitochondrial functioning, and destruction of neuronal survival are the common feature of many neurological disorders. Therefore, natural compounds with potent antioxidant properties are the relevant therapeutic compounds for the prevention and treatment of these diseases. Natural antioxidants not only alleviate oxidative stress through scavenging free radicals but also modulate various cellular signaling pathways that ultimately resulted in enhancing neuronal survival as demonstrated from various in vitro and in vivo neurodegenerative disease models. In this chapter, we described the pivotal neuroprotective role of various phytochemicals and non-phytochemicals including vitamins, prebiotics, and probiotics. These compounds by targeting the different cellular receptors and ligand restore mitochondrial functioning and inhibit the accumulation of abnormal protein that leads to a healthy nervous system. Dysregulation of miRNA homeostasis also participates in the progression of several neurodegenerative diseases and certain nutraceuticals exert their neuroprotective potential by regulating the expression of miRNAs. A substantial number of clinical studies have also proven the neuroprotective functioning of certain nutraceuticals specifically in AD and PD disease. Thus, a healthy lifestyle with dietary supplements of nutraceuticals can slow the progression of neurological diseases. The major drawbacks that limit the widespread application of nutraceuticals are their poor bioavailability and brain permeability. To overcome these difficulties, nanocarrier systems have been used and found to be more effective than natural form, though need concern for their toxic aspect. Altogether, various studies provided a great insight into the potential of nutraceuticals for the cure and management of neurological disorders, though strong holistic efforts should be made to address the underlying detailed molecular mechanism, better availability, and target delivery. Furthermore, large-scale studies should be conducted to strengthen the clinical efficacy of nutraceuticals and their active compound on neurological disorders.

References

Agostinho, P., Lopes, J.P., Velez, Z., and Oliveira, C.R. (2008). Overactivation of calcineurin induced by amyloid-beta and prion proteins. *Neurochemistry International* 52 (6): 1226–1233.

Al-Alawi, A.A. and Laleye, L.C. (2008). Characterization of camel milk protein isolates as nutraceutical and functional ingredients. Collaborative Research Project SQU/UAEU.

Alghamdi, B.S. (2018). The neuroprotective role of melatonin in neurological disorders. *Journal of Neuroscience Research* 96 (7): 1136–1149.

Alghazwi, M., Qi Kan, Y., Zhang, W. et al. (2016). Neuroprotective activities of marine natural products from marine sponges. *Current Medicinal Chemistry* 23 (4): 360–382.

Amakiri, N., Kubosumi, A., Tran, J., and Reddy, P.H. (2019). Amyloid beta and microRNAs in Alzheimer's disease. *Frontiers in Neuroscience* 13: 430.

Ansari, M.A., Abdul, H.M., Joshi, G. et al. (2009). Protective effect of quercetin in primary neurons against Aβ (1–42): relevance to Alzheimer's disease. *The Journal of Nutritional Biochemistry* 20 (4): 269–275.

Araque, A., Parpura, V., Sanzgiri, R.P., and Haydon, P.G. (1999). Tripartite synapses: glia, the unacknowledged partner. *Trends in Neurosciences* 22 (5): 208–215.

Aruoma, O.I., Bahorun, T., and Jen, L.S. (2003). Neuroprotection by bioactive components in medicinal and food plant extracts. *Mutation Research, Reviews in Mutation Research* 544 (2–3): 203–215.

Aseervatham, G.S.B., Sivasudha, T., Jeyadevi, R., and Arul Ananth, D. (2013). Environmental factors and unhealthy lifestyle influence oxidative stress in humans – an overview. *Environmental Science and Pollution Research International* 20 (7): 4356–4369.

Ashraf, S.A., Adnan, M., Patel, M. et al. (2020). Fish-based bioactives as potent nutraceuticals: exploring the therapeutic perspective of sustainable food from the Sea. *Marine Drugs* 18 (5): 265.

Asmat, U., Abad, K., and Ismail, K. (2016). Diabetes mellitus and oxidative stress – a concise review. *Saudi Pharmaceutical Journal* 24 (5): 547–553.

Awasthi, A., Matsunaga, Y., and Yamada, T. (2005). Amyloid-beta causes apoptosis of neuronal cells via caspase cascade, which can be prevented by amyloid-beta-derived short peptides. *Experimental Neurology* 196 (2): 282–289.

Ayaz, M., Sadiq, A., Junaid, M. et al. (2019). Flavonoids as prospective neuroprotectants and their therapeutic propensity in aging associated neurological disorders. *Frontiers in Aging Neuroscience* 11: 115.

Bakian, A.V., Huber, R.S., Scholl, L. et al. (2020). Dietary creatine intake and depression risk among US adults. *Translational Psychiatry* 10 (1): 1–11.

Bartel, D.P. (2004). MicroRNAs: genomics, biogenesis, mechanism, and function. *Cell* 116 (2): 281–297.

Bastow, E.L., Peswani, A.R., Tarrant, D.S.J. et al. (2016). New links between SOD1 and metabolic dysfunction from a yeast model of amyotrophic lateral sclerosis (ALS). *Journal of Cell Science*.

Bellows, L. and Moore, R. (2012). Water-soluble vitamins: B-complex and vitamin C. Fact sheet (Colorado State University. Extension). Food and nutrition series; no. 9.312.

Bender, A. and Klopstock, T. (2016). Creatine for neuroprotection in neurodegenerative disease: end of story? *Amino Acids* 48 (8): 1929–1940.

Bernstein, E., Kim, S.Y., Carmell, M.A. et al. (2003). Dicer is essential for mouse development. *Nature Genetics* 35 (3): 215–217.

Birben, E., Sahiner, U.M., Sackesen, C. et al. (2012). Oxidative stress and antioxidant defense. *World Allergy Organization Journal* 5 (1): 9–19.

Blautzik, J., Keeser, D., Paolini, M. et al. (2016). Functional connectivity increase in the default-mode network of patients with Alzheimer' s disease after long-term treatment with Galantamine. *European Neuropsychopharmacology* 26 (3): 602–613.

Block, M.L. (2008). NADPH oxidase as a therapeutic target in Alzheimer's disease. *BMC Neuroscience* 9 (SUPPL. 2): 1–8.

Bolisetty, S. and Jaimes, E.A. (2013). Mitochondria and reactive oxygen species: physiology and pathophysiology. *International Journal of Molecular Sciences* 14: 6306–6344.

Bonda, D.J., Wang, X., Perry, G. et al. (2010). Oxidative stress in Alzheimer disease: a possibility for prevention. *Neuropharmacology* 59 (4–5): 290–294.

Bonora, M., Wieckowski, M.R., Chinopoulos, C. et al. (2015). Molecular mechanisms of cell death: central implication of ATP synthase in mitochondrial permeability transition. *Oncogene* 34 (12): 1475–1486.

Bossy-Wetzel, E., Petrilli, A., and Knott, A.B. (2008). Mutant huntingtin and mitochondrial dysfunction. *Trends in Neurosciences* 31 (12): 609–616.

Boukhenouna, S., Wilson, M.A., Bahmed, K., and Kosmider, B. (2018). Reactive oxygen species in chronic obstructive pulmonary disease. *Oxidative Medicine and Cellular Longevity* 2018.

Brown, L.A., Riby, L.M., and Reay, J.L. (2009). Supplementing cognitive aging: a selective review of the effects of ginkgo biloba and a number of everyday nutritional substances. *Experimental Aging Research* 36 (1): 105–122.

Bu, Y., Rho, S., Kim, J. et al. (2007). Neuroprotective effect of tyrosol on transient focal cerebral ischemia in rats. *Neuroscience Letters* 414 (3): 218–221.

Bulat, N. and Widmann, C. (2009). Caspase substrates and neurodegenerative diseases. *Brain Research Bulletin* 80: 251–267.

Butterfield, D.A. (2014). The 2013 SFRBM discovery award: selected discoveries from the Butterfield laboratory of oxidative stress and its sequela in brain in cognitive disorders exemplified by Alzheimer disease and chemotherapy induced cognitive impairment. *Free Radical Biology and Medicine* 74: 157–174.

Caggiu, E., Paulus, K., Mameli, G. et al. (2018). Differential expression of miRNA 155 and miRNA 146a in Parkinson's disease patients. *eNeurologicalSci* 13: 1–4.

Carafoli, E. and Krebs, J. (2016). Why calcium? How calcium became the best communicator. *Journal of Biological Chemistry* 291 (40): 20849–20857.

Cario, E. and Podolsky, D.K. (2005). Intestinal epithelial TOLLerance versus inTOLLerance of commensals. *Molecular Immunology* 42 (8): 887–893.

Castelli, V., d'Angelo, M., Lombardi, F. et al. (2020a). Effects of the probiotic formulation SLAB51 in in vitro and in vivo Parkinson's disease models. *Aging (Albany NY)* 12 (5): 4641.

Castelli, V., Melani, F., Ferri, C. et al. (2020b). Neuroprotective activities of bacopa, lycopene, astaxanthin, and vitamin B12 combination on oxidative stress-dependent neuronal death. *Journal of Cellular Biochemistry* https://doi.org/10.1002/jcb.29722.

Chauhan, B., Kumar, G., Kalam, N., and Ansari, S.H. (2013). Current concepts and prospects of herbal nutraceutical: a review. *Journal of Advanced Pharmaceutical Technology & Research* 4 (1): 4.

Chen, T.J., Jeng, J.Y., Lin, C.W. et al. (2006). Quercetin inhibition of ROS-dependent and-independent apoptosis in rat glioma C6 cells. *Toxicology* 223 (1–2): 113–126.

Chiu, H.F., Venkatakrishnan, K., and Wang, C.K. (2020). The role of nutraceuticals as a complementary therapy against various neurodegenerative diseases: a mini-review. *Journal of Traditional and Complementary Medicine*.

Cho, K.S., Shin, M., Kim, S., and Lee, S.B. (2018). Recent advances in studies on the therapeutic potential of dietary carotenoids in neurodegenerative diseases. *Oxidative Medicine and Cellular Longevity* 2018: 4120458.

Chonpathompikunlert, P., Wattanathorn, J., and Muchimapura, S. (2010). Piperine, the main alkaloid of Thai black pepper, protects against neurodegeneration and cognitive impairment in animal model of cognitive deficit like condition of Alzheimer's disease. *Food and Chemical Toxicology* 48 (3): 798–802.

Chopra, N., Wang, R., Maloney, B. et al. (2020). MicroRNA-298 reduces levels of human amyloid-β precursor protein (APP), β-site APP-converting enzyme 1 (BACE1) and specific tau protein moieties. *Molecular Psychiatry*: 1–22.

Chung, M.J., Lee, S., Park, Y.I. et al. (2016). Neuroprotective effects of phytosterols and flavonoids from Cirsiumsetidens and Aster scaber in human brain neuroblastoma SK-N-SH cells. *Life Sciences* 148: 173–182.

Cotas, J., Leandro, A., Pacheco, D. et al. (2020). A comprehensive review of the nutraceutical and therapeutic applications of red seaweeds (Rhodophyta). *Lifestyles* 10 (3): 19.

Covarrubias-Pinto, A., Moll, P., Solís-Maldonado, M. et al. (2015). Beyond the redox imbalance: oxidative stress contributes to an impaired GLUT3 modulation in Huntington's disease. *Free Radical Biology and Medicine* 89: 1085–1096.

Coyle, J.T. and Puttfarcken, P. (1993). Lungenmetastase eines gutartigen Riesenzelltumors des Skeletts 27 Jahre nach Resektion eines Tumorrezidivs. *Science* 262: 689–695.

Cuellar, T.L., Davis, T.H., Nelson, P.T. et al. (2008). Dicer loss in striatal neurons produces behavioral and neuroanatomical phenotypes in the absence of neurodegeneration. *Proceedings of the National Academy of Sciences* 105 (14): 5614–5619.

Cui, K., Luo, X., Xu, K., and Murthy, M.V. (2004). Role of oxidative stress in neurodegeneration: recent developments in assay methods for oxidative stress and nutraceutical antioxidants. *Progress in Neuro-Psychopharmacology and Biological Psychiatry* 28 (5): 771–799.

Cunha, M.P., Martín-de-Saavedra, M.D., Romero, A. et al. (2014). Both creatine and its product phosphocreatine reduce oxidative stress and afford neuroprotection in an in vitro Parkinson's model. *ASN Neuro* 6 (6): 1759091414554945.

Dasari, K., Mandu, C.O., and Lu, Y. (2020). The role of oxidative stress in cancer. *Novel Approaches in Cancer Study* 4 (2): 350–355.

De Moura Linck, V., Herrmann, A.P., Goerck, G.C. et al. (2008). The putative antipsychotic alstonine reverses social interaction withdrawal in mice. *Progress in Neuro-Psychopharmacology and Biological Psychiatry* 32 (6): 1449–1452.

Del Bano, M.J., Lorente, J., Castillo, J. et al. (2003). Phenolic diterpenes, flavones, and rosmarinic acid distribution during the development of leaves, flowers, stems, and roots of *Rosmarinus officinalis*. Antioxidant activity. *Journal of Agricultural and Food Chemistry* 51 (15): 4247–4253.

Del Bano, M.J., Lorente, J., Castillo, J. et al. (2003). Phenolic diterpenes, flavones, and rosmarinic acid distribution during the development of leaves, flowers, stems, and roots of Rosmarinus officinalis. Antioxidant activity. *Journal of Agricultural and Food Chemistry* 51 (15): 4247–4253.

Deng, H., Wang, P., and Jankovic, J. (2018). The genetics of Parkinson disease. *Ageing Research Reviews* 42: 72–85.

Dey, A. and Mukherjee, A. (2018). Plant-derived alkaloids: a promising window for neuroprotective drug discovery. In: *Discovery and Development of Neuroprotective Agents from Natural Products* (ed. G. Brahmachari), 237–320. Elsevier.

Dey, A., Nandy, S., Mukherjee, A., and Pandey, D.K. (2020). Plant natural products as neuroprotective nutraceuticals: preclinical and clinical studies and future implications. *Proceedings of the National Academy of Sciences, India Section B: Biological Sciences* 90: 1–15.

Dias, V., Junn, E., and Mouradian, M.M. (2013). The role of oxidative stress in parkinson's disease. *Journal of Parkinson's Disease* 3 (4): 461–491.

Dogru, M., Kojima, T., Simsek, C., and Tsubotav, K. (2018). Potential role of oxidative stress in ocular surface inflammation and dry eye disease. *Investigative Ophthalmology and Visual Science* 59 (14 Special Issue): DES163–DES168.

Droge, W. (2002). Free radicals in the physiological control of cell function. *Physiological Reviews* 82 (1): 47–95.

Durairajan, S.S.K., Liu, L.F., Lu, J.H. et al. (2012). Berberine ameliorates β-amyloid pathology, gliosis, and cognitive impairment in an Alzheimer's disease transgenic mouse model. *Neurobiology of Aging* 33 (12): 2903–2919.

Dutta, K., Ghosh, D., and Basu, A. (2009). Curcumin protects neuronal cells from Japanese encephalitis virus-mediated cell death and also inhibits infective viral particle formation by dysregulation of ubiquitin–proteasome system. *Journal of Neuroimmune Pharmacology* 4 (3): 328–337.

Eckert, G.P., Lipka, U., and Muller, W.E. (2013). Omega-3 fatty acids in neurodegenerative diseases: focus on mitochondria. *Prostaglandins, Leukotrienes and Essential Fatty Acids* 88 (1): 105–114.

Egea, J., Martin-de-Saavedra, M.D., Parada, E. et al. (2012). Galantamine elicits neuroprotection by inhibiting iNOS, NADPH oxidase and ROS in hippocampal slices stressed with anoxia/reoxygenation. *Neuropharmacology* 62 (2): 1082–1090.

Emde, A. and Hornstein, E. (2014). mi RNA s at the interface of cellular stress and disease. *The EMBO Journal* 33 (13): 1428–1437.

Engedal, N., Žerovnik, E., Rudov, A. et al. (2018). From oxidative stress damage to pathways, networks, and autophagy via microRNAs. *Oxidative Medicine and Cellular Longevity* 2018.

Fadaeinasab, M., Basiri, A., Kia, Y. et al. (2015). New indole alkaloids from the bark of Rauvolfiareflexa and their cholinesterase inhibitory activity. *Cellular Physiology and Biochemistry* 37 (5): 1997–2011.

Ferreiro, E., Oliveira, C.R., and Pereira, C.M.F. (2008). The release of calcium from the endoplasmic reticulum induced by amyloid-beta and prion peptides activates the mitochondrial apoptotic pathway. *Neurobiology of Disease* 30 (3): 331–342.

Fiedor, J. and Burda, K. (2014). Potential role of carotenoids as antioxidants in human health and disease. *Nutrients* 6 (2): 466–488.

Foran, E., Bogush, A., Goffredo, M. et al. (2011). Motor neuron impairment mediated by a sumoylated fragment of the glial glutamate transporter EAAT2. *Glia* 59 (11): 1719–1731.

Furukawa, S., Yang, L., and Sameshima, H. (2014). Galantamine, an acetylcholinesterase inhibitor, reduces brain damage induced by hypoxia-ischemia in newborn rats. *International Journal of Developmental Neuroscience* 37: 52–57.

Gamez, J., Corbera-Bellalta, M., Nogales, G. et al. (2006). Mutational analysis of the Cu/Zn superoxide dismutase gene in a Catalan ALS population: should all sporadic ALS cases also be screened for SOD1? *Journal of the Neurological Sciences* 247 (1): 21–28.

Gandhi, S. and Abramov, A.Y. (2012). Mechanism of oxidative stress in neurodegeneration. *Oxidative Medicine and Cellular Longevity* 2012.

Ganguli, M., Chandra, V., Kamboh, M.I. et al. (2000). Apolipoprotein E polymorphism and Alzheimer disease: the Indo-US cross-national dementia study. *Archives of Neurology* 57 (6): 824–830.

Ganguly, K. and Poo, M. (2013). Activity-dependent neural plasticity from bench to bedside. *Neuron* 80 (3): 729–741.

Ganguly, G., Chakrabarti, S., Chatterjee, U., and Saso, L. (2017). Proteinopathy, oxidative stress and mitochondrial dysfunction: cross talk in alzheimer's disease and parkinson's disease. *Drug Design, Development and Therapy* 11: 797–810.

Gil-Mohapel, J., Brocardo, P., and Christie, B. (2014). The role of oxidative stress in Huntington's disease: are antioxidants good therapeutic candidates? *Current Drug Targets* 15 (4): 454–468.

Giraldo, E., Lloret, A., Fuchsberger, T., and Viña, J. (2014). Aβ and tau toxicities in Alzheimer's are linked via oxidative stress-induced p38 activation: protective role of vitamin E. *Redox Biology* 2 (1): 873–877.

Gitler, A.D., Dhillon, P., and Shorter, J. (2017). *Neurodegenerative Disease: Models, Mechanisms, and a New Hope*. The Company of Biologists.

Gomes, B.A.Q., Silva, J.P.B., Romeiro, C.F.R. et al. (2018). Neuroprotective mechanisms of resveratrol in Alzheimer's disease: role of SIRT1. *Oxidative Medicine and Cellular Longevity* 2018: 30510627.

Gong, J. and Sun, D. (2020). Study on the mechanism of curcumin to reduce the inflammatory response of temporal lobe in Alzheimer's disease by regulating miR-146a. *Minerva Medica* https://doi.org/10.23736/S0026-4806.20.06463-0.

Goozee, K.G., Shah, T.M., Sohrabi, H.R. et al. (2016). Examining the potential clinical value of curcumin in the prevention and diagnosis of Alzheimer's disease. *British Journal of Nutrition* 115 (3): 449–465.

Goyal, M.S., Hawrylycz, M., Miller, J.A. et al. (2014). Aerobic glycolysis in the human brain is associated with development and neotenous gene expression. *Cell Metabolism* 19 (1): 49–57.

Guo, S.Y., Yang, G.P., Jiang, D.J. et al. (2008). Protection of capsaicin against hypoxia–reoxygenation-induced apoptosis of rat hippocampal neurons. *Canadian Journal of Physiology and Pharmacology* 86 (11): 785–792.

Guo, J.D., Zhao, X., Li, Y. et al. (2018). Damage to dopaminergic neurons by oxidative stress in Parkinson's disease. *International Journal of Molecular Medicine* 41 (4): 1817–1825.

Gutierrez-Merino, C., Lopez-Sanchez, C., Lagoa, R. et al. (2011). Neuroprotective actions of flavonoids. *Current medicinal Chemistry* 18 (8): 1195–1212.

Habtemariam, S. (2019). Antioxidant and anti-inflammatory mechanisms of neuroprotection by ursolic acid: addressing brain injury, cerebral ischemia, cognition deficit, anxiety, and depression. *Oxidative Medicine and Cellular Longevity* 2019: 8512048.

Hakonen, A.H., Goffart, S., Marjavaara, S. et al. (2008). Infantile-onset spinocerebellar ataxia and mitochondrial recessive ataxia syndrome are associated with neuronal complex I defect and mtDNA depletion. *Human Molecular Genetics* 17 (23): 3822–3835.

Halliwell, B. (1992). Reactive oxygen species and the central nervous system. *Journal of Neurochemistry* 59 (5): 1609–1623.

Halliwell, B. (2001). Role of free radicals in the neurodegenerative diseases. *Drugs & Aging* 18 (9): 685–716.

Halliwell, B. (2006). Oxidative stress and neurodegeneration : where are we now ? *Journal of Neurochemistry* 97: 1634–1658.

Hamilton, A. and Holscher, C. (2012). The effect of ageing on neurogenesis and oxidative stress in the APP swe/PS1 deltaE9 mouse model of Alzheimer's disease. *Brain Research* 1449 (2012): 83–93.

Han, D., Antunes, F., Canali, R. et al. (2003). Voltage-dependent anion channels control the release of the superoxide anion from mitochondria to cytosol. *Journal of Biological Chemistry* 278 (8): 5557–5563.

Harnly, J.M., Doherty, R.F., Beecher, G.R. et al. (2006). Flavonoid content of US fruits, vegetables, and nuts. *Journal of Agricultural and Food Chemistry* 54 (26): 9966–9977.

Held, P. (2015). An introduction to reactive oxygen species measurement of ROS in yeast cells. BioTek White Paper, 1–21.

Hensley, K., Mhatre, M., Mou, S. et al. (2006). On the relation of oxidative stress to Neuroinflammation : lessons learned from the G93A-SOD1 mouse model of amyotrophic lateral sclerosis. *Antioxidants & Redox Signaling* 11 (12): 2075–2087.

Herrmann, A.P., Lunardi, P., Pilz, L.K. et al. (2012). Effects of the putative antipsychotic alstonine on glutamate uptake in acute hippocampal slices. *Neurochemistry International* 61 (7): 1144–1150.

Hong, J.T., Yen, J.H., Wang, L. et al. (2009). Regulation of heme oxygenase-1 expression and MAPK pathways in response to kaempferol and rhamnocitrin in PC12 cells. *Toxicology and Applied Pharmacology* 237 (1): 59–68.

Hong, H., Li, Y., and Su, B. (2017). Identification of circulating miR-125b as a potential biomarker of Alzheimer's disease in APP/PS1 transgenic mouse. *JAD* 59 (4): 1449–1458.

Hung, M.D. and Fraguela, M.G. (2014). El estrésoxidativoen las enfermedadesneurológicas:¿ causa o consecuencia? *Neurología: Publicaciónoficial de la Sociedad Española de Neurología* 29 (8): 451–452.

Hussain, G., Rasul, A., Anwar, H. et al. (2018). Role of plant derived alkaloids and their mechanism in neurodegenerative disorders. *International Journal of Biological Sciences* 14 (3): 341.

Hwang, E.M., Ryu, Y.B., Kim, H.Y. et al. (2008). BACE1 inhibitory effects of lavandulyl flavanones from Sophoraflavescens. *Bioorganic & Medicinal Chemistry* 16 (14): 6669–6674.

Ingre, C., Roos, P.M., Piehl, F. et al. (2015). Risk factors for amyotrophic lateral sclerosis. *Clinical Epidemiology* 7: 181–193.

Jain, N. and Ramawat, K.G. (2013). *Nutraceuticals and Antioxidants in Prevention of Diseases. Natural Products*, 2559–2580. Berlin: Springer.

Jia, X., Wang, F., Han, Y. et al. (2016). miR-137 and miR-491 negatively regulate dopamine transporter expression and function in neural cells. *Neuroscience Bulletin* 32 (6): 512–522.

Jiang, X., Jia, L.W., Li, X.H. et al. (2013). Capsaicin ameliorates stress-induced Alzheimer's disease-like pathological and cognitive impairments in rats. *Journal of Alzheimer's Disease* 35 (1): 91–105.

Jiang, W., Wei, W., Gaertig, M.A. et al. (2015). Therapeutic effect of berberine on Huntington's disease transgenic mouse model. *PLoS One* 10 (7): e0134142.

Kabaria, S., Choi, D.C., Chaudhuri, A.D. et al. (2015). MicroRNA-7 activates Nrf2 pathway by targeting Keap1 expression. *Free Radical Biology and Medicine* 89: 548–556.

Kelsey, N.A., Wilkins, H.M., and Linseman, D.A. (2010). Nutraceutical antioxidants as novel neuroprotective agents. *Molecules* 15 (11): 7792–7814.

Kiernan, M.C., Vucic, S., Cheah, B.C. et al. (2011). Amyotrophic lateral sclerosis. *The Lancet* 377 (9769): 942–955.

Kim, S. and Dewapriya, P. (2012). Bioactive compounds from marine sponges and their symbiotic microbes: a potential source of nutraceuticals. *Advances in Food and Nutrition Research* 65: 137–151.

Kim, S.J. and Linden, D.J. (2007). Ubiquitous plasticity and memory storage. *Neuron* 56 (4): 582–592.

Kim, J., Inoue, K., Ishii, J. et al. (2007). A MicroRNA feedback circuit in midbrain dopamine neurons. *Science* 317 (5842): 1220–1224.

Kim, M., Cho, K.H., Shin, M.S. et al. (2014). Berberine prevents nigrostriatal dopaminergic neuronal loss and suppresses hippocampal apoptosis in mice with Parkinson's disease. *International Journal of Molecular Medicine* 33 (4): 870–878.

Konovalova, J., Gerasymchuk, D., Parkkinen, I. et al. (2019). Interplay between MicroRNAs and oxidative stress in neurodegenerative diseases. *International Journal of Molecular Sciences* 20 (23): 6055.

Kulkarni, S.K. and Dhir, A. (2008). On the mechanism of antidepressant-like action of berberine chloride. *European Journal of Pharmacology* 589 (1–3): 163–172.

Kumar, H., Kim, I.S., More, S.V. et al. (2013). Gastrodin protects apoptotic dopaminergic neurons in a toxin-induced Parkinson's disease model. *Evidence-based Complementary and Alternative Medicine* 2013: 514095.

Kundu, P., Das, M., Tripathy, K., and Sahoo, S.K. (2016). Delivery of dual drug loaded lipid based nanoparticles across the blood–brain barrier impart enhanced neuroprotection in a rotenone induced mouse model of Parkinson's disease. *ACS Chemical Neuroscience* 7 (12): 1658–1670.

Labbadia, J. and Morimoto, R.I. (2013). Huntington's disease: underlying molecular mechanisms and emerging concepts. *Trends in Biochemical Sciences* 38 (8): 378–385.

Lama, A., Pirozzi, C., Avagliano, C. et al. (2020). Nutraceuticals: an integrative approach to starve Parkinson's disease. *Brain, Behavior, & Immunity-Health* 2: 100037.

Lau, F.C., Bielinski, D.F., and Joseph, J.A. (2007). Inhibitory effects of blueberry extract on the production of inflammatory mediators in lipopolysaccharide-activated BV2 microglia. *Journal of Neuroscience Research* 85 (5): 1010–1017.

Lee, Y.B., Lee, H.J., Won, M.H. et al. (2004). Soy isoflavones improve spatial delayed matching-to-place performance and reduce cholinergic neuron loss in elderly male rats. *The Journal of Nutrition* 134 (7): 1827–1831.

Lee, J., Hyeon, S.J., Im, H. et al. (2016). Astrocytes and microglia as non-cell autonomous players in the pathogenesis of ALS. *Experimental Neurobiology* 25 (5): 233–240.

Lei, X., Lei, L., Zhang, Z., and Cheng, Y. (2016). Neuroprotective effects of lycopene pretreatment on transient global cerebral ischemia reperfusion in rats: the role of the Nrf2/HO-1 signaling pathway. *Molecular Medicine Reports* 13: 412–418.

Li, Q., Spencer, N.Y., Pantazis, N.J., and Engelhardt, J.F. (2011). Alsin and SOD1 G93A proteins regulate endosomal reactive oxygen species production by glial cells and proinflammatory pathways responsible for neurotoxicity. *Journal of Biological Chemistry* 286 (46): 40151–40162.

Li, J.J., Dolios, G., Wang, R., and Liao, F.F. (2014). Soluble beta-amyloid peptides, but not insoluble fibrils, have specific effect on neuronal microRNA expression. *PLoS One* 9 (3): e90770.

Li, K., Hala, T.J., Seetharam, S. et al. (2015). GLT1 overexpression in SOD1G93A mouse cervical spinal cord does not preserve diaphragm function or extend disease. *Neurobiology of Disease* 78: 12–23.

Limanaqi, F., Biagioni, F., Busceti, C.L. et al. (2019). Phytochemicals bridging autophagy induction and alpha-Synuclein degradation in parkinsonism. *International Journal of Molecular Sciences* 20 (13): 3274.

Lin, M.T. and Beal, M.F. (2006). Mitochondrial dysfunction and oxidative stress in neurodegenerative diseases. *Nature Reviews* 443: 787–795.

Linck, V.M., Herrmann, A.P., Piato, Â.L. et al. (2011). Alstonine as an antipsychotic: effects on brain amines and metabolic changes. *Evidence-based Complementary and Alternative Medicine: Ecam* 2011: 19189988.

Liot, G., Valette, J., Pépin, J. et al. (2017). Energy defects in Huntington's disease: why "in vivo" evidence matters. *Biochemical and Biophysical Research Communications* 483 (4): 1084–1095.

Liu, C.G., Wang, J.L., Li, L. et al. (2014). MicroRNA-135a and-200b, potential biomarkers for Alzheimer' s disease, regulate β secretase and amyloid precursor protein. *Brain Research* 1583: 55–64.

Liu, Q., Xu, X., Zhao, M. et al. (2015). Berberine induces senescence of human glioblastoma cells by downregulating the EGFR–MEK–ERK signaling pathway. *Molecular Cancer Therapeutics* 14 (2): 355–363.

Liu, T., Liu, W.H., Zhao, J.S. et al. (2017). Lutein protects against β-amyloid peptide-induced oxidative stress in cerebrovascular endothelial cells through modulation of Nrf-2 and NF-κb. *Cell Biology and Toxicology* 33 (1): 57–67.

Liu, H.Y., Fu, X., Li, Y.F. et al. (2019). miR-15b-5p targeting amyloid precursor protein is involved in the anti-amyloid eflect of curcumin in swAPP695-HEK293 cells. *Neural Regeneration Research* 14 (9): 1603–1609.

Long, J.M. and Holtzman, D.M. (2019). Alzheimer disease: an update on pathobiology and treatment strategies. *Cell* 179 (2): 312–339.

Losi, G., Puia, G., Garzon, G. et al. (2004). Apigenin modulates GABAergic and glutamatergic transmission in cultured cortical neurons. *European Journal of Pharmacology* 502 (1–2): 41–46.

Lu, J., Cao, Y., Cheng, K. et al. (2015). Berberine regulates neurite outgrowth through AMPK-dependent pathways by lowering energy status. *Experimental Cell Research* 334 (2): 194–206.

Ma, J., Fang, B., Zeng, F. et al. (2014). Curcumin inhibits cell growth and invasion through up-regulation of miR-7 in pancreatic cancer cells. *Toxicology Letters* 231 (1): 82–91.

Ma, N.T., Zhou, R., Chang, R.Y. et al. (2015). Protective effects of aloperine on neonatal rat primary cultured hippocampal neurons injured by oxygen–glucose deprivation and reperfusion. *Journal of Natural Medicines* 69 (4): 575–583.

Magistretti, P.J. and Allaman, I. (2015). A cellular perspective on brain energy metabolism and functional imaging. *Neuron* 86 (4): 883–901.

Manach, C., Scalbert, A., Morand, C. et al. (2004). Polyphenols: food sources and bioavailability. *The American Journal of Clinical Nutrition* 79 (5): 727–747.

Manto, M.U. (2005). The wide spectrum of spinocerebellar ataxias (SCAs). *Cerebellum* 4 (1): 2–6.

Mao, Q.Q., Huang, Z., Ip, S.P. et al. (2012). Protective effects of piperine against corticosterone-induced neurotoxicity in PC12 cells. *Cellular and Molecular Neurobiology* 32 (4): 531–537.

Mao, X.Y., Jin, M.Z., Chen, J.F. et al. (2018). Live or let die: neuroprotective and anti-cancer effects of nutraceutical antioxidants. *Pharmacology & Therapeutics* 183: 137–151.

Masoud, S.T., Vecchio, L.M., Bergeron, Y. et al. (2015). Increased expression of the dopamine transporter leads to loss of dopamine neurons, oxidative stress and l-DOPA reversible motor deficits. *Neurobiology of Disease* 74: 66–75.

Mathew, A., Aravind, A., Fukuda, T. et al. (2011). Curcumin nanoparticles-a gateway for multifaceted approach to tackle Alzheimer's disease. *2011 11th IEEE International Conference on Nanotechnology* (pp. 833–836). IEEE.

Mayer, A.M., Rodríguez, A.D., Berlinck, R.G., and Fusetani, N. (2011). Marine pharmacology in 2007–8: marine compounds with antibacterial, anticoagulant, antifungal, anti-inflammatory, antimalarial, antiprotozoal, antituberculosis, and antiviral activities; affecting the immune and nervous system, and other miscellaneous mechanisms of action. *Comparative Biochemistry and Physiology Part C: Toxicology & Pharmacology* 153 (2): 191–222.

McCormack, A.L., Thiruchelvam, M., Manning-Bog, A.B. et al. (2002). Environmental risk factors and Parkinson's disease: selective degeneration of nigral dopaminergic neurons caused by the herbicide paraquat. *Neurobiology of Disease* 10 (2): 119–127.

McGregor, M.M. and Nelson, A.B. (2019). Circuit mechanisms of Parkinson's disease. *Neuron* 101 (6): 1042–1056.

McMillan, K.J., Murray, T.K., Bengoa-Vergniory, N. et al. (2017). Loss of microRNA-7 regulation leads to α-synuclein accumulation and dopaminergic neuronal loss in vivo. *Molecular Therapy* 25 (10): 2404–2414.

Mecocci, P., Tinarelli, C., Schulz, R.J., and Polidori, M.C. (2014). Nutraceuticals in cognitive impairment and Alzheimer's disease. *Frontiers in Pharmacology* 5: 147.

Mehbub, M.F., Lei, J., Franco, C., and Zhang, W. (2014). Marine sponge derived natural products between 2001 and 2010: trends and opportunities for discovery of bioactives. *Marine Drugs* 12 (8): 4539–4577.

Meiser, J., Weindl, D., and Hiller, K. (2013). Complexity of dopamine metabolism. *Cell Communication and Signaling: CCS* 11 (1): 1–18.

Melo, J.B., Sousa, C., Garçao, P. et al. (2009). Galantamine protects against oxidative stress induced by amyloid-beta peptide in cortical neurons. *European Journal of Neuroscience* 29 (3): 455–464.

Meng, X., Li, Y., Li, S. et al. (2017). Dietary sources and bioactivities of melatonin. *Nutrients* 9 (4): 367.

Mink, J.W., Blumenschine, R.J., and Adams, D.B. (1981). Ratio of central nervous system to body metabolism in vertebrates: its constancy and functional basis. *American Journal of Physiology. Regulatory, Integrative and Comparative Physiology* 10 (2): 203–212.

Mishra, A., Punia, J.K., Bladen, C. et al. (2015). Anticonvulsant mechanisms of piperine, a piperidine alkaloid. *Channels* 9 (5): 317–323.

Mochel, F., Haller, R.G., Mochel, F., and Haller, R.G. (2011). Energy deficit in Huntington disease : why it matters find the latest version : review series energy deficit in Huntington disease : why it matters. *The Journal of Clinical Investigation* 121 (2): 493–499.

Moreira, P.I., Nunomura, A., Honda, K. et al. (2007). The key role of oxidative stress in alzheimer's disease. In: *Oxidative Stress and Neurodegenerative Disorders* (eds. G.A. Qureshi and S.H. Parvez), 267–281. Elsevier.

Moussa, C., Hebron, M., Huang, X. et al. (2017). Resveratrol regulates neuro-inflammation and induces adaptive immunity in Alzheimer's disease. *Journal of Neuroinflammation* 14 (1): 1.

Munro, D. and Treberg, J.R. (2017). A radical shift in perspective: mitochondria as regulators of reactive oxygen species. *Journal of Experimental Biology* 220 (7): 1170–1180.

Murphy, M.P., Holmgren, A., Larsson, N.G. et al. (2011). Unraveling the biological roles of reactive oxygen species. *Cell Metabolism* 13 (4): 361–366.

Nagai, M., Re, D.B., Nagata, T. et al. (2007). Astrocytes expressing ALS-linked mutated SOD1 release factors selectively toxic to motor neurons. *Nature Neuroscience* 10 (5): 615–622.

Nakamura, T. and Lipton, S.A. (2010). Preventing Ca2+−mediated nitrosative stress in neurodegenerative diseases: possible pharmacological strategies. *Cell Calcium* 47 (2): 190–197.

Nakamura, T. and Lipton, S.A. (2011). Redox modulation by S-nitrosylation contributes to protein misfolding, mitochondrial dynamics, and neuronal synaptic damage in neurodegenerative diseases. *Cell Death and Differentiation* 18 (9): 1478–1486.

Narasimhan, M., Patel, D., Vedpathak, D. et al. (2012). Identification of novel microRNAs in post-transcriptional control of Nrf2 expression and redox homeostasis in neuronal, SH-SY5Y cells. *PLoS One* 7 (12): e51111.

Nasri, H., Baradaran, A., Shirzad, H., and Rafieian-Kopaei, M. (2014). New concepts in nutraceuticals as alternative for pharmaceuticals. *International Journal of Preventive Medicine* 5 (12): 1487.

Nedergaard, M., Ransom, B., and Goldman, S.A. (2003). New roles for astrocytes: redefining the functional architecture of the brain. *Trends in Neurosciences* 26 (10): 523–530.

Nehlig, A. (2013). The neuroprotective effects of cocoa flavanol and its influence on cognitive performance. *British Journal of Clinical Pharmacology* 75 (3): 716–727.

Nieves, J.W., Gennings, C., Factor-Litvak, P. et al. (2016). Association between dietary intake and function in amyotrophic lateral sclerosis. *JAMA Neurology* 73 (12): 1425–1432.

Ogle, W.O., Speisman, R.B., and Ormerod, B.K. (2013). Potential of treating age-related depression and cognitive decline with nutraceutical approaches: a mini-review. *Gerontology* 59 (1): 23–31.

Paiva, I.H.R., Duarte-Silva, E., and Peixoto, C.A. (2020). The role of prebiotics in cognition, anxiety, and depression. *European Neuropsychopharmacology* 34: 1–18.

Paladino, S., Conte, A., Caggiano, R. et al. (2018). Nrf2 pathway in age-related neurological disorders: insights into MicroRNAs. *Cellular Physiology and Biochemistry* 47 (5): 1951–1976.

Pandey, K.R., Naik, S.R., and Vakil, B.V. (2015). Probiotics, prebiotics and synbiotics-a review. *Journal of Food Science and Technology* 52 (12): 7577–7587.

Panov, A.V., Gutekunst, C.A., Leavitt, B.R. et al. (2002). Early mitochondrial calcium defects in Huntington's disease are a direct effect of polyglutamines. *Nature Neuroscience* 5 (8): 731–736.

Paredes, S.D., Rancan, L., Kireev, R. et al. (2015). Melatonin counteracts at a transcriptional level the inflammatory and apoptotic response secondary to ischemic brain injury induced by middle cerebral artery blockade in aging rats. *BioResearch Open Access* 4 (1): 407–416.

Patel, M. (2016). Targeting oxidative stress in central nervous system disorders. *Physiology & Behavior* 37 (9): 1–17.

Patten, D.A., Germain, M., Kelly, M.A., and Slack, R.S. (2010). Reactive oxygen species: stuck in the middle of neurodegeneration. *Journal of Alzheimer's Disease* 20: s357–s367.

Pearson, V.E. (2001). Galantamine: a new Alzheimer drug with a past life. *Annals of Pharmacotherapy* 35 (11): 1406–1413.

Perfeito, R., Cunha-Oliveira, T., and Rego, A.C. (2012). Revisiting oxidative stress and mitochondrial dysfunction in the pathogenesis of Parkinson disease – resemblance to the effect of amphetamine drugs of abuse. *Free Radical Biology and Medicine* 53 (9): 1791–1806.

Phaniendra, A., Jestadi, D.B., and Periyasamy, L. (2015). Free radicals: properties, sources, targets, and their implication in various diseases. *Indian Journal of Clinical Biochemistry* 30 (1): 11–26.

Poewe, W., Seppi, K., Tanner, C.M. et al. (2017). Parkinson disease. *Nature Reviews. Disease Primers* 3 (1): 1–21.

Polanco, J.C., Li, C., Bodea, L.G. et al. (2018). Amyloid-β and tau complexity – towards improved biomarkers and targeted therapies. *Nature Reviews Neurology* 14 (1): 22.

Poljsak, B., Šuput, D., and Milisav, I. (2013). Achieving the balance between ROS and antioxidants: when to use the synthetic antioxidants. *Oxidative Medicine and Cellular Longevity* 2013: 1–11.

Poyton, R.O., Ball, K.A., and Castello, P.R. (2009). Mitochondrial generation of free radicals and hypoxic signaling. *Trends in Endocrinology and Metabolism* 20 (7): 332–340.

Prasad, K.N. (2016). Simultaneous activation of Nrf2 and elevation of antioxidant compounds for reducing oxidative stress and chronic inflammation in human Alzheimer's disease. *Mechanisms of Ageing and Development* 153: 41–47.

Prins, N.D., van der Flier, W.A., Knol, D.L. et al. (2014). The effect of galantamine on brain atrophy rate in subjects with mild cognitive impairment is modified by apolipoprotein E genotype: post-hoc analysis of data from a randomized controlled trial. *Alzheimer's Research & Therapy* 6 (4): 47.

Qin, L.X., Tan, J.Q., Zhang, H.N. et al. (2017). BAG5 interacts with DJ-1 and inhibits the neuroprotective effects of DJ-1 to combat mitochondrial oxidative damage. *Oxidative Medicine and Cellular Longevity* 2017: 1–10.

Querfurth, H.W. and Laferla, F.M. (2018). Alzheimer's disease. *The New England Journal of Medicine* 362 (4): 329–344.

Reagan, L.P., Magariños, A.M., Yee, D.K. et al. (2000). Oxidative stress and HNE conjugation of GLUT3 are increased in the hippocampus of diabetic rats subjected to stress. *Brain Research* 862: 292–300.

Reynolds, I.J. and Hastings, T.G. (1995). Glutamate induces the production of reactive oxygen species in cultured forebrain neurons following NMDA receptor activation. *Journal of Neuroscience* 15 (5 I): 3318–3327.

Ríos-Covián, D., Ruas-Madiedo, P., Margolles, A. et al. (2016). Intestinal short chain fatty acids and their link with diet and human health. *Frontiers in Microbiology* 7: 185.

Ritter, S. (2017). Monitoring and maintenance of brain glucose supply: importance of hindbrain catecholamine neurons in this multifaceted task. In: *Appetite and Food Intake: Central Control*, 2e, 177–205. Boca Raton (FL): CRC Press/Taylor & Francis.

Robles, L. (2013). Role of oxidative stress in the pathogenesis of pancreatitis: effect of antioxidant therapy. *Pancreatic Disorders & Therapy* 03 (01): 1–8.

Rossi, M., Perez-Lloret, S., Doldan, L. et al. (2013). Autosomal dominant cerebellar ataxias: a systematic review of clinical features. *Journal of the Neurological Sciences* 333: e610.

Rubattu, S., Forte, M., and Raffa, S. (2019). Circulating leukocytes and oxidative stress in cardiovascular diseases: a state of the art. *Oxidative Medicine and Cellular Longevity* 2019: 2650429.

Saccon, R.A., Bunton-Stasyshyn, R.K.A., Fisher, E.M.C., and Fratta, P. (2013). Is SOD1 loss of function involved in amyotrophic lateral sclerosis? *Brain* 136 (8): 2342–2358.

Salim, S. (2017). Oxidative stress and the central nervous system. *Journal of Pharmacology and Experimental Therapeutics* 360 (1): 201–205.

Sandhir, R., Yadav, A., Mehrotra, A. et al. (2014). Curcumin nanoparticles attenuate neurochemical and neurobehavioral deficits in experimental model of Huntington's disease. *Neuromolecular Medicine* 16 (1): 106–118.

Satoh, T., Kosaka, K., Itoh, K. et al. (2008). Carnosic acid, a catechol-type electrophilic compound, protects neurons both in vitro and in vivo through activation of the Keap1/Nrf2 pathway via S-alkylation of targeted cysteines on Keap1. *Journal of Neurochemistry* 104 (4): 1116–1131.

Saudou, F. and Humbert, S. (2016). The biology of huntingtin. *Neuron* 89 (5): 910–926.

Schachter, J., Martel, J., Lin, C.S. et al. (2018). Effects of obesity on depression: a role for inflammation and the gut microbiota. *Brain, Behavior, and Immunity* 69: 1–8.

Schepers, M., Martens, N., Tiane, A. et al. (2020). Edible seaweed-derived constituents: an undisclosed source of neuroprotective compounds. *Neural Regeneration Research* 15 (5): 790.

Schratt, G. (2009). microRNAs at the synapse. *Nature Reviews Neuroscience* 10 (12): 842–849.

Sestili, P., Martinelli, C., Colombo, E. et al. (2011). Creatine as an antioxidant. *Amino Acids* 40 (5): 1385–1396.

Shelat, P.B., Chalimoniuk, M., Wang, J.H. et al. (2008). Amyloid beta peptide and NMDA induce ROS from NADPH oxidase and AA release from cytosolic phospholipase A2 in cortical neurons. *Journal of Neurochemistry* 106 (1): 45–55.

Shukla, V., Mishra, S.K., and Pant, H.C. (2011). Oxidative stress in neurodegeneration. *Advances in Pharmacological Sciences* 2011: 1–13.

Singh, A., Kukreti, R., Saso, L., and Kukreti, S. (2019). Oxidative stress: a key modulator in neurodegenerative diseases. *Molecules* 24 (8): 1583.

Smith, M.A., Zhu, X., Tabaton, M. et al. (2010). Increased iron and free radical generation in preclinical Alzheimer disease and mild cognitive impairment. *Journal of Alzheimer's Disease* 19 (1): 353–372.

Soares, R.O.S., Losada, D.M., Jordani, M.C. et al. (2019). Ischemia/reperfusion injury revisited: an overview of the latest pharmacological strategies. *International Journal of Molecular Sciences* 20 (20): 5034.

Song, P. and Zou, M.-H. (2015). Atherosclerosis: risks, mechanisms, and therapies. *Risks, Mechanisms, and Therapies* 1: 379–392.

Spencer, J.P., Abd El Mohsen, M.M., Minihane, A.M., and Mathers, J.C. (2008). Biomarkers of the intake of dietary polyphenols: strengths, limitations and application in nutrition research. *British Journal of Nutrition* 99 (1): 12–22.

Squillaro, T., Cimini, A., Peluso, G. et al. (2018). Nano-delivery systems for encapsulation of dietary polyphenols: an experimental approach for neurodegenerative diseases and brain tumors. *Biochemical Pharmacology* 154: 303–317.

Stucki, D.M., Ruegsegger, C., Steiner, S. et al. (2016). Mitochondrial impairments contribute to spinocerebellar ataxia type 1 progression and can be ameliorated by the mitochondria-targeted antioxidant MitoQ. *Free Radical Biology and Medicine* 97: 427–440.

Sun, Y., Lu, C.J., Chien, K.L. et al. (2007). Efficacy of multivitamin supplementation containing vitamins B6 and B12 and folic acid as adjunctive treatment with a cholinesterase inhibitor in Alzheimer's disease: a 26-week, randomized, double-blind, placebo-controlled study in Taiwanese patients. *Clinical Therapeutics* 29 (10): 2204–2214.

Sun, Y.M., Lu, C., and Wu, Z.Y. (2016). Spinocerebellar ataxia: relationship between phenotype and genotype–a review. *Clinical Genetics* 90 (4): 305–314.

Sun, J., Liu, S., Ling, Z. et al. (2019). Fructooligosaccharides ameliorating cognitive deficits and neurodegeneration in APP/PS1 transgenic mice through modulating gut microbiota. *Journal of Agricultural and Food Chemistry* 67 (10): 3006–3017.

Taram, F., Ignowski, E., Duval, N., and Linseman, D.A. (2018). Neuroprotection comparison of rosmarinic acid and carnosic acid in primary cultures of cerebellar granule neurons. *Molecules* 23 (11): 2956.

Taylor, M., Moore, S., Mourtas, S. et al. (2011). Effect of curcumin-associated and lipid ligand-functionalized nanoliposomes on aggregation of the Alzheimer's Aβ peptide. *Nanomedicine: Nanotechnology, Biology and Medicine* 7 (5): 541–550.

Taylor, J.P., Brown, R.H., and Cleveland, D.W. (2016). Decoding ALS: from genes to mechanism. *Nature* 539 (7628): 197–206.

Tiwari, S.K., Agarwal, S., Seth, B. et al. (2014). Curcumin-loaded nanoparticles potently induce adult neurogenesis and reverse cognitive deficits in Alzheimer's disease model via canonical Wnt/β-catenin pathway. *ACS Nano* 8 (1): 76–103.

Toden, S., Okugawa, Y., Buhrmann, C. et al. (2015). Novel evidence for curcumin and boswellic acid–induced chemoprevention through regulation of miR-34a and miR-27a in colorectal cancer. *Cancer Prevention Research* 8 (5): 431–443.

Toler, S.M. (1997). Creatine is an ergogen for anaerobic exercise. *Nutrition Reviews* 55 (1): 21–23.

Touyz, R.M., Rios, F.J., Alves-Lopes, R. et al. (2020). Oxidative stress: a unifying paradigm in hypertension. *The Canadian Journal of Cardiology* 36 (5): 659–670.

Turner, R.J. and Vink, R. (2014). NK1 tachykinin receptor treatment is superior to capsaicin pre-treatment in improving functional outcome following acute ischemic stroke. *Neuropeptides* 48 (5): 267–272.

Turrens, J.F. (2003). Mitochondrial formation of reactive oxygen species. *The Journal of Physiology* 552 (2): 335–344.

Valente, E.M., Abou-Sleiman, P.M., Caputo, V. et al. (2016). American association for the advancement of science. *Science* 304: 1158–1160.

Velagapudi, R., Jamshaid, F., Lepiarz, I. et al. (2019). The tiliroside derivative, 3-O-[(E)-2-oxo-4-(p-tolyl) but–3–en–1–yl] kaempferol produced inhibition of neuroinflammation and activation of AMPK and Nrf2/HO-1 pathways in BV-2 microglia. *International Immunopharmacology* 77: 105951.

Verghese, P.B., Castellano, J.M., and Holtzman, D.M. (2011). Apolipoprotein E in Alzheimer's disease and other neurological disorders. *The Lancet Neurology* 10 (3): 241–252.

Wang, S., Ding, L., and Zhou, R.Q. (2005a). Determination of isoflavones in soybean meal by HPLC. *Chemical Industry and Engineering Progress* 24 (2): 196.

Wang, X., Wang, R., Xing, D. et al. (2005b). Kinetic difference of berberine between hippocampus and plasma in rat after intravenous administration of Coptidisrhizoma extract. *Life Sciences* 77 (24): 3058–3067.

Wang, D., Noda, Y., Zhou, Y. et al. (2007). The allosteric potentiation of nicotinic acetylcholine receptors by galantamine ameliorates the cognitive dysfunction in beta amyloid 25–35 icv-injected mice: involvement of dopaminergic systems. *Neuropsychopharmacology* 32 (6): 1261–1271.

Wang, W.X., Rajeev, B.W., Stromberg, A.J. et al. (2008). The expression of microRNA miR-107 decreases early in Alzheimer's disease and may accelerate disease progression through regulation of β-site amyloid precursor protein-cleaving enzyme 1. *Journal of Neuroscience* 28 (5): 1213–1223.

Wang, M.H., Chang, W.J., Soung, H.S., and Chang, K.C. (2012). (−)-Epigallocatechin-3-gallate decreases the impairment in learning and memory in spontaneous hypertension rats. *Behavioural Pharmacology* 23 (8): 771–780.

Wang, Z.H., Zhang, J.L., Duan, Y.L. et al. (2015). MicroRNA-214 participates in the neuroprotective effect of resveratrol via inhibiting α-synuclein expression in MPTP-induced Parkinson's disease mouse. *Biomedicine & Pharmacotherapy* 74: 252–256.

Wang, Z., Fan, J., Wang, J. et al. (2016). Protective effect of lycopene on high-fat diet-induced cognitive impairment in rats. *Neuroscience Letters* 627: 185–191.

Wang, L., Liu, J., Wang, Q. et al. (2019). MicroRNA-200a-3p mediates neuroprotection in Alzheimer-related deficits and attenuates amyloid-beta overproduction and tau hyperphosphorylation via co-regulating BACE1 and PRKACB. *Frontiers in Pharmacology* 10: 806.

Wheeler, D.B., Randall, A., and Tsien, R.W. (1993). Roles of N-type and Q-type Ca2+ channels inSupporting hippocampal synaptic transmission. *Science* 264: 107–111.

World Health Organization. (2016). Neurological disorders.

Wu, F., Xu, K., Liu, L. et al. (2019). Vitamin B12 enhances nerve repair and improves functional recovery after traumatic brain injury by inhibiting ER stress-induced neuron injury. *Frontiers in Pharmacology* 10: 406.

Wu, W., Zhang, Z., Li, F. et al. (2020). A network-based approach to explore the mechanisms of Uncaria Alkaloids in treating hypertension and alleviating Alzheimer's disease. *International Journal of Molecular Sciences* 21 (5): 1766.

Xia, D., Sui, R., and Zhang, Z. (2019). Administration of resveratrol improved Parkinson's disease-like phenotype by suppressing apoptosis of neurons via modulating the MALAT1/miR-129/SNCA signaling pathway. *Journal of Cellular Biochemistry* 120 (4): 4942–4951.

Xie, Y. and Chen, Y. (2016). microRNAs: emerging targets regulating oxidative stress in the models of Parkinson's disease. *Frontiers in Neuroscience* 10: 298.

Xu, Y., Wang, Z., You, W. et al. (2010). Antidepressant-like effect of trans-resveratrol: involvement of serotonin and noradrenaline system. *European Neuropsychopharmacology* 20 (6): 405–413.

Yang, X., Li, Y., Li, Y. et al. (2017). Oxidative stress-mediated atherosclerosis: mechanisms and therapies. *Frontiers in Physiology* 8: 1–16.

Ye, X., Luo, H., Chen, Y. et al. (2015). MicroRNAs 99b-5p/100-5p regulated by endoplasmic reticulum stress are involved in a beta-induced pathologies. *Frontiers in Aging Neuroscience* 7: 210.

Zhang, Z.C., Su, G., Li, J. et al. (2013). Two new neuroprotective phenolic compounds from Gastrodiaelata. *Journal of Asian Natural Products Research* 15 (6): 619–623.

Zhao, J., Yue, D., Zhou, Y. et al. (2017). The role of microRNAs in Aβ deposition and tau phosphorylation in Alzheimer's disease. *Frontiers in Neurology* 8: 342.

Zhao, J., Zhang, G., Li, M. et al. (2018). Neuro-protective effects of aloperine in an Alzheimer's disease cellular model. *Biomedicine & Pharmacotherapy* 108: 137–143.

Zoghbi, H.Y. and Orr, H.T. (2009). Pathogenic mechanisms of a polyglutamine-mediated neurodegenerative disease, spinocerebellar ataxia type 1. *Journal of Biological Chemistry* 284 (12): 7425–7429.

Zorov, D.B., Juhaszova, M., and Sollott, S.J. (2014). Mitochondrial reactive oxygen species (ROS) and ROS-induced ROS release. *Physiological Reviews* 94 (3): 909–950.

Zucker, R.S. (1999). Calcium- and activity-dependent synaptic plasticity. *Current Opinion in Neurobiology* 9 (3): 305–313.

Zuo, L. and Motherwell, M.S. (2013). The impact of reactive oxygen species and genetic mitochondrial mutations in Parkinson's disease. *Gene* 532 (1): 18–23.

Zuo, L., Zhou, T., Pannell, B.K. et al. (2015a). Biological and physiological role of reactive oxygen species – the good, the bad and the ugly. *Acta Physiologica* 214 (3): 329–348.

Zuo, L., Hemmelgarn, B.T., Chuang, C.C., and Best, T.M. (2015b). The role of oxidative stress-induced epigenetic alterations in amyloid-β production in Alzheimer's disease. *Oxidative Medicine and Cellular Longevity* 2015: 1–13.

9

Flavonoids as Nutraceuticals

Shreya C. Adangale, Ritushree Ghosh, and Sarika Wairkar

Shobhaben Pratapbhai Patel School of Pharmacy & Technology Management, SVKM's NMIMS, Mumbai, Maharashtra, India

9.1 Nutraceuticals

The phrase "Let thy food be thy medicine and medicine be thy food" is said by Hippocrates, the father of medicine, and it perfectly explains the significance of nutrition to prevent or cure diseases. He has identified the relationship between food and health and emphasized that "differences of diseases depend on nutriment." This clearly meant that food is linked to the treatment of various ailments or, in other words, food is medicine. The term "nutraceuticals" was first coined by Stephen DeFelice from the combination of "nutrition" and "pharmaceuticals" in 1989. According to DeFelice, a nutraceutical is "a food (or a part of food) that provides medical or health benefits, including the prevention and/or treatment of a disease." Nutraceuticals may include isolated nutrients, dietary supplements to genetically engineered "designer" foods, herbal products, and processed products such as cereals, soups, and beverages (Andlauer and Fürst 2002). Nutraceuticals can have a variety of therapeutic effects in metabolic disorders like diabetes and indigestion, cardiovascular disorders like blood pressure and cholesterol control, prevention of certain cancers, in cold and cough, sleeping disorders, osteoporosis, pain, and neurological disorders like depression (Dillard and German 2000; Andlauer and Fürst 2002). Nutraceuticals can be classified based on various criteria; traditional nutraceuticals are classified in the following ways (Singh and Sinha 2012):

1) Chemical constituents like nutrients, herbals, and phytochemicals
2) Probiotic microorganisms
3) Nutraceutical enzymes

Phytochemicals are an important class of nutraceuticals which are further classified based on their chemical classes as follows (Vincken et al. 2007; Cheung and Kong 2010; Agerbirk and Olsen 2012; Da Costa 2017):

1) Polyphenolic compounds – flavone, isoflavone, flavonoids, flavonols, phenolic acids, anthocyanins, proanthocyanidins, resveratrol, curcumin, ellagic acid, and ellagitannins
2) Carotenoids – lutein, lycopene, α and β carotene, α cryptoxanthin, zeaxanthin, and fucoxanthin
3) Anthraquinones – barbaloin, capsaicin, hypericin, and piperine
4) Terpenes – borneol, santonin, gossypol, and menthol

Handbook of Nutraceuticals and Natural Products: Biological, Medicinal, and Nutritional Properties and Applications, Volume 1, First Edition. Edited by Sreerag Gopi and Preetha Balakrishnan.
© 2022 John Wiley & Sons, Inc. Published 2022 by John Wiley & Sons, Inc.

5) Alkaloids – quine, morphine, ergot alkaloids, and coumarin
6) Glucosinolates – allyl glucosinolate (sinigrin), and benzyl glucosinolate
7) Saponins – triterpenoid, spirostanol, and furostanol
8) Isothiocyanates – phenethyl isothiocyanate, and sulforaphane

One of the most important classes of phytochemicals is flavonoids. This chapter summarizes the various flavonoids useful as nutraceuticals, their physicochemical properties, and various pharmacological actions.

9.2 Flavonoids

In 1930, Albert Szent-Gyorgyi isolated a new compound from lemon juice and named it vitamin P. Later, this compound was termed as a flavonoid (Kozłowska and Szostak-Węgierek 2017). Up till now, there were at least 9000 different types of naturally occurring flavonoids that have been discovered (Wang et al. 2011). Flavonoids are polyphenolic compounds consisting of nonvolatile secondary plant metabolites with a basic structure of diphenylpropane (C6–C3–C6), showing numerous therapeutic activities (Hollman 2004). Flavonoids with biological activity are often referred to as bioflavonoids and have the exceptional ability to capture superoxide, hydroxyl, and lipid radicals (Brodowska 2017). Flavonoids are found mostly in all parts of plants. They are mainly responsible for color, taste, prevention of fat oxidation, and protection of vitamins and enzymes in plants. Edible sources of flavonoids in the human diet include tea, wine, berries, vegetables, fruits, nuts, and many more (Kaleem and Ahmad 2018). Flavonoids occur as glycosides, aglycones, and methylated derivatives. In plants, flavonoid aglycones show a variety of structural forms. All of them contain fifteen carbon atoms in their basic nucleus: two aromatic rings labeled as rings A and B linked via a heterocyclic pyran ring C (Kumar and Pandey 2013).

9.2.1 Structure and Classification of Flavonoids

Flavonoids can be classified into different classes based on their chemical structure and their classification as shown in Figure 9.1.

1) **Flavone:** Flavones are one of the important classes of flavonoids characterized by a double bond between the second and third carbon of ring C and a carbonyl group present at the fourth position. Generally, flavones have a hydroxyl group present in carbon 5 of ring A, e.g. apigenin and luteolin.
2) **Flavonol:** Flavonols have structural similarity with flavone, the only difference being the presence of hydroxyl group at the third position of ring C, e.g. quercetin and kaempferol (Ruiz-Cruz et al. 2017).
3) **Flavanone:** Flavanone lacks a double bond between the second and third carbon atom of the ring C which is accompanied by an absence of the hydroxyl group. This unique feature makes them easily distinguished from flavones and flavonols (Barreca et al. 2017). They play an important role in the metabolic pathway of other flavonoids and their precursors are chalcones, flavones, isoflavones, and dihydroxyflavonols that are biosynthesized from flavanones, e.g. naringenin and hesperetin (Ruiz-Cruz et al. 2017).
4) **Isoflavone:** It consists of a phenyl chromen B skeleton which is linked to the third position of the C ring instead of the second position like the other flavonoids. Isoflavones are found widely in Soybean in three forms – genistin, daidzin, and glycitein. They abundantly belong to the

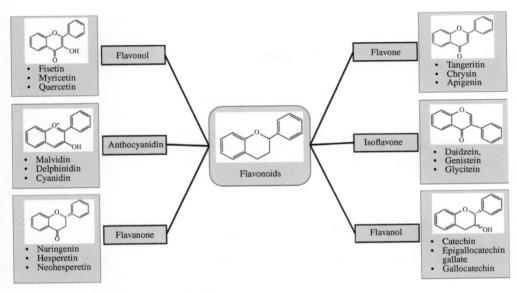

Figure 9.1 Structural classification of flavonoids.

family *Leguminosae*. They are characterized by their unique phytoestrogenic properties (Corradini et al. 2011).

5) **Flavanol:** Flavanols are colorless compounds and also known as flavan-3-ols with a hydroxyl group in the third position of ring C which lacks the carbonyl group. No double bond is present between the second and third carbon of ring B, e.g. epigallocatechin and catechin.

6) **Anthocyanidin:** Anthocyanidins are water-soluble pigments responsible for color in plants, fruits, and flowers. They have a hydroxyl group on third carbon and also exhibit a double bond between the third and fourth carbon of ring C, e.g. cyanidin and delphinidin (Ruiz-Cruz et al. 2017).

9.2.2 Physicochemical and Pharmacokinetic Properties of Flavonoids

Solubility plays an important role in the pharmacological activity of flavonoids. Generally, the aqueous solubility of flavonoids is low and therefore to increase its solubility, semisynthetic water-soluble flavonoids have been developed such as hydroxyethylrutosides and inositol-2-phosphatequercetin (Havsteen 2002). Another important parameter is lipophilicity that plays an important role in helping molecules to cross the cell membrane and reach their target site. Although flavonoids are low molecular weight lipophilic compounds, many of them have poor oral bioavailability due to extensive first-pass metabolism and hydrolyzation by bacterial enzymes (Nagula and Wairkar 2019).

The absorption of flavonoids plays an important role in deciding their bioavailability. The absorption of flavonoids depends on their physicochemical properties such as their solubility, pK_a, lipophilicity, molecular size, and configuration. The two important places for the yabsorption of flavonoids are the intestine and the colon. Dietary flavanols having glycosides show a very rapid to seemingly slow absorption in humans whereas catechins are rapidly absorbed from the small intestine. Out of all the flavonoid, isoflavones are more bioavailable and anthocyanins show the lowest bioavailability.

Flavonoids are metabolized in two compartments in which the first compartment consists of the small intestine, kidneys, and liver and the second compartment is the colon that contains unmetabolized or unabsorbed flavonoids previously. The liver is the chief organ involved in the metabolism of these secondary plant metabolites but the role of kidneys and intestines cannot be overlooked. Flavonoids are conjugated in the liver by glucuronidation, methylation, or sulfation process. Apart from that, glycoside degradation enzymes like glycosidases, sulfatases, and glucuronidases can separate or break flavonoid conjugates (Hollman 2004). Polar water-soluble flavonoid glucuronides in mammals either go through biliary excretion or are expelled through urine. Factors like molecular weight, chemical substitution, and degree of polarity determine the extent of biliary excretion. Flavonoids are also eliminated by renal excretion after conjugation in the liver (Aherne and O'Brien 2002).

9.3 Pharmacological Actions

Flavonoids possess several vital pharmacological actions like antioxidants, anti-inflammatory, neuroprotective, antidiabetic, cardioprotective, anticancer, and hepatoprotective activity, etc. These activities along with *in vitro* and *in vivo* studies and few delivery systems of flavonoids are described in detail in the following section.

9.3.1 Antioxidant Activity

Flavonoids have a very prominent antioxidant activity that is shown by almost all groups of flavonoids. The extent of antioxidant action varies with the arrangement and type of the functional group around the basic skeleton. Several mechanisms such as free radical scavenging and transition metal ion chelating ability would be influenced by the configuration, substitution, and presence of a total number of hydroxyl groups (Pandey et al. 2012). Oxidative stress is induced by lipid peroxidation (Kumar et al. 2013) and reactive oxygen species (ROS) or due to inhibition of antioxidants (Pietta 2000; Procházková et al. 2011) as shown in Figure 9.2. Mechanism of antioxidant activity includes: (i) ROS formation which can be suppressed either by enzyme inhibition or chelating trace elements that are involved in free radical production; (ii) scavenging ROS; (iii) upregulating or protecting antioxidant defences (Kumar and Pandey 2013). Flavonoids such as kaempferol, quercetin, catechin, apigenin, etc., exhibit prominent antioxidant properties against DNA damage.

In this study, apigenin existed in the form of apiin, isolated from celery leaf studied for antioxidant activity with rutin as a positive control. In an *in vitro* study, 1,1-diphenyl-2-picrylhydrazyl (DPPH), superoxide and hydroxyl radical scavenging assays were performed. In the case of apiin, DPPH and superoxide radical scavenging activities, IC50 values were found to be 68.0 μg/ml and 0.39 mg/ml, respectively, whereas, in the case of rutin, those values were 45.6 μg/ml and 0.19 mg/ml. But in the case of hydroxyl radical scavenging assay, both apiin and rutin showed maximum antioxidant activities at lower concentrations. Also, *in vivo* studies were performed using the mice model (50 mg/kg) to measure the activities of superoxide dismutase (SOD), catalase (CAT), and glutathione peroxidase (GSH-Px) in the serum, brain, kidney, liver, and heart. It was observed that apiin showed the strongest *in vivo* antioxidant activities by improving SOD, CAT, and GSH-Px contents which were due to increased mRNA expression that provides defence for the damage of free radicals and was also useful in preventing brain oxidative state and provides protection for liver, kidney, and heart against DNA damage (Li et al. 2014). A similar *in vitro* and *in vivo* study was

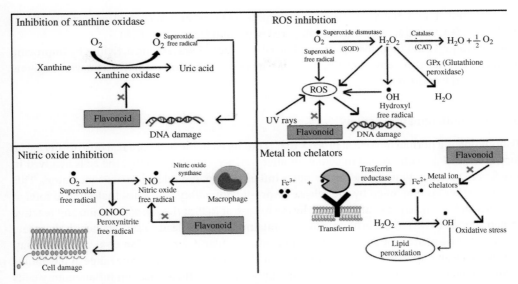

Figure 9.2 Mechanism of antioxidant activity of flavonoids.

conducted for antioxidant activity of Assam black tea extract and results demonstrated the efficacy of black tea and its polyphenols in scavenging free radicals and improving aforesaid antioxidant enzymes (Sun et al. 2012). Flavonoids were extracted from berries and *in vitro* antioxidant studies were performed to determine free radical scavenging assays along with ferric ion reducing antioxidant power (FRAP) assay. The results found that EC50 values of flavonoids showing DPPH, superoxide, hydroxyl, and FRAP activities were 10.97 ± 0.18, 214.83 ± 6.54, 217.73 ± 3.46, and $28.67 \pm 1.37 \, \mu g/ml$ respectively. The *in vivo* study carried out using Kunming mice model (5, 25, 125 mg/kg) and maximum antioxidant activity was observed at 125 mg/kg dose with 282.1 ± 19.6 and $52.1 \pm 2.23 \, U/ml$ SOD and GSH-Px contents, respectively (Wu et al. 2015). Similar observations were reported by Sobeh et al. for proanthocyanidin extracted from the Cassia root (Sobeh et al. 2018).

Another study was conducted to determine the antioxidant activity of isoquercitrin (5–2000 μM) that opposes oxidative damage induced by cadmium in the kidney and liver of mouse. In an *in vitro* study, high levels of scavenging were seen for superoxide, hydroxyl, and nitrite radicals with increasing concentrations of isoquercitrin. The *in vivo* study carried out using Kunming albino mice (2.5 mg/kg) revealed elevated levels of SOD and CAT (Li et al. 2011). Hibatallah et al. studied *Ginkgo* extract containing quercetin and kaempferol to evaluate antioxidant activities. In an *in vitro* study, electron-spin resonance (ESR) assay was performed and results showed that inhibition rates of quercetin and *Ginkgo* extracts were 28 and 22%, respectively. But when kaempferol and *Ginkgo* extract were compared, the latter was better than kaempferol (Hibatallah et al. 1999).

Flavonoids are formulated and evaluated into novel delivery systems. Here, the phospholipid complex of hesperidin was prepared to improve dissolution. The *in vitro* release study in pH 7.4 buffer showed greater release from phospholipid-complex (78.2%) than plain hesperidin (46.9%) after seven hours. The reducing power method was used to study the antioxidant activity of the formulation that disclosed the concentration-dependent antioxidant effect (Kalita and Patwary 2020). Also, rutin nano-lipid complexes were prepared and comparative *in vitro* antioxidant activities for free rutin and rutin nano-complexes (50 μg/ml) showed better antioxidant activity of the latter by DPPH assay. In addition, *in vivo* study in a rat model (200 mg/kg) demonstrated improved SOD,

CAT, GSH, and glutathione *S*-transferase (GST) contents for rutin-nano complexes against carbon tetrachloride (CCl_4)-induced toxicity as compared with rutin (Ravi et al. 2018).

Thus, flavonoids and their formulations showed free radical scavenging activities by improving antioxidant enzymes, thereby providing a defence mechanism against oxidative damage and giving protection to the entire body.

9.3.2 Anti-inflammatory Activity

Inflammation is a normal biological process that is produced in the body as a response to any tissue injury, microbial or pathological infection, or allergy. Once an injury occurs, the cells involved in the defence system migrate to the site to cause inflammation and release various mediators. This action is further accompanied by the release of pro-inflammatory cytokines that remove foreign pathogens and normalize the infected site, by the release of ROS at the site of infection and reactive nitrogen species (RNS). Furthermore, chronic inflammation can lead to serious health disorders like cancers, and neurological, metabolic, and cardiovascular disorders (Pan et al. 2010). Dietary flavonoids play an important role in maintaining one's immune system. A wide range of flavonoids including apigenin, luteolin, and quercetin are known to show their effect on inflammatory cells and the immune system. Flavonoids selectively bind to cyclooxygenase-2 (COX-2) enzymes and decrease the process of inflammation (Panche et al. 2016). Their anti-inflammatory action is also linked to the inhibition of tumor necrosis factor-alpha (TNF-α), a typical cell signaling pro-inflammatory cytokine produced majorly by the macrophage which is known to primarily act by NF-kb pathway. Flavonoids have thereby shown to inhibit COX-2, 5-LOX, iNOS, and matrix metalloproteinases (MMPS) as they are key role players in inflammation as shown in Figure 9.3.

The soy isoflavone, genistein found in soybean was studied *in vivo* in high-fat diet-induced rats against nonalcoholic steatohepatitis (NASH) disease of the liver which is particularly characterized by fat accumulation in the liver, necroinflammation and hepatocellular injury. It was seen that genistein lowered the levels of alanine aminotransferase (ALT) and aspartate aminotransaminase (AST) which are involved in damage to the liver cells in NASH. Enzyme-linked immunosorbent assay (ELISA) used liver homogenates to determine that genistein downregulated the liver and serum cytokines like TNF-α, Interleukin-6 (IL-6) and Transforming Growth Factor Beta 1 (TGF-β 1) which are biomarkers of inflammation. Western blot revealed that genistein mediated its

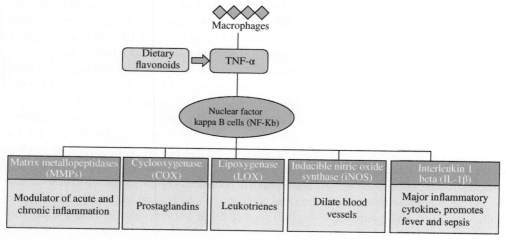

Figure 9.3 Anti-inflammatory action of flavonoids.

anti-inflammatory effect in the liver by blocking the proteins involved in signal transduction pathways, namely mitogen-activated protein kinase (MAPKs) and nuclear factor-kappa B (NF-κB) pathways (Ji et al. 2011). Puerarin extracted from *Radix puerariae* is an isoflavone-c-glycoside that is reported to show its anti-inflammatory activity in atherosclerosis, an inflammatory disease that involves the adhesion of monocytes in the walls of blood vessels. Puerarin majorly suppresses NF-κB which is responsible for controlling various inflammatory activities. In this study, high-lipid diet-induced rabbits were treated with puerarin. Western blot analysis confirmed that puerarin (20 mg/kg) suppressed the phosphorylation of Ik-b, which causes suppression or inactivation of NF-κB. These results thus confirmed puerarin's role in the reduction of adhesion molecule levels and inflammatory response, thereby leading to antiatherogenic effects (Ji et al. 2016). Apigenin is widely found in parsley (*Petroselinum crispum*) and celery (*Apium graveolens*). The *in vivo* studies performed in mice by orally administering apigenin displayed attenuation of neuroinflammation. It was seen that apigenin was involved in the deactivation or downregulation of TLR4/NF-κB signalling pathways that are the key mediators of inflammation. ELISA results showed that apigenin decreased the pro-inflammatory cytokines like IL-β, IL-6, and TNF-α (Zhao et al. 2019).

Cyanidin-3-β-D-glucoside (C3G) occurs in black rice that exhibits antioxidant, anaphylactic, antiallergic, and anti-inflammatory effects. Sung-Won Mi et al. carried out *in vivo* and *in vitro* anti-inflammatory studies to examine the effects of C3G and its main metabolites, namely cyanidin and protocatechuic acid (PA). In *in vitro* study on lipopolysaccharide (LPS)-stimulated RAW 264.7 cells, ELISA and immunoblot analyses suggested that C3G, cyaniding, and PA co-treatment inhibited the protein expression of pro-inflammatory cytokines like TNF-α and IL-1β in LPS-induced macrophages and also brought down the levels of inflammatory mediators like NO, and prostaglandins (PGE2) and inhibited enzymes like COX-2 and inducible nitric oxide synthase (iNOS) expression in a dose-dependent manner. In *in vivo* studies on carrageenan-induced inflammation in air pouches on BALB/c mice, it was revealed that the exudates of the air pouch in mice that C3G along with its metabolites inhibited the number of leukocytes, TNF-α, IL-1β, PGE2, COX-2 expression, and NF-κB activation. It is important to note that out of two metabolites, PA most potently inhibited all the mediators of inflammation *in vivo* and *in vitro* (Min et al. 2010).

Fisetin found in many fruits and vegetables such as strawberry, apple, onion, and cucumber was investigated for attenuating acute renal sepsis. A study was performed on endotoxin lipopolysaccharide-induced septic acute kidney infection in male C57BL/6 mice that were pretreated with fisetin (100 mg/kg) for three days. PCR was employed to check the expression of pro-inflammatory factors (IL-6, IL-1β, and TNF-α), thereby establishing evidence that fesitin decreased these factors in the renal tissues. It was also seen that fesitin decreased the inflammation-related proteins in the kidneys, namely IL-6, IL-1β, TNF-α, iNOS, and COX-2 to reduce the inflammatory response. Western blot analysis further revealed that fesitin showed its anti-inflammatory effects by blocking the phosphorylation of NF-κB p65 and kinases-belonging group to MAPK like p38, extracellular-signal-regulated kinase (ERK1/2) and c-Jun N-terminal kinase (JNK) (Ren et al. 2020).

These studies thus suggest that dietary intake of flavonoids is highly effective in reducing both acute and chronic inflammation associated with various diseases, organs, and disorders, and is thereby one of the most pronounced and discussed flavonoid bioactivities.

9.3.3 Neuroprotective Activity

Flavonoids have a major potential to modulate neuronal function and to prevent age-related neurodegeneration. The brain is a complex organ and the effectiveness of a flavonoid in the brain largely depends upon its bioavailability. Generally, most of the neuroprotective flavonoids undergo metabolic transformation by various pathways, which leads to poor bioavailability. Another major obstacle in brain delivery is the blood–brain barrier (BBB) (Dajas et al. 2003). Flavanones like naringenin and hesperidin and dietary anthocyanins have been shown to traverse the BBB in relevant *in vitro* and *in situ* models. The lesser polar compounds can cross BBB easily as compared to the polar ones due to more lipophilicity. Certainly, one of the benefits of flavonoid supplementation revolves around improved cognitive effects as a result of enhanced protection of neurons by stimulating or enhancing neuronal regeneration or enhancing the functions of existing neurons (Vauzour et al. 2008). It is important to note that this neuroprotective activity of flavonoids can't solely be attributed to their ability to act as antioxidant agents and scavengers of ROS. This means flavonoids show their neuroprotective potential (at low concentration) by interacting with important neuronal intracellular signaling pathways that are very critical in controlling the survival as well as differentiation of neurons. Flavonoids also play an important role in neuroinflammation which is involved with most neurodegenerative diseases like Alzheimer's and Parkinson's by reducing inflammatory mediators like cytokines, TNF-α, and IL-1β. Their action is also reported on other inflammatory mediators like iNOS and NO·, and are known to increase nicotinamide adenine dinucleotide phosphate hydrogen (NADPH) oxidase activation through MAPK signaling pathway (Figure 9.4). Flavonoids act on cognitive behavior, memory, and learning functions by binding to adenosine triphosphate (ATP) sites on enzymes and receptors, modulating the activity of kinases directly, acting on calcium homeostasis and binding to promoter sequences. This leads to dendritic spine growth, neuronal communication, and synaptic plasticity, thereby showing cognitive effects (Spencer 2009). Some of the studies of neuroprotective flavonoids are presented below.

Alzheimer's disease (AD) is mainly characterized by the accumulation of amyloid β plaques in the brain, which are formed by the conversion of the β-amyloid (Aβ) peptide into amyloid plaques. Preventing the aggregation of Aβ and neurofibrillary tangles is said to be a therapeutic strategy for treating AD. In a study, rutin and quercetin were tested together to check their effects in AD. Electron microscopic studies revealed that when Aβ25–35 fibrils were co-incubated with quercetin (10 μM) and rutin (10 μM), the number of fibrils were decreased and there was a significant reduction of Thio-T binder, thus showing anti-amyloidogenic effects *in vitro*. Also, quercetin and rutin (100 μM) had a significant β-secretase enzyme (BACE) inhibitory activity in a cell-free assay system by 11.85 and 50.67%, respectively. The H_2O_2-treated Swedish mutant APP stable cell line was used to examine cytoprotective effects and it was seen that both flavonoids decreased ROS, increased GSH content and redox potential, and decreased lipid peroxidation, thereby showing effect against Aβ25–35 fibrillogenesis and having antiamyloidogenic properties (Jiménez-Aliaga et al. 2011). The neuroprotective activity of epicatechin gallate (ECG) and epigallocatechin gallate (EGCG) on acrylamide (ACR) neurotoxicity was performed *in vivo* and *in vitro*. It was seen that

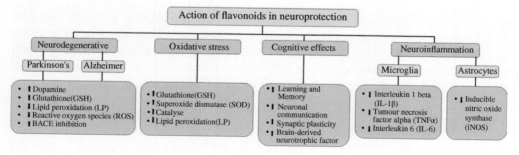

Figure 9.4 Neuroprotective actions of flavonoids.

both these catechins increased the GSH and malondialdehyde (MDA) and decreased lipid peroxidation in the cerebral cortex of rats, thereby overcoming all neurotoxic effects (Esmaeelpanah et al. 2018). For the same flavonoid, Adachi et al. showed that EGCG was alone responsible for sedative effects and in attenuation of the acute stress response. It was hypothesized that the presence of the gallate group as a substitute to the carbonyl group on the EGCG was responsible for its binding to the GABAergic neurons of the brain (Adachi et al. 2006). Another study concluded that catechins (0.05%) found in green tea show promising effects on aging of the brain in a mouse model by inhibiting various oxidative stress-promoting mechanisms (Li et al. 2010).

Parkinson's disease is another second most common neurodegenerative disease that is marked by loss of dopamine-producing neurons of the nigrostriatal region of the midbrain and accumulation of α-synuclein in the form of Lewy bodies which results in motor and cognitive defects. Studies show that flavonoids reduce markers of inflammation, oxidative stress, increase markers of neurotrophic factor signaling and prevent an increase in α-synuclein in Parkinson's (Maher 2019). Flavonoid chrysin exhibited anti-Parkinson's activity in 6-Hydroxy dopamine (6-OHDA)-induced mice by protecting against impairment of age-related memory and reducing oxidative stress by preventing neurochemical biomarkers like NO, 4-Hydroxynonenal (HNE) which contribute to the degeneration of neurons. Chrysin helped in improving GSH levels in the stratum of the mouse and also reducing the activities of NADPH oxidase and ATPase in the stratum, thereby partially restoring the dopamine in the stratum of the mouse (Del Fabbro et al. 2019). Hesperidin is a flavanone that occurs naturally in citrus fruits like oranges. The evidence of hesperidin as a neuroprotective agent in Parkinson's disease is reported by Tamilselvam et al. Hesperidin through 3-[4,5-Dimethylthiazol-2-yl]-2,5-Diphenyltetrazolium Bromide (MTT) assay showed dose-dependent proapoptotic effects on rotenone-induced apoptosis in human neuroblastoma SK-N-SH cell lines with almost 85% protection after 24 hours. At a similar dose, there was a reduction in ROS generation in the brain, an increase in GSH levels, and other enzymes like CAT, SOD (Tamilselvam et al. 2013).

Flavonoids are thus key role players and act as neuroprotective agents in multiple neuronal disorders by acting on several pathways in therapeutics of neurodegenerative disorders.

9.3.4 Antidiabetic Activity

Diabetes is a chronic, metabolic disorder characterized by elevated levels of blood glucose, which lead to serious complications like cardiac dysfunction, nephropathy, neuropathy, etc. The number of plant-derived phytochemicals and flavonoids are used in the treatment and management of diabetes and related complications (Al-Ishaq et al. 2019). Flavonoids show antidiabetic effects by acting on uptake of glucose, secretion of insulin, insulin-signaling mechanisms, promoting carbohydrate digestion, and also by regulating adipose deposition. Apart from these, they show evidence in lowering glucose levels by acting on key molecules that are involved in the regulation of beta-cell proliferation, reducing the apoptosis of beta cells and also by regulating the breakdown of glucose in the liver. It is hypothesized that the majority of flavonoid bioactivities occur due to their hydroxyl group α and β ketones (Kulkarni et al. 2016).

The study was performed to check the relation between antidiabetic effects and flavonoids in the US involving 200 000 women and men between 26 and 75 years of age. Data from three different prospective cohort studies were considered to check the association of each subclass of flavonoid with type-2 diabetes (T2D). There were only 12 611 incidences of T2D out of the 3 645 585 person-years of follow-up under evaluation who had flavonoids as part of their diet. It was observed that anthocyanin, flavanols, flavonols, flavan-3-ols, anthocyanins, and total flavonoids were positively associated with lower instances of T2D in these individuals. Moreover, pooled data indicated that out of all these flavonoids, anthocyanin supplementation showed the least number of incidences of T2D. It appeared that blueberries, pears, and apples were the major anthocyanin-rich food consumed by these cohorts. Further analysis revealed that it was cyanidin, an individual from the anthocyanin group, who showed the strongest effects against T2D (Willett 2010).

Various *in vitro* and *in vivo* studies of flavonoids were reported in the last few decades. Genistein, an isoflavonoid with different biological actions, is found in legumes. *In vitro* studies were conducted by cell proliferation assay on INS1 cells or human islet cells and genistein was found to be effective in the range of 0.1–5 μM on β-cell proliferation. Genistein mainly worked by the expression of a cell cycle regulator for β islet cell growth called cyclin D1 protein. Genistein ameliorates hyperglycemia in streptozotocin (STZ)-induced diabetic mice (0.25 g/kg) and only 13% of rats remained diabetic in the treatment group as compared to the disease control group at the en d of 28 days. Mice fed with genistein showed higher levels of blood insulin with improved glucose tolerance (Fu et al. 2010). In another study, the role of rutin was checked for its carbohydrate metabolism activity in STZ-induced diabetic rats. Oral administration of rutin to diabetic rats (100 mg/kg) for 45 days lead to a significant decrease in plasma glucose as well as an increase in insulin levels, accompanied by a decrease in glycogen with various activities related to enzymes that metabolize carbohydrates (Prince and Kamalakkannan 2006). Similarly, kaempferol acts by reducing fasting blood glucose, haemoglobin A1c levels, and increased insulin resistance in C57BL/6J mice when treated with a dose of 0.15% kaempferol (Zang et al. 2015). Hesperidin is a flavonoid found in citrus fruits and showed a dose-dependent antidiabetic effect by preventing the reversal of the high levels of plasma insulin. It also increases the activity of hexokinase and glucose-6-phosphate dehydrogenase and decreases the activity of glucose-6-phosphatase and fructose-1,6-bisphosphatase (Sundaram et al. 2019). Diosmin is a natural flavone glycoside obtained by dehydrogenation of it's flavanone glycoside, hesperidin. *in vivo* study performed on STZ-induced male albino Wistar rats treated with diosmin (100 mg/kg) showed its antidiabetic activity by acting on key enzymes related to the metabolism of carbohydrates and levels of total hemoglobin and glycosylated hemoglobin were extensively reversed by the administration of diosmin (Pari and Srinivasan 2010). Tangeretin is a polymethoxylated flavone found in the citrus fruit rinds including mandarin orange. An *in vivo* study was performed on male albino Wistar rats with tangeretin (100 mg/kg) which resulted in a reduction in the levels of plasma glucose, glycosylated hemoglobin and an increase in the levels of insulin and hemoglobin (Sundaram et al. 2014).

From the afore-discussed studies, it can be concluded that flavonoids show their antidiabetic actions by acting on increased glucose levels and different glucose-regulating parameters and are, hence, associated with a lower risk of diabetes.

9.3.5 Cardioprotective Activity

There are evidences that significant dietary intake of flavonoid-rich diet protects against various causes of cardiovascular diseases. Apart from the main antioxidant property, flavonoids also play important roles in cardioprotection including anti-inflammatory action, lowering of cholesterol, antihypertensive effect, antiplatelet action as well as inhibition of smooth muscle cell proliferation with improved blood vessel function (Gross 2004). Few flavonoids might prevent stroke by regulating endothelial-derived nitric oxide level or by reducing the peroxidation of mitochondrial lipids. Catechins and pro-anthocyanins show their cardioprotective effects against stroke by acting on cellular proliferation, hypertension, thrombogenesis, inflammation as well as hypercholesterolemia, and hyperglycemia (Vazhappilly et al. 2019). A study shows that wogonin, a flavonoid of *Scutellaria Baicalensis Georgi*, prevents ventricular arrhythmias due to ischemia–reperfusion by reducing the levels of biomarkers of cardiac death (Siasos et al. 2013).

Flavanols have a major role in preventing hypertension. Rutin and quercetin were investigated for their antihypertensive effects and compared with antihypertensive drug Nifedipine. In *in vivo* studies, salt-induced hypertension in Wister albino rats was treated with both the flavonoids for about two weeks that showed dose-dependent reductions in the systolic and diastolic pressure, heart rate, and arterial blood pressure. There was also an effect on the lipid profile showing a decreased level of serum triglyceride, cholesterol, and low-density lipoprotein (LDL) in the hypertensive rats (Olaleye et al. 2014).

Atherosclerosis is a condition that results from the deposition of cholesterol plaques in the blood vessel, thereby leading to blockages in the heart. In a study, chrysin isolated from fruits of *Pandanus tectorius* was checked for effects against atherosclerosis *in vitro*, in RAW 264.7 macrophages. The cells were supplemented with rosiglitazone, a cholesterol efflux stimulator and it was seen that treatment with chrysin dose-dependently increases cholesterol efflux with efficiency comparable to that of rosiglitazone. Chrysin showed a higher cholesterol efflux rate than that of rosiglitazone ($1 \mu M$) at $10 \mu M$ but lower at $1 \mu M$ by fluorescent assays. The formation of foam cells, i.e. cholesterol-containing macrophages in the arterial wall was induced by oxidized LDL cholesterol in RAW 264.7 macrophages. Hence, it is proved that chrysin inhibits foam cell formation by promoting cholesterol efflux from RAW 264.7 macrophages (Wang et al. 2015).

Malvidin (Malvidin-3-glucoside) is a polyphenol belonging to the anthocyanin class. It is widely present in wine, skin of red grapes, and colored fruits and shows activity in isoproterenol-induced myocardial infarction in rats. One of the main causes of the myocardial infarct is ischemia due to an imbalance between myocardial blood demand and coronary blood delivery. An *in vivo* study that was carried on albino Wister rats showed that malvidin (100 and 200 mg/kg) acts by alleviating various key factors like histopathology of cardiac tissues and biochemical alterations associated with mitochondrial impairment, lipid peroxidation, and changes in the endogenous antioxidants in the myocardium of the rats. Immunosorbent assay showed that malvidin also acted on serum levels of pro-inflammatory cytokines like TNF-α and IL-6 (Wei et al. 2017).

Baicalein is flavone extracted from Labiatae plant *S. baicalensis Georgi's* dry root. Out of the several properties that baicalein possesses, a recent study was conducted to evaluate its effects on heart failure. The *in vitro* studies were performed by treating H9C2 cells with isoproterenol and *in vivo* studies were conducted by establishing heart failure in a rat model with abdominal aortic constriction. It was seen that baicalein alleviated heart failure both *in vitro* and *in vivo*. Additionally, treatment with baicalein inhibited myocardial fibrosis, and suppressed the expression and activity of matrix metalloproteinases (MMP2 and MMP9), thereby suppressing apoptosis in heart tissue. Moreover, baicalein could inhibit cardiac myocyte hypertrophy and apoptosis induced by isoproterenol *in vitro*. It effectively inhibited all the increased levels of chemokines like TNF-α, angiotensin-ll, and brain natriuretic peptide induced by heart failure (Zhao et al. 2016).

An important flavonoid that shows a diverse beneficial activity in cardiovascular diseases is flavone luteolin found in thyme as well as foods like cauliflower, celery, cabbage, chamomile tea, etc. As per a study, luteolin ameliorated contractile function in ischemic reperfusion injury-induced culture of cardiomyocytes that were pretreated with different doses (0.5, 1.5, 2.5, and 50 μg/ml) of the flavonoid. Luteolin (0.5–2.5 μg/ml) enhanced cell viability in a concentration-dependent manner and decreased the release of lactate dehydrogenase (LDH), thereby declining the cardiomyocyte damage to prevent necrosis. It was also seen that luteolin further attenuated ischemic reperfusion injury and cardiomyocyte apoptosis by suppressing the activity of Caspase3,

Bcl-2, and Bax as well as Cytochrome C which is a very important contributor for myocardial infarcts and heart failures (Qi et al. 2011).

Therefore, there is growing evidence that flavonoids can show cardioprotective actions by acting on various precursors and mediators of cardiovascular diseases.

9.3.6 Antimicrobial Activity

The development of new antimicrobial agents is important at the present time due to the increasing resistance of microorganisms against the existing therapeutic agents. Few flavonoids possess a strong antibacterial activity by varying membrane fluidity (Kaleem and Ahmad 2018). Antibacterial activities of flavonoids can be utilized in three ways: killing the bacteria directly, synergistically activating the antibiotics, and reducing bacterial pathogenicity (Cushnie and Lamb 2011; Xie et al. 2015). Flavonoids such as quercetin, catechins, and naringenin exhibit antibacterial activities against *Streptococcus* and *Staphylococcus aureus* whereas apigenin and quercetin were effective against *Escherichia coli* (Kaleem and Ahmad 2018). Flavonoids which are extracted from different plant sources are gaining a lot of interest for the development of antiviral drugs with lesser side effects and are used for viruses like Herpes simplex virus type 1, poliovirus type 1, parainfluenza virus type 3, and adenovirus (Kaul et al. 1985). Flavonoids in their glycone form are showing more inhibitory mechanism as compared to their aglycone form (Bae et al. 2000; Agrawal 2011). Flavonoids such as quercetin exhibit anti-infective and antireplicative activities (Agrawal 2011). Other flavonoids like naringenin, hesperidin, and kaempferol were effective against various types of viruses.

Phenolic compounds have been extracted from cranberry fruits showed antibacterial activities against *S. aureus* alone or in the presence of the β-lactam antibiotic. The *in vitro* study was performed using a mixture of amoxicillin and fragment crystallizable portion of cranberry (FC111) with the help of checkerboard assay and the result stated that the fraction FC111 enhanced the inhibitory effect of amoxicillin against tested *S. aureus* [American Type Culture Collection (ATCC) 29213 and Methicillin-resistant *S. aureus* (MRSA) COL] strains. Also, *in vivo* study carried out using a mouse mastitis model of infected *S. aureus* treated with amoxicillin, FC111, or in the combination of both. Combination treatment displayed a synergistic effect to decrease bacterial counts significantly as compared to FC111 and amoxicillin alone. This antibacterial activity is attributed to disruption of the cell wall and also has an application in the agri-food industry and animal food production (Diarra et al. 2013).

EGCG was evaluated for antibacterial activity against *Helicobacter pylori* (*H. pylori*) for treating the gastric mucosal injury. It was observed that epigallocatechin gallate was more effective than the other six catechins present in the tea. The *in vitro* killing assay was performed to determine bacteriostatic and bactericidal activities of *H. pylori* and the result showed that the minimum inhibitory concentration (MIC) value for 50% of the strains tested was at 8 μg/ml. Also *in vivo* study carried out using a Mongolian gerbil model and when treated with catechin, *H. pylori* was destroyed at a lower eradication rate (10–36.4%) due to lesser gastric transit time of catechin. Thus, catechin may be combined with a proton pump inhibitor to prolong gastric transit time and better antibacterial effect against *H. pylori* (Mabe et al. 1999).

Quercetin antibacterial activity was explored against various bacterial strains by Wang et al. Oxford cup assay method was used to perform study and MIC values of quercetin for *E. coli*, *Salmonella enterica*, *S. aureus*, and *Pseudomonas aeruginosa* strains were 0.0082, 0.0072, 0.0068, and 0.0085 μmol/ml, respectively which implied that gram-positive bacteria showed the highest bacteriostatic activity than gram-negative bacteria. Also, *in vivo* study carried out at a dose of 0.2, 0.4, or 0.6 g/kg using AA broilers and found that 0.6 g/kg dose displayed maximum effects of quercetin on DNA copies of *cecal microbiota*. It was observed that the bacterial cell wall has been damaged which causes increased permeability after treatment with quercetin, thus inhibiting the growth of *E. coli* and *S. aureus* (Wang et al. 2018).

Another study demonstrated anti-HIV activities of kaempferol and kaempferol-7-*O*-glucoside isolated from *Securigera securidaca* using HIV-1 p24 antigen kit. The results found that at concentration, 100 μg/ml kaempferol and kaempferol-7-*O*-glucoside showed inhibition rate of 82 ± 3.1 and $95 \pm 1.2\%$, respectively with IC50 values 50 and 32 μg/ml, respectively. The *in vitro* antiviral activity of kaempferol-7-*O*-glucoside was stronger than kaempferol due to its potent inhibitory effect (Behbahani et al. 2014).

The abovesaid studies of flavonoids indicated their effective antimicrobial, antibacterial, and antiviral actions and provided protection against various microorganisms effectively.

9.3.7 Anticancer Activity

Cancer is a large group of diseases characterized by the uncontrolled multiplication of numerous cells leading to abnormal growth (Kroemer and Pouyssegur 2008; Neagu et al. 2019). The ability of an ideal anticancer agent is to prevent the growth of tumor or kill cancerous cells without any side effects (Zhao et al. 2012). The major problem of chemotherapy is the toxicity and destruction of healthy cells whereas natural products like flavonoids are considered to be safe and promising candidates for chronic therapy (Zhao et al. 2012; Sak 2014). Flavonoids consist of polyphenolic aromatic rings which exhibit pro- and antioxidant properties (Leung et al. 2007). In cancerous cells, higher oxidative stress is observed which can be combated by flavonoids (Valdameri et al. 2011). They show binary mechanisms that are responsible for activating cell death signaling pathways in cancerous cells either by activating antiapoptotic proteins or by suppressing proapoptotic proteins and caspases (Abotaleb et al. 2019; Kopustinskiene et al. 2020). Flavonoids behave as pro-oxidants that subdue the proliferation of cancer cells by inhibiting EGFR, protein kinase B (Akt), phosphatidylinositide 3-kinases (PT3K) along with nuclear factor kappa-light-chain-enhancer of activated B cells (NF-κB) (Kopustinskiene et al. 2020). Flavonoids like kaempferol, hesperidin, genistein exhibit anticancer effects that suppress cell growth.

Kaempferol hinders the growth of gastric tumors and it was observed that it (120 μM) prevented the proliferation of gastric cancer cell lines and induced apoptosis in MKN28 and SGC7901 cells. The *in vitro* data showed a decrease in expression levels of COX-2, p-AKT, and p-ERK. Also, *in vivo* study was carried (20 mg/kg) in mice which revealed that kaempferol stopped the tumor growth without any alteration in the body, spleen, and liver weight of mice (Song et al. 2015). Du et al. studied antitumor activities of hesperidin against human osteosarcoma MG-63 cells confirmed its dose-dependent cytotoxic effect. Antitumor effects of hesperidin using a nude xenograft mouse model showed reduced tumor growth after treatment for 14 days. Hesperidin possesses antitumor and apoptotic effects through inhibition of cell migration, cell cycle arrest, and induction of mitochondria-mediated apoptosis (Du et al. 2018). Similar antitumor activity was shown by genistein against human leukemia HL-60 cells and morusin against human hepatocellular carcinoma cells (HepG2 and Hep3B) and human umbilical vein endothelial cells (HUVECs) (Gao et al. 2017; Hsiao et al. 2019).

Anticancer activity of luteolin-loaded long-circulating micelles were carried out by MTT assay and results showed that IC50 values for free luteolin and luteolin-micelles were 9.83 and 3.11 μg/ml, respectively which implied potent cytotoxic effect of the latter against A549 cells. The *in vivo* study carried out in nude mice (5.0 mg/kg) demonstrated decreased tumor growth along with reduced toxicity when treated with luteolin micelles (Yan et al. 2016). Similarly, quercetin-loaded chitosan nanoparticles were evaluated for anticancer activity using tumor xenograft mice model (25 mg/kg) exhibited reduced tumor growth along with a reduction in tumor volume by 62.86 and

49.96% in A549 and MDA MB 468 cell lines, respectively when compared with free quercetin and confirmed enhanced bioavailability of quercetin in its nanoformulation (Baksi et al. 2018).

It can be concluded that flavonoids and their formulations demonstrated strong anticancer activities by acting on various mediators to prevent the growth of tumor or kill cancerous cells.

9.3.8 Hepatoprotective Activity

Liver is one of the largest organs in the human body that plays a major role in metabolism, storage, and excretion, thereby maintaining and regulating homeostasis in the body. Toxic chemical substances which get accumulated and deposited in the liver, thereby cause serious injury that can be cured with natural hepatoprotective agents. Oxidative stress and lipid peroxidation are the elements that are leading to hepatotoxin-associated liver damage and, thus, the use of antioxidants can be recommended for its cure (Arige et al. 2017). Flavonoids like kaempferol, apigenin, silymarin, etc., are potential hepatoprotective agents. In all below-described studies, researchers used CCl_4-induced hepatotoxicity model to determine the activity.

The hepatoprotective activity of apigenin-O/C-diglucoside saponarin isolated from *Gypsophila* plant was studied. The *in vitro* study of saponarin (0.006–60 µg/ml) was performed using isolated rat hepatocytes which showed concentration-dependent hepatoprotective activity by increasing cell viability and GSH levels followed by decreasing LDH activity and MDA levels. Also, increased levels of GSH, SOD, CAT, and GPx were observed in saponarin-treated Wistar rats (Simeonova et al. 2014).

Quercetin 7-rhamnoside obtained from *Hypericum* herb indicated both hepatoprotective as well as antioxidant activities. DPPH, (2,2'-Azino-bis(3-ethylbenzothiazoline-6-sulfonic acid)) (ABTS), and FRAP assays showed better antioxidant activities against H_2O_2-induced *in vitro* cytotoxicity in L-02 cells. The *in vivo* study was carried out using a mice model and quercetin 7-rhamnoside (20 mg/kg) showed reduced serum activities of ALT, AST, LDH, and triglyceride (TG) levels suggesting its distinct hepatoprotective activity (Huang et al. 2018). Hermenean et al. studied the hepatoprotective activity of chrysin mediated via TNF-α. The *in vivo* study in mice showed a reduction in serum ALT and AST levels when mice were pretreated with chrysin with retention of the structural integrity of membranes. Molecular modeling was performed to study the interaction between chrysin and TNF-α-converting enzyme (TACE) and chrysin showed a reduction in soluble TNF-α expression by inhibiting TACE, thus showing hepatoprotection (Hermenean et al. 2017).

To determine hepatoprotective activity, silymarin-loaded bilosomes were prepared using thin-film hydration method. The results of *in vitro* drug release study showed 64.72% release for free silymarin and silymarin bilosomes showed slower release reaching up to 40–44% after 24 hours due to hydrophobic constituents. The *in vivo* study carried out using the albino Wistar rat model (50 mg/kg) showed better hepatoprotective activity by bilosomes by reducing ALT and AST levels in the serum when compared with free silymarin (Mohsen et al. 2017).

Hence, it was concluded that flavonoids showed potential hepatoprotective activities against CCl_4-induced liver injury by acting on enzyme inhibitors and mediators of liver diseases.

9.4 Conclusion

The scope of this chapter was to highlight the therapeutic properties of flavonoids. The aforesaid studies make it clear that flavonoids are a boon to mankind from nature. Over 9000 flavonoids are discovered till date which needs to be explored in terms of their physicochemical properties, pharmacokinetic and pharmacodynamic behaviour to cure several ailments. Furthermore, research should be focused on emphasis to develop sensitive analytical methods to analyze these phenolic compounds precisely in the blood. In recent years, there have been major breakthroughs to overcome problems associated with their lower bioavailability. Although various delivery systems have been reported for many flavonoids, they can be further studied with novel formulation and process technologies. Besides, extensive clinical evaluation is need of the hour to commercialize this important sector of nutraceuticals.

References

Abotaleb, M., Samuel, S.M., Varghese, E. et al. (2019). Flavonoids in cancer and apoptosis. *Cancers* 11 (1): 28.

Adachi, N., Tomonaga, S., Tachibana, T. et al. (2006). (−)-Epigallocatechin gallate attenuates acute stress responses through GABAergic system in the brain. *European Journal of Pharmacology* 531 (1–3): 171–175.

Agerbirk, N. and Olsen, C.E. (2012). Glucosinolate structures in evolution. *Phytochemistry.* 77: 16–45.

Agrawal, A.D. (2011). Pharmacological activities of flavonoids: a review. *International Journal of Pharmaceutical Sciences and Nanotechnology* 4 (2): 1394–1398.

Aherne, S.A. and O'Brien, N.M. (2002). Dietary flavonols: chemistry, food content, and metabolism. *Nutrition* 18 (1): 75–81.

Al-Ishaq, R.K., Abotaleb, M., Kubatka, P. et al. (2019). Flavonoids and their anti-diabetic effects: cellular mechanisms and effects to improve blood sugar levels. *Biomolecules* 9 (9): 430.

Andlauer, W. and Fürst, P. (2002). Nutraceuticals: a piece of history, present status and outlook. *Food Research International* 35 (2–3): 171–176.

Arige, S.S., Arige, S.D., and Rao, L.A. (2017). A review on hepatoprotective activity. *International Journal of Current Research* 9 (6): 51876–51881.

Bae, E.A., Han, M.J., Lee, M., and Kim, D.H. (2000). in vitro inhibitory effect of some flavonoids on rotavirus infectivity. *Biological and Pharmaceutical Bulletin* 23 (9): 1122–1124.

Baksi, R., Singh, D.P., Borse, S.P. et al. (2018). in vitro and in vivo anticancer efficacy potential of Quercetin loaded polymeric nanoparticles. *Biomedicine and Pharmacotherapy* 106: 1513–1526.

Barreca, D., Gattuso, G., Bellocco, E. et al. (2017). Flavanones: citrus phytochemical with health-promoting properties. *BioFactors* 43 (4): 495–506.

Behbahani, M., Sayedipour, S., Pourazar, A., and Shanehsazzadeh, M. (2014). in vitro anti-HIV-1 activities of kaempferol and kaempferol-7-O-glucoside isolated from *Securigera securidaca*. *Research in Pharmaceutical Sciences* 9 (6): 463.

Brodowska, K.M. (2017). Natural flavonoids: classification, potential role, and application of flavonoid analogues. *European Journal of Biological Research* 7 (2): 108–123.

Cheung, K.L. and Kong, A.N. (2010). Molecular targets of dietary phenethyl isothiocyanate and sulforaphane for cancer chemoprevention. *The AAPS Journal* 12 (1): 87–97.

Corradini, E., Foglia, P., Giansanti, P. et al. (2011). Flavonoids: chemical properties and analytical methodologies of identification and quantitation in foods and plants. *Natural Product Research* 25 (5): 469–495.

Cushnie, T.T. and Lamb, A.J. (2011). Recent advances in understanding the antibacterial properties of flavonoids. *International Journal of Antimicrobial Agents* 38 (2): 99–107.

Da Costa, J.P. (2017). A current look at nutraceuticals – key concepts and future prospects. *Trends in Food Science and Technology* 62: 68–78.

Dajas, F., Rivera-Megret, F., Blasina, F. et al. (2003). Neuroprotection by flavonoids. *Brazilian Journal of Medical and Biological Research* 36 (12): 1613–1620.

Del Fabbro, L., Goes, A.R., Jesse, C.R. et al. (2019). Chrysin protects against behavioral, cognitive and neurochemical alterations in a 6-hydroxydopamine model of Parkinson's disease. *Neuroscience Letters* 706: 158–163.

Diarra, M.S., Block, G., Rempel, H. et al. (2013). in vitro and in vivo antibacterial activities of cranberry press cake extracts alone or in combination with β-lactams against *Staphylococcus aureus*. *BMC Complementary and Alternative Medicine* 13 (1): 90.

Dillard, C.J. and German, J.B. (2000). Phytochemicals: nutraceuticals and human health. *Journal of the Science of Food and Agriculture* 80 (12): 1744–1756.

Du, G.Y., He, S.W., Zhang, L. et al. (2018). Hesperidin exhibits in vitro and in vivo antitumor effects in human osteosarcoma MG-63 cells and xenograft mice models via inhibition of cell migration and invasion, cell cycle arrest and induction of mitochondrial-mediated apoptosis. *Oncology Letters* 16 (5): 6299–6306.

Esmaeelpanah, E., Razavi, B.M., Vahdati Hasani, F., and Hosseinzadeh, H. (2018). Evaluation of epigallocatechin gallate and epicatechin gallate effects on acrylamide-induced neurotoxicity in rats and cytotoxicity in PC 12 cells. *Drug and Chemical Toxicology* 41 (4): 441–448.

Fu, Z., Zhang, W., Zhen, W. et al. (2010). Genistein induces pancreatic β-cell proliferation through activation of multiple signaling pathways and prevents insulin-deficient diabetes in mice. *Endocrinology* 151 (7): 3026–3037.

Gao, L., Wang, L., Sun, Z. et al. (2017). Morusin shows potent antitumor activity for human hepatocellular carcinoma in vitro and in vivo through apoptosis induction and angiogenesis inhibition. *Drug Design, Development and Therapy* 11: 1789.

Gross, M. (2004). Flavonoids and cardiovascular disease. *Pharmaceutical Biology* 42 (sup1): 21–35.

Havsteen, B.H. (2002). The biochemistry and medical significance of the flavonoids. *Pharmacology and Therapeutics* 96 (2–3): 67–202.

Hermenean, A., Mariasiu, T., Navarro-González, I. et al. (2017). Hepatoprotective activity of chrysin is mediated through TNF-α in chemically-induced acute liver damage: an in vivo study and molecular modeling. *Experimental and Therapeutic Medicine* 13 (5): 1671–1680.

Hibatallah, J., Carduner, C., and Poelman, M.C. (1999). In-vivo and in-vitro assessment of the free-radical-scavenger activity of Ginkgo flavone glycosides at high concentration. *Journal of Pharmacy and Pharmacology* 51 (12): 1435–1440.

Hollman, P.C. (2004). Absorption, bioavailability, and metabolism of flavonoids. *Pharmaceutical Biology* 42 (sup1): 74–83.

Hsiao, Y.C., Peng, S.F., Lai, K.C. et al. (2019). Genistein induces apoptosis in vitro and has antitumor activity against human leukemia HL-60 cancer cell xenograft growth in vivo. *Environmental Toxicology* 34 (4): 443–456.

Huang, Z.Q., Chen, P., Su, W.W. et al. (2018). Antioxidant activity and hepatoprotective potential of quercetin 7-rhamnoside in vitro and in vivo. *Molecules* 23 (5): 1188.

Ji, G., Yang, Q., Hao, J. et al. (2011). Anti-inflammatory effect of genistein on non-alcoholic steatohepatitis rats induced by high fat diet and its potential mechanisms. *International Immunopharmacology* 11 (6): 762–768.

Ji, L., Du, Q., Li, Y., and Hu, W. (2016). Puerarin inhibits the inflammatory response in atherosclerosis via modulation of the NF-κB pathway in a rabbit model. *Pharmacological Reports* 68 (5): 1054–1059.

Jiménez-Aliaga, K., Bermejo-Bescós, P., Benedí, J., and Martín-Aragón, S. (2011). Quercetin and rutin exhibit antiamyloidogenic and fibril-disaggregating effects in vitro and potent antioxidant activity in APPswe cells. *Life Sciences* 89 (25–26): 939–945.

Kaleem, M. and Ahmad, A. (2018). Flavonoids as nutraceuticals. In: *Therapeutic, Probiotic, and Unconventional Foods*, 137–155. Academic Press.

Kalita, B. and Patwary, B.N. (2020). Formulation and in vitro evaluation of hesperidin-phospholipid complex and its antioxidant potential. *Current Drug Therapy* 15 (1): 28–36.

Kaul, T.N., Middleton, E. Jr., and Ogra, P.L. (1985). Antiviral effect of flavonoids on human viruses. *Journal of Medical Virology* 15 (1): 71–79.

Kopustinskiene, D.M., Jakstas, V., Savickas, A., and Bernatoniene, J. (2020). Flavonoids as anticancer agents. *Nutrients* 12 (2): 457.

Kozłowska, A. and Szostak-Węgierek, D. (2017). Flavonoids – food sources, health benefits, and mechanisms involved. In: *Bioactive Molecules in Food* (eds. J.-M. Mérillon and K.G. Ramawat), 1–27. Cham: Springer.

Kroemer, G. and Pouyssegur, J. (2008). Tumor cell metabolism: cancer's Achilles' heel. *Cancer Cell* 13 (6): 472–482.

Kulkarni, Y.A., Garud, M.S., Oza, M.J. et al. (2016). Diabetes, diabetic complications, and flavonoids. In: *Fruits, Vegetables, and Herbs*, 77–104. Academic Press.

Kumar, S. and Pandey, A.K. (2013). Chemistry and biological activities of flavonoids: an overview. *The Scientific World Journal* 2013: 1–16.

Kumar, S., Mishra, A., and Pandey, A.K. (2013). Antioxidant mediated protective effect of *Parthenium hysterophorus* against oxidative damage using in vitro models. *BMC Complementary and Alternative Medicine* 13 (1): 120.

Leung, H.W., Lin, C.J., Hour, M.J. et al. (2007). Kaempferol induces apoptosis in human lung non-small carcinoma cells accompanied by an induction of antioxidant enzymes. *Food and Chemical Toxicology* 45 (10): 2005–2013.

Li, Q., Zhao, H., Zhao, M. et al. (2010). Chronic green tea catechins administration prevents oxidative stress-related brain aging in C57BL/6J mice. *Brain Research* 1353: 28–35.

Li, R., Yuan, C., Dong, C. et al. (2011). in vivo antioxidative effect of isoquercitrin on cadmium-induced oxidative damage to mouse liver and kidney. *Naunyn–Schmiedeberg's Archives of Pharmacology* 383 (5): 437–445.

Li, P., Jia, J., Zhang, D. et al. (2014). in vitro and in vivo antioxidant activities of a flavonoid isolated from celery (*Apium graveolens* L. var. dulce). *Food and Function* 5 (1): 50–56.

Mabe, K., Yamada, M., Oguni, I., and Takahashi, T. (1999). in vitro and in vivo activities of tea catechins against *Helicobacter pylori*. *Antimicrobial Agents and Chemotherapy* 43 (7): 1788–1791.

Maher, P. (2019). The potential of flavonoids for the treatment of neurodegenerative diseases. *International Journal of Molecular Sciences* 20 (12): 3056.

Min, S.W., Ryu, S.N., and Kim, D.H. (2010). Anti-inflammatory effects of black rice, cyanidin-3-*O*-β-d-glycoside, and its metabolites, cyanidin and protocatechuic acid. *International Immunopharmacology* 10 (8): 959–966.

Mohsen, A.M., Asfour, M.H., and Salama, A.A. (2017). Improved hepatoprotective activity of silymarin via encapsulation in the novel vesicular nanosystem bilosomes. *Drug Development and Industrial Pharmacy* 43 (12): 2043–2054.

Nagula, R.L. and Wairkar, S. (2019). Recent advances in topical delivery of flavonoids: a review. *Journal of Controlled Release* 296: 190–201.

Neagu, M., Constantin, C., Popescu, I.D. et al. (2019). Inflammation and metabolism in cancer cell – mitochondria key player. *Frontiers in Oncology* 9: 348.

Olaleye, M.T., Crown, O.O., Akinmoladun, A.C., and Akindahunsi, A.A. (2014). Rutin and quercetin show greater efficacy than nifedipin in ameliorating hemodynamic, redox, and metabolite imbalances in sodium chloride-induced hypertensive rats. *Human and Experimental Toxicology* 33 (6): 602–608.

Pan, M.H., Lai, C.S., and Ho, C.T. (2010). Anti-inflammatory activity of natural dietary flavonoids. *Food and Function* 1 (1): 15–31.

Panche, A.N., Diwan, A.D., and Chandra, S.R. (2016). Flavonoids: an overview. *Journal of Nutritional Science* 5: 1–15.

Pandey, A.K., Mishra, A.K., and Mishra, A. (2012). Antifungal and antioxidative potential of oil and extracts derived from leaves of Indian spice plant *Cinnamomum tamala*. *Cellular and Molecular Biology* 58 (1): 142–147.

Pari, L. and Srinivasan, S. (2010). Antihyperglycemic effect of diosmin on hepatic key enzymes of carbohydrate metabolism in streptozotocin–nicotinamide-induced diabetic rats. *Biomedicine and Pharmacotherapy* 64 (7): 477–481.

Pietta, P.G. (2000). Flavonoids as antioxidants. *Journal of Natural Products* 63 (7): 1035–1042.

Prince, P.S. and Kamalakkannan, N. (2006). Rutin improves glucose homeostasis in streptozotocin diabetic tissues by altering glycolytic and gluconeogenic enzymes. *Journal of Biochemical and Molecular Toxicology* 20 (2): 96–102.

Procházková, D., Boušová, I., and Wilhelmová, N. (2011). Antioxidant and prooxidant properties of flavonoids. *Fitoterapia* 82 (4): 513–523.

Qi, L., Pan, H., Li, D. et al. (2011). Luteolin improves contractile function and attenuates apoptosis following ischemia–reperfusion in adult rat cardiomyocytes. *European Journal of Pharmacology* 668 (1–2): 201–207.

Ravi, G.S., Charyulu, R.N., Dubey, A. et al. (2018). Nano-lipid complex of rutin: development, characterization and in vivo investigation of hepatoprotective, antioxidant activity and bioavailability study in rats. *AAPS PharmSciTech* 19 (8): 3631–3649.

Ren, Q., Guo, F., Tao, S. et al. (2020). Flavonoid fisetin alleviates kidney inflammation and apoptosis via inhibiting Src-mediated NF-κB p65 and MAPK signaling pathways in septic AKI mice. *Biomedicine and Pharmacotherapy* 122: 109772.

Ruiz-Cruz, S., Chaparro-Hernández, S., Hernández-Ruiz, K.L. et al. (2017). Flavonoids: important biocompounds in food. Flavonoids: from biosynthesis to human health, London. *IntechOpen* 23: 353–370.

Sak, K. (2014). Cytotoxicity of dietary flavonoids on different human cancer types. *Pharmacognosy Reviews* 8 (16): 122.

Siasos, G., Tousoulis, D., Tsigkou, V. et al. (2013). Flavonoids in atherosclerosis: an overview of their mechanisms of action. *Current Medicinal Chemistry* 20 (21): 2641–2660.

Simeonova, R., Kondeva-Burdina, M., Vitcheva, V. et al. (2014). Protective effects of the apigenin-O/C-diglucoside saponarin from *Gypsophila trichotoma* on carbone tetrachloride-induced hepatotoxicity in vitro/in vivo in rats. *Phytomedicine* 21 (2): 148–154.

Singh, J. and Sinha, S. (2012). Classification, regulatory acts and applications of nutraceuticals for health. *International Journal of Pharma and Bio Sciences* 2 (1): 177–187.

Sobeh, M., Mahmoud, M.F., Abdelfattah, M.A. et al. (2018). A proanthocyanidin-rich extract from *Cassia abbreviata* exhibits antioxidant and hepatoprotective activities in vivo. *Journal of Ethnopharmacology* 213: 38–47.

Song, H., Bao, J., Wei, Y. et al. (2015). Kaempferol inhibits gastric cancer tumor growth: an in vitro and in vivo study. *Oncology Reports* 33 (2): 868–874.

Spencer, J.P. (2009). Flavonoids and brain health: multiple effects underpinned by common mechanisms. *Genes and Nutrition* 4 (4): 243–250.

Sun, S., Pan, S., Ling, C. et al. (2012). Free radical scavenging abilities in vitro and antioxidant activities in vivo of black tea and its main polyphenols. *Journal of Medicinal Plants Research* 6 (1): 114–121.

Sundaram, R., Shanthi, P., and Sachdanandam, P. (2014). Effect of tangeretin, a polymethoxylated flavone on glucose metabolism in streptozotocin-induced diabetic rats. *Phytomedicine* 21 (6): 793–799.

Sundaram, R., Nandhakumar, E., and Haseena, B.H. (2019). Hesperidin, a citrus flavonoid ameliorates hyperglycemia by regulating key enzymes of carbohydrate metabolism in streptozotocin-induced diabetic rats. *Toxicology Mechanisms and Methods* 29 (9): 644–653.

Tamilselvam, K., Braidy, N., Manivasagam, T. et al. (2013). Neuroprotective effects of hesperidin, a plant flavanone, on rotenone-induced oxidative stress and apoptosis in a cellular model for Parkinson's disease. *Oxidative Medicine and Cellular Longevity* 2013: 1–11.

Valdameri, G., Trombetta-Lima, M., Worfel, P.R. et al. (2011). Involvement of catalase in the apoptotic mechanism induced by apigenin in HepG2 human hepatoma cells. *Chemico-biological Interactions* 193 (2): 180–189.

Vauzour, D., Vafeiadou, K., Rodriguez-Mateos, A. et al. (2008). The neuroprotective potential of flavonoids: a multiplicity of effects. *Genes and Nutrition* 3 (3–4): 115–126.

Vazhappilly, C.G., Ansari, S.A., Al-Jaleeli, R. et al. (2019). Role of flavonoids in thrombotic, cardiovascular, and inflammatory diseases. *Inflammopharmacology* 15: 1–7.

Vincken, J.P., Heng, L., de Groot, A., and Gruppen, H. (2007). Saponins, classification and occurrence in the plant kingdom. *Phytochemistry* 68 (3): 275–297.

Wang, Y., Chen, S., and Yu, O. (2011). Metabolic engineering of flavonoids in plants and microorganisms. *Applied Microbiology and Biotechnology* 91 (4): 949.

Wang, S., Zhang, X., Liu, M. et al. (2015). Chrysin inhibits foam cell formation through promoting cholesterol efflux from RAW264. 7 macrophages. *Pharmaceutical Biology* 53 (10): 1481–1487.

Wang, S., Yao, J., Zhou, B. et al. (2018). Bacteriostatic effect of quercetin as an antibiotic alternative in vivo and its antibacterial mechanism in vitro. *Journal of Food Protection* 81 (1): 68–78.

Wei, H., Li, H., Wan, S.P. et al. (2017). Cardioprotective effects of Malvidin against isoproterenol-induced myocardial infarction in rats: a mechanistic study. *Medical Science Monitor: International Medical Journal of Experimental and Clinical Research* 23: 2007.

Willett, W.C. (2010). The WHI joins MRFIT: a revealing look beneath the covers. *The American Journal of Clinical Nutrition* 91 (4): 829.

Wu, P., Ma, G., Li, N. et al. (2015). Investigation of in vitro and in vivo antioxidant activities of flavonoids rich extract from the berries of *Rhodomyrtus tomentosa* (Ait.) Hassk. *Food Chemistry* 173: 194–202.

Xie, Y., Yang, W., Tang, F. et al. (2015). Antibacterial activities of flavonoids: structure-activity relationship and mechanism. *Current Medicinal Chemistry* 22 (1): 132–149.

Yan, H., Wei, P., Song, J. et al. (2016). Enhanced anticancer activity in vitro and in vivo of luteolin incorporated into long-circulating micelles based on DSPE-PEG2000 and TPGS. *Journal of Pharmacy and Pharmacology* 68 (10): 1290–1298.

Zang, Y., Zhang, L., Igarashi, K., and Yu, C. (2015). The anti-obesity and anti-diabetic effects of kaempferol glycosides from unripe soybean leaves in high-fat-diet mice. *Food and Function* 6 (3): 834–841.

Zhao, X., Shu, G., Chen, L. et al. (2012). A flavonoid component from *Docynia delavayi* (Franch.) Schneid represses transplanted H22 hepatoma growth and exhibits low toxic effect on tumor-bearing mice. *Food and Chemical Toxicology* 50 (9): 3166–3173.

Zhao, F., Fu, L., Yang, W. et al. (2016). Cardioprotective effects of baicalein on heart failure via modulation of Ca^{2+} handling proteins in vivo and in vitro. *Life Sciences* 145: 213–223.

Zhao, F., Dang, Y., Zhang, R. et al. (2019). Apigenin attenuates acrylonitrile-induced neuro-inflammation in rats: Involved of inactivation of the TLR4/NF-κB signaling pathway. *International Immunopharmacology* 75: 105697.

10

Current Concepts and Prospects of Herbal Nutraceutical

Sunil Bishnoi[1] and Deepak Mudgil[2]

[1] Department of Food Technology, Guru Jambheshwar University of Science and Technology, Hisar, Haryana, India
[2] Department of Dairy & Food Technology, Mansinhbhai Institute of Dairy & Food Technology, Mehsana, Gujarat, India

10.1 Introduction

Food is necessary for human life, but nowadays, the interest of people is increasing in healthy foods which are considered to be beneficial to well-being in ways beyond a normal healthy diet required for human nutrition. In the current world, diseases such as cancer, obesity, hypertension, diabetes, inflammatory and autoimmune conditions, psychoneurological issues, etc., are increasing due to unhealthy eating habits and sedentary lifestyle (Kapoor et al. 2020; Prasad et al. 2012). Nutraceutical is a portmanteau of the word "nutrition" and "pharmaceutical" where "nutrition" means food constituents that provide health benefits and help in curing diseases and pharmaceutical deals with chemical compounds that target directly to diseases. Nutraceuticals are also described as medical foods, designer foods, functional foods, nutritional supplements, and phytochemicals that are present in large amount in plant-based sources (Bishnoi 2017). The term "nutraceutical" was coined in 1989 by Stephen Defelice MD and founder of the Foundation for Innovation in Medicine (FIM), Cranford, New Jersey. According to Defelice, "nutraceuticals are food constituents or part of food that has medicinal properties which provide health benefits to prevent or treat the various diseases." The father of medicines says, "Let food be your medicine." "Nutraceutical" is defined in the Oxford English Dictionary as "a foodstuff, food additive, or dietary supplement that has beneficial physiological effects but is not essential to the diet." In the proposed US Nutraceutical Research and Education Act (106th Congress of 1999–2000), it was defined as "a dietary supplement, food, or medical food that has a benefit, which prevents or reduces the risk of a disease or health condition, including the management of a disease or health condition or the improvement of health, and is safe for human consumption in the quantity, and with the frequency required to realize such properties" (Congress.gov 2020). The European Nutraceutical Association defines nutraceuticals as "nutritional products which have effects that are relevant to health, which are not synthetic substances or chemical compounds formulated for specific indications, containing nutrients (partly in concentrated form)." Health Canada has defined a nutraceutical as "a product isolated or purified from foods that are generally sold in medicinal forms not usually associated with food. A nutraceutical is demonstrated to have a physiological benefit or provide protection against chronic disease." (ARCHIVED 2020). An accompanying definition says that a nutraceutical is "a product isolated or purified from foods that are generally sold in medicinal forms not usually associated with food, demonstrated to have a physiological benefit or provide protection against chronic disease." This seems to differentiate the two terms "functional food" and "nutraceutical" (Corzo et al. 2020). Functional foods include vitamins, fats, proteins, and carbohydrates for the survival of health whereas when food is providing prevention and/or cure from the disease, it is called a nutraceutical. When food is used as a therapeutic agent meant for the nutritional management of disease such as food for managing inborn amino acid metabolism errors, it is called medical food. Nutraceuticals are partly nutritional and partly pharmaceutical, for example, probiotics, which is found in yoghurt, includes other fortified or modified food products and supplements. They act as medicine for improving health (Ruchi et al. 2017).

Herbals are basically biologically active natural products that contain plants, specific parts of plants, minerals such as kaolin, bentonite, etc., herbal materials, fungal, insects, shells, etc., are used for health benefits and help in managing various chronic diseases. Herbal products contain phytochemicals or bioactive compounds that exhibit numerous disease-preventing effects. Bioactive compounds include phenols, alkaloids, flavonoids, and carotenoids, which impart favorable health-related effects. Therefore, nutraceutical has an advantage over the medicines because medicines somehow give side effects on the human body but nutraceuticals avoid side effects. Nutraceuticals are categorized as a natural dietary supplement, dietary fiber, herbal nutrients, etc. (Mosihuzzaman 2012).

The current situation of COVID-19 has also increased the need for nutraceuticals that can improve the immunity of an individual to combat the current situation. Recently, in India, FSSAI (Food Safety and Standard Authority of India) was urged to promote plant-based food as an immunity builder, which is vital against novel coronavirus by improving the immunity of all age groups and seeking food hygiene and safety guidelines for meat shops and slaughterhouses during the COVID-19 pandemic (World Health Organization 2020). In a recent review (Jayawardena et al. 2020), it is clearly depicted that herbal extracts in the form of nutraceuticals can play an important role as an immunity enhancer to fight against novel coronavirus/COVID-19 situation.

Currently, the worldwide interest is in finding the mechanism of action and safety of nutraceuticals so that they could complement a pharmacological therapy and could be helpful in preventing a cluster of conditions that occur together such as diabetes, stroke, and heart attack. Nanotechnological approaches are being studied as a new delivery system for nutraceuticals and to improve their bioavailability (Durazzo et al. 2020).

10.2 Global Market of Nutraceuticals

Globally, the demand for nutraceuticals has increased hugely in the past two decades due to increased awareness in people regarding preventive healthcare measures and also due to the increased prevalence of lifestyle disorders. The global nutraceutical market size was valued at USD 382.51 billion in 2019 and is expected to expand at a compound annual growth rate (CAGR) of 8.3% over the period of 2020–2027 (Global Nutraceutical Market 2020). 31.01% of market share was held by the Asia-Pacific in 2019 and it would be likely to maintain the lead till 2027. Brazil, China, and India would likely expand at faster CAGR in the near future due to changing lifestyle, rising disposable income, rapid urbanization, and preference shift toward healthier dietary intake in these growing economies whereas vast product portfolio and government regulations on nutraceutical products are a few factors suppressing the nutraceutical industry growth. In product categorization, the functional beverage sector is leading the overall market followed by functional foods and dietary supplements in the year 2019 (Global Nutraceutical Market 2020). In a study by The

Associated Chambers of Commerce and Industry of India (ASSOCAM-India) and RNCOS, the nutraceutical industry in India is expected to touch the value of USD 8.5 billion by 2022 with approximately 3% share in the global nutraceutical market (Assocham India 2020).

High margins and minimal regulatory requirements have made these nutraceuticals attractive to food and beverage companies. They do not easily fall into the legal categories of food or drug and often reside in a gray area between the two (Ghosh et al. 2019). The key international players in the nutraceutical industry are Cargill, Incorporated, Archer Daniels Midland Company, DuPont, Nestle S.A, Danone, General Mills, Innophos, WR Grace, and Amway Corporation.

With such a huge potential and market for nutraceuticals, there are some limitations as well. The lack of specific regulations such as unclear definition due to which nutraceuticals are generally sold in the form of medicines and not associated with foods (Boccia and Covino 2016). Research demonstrated that nutraceuticals are in a competitive position with pharmaceuticals in the areas of blood pressure, diabetes, gastroenteritis, obesity, and osteoarthritis, and that can alleviate some pathologies, e.g. cholesterol. If we compare these two terms, pharmaceuticals include drugs made for the treatment of diseases, whereas nutraceuticals prevent the occurrence of diseases. Pharmaceuticals enjoy patent protection and government sanctioning whereas nutraceuticals never receive government appreciation and cannot be patented (Rajasekaran et al. 2008).

10.3 Classification of Nutraceutical Herbal Products

Classifications of functional foods, nutraceuticals, and dietary supplements have been attempted by the researches but not for nutraceutical herbal products. Previously, the categorization of nutraceuticals has been done on the basis of either potential or established nutraceuticals (Pandey et al. 2010), on the basis of the food material and nutrients (Kokate et al. 2002; Singh and Sinha 2012), or in terms of their effects on the body (Hänninen and Sen 2008; Prabu et al. 2012), on the chemical constituents and/or active ingredients (Espín et al. 2007; Pinto 2017; Shinde et al. 2014; Tapas et al. 2008).

Nutraceutical herbal products are classified as:

1) On the basis of natural sources they obtain from plants (Table 10.1), animals (Table 10.2), minerals, or microbial sources.
2) On the basis of chemical groupings, such as vitamins, minerals, amino acids, or other bioactive chemicals (Table 10.3) that are obtained from different sources.

Herbals are extracts of herbs or other botanical sources. They contain a broad spectrum of phytochemicals and the chemicals are derived from different sources such as shikimic, phenylpropanoids, pyruvate pathways, chondroitin sulfate, steroid hormone precursors, etc.

Botanical products in the form of nutraceuticals are vastly used for disease prevention and health promotion. In India, the traditional medicinal systems like Ayurveda/Unani have regulatory status as Ayurvedic/Unani drugs. Various extracts from herbs got the status to be sold as drugs by these regulatory bodies from time to time such as *Guglip* extract from *Cammiphora mukul* for cholesterol reduction, ginger capsules for treating chemotherapy-induced nausea, Ginseng tablet for immunity and energy, etc. (Ray et al. 2016). There are technological advancements over time but according to the WHO, there is 80% of the Indian and African population that still depends on traditional treatments for primary health care (WHO 2020). Recent developments in extraction, chromatography, electrophoresis, and spectroscopy techniques have enhanced the importance and value of plant-based foods and drugs (Srivastava and Mishra 2009). There are around 120 distinct chemical

Table 10.1 List of bioactive compounds and their health benefits derived from herbal plants.

Bioactive chemical	Health benefits	References
Carotenoids	Scavenge free radicals to prevent cell damage	Pinto (2017))
Lutein	Reduce the risk of macular degeneration	Bian et al. (2012)
Dietary fibers (soluble, insoluble, and glucan)	Reduce the risk of breast or colon cancer, cardiovascular diseases	Gul et al. (2016)
Plant-based fatty acids (DHA, linoleic acid)	Improve mental health, heart problems, and visual functions	Dolkar et al. (2017)
Phenolic compounds (flavonones, anthocyanidins, tannins, lignans, etc.)	Reduce the risk of the cancer-causing cell and neutralize free radicals	Pinto (2017) and Kasala et al. (2016)
Plant-based sterols	Maintain blood cholesterol level	Ghosh et al. (2019)

Table 10.2 List of bioactive compounds and their health benefits derived from animal sources (Hamed et al. 2015; Hooper and Cassidy 2006).

Bioactive compounds	Health benefits
Fatty acids (omega 3 fatty acids, conjugated linoleic acid)	Balance cholesterol, improve mental health, and cardiovascular problem
Probiotics (lactobacillus yogurt)	Improve intestine microflora, gastrointestinal health
Phenolic compounds (algae sources)	Scavenge free radicals

Table 10.3 List of various active ingredients, their sources, and health benefits (Dai and Koh 2015; Kennedy 2016; Moldes et al. 2017; Reid et al. 2015).

Active ingredients	Source	Health benefits
Vitamin A	Fish oil, orange and yellow fruits and vegetables, and fortified products	Maintain vision, skin problems, antioxidant, and treat cancer and skin disorder
Vitamin D	Egg yolk and milk	Help in the absorption of calcium and formation of bones
Vitamin E	Cottonseed oil and peanut oil	Antioxidant, boost the immune system, and blood cell formation
Vitamin K	Mustard greens, parsley, and green leaf lettuce	Essential for blood clotting
Vitamin C	Broccoli, guava, and coriander	Antioxidant, necessary for healthy bones, gums, teeth and skin, and helps in wound healing
Vitamin B_1	Sunflower seed and brown rice	Essential in neurologic functions
Vitamin B_2	Avocado, almonds, wild rice, and mushrooms	Chemical processes in the body help maintain healthy eyes, skin, and nerve function
Vitamin B_3	Yeast, meat, poultry, and coffee	Maintain proper brain functioning

Table 10.3 (Continued)

Active ingredients	Source	Health benefits
Vitamin B_{12}	Animal products and fortified products	Helps produce the genetic material of cells and also helps with the formation of the red blood cells
Folic acid	Beans, peanuts, and green vegetables	Produces the genetic materials of cells, essential in the first three months of pregnancy
Pantothenic acid	Poultry product, milk, and mushroom	Synthesis of cholesterol, steroids, and fatty acids
Magnesium	Dark chocolate, tofu, and avocado	Essential for healthy nerve and muscle functioning and bone formation and may help prevent premenstrual syndrome (PMS)
Copper	Dry berries, nuts, lobster, and oyster	Essential for hemoglobin and collagen production, and healthy functioning of the heart
Zinc	Chickpea, almond, and cashew	Essential for cell reproduction, normal growth, and development in children
Quinic acid	Cranberries	Remove toxins from the bladder, kidneys, prostate, and testicles
Glucosinolates and isothiocyanates	Broccoli, cabbage, cauliflower, collards, kale, and Brussels sprouts	Help detoxify organisms, exert a protective effect against cancer in the respiratory, gastrointestinal, and genitourinary systems and reproductive organs

substances derived from plants that are considered as in drugs (Bahorun et al. 2019). Herbs such as ginger, turmeric, green tea, etc., containing bioflavonoids, polyphenols, carotenoids (Table 10.4) act as nutraceuticals (Shen et al. 2012). In the market, various nutraceutical products containing herbs are available (Table 10.5) in the form of capsules, powder, tablets, extract, syrup, etc., like chyawanprash, green tea, psyllium husk, brahmi, mucuna, etc. Traditionally, ginger, ashwagandha, amla, neem, *Ginkgo biloba*, *Kava kava*, *Passionflower*, *Valerian*, *St. John's wort*, etc., have been used for centuries for their nutraceutical properties (Bishnoi 2017).

10.4 Health Benefits of Herbal-Based Nutraceuticals

Uses of herbal-based nutraceuticals avoid unpleasant side effects in the body and increase the health-beneficial effect. They are purely natural, have dietary supplements, are easily available, and affordable that improve the health value or medical condition of human beings. Herbal nutraceuticals possess nutritional therapeutic properties which have a healing system toward chronic diseases. This therapy is based on the herbal system and its goal to detoxifying the body by maintaining vitamins and minerals, restoring the digestion system, and also improving dietary habits.

Broadly, nutraceutical products focus on:

1) Cellular-based health improvements
2) Immune-based health improvements
3) Biochemical or neuroendocrine support
4) Nutritional-based supports because herbal-based nutraceuticals are rich in phytonutrients

Herbal nutraceuticals arise from plant sources and plants consist of a lot of phytochemicals or phytonutrients that have a particular biological impact on human health. These nutraceutical

Table 10.4 List of herbs as nutraceuticals with their active constituent and health benefits.

Herb	Constituent	Health benefits	References
Garlic – *Allium sativum* (Liliaceae)	Alliin and allicin	Anti-inflammatory, antibacterial, antigout, nervine tonic	Arreola et al. (2015)
Ginger – *Zingiber officinale* (Zingiberaceae)	Zingiberene and gingerols	Stimulant, chronic bronchitis, antiemetic, carminative hyperglycemia, and throat ache	Malhotra and Singh (2003), Palatty et al. (2013), Funk et al. (2016) and Sharma (2017)
Maiden – *Ginkgo biloba* (Ginkgoaceae)	Ginkgolide and bilobalide	PAF antagonist, memory enhancer, Antioxidant, improvement in blood circulation, neurodegenerative diseases such as Alzheimer's disease	(Maclennan et al. (2002), Wąsik and Antkiewicz-Michaluk (2017) and McKeage and Lyseng-Williamson (2018)
Echinacea – *Echinacea purpurea* (Asteraceae)	Alkylamide and echinacoside	Anti-inflammatory, immunomodulator, and antiviral	Manayi et al. (2015)
Ginseng – *Panax ginseng* (Araliaceae)	Ginsenosides and Panaxosides	Stimulating immune, anti-inflammatory, and nervous system and adaptogenic properties	Kang and Min (2012) and Kim et al. (2017)
Liquorice – *Glycyrrhiza glabra* (leguminosae)	Glycyrrhizin and liquirtin	Anti-inflammatory and anti-allergic, expectorant, free radical scavenger, anti-allergy	Kalsi et al. (2016)
St. John's wort – *Hypericum perforatum* (Hypericaceae)	Hypericin and hyperforin	Antidepressant, against HIV and hepatitis C virus	Bishnoi (2017)
Turmeric – *Curcuma longa* (Zingiberacae)	Curcumin	Anti-inflammatory, antiarthritic, anticancer, and antiseptic	Kohli et al. (2005) and Hewlings and Kalman (2017)
Onion – *Allium cepa* Linn. (Liliaceae)	Allicin and alliin	Hypoglycemic activity, antibiotic and antiatherosclerotic	Bishnoi (2017)
Valeriana – *Valeriana officinalis* Linn. (Valerianaceae)	Valerenic acid and valerate	Tranquillizer, migraine, menstrual pain, intestinal cramps, and bronchial spasm	Pilerood and Prakash (2013)
Aloes – *Aloe barbadensis* Mill. (Liliaceae)	Aloins and aloesin	Dilates capillaries, anti-inflammatory, emollient, wound healing properties	Chauhan et al. (2013)
Goldenseal – *Hydrastis canadensis* (Ranunculaceae)	Hydrastine and berberine	Antimicrobial, astringent, antihemorrhagic, and treatment of mucosal inflammation	Builders (2019)
Senna – *Cassia angustifolia* (Leguminosae)	Sennosides	Purgative	Ramchander and Middha (2017)

Table 10.4 (Continued)

Herb	Constituent	Health benefits	References
Asafetida – *Ferula assafoetida* L. (Umbelliferae)	Ferulic acid and umbellic acid	Stimulant, carminative, and expectorant	Lewis (1992)
Bael – *Aeglemarmelos Corr.* (Rutaceae)	Marmelosin	Digestive, appetizer, and treatment of diarrhea and dysentery	Phogat et al. (2017)
Brahmi – *Centella asiatica* (Umbelliferae)	Asiaticoside and madecassoside	Nerve tonic, antianxiety, and spasmolytic	Chauhan et al. (2013)
Hawthorn – *Crataegus monogyna*	Oligomeric procyanidins and flavonoids	Used for several heart-related conditions, heart failure, and high blood pressure	Builders (2019)
Feverfew – *Tanacetum parthenium*	Parthenolide	Pain-relieving properties, migraine headaches, and menstrual cramps	Wąsik and Antkiewicz-Michaluk (2017)
Ashwagandha – *Withania somnifera*	Withanolides and withaferins	Restorative and rejuvenating benefits, stress management, and blood formation	Lopresti et al. (2019) and Sharma et al. (2011)
Ocimum sanctum	Eugenol	Antimicrobial, antistress, antidiabetic, hepatoprotective, anti-inflammatory, neuroprotective, and cardioprotective	Prakash and Gupta (2005) and Baliga et al. (2013)
Scutellaria baicalensis	Baicalein	Antioxidant and anti-inflammatory	Shieh et al. (2000)
Larrea tridentate	Nordihydroguaiare-tic acid	Antioxidant, antiviral, and anti-inflammatory	Rahman et al. (2011)
Tinospora cordifolia, Giloy or guduchi	Diterpenoid lactones, glycosides, steroids, sesquiterpenoids, and phenolics	Treatment of stress, mood elevation, and mental well-being, anti-inflammatory, and antipyretic properties, and is often used in conditions like dengue, swine flu, malaria, and urinary tract infections	Kumar et al. (2020) and Ghosh and Saha (2012)
Emblica officinalis, Indian gooseberry (Phyllanthaceae) (Amla)	Tannins and flavonoids	Anti-inflammatory, fever, anemia, digestion, and relieving constipation	Yadav et al. (2017), Lanka (2018) and Kalaiselvan and Rasool (2015)
Agathosma betulina Rutaceae	Diosphenol and menthone	Diuretic, urinary pain reliever, hypertension, and heart diseases	Cunningham (1993) and Nwaka (2005)
Cinchona succirubra	Quinine	Antimalarial agent	Ferreira Júnior et al. (2012)
Catharanthus roseus	Vincristine and vinblastine	Antileukemic	Elujoba et al. (2005)
Plantago ovata (Plantaginaceae)	Psyllium husk	Laxative properties, reducing cholesterol, and treatment of constipation	Xing et al. (2017)

(Continued)

Table 10.4 (Continued)

Herb	Constituent	Health benefits	References
Brahmi – *Bacopa monnieri* (Scrophulariaceae)	Triterpenoidsaponins: asiaticoside, madecassoside, and bacosides A and B	Mental health, memory enhancement, and antidepressant	Bai Kunte and Kuna (2013), Gohil and Patel (2010) and Kadali et al. (2014)
Mucuna pruriens (Fabaceae)	L-dopa	Nervous disorders and Parkinson's disease	Patil et al. (2014)
Camellia sinensis (Theaceae)	Epigallocatechin 3-gallate	Cardiovascular protection, weight maintenance, skin care, allergy inhibition, and protection from osteoarthritis	Katiyar and Raman (2011), Wu et al. (2012) and Zink and Traidl-Hoffmann (2015)
Azadirachta indica (Meliaceae) neem	Nimbidin, octadecanoic acid-3,4-tetrahydrofuran diester	Purifies blood, detoxifies the body, and neutralizes free radicals, supports the immune system, provides radiant skin, supports healthy digestion, and boosts liver function	Bhowmik et al. (2010) and Ishita et al. (2007)

Table 10.5 List of marketed nutraceutical products (Chaddha et al. 2013).

Product	Category	Contents	Manufacturer
Calcirol	D-3 Calcium supplement	Calcium and vitamins	Cadila Healthcare Limited, Ahmedabad, India
GRD (Pinto 2017; Shinde et al. 2014; Tapas et al. 2008)	Nutritional supplement Proteins	Vitamins, minerals, and carbohydrates	Zydus Cadila Ltd., Ahmedabad, India
Proteinex®	Protein supplement	Predigested proteins, vitamins, minerals, and carbohydrates	Pfizer Ltd., Mumbai, India
Coral calcium	Calcium supplement	Calcium and trace minerals	Nature's answer, Hauppauge, NY, USA
Chyawanprash	Immune booster	Amla, ashwagandha, and pippali	Dabur India Ltd.
Omega woman	Immune supplement	Antioxidants, vitamins, and phytochemicals (e.g. Lycopene and resveratrol)	Wassen, Surrey, UK
Celestial Healthtone	Immune booster	Dry fruit extract	Celestial Biolabs Limited
Amiriprash (Gold)	Good immunomodulator	Chyawanprash Avaleha, Swarnabhasma, and Ras	Sindur Uap Pharma Pvt. Ltd.

phytochemicals work in various ways such as they play the role of substrates or cofactors for biochemical or enzymatic reactions. They act as absorbents that bind, absorb, or stabilize essential nutrients in the intestine and eliminate undesirable constituents. They support beneficial bacteria in the intestine and scavenge the free reactive radicals or toxic chemicals from the body. Herbal nutraceuticals like *Ginkgo biloba*, green tea, garlic, etc., are used in the traditional system in medicine from very ancient time. *Ginkigo bibola* is used for the treatment of dementia (Chauhan et al. 2013), green tea for prevention of heart ailments, weight management, and for positive effects on metabolism (Ahmad et al. 2014; Shinde et al. 2014), whereas garlic is used worldwide as curative for fevers, swelling, antibacterial, reduction in blood sugar, and cholesterol (Bhagyalakshmi et al. 2005; Wang et al. 2017). Advancement in technology in the field of nutraceuticals is evolved with new methods for drug delivery systems. These novel drug delivery systems include nanoemulsions, liposomes, phytosomes, microspheres, and transfersomes (Ruchi et al. 2017). Nanoemulsion includes the nano-sized formulation of two immiscible liquids, mixed to form a single phase, whereas liposomes are composed of phospholipids consisting of a lipid bilayer. In phytosomes, a complex of phospholipid is formed with a biologically active ingredient. Ginseng is having low solubility and this problem was overcome by making Ginseng phytosomes which provide enhanced therapeutic effects by increased absorption in the body. Similarly, hawthorns and quercetin phytosomes are also used for their increased therapeutic efficacy (Şanlı et al. 2009). Microspheres are small (1–1000 μm), spherical vesicular particles that can be ingested or injected for site-specific as well as organ-targeted drug delivery. An example of a microsphere is the camptothecin microsphere used for their anticancer effect (Gavini et al. 2005; Patel et al. 2009; Zheng et al. 2006). Transfersomes consist of an aqueous phase and a core surrounded by the lipid bilayer complex which is capable of crossing several transport berries. Capsaicin and colchicine transfersomes are studied for their better therapeutic effects (Garti and McClements 2012).

Clearly, it is very important to study all aspects very carefully to develop a better drug delivery system because nutraceutical formulations are meant to be taken as a diet but not as a medicine. The requirement of formulation to be food-grade thus limits the choices of researchers (Ruchi et al. 2017).

Some medicinal plants are used as a traditional treatment for anti-infection, antimicrobial, and antiviral properties (Palombo 2011) and also used in nutraceuticals (Table 10.6).

10.5 Government Regulations

Nutraceutical products are directly natural products or their isolated components. For making a quality nutraceutical product, it is important to maintain the quality throughout, starting from collection of raw material, identification, and quantification of the active component, standardization of methods of extraction, safety, efficacy testing, and formulation of nutraceutical products. Nutraceutical products could be taken for a long time without the need for a prescription. So, their regulation becomes more important to judge their safety. Nutraceuticals are considered food products but their classification and regulatory requirements are different in different regions of the world. Dietary Supplement Health and Education Act (DSHEA) is the legislation for manufacturing and marketing of nutraceuticals in the United States. The safety of nutraceuticals before their marketing is ensured by Food and Drug Administration (FDA). The USFDA Modernization Act (1997) mentions that at least four months before a supplement is marketed, the FDA has to be notified about the health claims and/or the nutrient content claims on the product label of a dietary supplement (FDA 2020). In Canada, the regulation of nutraceuticals is more like a drug than a food category (L'Abbé et al. 2008). The European Food and Safety Authority (EFSA) regulates food legislation for food supplements according to Directive 2002/46/EC of the European Parliament and of the Council of 10 June 2002 in the European Union (EU) (EUR-Lex 2020). The EU have strict rules for product claims and a list of permitted vitamin or mineral substances. Unlike USFDA,

Table 10.6 List of herbal plants that exhibit antimicrobial properties (Builders 2019).

Herbal plants	Antimicrobial properties against
Drosera peltata (Droseraceae)	Act on oral bacteria, *S. mutans*, and *S. sobrinus*
Coptidis rhizoma (Ranunculacea)	Period onto pathogenic bacteria and bactericidal activity
Garlic, *Allium sativum* (Liliaceae)	Gram-negative pathogens
Abies canadensis (Pinaceae)	Gram-negative and gram-positive pathogens
Harungana madagascariensis (Hypericaceae)	*Actinomyces, Fusobacterium, Lactobacillus, Preotella, Propionibacterium*, and *Streptococcus* species
Pistacia lentiscus (Anacardiaceae) (mastic gum)	*Streptococci* species
Piper cubeba (Piperaceae)	Cariogenic pathogens
Breynia nivosus (Euphorbiaceae) and *Ageratum conyzoides* (Asteraceae)	*S. mutans*
Red grape seeds, green tea, and unfermented cocoa	*S. mutans*
Helichrysum italicum (Compositae)	*S. mutans, S. sanguis*, and *S. sobrinus*
Ziziphus joazeiro (Rhamnaceae), *Caesalpinia pyramidalis* (Fabaceae), and *Aristolochia cymbifera* (Aristolochiaceae)	*S. mutans* and *S. sanguis*
Tea – *Camelia sinensis* (Theaceae)	Anticariogenic effects
and *Psidium guajava* (Myrtaceae)	*S. mutans* biofilms, Gram-positive, yeast *Candida albicans*, fungicidal activity
Root, bark of *Morus alba* (Moraceae)	Food poisoning micro-organisms, *S. mutans*
Flavononephytoalexins from *Sophora exigua* (Leguminosae)	Cariogenic bacteria
Honeycomb of *Polistes olivaceous, Nidus Vespae*	*S. mutans* anti-acidogenic activity
Artocarpus heterophyllus (Moraceae)	Streptococci, actinomyces, lactobacilli, cariogenic, and oral bacteria
Naringin (polymethoxylated)	*Actinobacillus actinomycetemcomitans* and *P. gingivalis*
Psoralea corylifolia (Fabaceae)	Gram-positive and gram-negative bacteria

EFSA is not mandatory to take legal action against an unsafe product (Hasler 2005). In Korea, the regulator is the Ministry of Food and Drug Safety (MFDS) which crafted the Health Function Food Act in May 2004.

There are two segments for nutraceutical industries in Japan which are regulatory bodies under the Ministry of Health, Labor and Welfare (MHLW) (Shimizu 2003). The first segment is for foods with nutrient function claims (FNFC) including Standards for 12 vitamins and 5 minerals while another segment is for dietary ingredients having reported physiological benefits under Foods for Specified Health Uses (FOSHU) (Saito 2007; Santini et al. 2018). The government of China makes policies for nutraceutical industries in three segments. The first segment which is in charge of dietary supplements is China's State Food and Drug Administration (SFDA). Approval of new novel food ingredient comes under the second segment which is the Ministry of Health (MOH). The third segment, Administration of Quality Supervision Inspection and Quarantine (AQSIQ) controls all the imports and exports of the country. In Taiwan, there is the Taiwan Food and Drug Administration (TFDA).

In a country such as Australia, detailed evaluation of nutraceutical products with clinical trial as well as safety assessment studies should be carried out before their marketing (Tapsell 2008; Tee et al. 2002; Yang 2008). In India, the Food Safety and Standards Authority of India (FSSAI) made under Food Safety and Standards Regulation (2006) regulates the issues of food safety. Nutraceuticals and dietary supplements are regulated under The Food Safety and Standards (Health Supplements, Nutraceuticals, Food for Special Dietary Use, Food for Special Medical Purpose, Functional Foods and Novel Foods) Regulations, 2016 which have been notified on 23 December, 2016 and were effective from 1 January, 2018 (FSSAI 2016). Detailed definitions, requirements for a claim, labeling requirements, maximum, and minimum primitive limits for components, list of vitamins, minerals, amino acids, and their components, Recommended Daily Allowance (RDA), list of plants and botanical ingredients, formulation, prebiotic, probiotics were covered under these regulations and their update from time to time is being carried out. FSSAI has directed manufacturers to stop using 14 ingredients, namely raspberry ketone, silica, angelica sinensis, paullinia cupana, saw palmetto, notoginseing, chlorella growth factor, pine bark extracted from Pinus radiata, pine bark extracted from Pinus pinaster, Vitamin D3 (veg), Chaga extract, Oxalobacter formigenes, Phytavail iron, and tea tree oil lacking scientific data for safe usage (Maindola 2018), and recently directed to stop the use of PABA (Para Amino Benzoic Acid) due to safety concerns (FSSAI 2020).

10.6 Future Scope for Herbal Nutraceuticals

Increasing lifestyle disorders, ever-increasing medical cost, awareness, and increasing disposable income throughout the world are major drivers for the nutraceutical market all over the modern world. The trend of increasing demand will move upward with same or even with higher CAGR world specifically in developing economies. The interest of people toward herbal nutraceutical is an alternate form of treatment for a number of therapeutic purposes. Strong regulatory requirements for safe products to the public are the need of the hour and regulatory agencies over the globe are working positively.

References

Ahmad, M., Baba, W.N., Shah, U. et al. (2014). Nutraceutical properties of the green tea polyphenols. *J. Food Process. Technol.* 5 (11): 1–5.

ARCHIVED (2020). ARCHIVED – Policy Paper – Nutraceuticals/Functional Foods and Health Claims On Foods – Canada.ca [Internet]. https://www.canada.ca/en/health-canada/services/food-nutrition/food-labelling/health-claims/nutraceuticals-functional-foods-health-claims-foods-policy-paper.html (accessed 25 July 2020).

Arreola, R., Quintero-Fabián, S., Ivette López-Roa, R. et al. (2015). Immunomodulation and anti-inflammatory effects of garlic compounds. *J. Immunol. Res.*: 1–13. https://doi.org/10.1155/2015/401630.

Assocham India (2020) Assocham India [Internet]. https://www.assocham.org/newsdetail.php?id=6259 (accessed 26 July 2020).

Bahorun, T., Aruoma, O.I., and Neergheen-bhujun, V.S. (2019). Phytomedicines, nutraceuticals, and functional foods regulatory framework: the African context. In: *Nutraceutical and Functional Food Regulations in the United States and around the World*, 3e, 509–521. Elsevier Inc.

Bai Kunte, K. and Kuna, Y. (2013). Neuroprotective effect of *Bacopa monniera* on memory deficits and ATPase system in Alzheimer's disease (AD) induced mice. *J. Sci. Innov. Res.* 2 (4): 719–735.

Baliga, M.S., Jimmy, R., Thilakchand, K.R. et al. (2013). *Ocimum sanctum* L. (holy basil or tulsi) and its phytochemicals in the prevention and treatment of cancer. *Nutr. Cancer* 65 (1): 26–35.

Bhagyalakshmi, N., Thimmaraju, R., Venkatachalam, L. et al. (2005). Nutraceutical applications of garlic and the intervention of biotechnology. *Crit. Rev. Food Sci. Nutr.* 45 (7–8): 607–621.

Bhowmik, D., Yadav, J., Tripathi, K.K., and Sampath Kumar, K.P. (2010). Herbal remedies of *Azadirachta indica* and its medicinal application. *J. Chem. Pharm. Res.* 2 (1): 62–72.

Bian, Q., Gao, S., Zhou, J. et al. (2012). Lutein and zeaxanthin supplementation reduces photooxidative damage and modulates the expression of inflammation-related genes in retinal pigment epithelial cells. *Free Radic. Biol. Med.* 53 (6): 1298–1307.

Bishnoi, S. (2017). Herbs as functional foods. In: *Functional Foods: Sources and Health Benefits* (eds. D. Mudgil and S. Barak), 141–172. Scientific Publishers.

Boccia, F. and Covino, D. (2016). Innovation and sustainability in agri-food companies: the role of quality. *Riv. di Stud. sulla Sostenibilita.* 1: 131–141.

Builders, F.P. (ed.) (2019). Introduction to herbal medicine. In: *Herbal Medicine*. IntechOpen.

Chaddha, V., Kushwah, A.S., and Shrivastava, V. (2013). An importance of herbal drugs as anti diarrheal: a review. *Int. J. Res. Appl. Nat. Soc. Sci.* 1 (7): 25–28.

Chauhan, B., Kumar, G., Kalam, N., and Ansari, S.H. (2013). Current concepts and prospects of herbal nutraceutical: a review. *J. Adv. Pharm. Technol. Res.* 4 (1): 4–8.

Congress.gov (2020). H.R.3001 – 106th Congress (1999–2000): Nutraceutical Research and Education Act|Congress.gov|Library of Congress [Internet]. https://www.congress.gov/bill/106th-congress/house-bill/3001?s=4&r=2681 (accessed 25 July 2020).

Corzo, L., Fernández-novoa, L., Carrera, I. et al. (2020). Nutrition, health, and disease: role of selected marine and vegetal nutraceuticals. 12 (747): 1–28. https://doi.org/10.3390/nu12030747.

Cunningham, A.B. (1993). African medicinal plants setting priorities at the interface between conservation and primary healthcare. People and plants working paper 1.

Dai, Z. and Koh, W.-P. (2015). B-Vitamins and bone health – a review of the current evidence. *Nutrients* 7 (5): 3322–3346.

Dolkar, D., Bakshi, P., Wali, V.K. et al. (2017). Fruits as nutraceuticals. *Eco. Env. Cons.* 23: S113–S118.

Durazzo, A., Lucarini, M., and Santini, A. (2020). Nutraceuticals in human health. *Foods* 9: 18–20.

Elujoba, A.A., Odeleye, O.M., and Ogunyemi, C.M. (2005). Traditional medicine development for medical and dental primary health care delivery system in Africa. *Afr. J. Trad. CAM* 2: 46–61.

Espín, J.C., García-Conesa, M.T., and Tomás-Barberán, F.A. (2007). Nutraceuticals: facts and fiction. *Phytochemistry* 68 (22–24): 2986–3008.

EUR-Lex (2020). EUR-Lex – 32002L0046 – EN – EUR-Lex [Internet]. https://eur-lex.europa.eu/legal-content/EN/ALL/?uri=celex%3A32002L0046 (accessed 28 July 2020).

FDA (2020). Food and Drug Administration Modernization Act (FDAMA) of 1997|FDA [Internet]. https://www.fda.gov/regulatory-information/selected-amendments-fdc-act/food-and-drug-administration-modernization-act-fdama-1997 (accessed 28 July 2020).

Ferreira Júnior, W.S., Cruz, M.P., Dos Santos, L.L., and MFT, M. (2012). Use and importance of quina (*Cinchona* spp.) and ipeca (*Carapichea ipecacuanha* (Brot.) L. Andersson): plants for medicinal use from the 16th century to the present. *J. Herb. Med.* 2: 103–112.

FSSAI (2016). FSSAI Regulations 2016 [Internet]. https://www.fssai.gov.in/upload/uploadfiles/files/Nutraceuticals_Regulations.pdf (25 July 2020).

FSSAI (2020). FSSAI [Internet]. https://www.fssai.gov.in/upload/advisories/2020/07/5f1035178000aLetter_Surveillance_Enforcement_Sell_HealthSuppliments_16_07_2020.pdf (27 July 2020).

Funk, J.L., Frye, J.B., Oyarzo, J.N. et al. (2016). Anti-inflammatory effects of the essential oils of ginger (*Zingiber officinale* Roscoe) in experimental rheumatoid arthritis. *Pharma. Nutr.* 4 (3): 123–131.

Garti, N. and McClements, D. (2012). Encapsulation technologies and delivery systems for food ingredients and nutaceuticals. In: , 1e (eds. N. Garti and D. McClements), 23–30. Florida: Woodhead Publishing Series in Food Sciences, Technology and Nutrition.

Gavini, E., Alamanni, M.C., Cossu, M., and Giunchedi, P. (2005). Tabletted microspheres containing *Cynara scolymus* (var. *Spinoso sardo*) extract for the preparation of controlled release nutraceutical matrices. *J. Microencapsul.* 22 (5): 487–499.

Ghosh, S. and Saha, S. (2012). *Tinospora cordifolia*: one plant, many roles. *Anc. Sci. Life.* 31 (4): 151–159.

Ghosh, N., Das, A., and Sen, C.K. (2019). Nutritional supplements and functional foods: functional significance and global regulations. In: *Nutraceutical and Functional Food Regulations in the United States and around the World*, 3e, 13–35. Elsevier Inc.

Global Nutraceutical Market (2020). Global Nutraceutical Market Growth Analysis Report, 2020–2027 [Internet]. https://www.grandviewresearch.com/industry-analysis/nutraceuticals-market (accessed 25 July 2020).

Gohil, K.J. and Patel, J.A. (2010). A review on *Bacopa monniera*: current research and future prospects. *Int. J. Green. Pharm.* 4 (1): 1–9.

Gul, K., Singh, A.K., and Jabeen, R. (2016). Nutraceuticals and functional foods: the foods for the future world. *Crit. Rev. Food Sci. Nutr.* 56 (16): 2617–2627.

Hamed, I., Özogul, F., Özogul, Y., and Regenstein, J.M. (2015). Marine bioactive compounds and their health benefits: a review. *Compr. Rev. Food Sci. Food Saf.* 14 (4): 446–465.

Hänninen, O. and Sen, C.K. (2008). Nutritional supplements and functional foods: functional significance and global regulations. In: *Nutraceutical and Functional Food Regulations in the United States and Around the World*, 11–35. Elsevier Ltd.

Hasler, C. (2005). *Regulation of Functional Foods and Nutraceuticals: A Global Perspective* (ed. C. Hasler), 1–432. New Jersey: Wiley.

Hewlings, S. and Kalman, D. (2017). Curcumin: a review of its' effects on human health. *Foods* 6 (10): 92.

Hooper, L. and Cassidy, A. (2006). A review of the health care potential of bioactive compounds. *J. Sci. Food Agric.* 86 (12): 1805–1813.

Ishita, M.-G., Chattopadhyay, U., and Baral, R. (2007). Neem leaf preparation enhances Th1 type immune response and anti-tumor immunity against breast tumor associated antigen. *Cancer Immunol. Res.* 7 (1): 1–9.

Jayawardena, R., Sooriyaarachchi, P., Chourdakis, M. et al. (2020). Enhancing immunity in viral infections, with special emphasis on COVID-19: a review. *Diabetes Metab. Syndr. Clin. Res. Rev.* 14 (4): 367–382.

Kadali, R., Murty, S., Das, M.C. et al. (2014). Antidepressant activity of brahmi in albino mice. *J. Clin. Diagnostic Res.* 8 (3): 35–37.

Kalaiselvan, S. and Rasool, M.K. (2015). The anti-inflammatory effect of triphala in arthritic-induced rats. *Pharm. Biol.* 53 (1): 51–60.

Kalsi, S., Verma, S.K., Kaur, A., and Singh, N. (2016). A review on *Glycyrrhiza glabra* (Liquorice) and its pharmacological activities. *Int. J. Pharm. Drug Anal.* 4 (5): 234–239.

Kang, S. and Min, H. (2012). Ginseng, the "immunity boost": the effects of panax ginseng on immune system. *J. Ginseng Res.* 36 (4): 354–368.

Kapoor, N., Jamwal, V.L., Shukla, M.R., and Gandhi, S.G. (2020). Biotechnology business – concept to delivery. In: *Biotechnology Business – Concept to Delivery* (ed. A. Saxena), 67–92. Switzerland: Springer Nature.

Kasala, E.R., Bodduluru, L.N., Barua, C.C., and Gogoi, R. (2016). Antioxidant and antitumor efficacy of Luteolin, a dietary flavone on benzo(a)pyrene-induced experimental lung carcinogenesis. *Biomed. Pharmacother.* 82: 568–577.

Katiyar, S.K. and Raman, C. (2011). Green tea: a new option for the prevention or control of osteoarthritis. *Arthr. Res. Ther.* 13 (4): 121.

Kennedy, D. (2016). B Vitamins and the brain: mechanisms, dose and efficiency – a review. *Nutrients* 8 (2): 68.

Kim, J.H., Yi, Y.S., Kim, M.Y., and Cho, J.Y. (2017 Oct 1). Role of ginsenosides, the main active components of *Panax ginseng*, in inflammatory responses and diseases. *J. Ginseng Res.* 41 (4): 435–443.

Kohli, K., Ali, J., Ansari, M., and Raheman, Z. (2005). Curcumin: a natural antiinflammatory agent. *Indian J. Pharmacol.* 37 (3): 141.

Kokate, C.K., Purohit, A.P., and Gokhale, S.B. (2002). Nutraceutical and cosmaceutical. In: *Pharmacognosy*, 21e (eds. V.E. Tyler, L.R. Brady and J.E. Robbers), 542–549. Pune, India: Nirali Prakashan.

Kumar, P., Kamle, M., Mahato, D.K. et al. (2020). *Tinospora cordifolia* (Giloy): phytochemistry, ethnopharmacology. *Clin. Appl. Conserv. Strateg. Curr. Pharm. Biotechnol.* 30: 21.

L'Abbé, M.R., Dumais, L., Chao, E., and Junkins, B. (2008). Health claims on foods in Canada. *J. Nutr.* 138 (6): 1221S–1227S.

Lanka, S. (2018). A review on pharmacological, medicinal and ethnobotanical important plant: *Phyllanthus emblica* linn. (*Syn. emblica officinalis*). *World J. Pharm. Res.* 7 (4): 380–396.

Lewis, W.H. (ed.) (1992). Plants used medically by indigenous peoples. In: *Phytochemical Resources for Medicine and Agriculture*, 33–74. Springer US.

Lopresti, A.L., Drummond, P.D., and Smith, S.J. (2019). A randomized, double-blind, placebo-controlled, crossover study examining the hormonal and vitality effects of ashwagandha (*Withania somnifera*) in aging, overweight males. *Am. J. Mens Health.* 13 (2): 1–15.

Maclennan, K.M., Darlington, C.L., and Smith, P.F. (2002). The CNS effects of *Ginkgo biloba* extracts and ginkgolide B. *Prog. Neurobiol.* 67 (3): 235–257.

Maindola, A. (2018). FSSAI prohibits use of 14 ingredients under Nutraceutical Regulations. https://www.fssai.gov.in/upload/media/5b44564e06c36FSSAI_News_Nutraceutical_FNB_03_07_2018.pdf (accessed 27 July 2020).

Malhotra, S. and Singh, A.P. (2003). *Medicinal Properties of Ginger (Zingiber officinale Rosc.)*, vol. 2. Natural Product Radiance.

Manayi, A., Vazirian, M., and Saeidnia, S. (2015). *Echinacea purpurea*: pharmacology, phytochemistry and analysis methods. *Pharmacogn. Rev.* 9 (17): 63–72.

McKeage, K. and Lyseng-Williamson, K.A. (2018). Ginkgo biloba extract EGb 761® in the symptomatic treatment of mild-to-moderate dementia: a profile of its use. *Drugs Ther. Perspect.* 34 (8): 358–366.

Moldes, A.B., Vecino, X., and Cruz, J.M. (2017). Nutraceuticals and food additives. In: *Current Developments in Biotechnology and Bioengineering*, 143–164. Elsevier B.V.

Mosihuzzaman, M. (2012). Herbal medicine in healthcare – an overview. *Nat. Prod. Commun.* 7 (6): 807–812.

Nwaka, S. (2005). Drug discovery and beyond: the role of public–private partnerships in improving access to new malaria medicines. *Trans. R. Soc. Trop. Med. Hyg.* 99 (1): 20–29.

Palatty, P.L., Haniadka, R., Valder, B. et al. (2013). Ginger in the prevention of nausea and vomiting: a review. *Crit. Rev. Food Sci. Nutr.* 53 (7): 659–669.

Palombo, E.A. (2011). Traditional medicinal plant extracts and natural products with activity against oral bacteria: potential application in the prevention and treatment of oral diseases. *Evid. Based Compl. Altern. Med.*: 1–15. https://doi.org/10.1093/ecam/nep067.

Pandey, M., Verma, R.K., and Saraf, S.A. (2010). Nutraceuticals: new era of medicine and health. *Asian J. Pharm. Clin. Res.* 3 (1): 11–15.

Patel, R., Singh, S., Singh, S. et al. (2009). Development and characterization of curcumin loaded transfersome for transdermal delivery. *J. Pharm. Sci. Res.* 1 (4): 71–80.

Patil, R.R., Gholave, A.R., Jadhav, J.P. et al. (2014). Mucuna sanjappae Aitawade et Yadav: a new species of Mucuna with promising yield of anti-Parkinson's drug l-DOPA. *Genet. Resour. Crop Evol.* 62 (1): 155–162.

Phogat, N., Bisht, V., and Johar, V. (2017). Bael (*Aegle marmelos*) extraordinary species of India: a review. *Int. J. Curr. Microbiol. Appl. Sci.* 6 (3): 1870–1887.

Pilerood, S.A. and Prakash, J. (2013). Nutritional and medicinal properties of valerian (*Valeriana officinalis*) Herb: a review. *Int. J. Food Nutr. Diabetes.* 1 (1): 25–32.

Pinto, J. (2017). A current look at nutraceuticals – key concepts and future prospects. *Trends Food Sci. Technol.* https://doi.org/10.1016/j.tifs.2017.02.010.

Prabu, S.L., Suriyaprakash, T.N.K., Kumar, C.D. et al. (2012). Nutraceuticals: a review. *Elixir Pharm.* 46: 8372–8377.

Prakash, P. and Gupta, N. (2005). Therapeutic uses of *Ocimum sanctum* Linn (Tulsi) with a note on eugenol and its pharmacological actions: a short review. *Indian J. Physiol. Pharmacol.* 49 (2): 125–131.

Prasad, S., Sung, B., and Aggarwal, B.B. (2012). Age-associated chronic diseases require age-old medicine: role of chronic inflammation. *Prev. Med. (Baltim)* 54: S29–S37.

Rahman, S., Ansari, R.A., Rehman, H. et al. (2011). Nordihydroguaiaretic acid from creosote bush (*Larrea tridentata*) mitigates 12-O-tetradecanoylphorbol-13-acetate-induced inflammatory and oxidative stress responses of tumor promotion cascade in mouse skin. *Evid. Based Compl. Altern. Med.* 2009: 1–10.

Rajasekaran, A., Sivagnanam, G., and Xavier, R. (2008). Nutraceuticals as therapeutic agents: a review. *Res. J. Pharm. Technol.* 4: 328–340.

Ramchander, J.P. and Middha, A. (2017). Recent advances on senna as a laxative: a comprehensive review. *J. Pharmacogn. Phytochem.* 6 (2): 349–353.

Ray, A., Joshi, J., and Gulati, K. (2016). *Regulatory Aspects of Nutraceuticals: An Indian Perspective.* *Nutraceuticals*, 941–946. Elsevier Inc.

Reid, I.R., Bristow, S.M., and Bolland, M.J. (2015). Calcium supplements: benefits and risks. *J. Intern. Med.* 278 (4): 354–368.

Ruchi, S., Amanjot, K., Sourav, T. et al. (2017). Role of nutraceuticals in health care: a review. *Int. J. Green Pharm.* 11 (3): S385–S394.

Saito, M. (2007). Role of FOSHU (food for specified health uses) for healthier life. *Yakugaku Zasshi.* 127 (3): 407–416.

Şanlı, O., Karaca, I., and Işıklan, N. (2009). Preparation, characterization, and salicylic acid release behavior of chitosan/poly(vinyl alcohol) blend microspheres. *J. Appl. Polym. Sci.* 111 (6): 2731–2740.

Santini, A., Cammarata, S.M., Capone, G. et al. (2018). Nutraceuticals: opening the debate for a regulatory framework. *Br. J. Clin. Pharmacol.* 84 (4): 659–672.

Sharma, Y. (2017). Ginger (*Zingiber officinale*)-an elixir of life a review. *Pharma. Innov. J.* 6 (10): 22–27.

Sharma, V., Sharma, S., Pracheta, and Paliwal, R. (2011). *Withania somnifera*: a rejuvenating ayurvedic medicinal herb for the treatment of various human ailments. *Int. J. Pharm. Tech. Res.* 3 (1): 187–192.

Shen, C.L., Smith, B.J., Lo, D.F. et al. (2012). Dietary polyphenols and mechanisms of osteoarthritis. *J. Nutr. Biochem.* 23 (11): 1367–1377.

Shieh, D.E., Liu, L.T., and Lin, C.C. (2000). Antioxidant and free radical scavenging effects of baicalein, baicalin and wogonin. *Anticancer Res.* 20 (5A): 2861–2865.

Shimizu, T. (2003). Health claims on functional foods: the Japanese regulations and an international comparison. *Nutr. Res. Rev.* 16 (2): 241–252.

Shinde, N., Bhaskar, B., Deshmukh, S., and Pratik, K. (2014). Nutraceuticals: a review on current status. *Res. J. Pharm. Tech.* 7 (1): 110–113.

Singh, J. and Sinha, S. (2012). Classification, regulatory acts and application of nutraceuticals for health. *Int. J. Pharm. Biol. Sci.* 2: 177–187.

Srivastava, S. and Mishra, N. (2009). Genetic markers – a cutting-edge technology in herbal drug research. *J. Chem. Pharm. Res.* 1 (1): 1–18.

Tapas, A., Sakarkar, D., and Kakde, R. (2008). Flavonoids as nutraceuticals. *Trop. J. Pharm. Res.* 7 (3): 1089–1099.

Tapsell, L.C. (2008). Evidence for health claims: a perspective from the Australia–New Zealand Region. *J. Nutr.* 138 (6): 1206–1209.

Tee, E.-S., Tamin, S., Ilyas, R. et al. (2002). Current status of nutrition labelling and claims in the South-East Asian region: are we in harmony? *Asia Pac. J. Clin. Nutr.* 11 (2): S80–S86.

Wang, J., Zhang, X., Lan, H., and Wang, W. (2017). Effect of garlic supplement in the management of type 2 diabetes mellitus (T2DM): a meta-analysis of randomized controlled trials. *Food Nutr. Res.* 61 (1): 1–9.

Wąsik, A. and Antkiewicz-Michaluk, L. (2017). The mechanism of neuroprotective action of natural compounds. *Pharmacol. Rep.* 69 (5): 851–860.

WHO (2020). Traditional, complementary and integrative medicine [Internet]. https://www.who.int/health-topics/traditional-complementary-and-integrative-medicine#tab=tab_2 (accessed 27 July 2020).

World Health Organization (2020). Coronavirus: FSSAI urged to promote plant–based food as immunity builder. *The Times of India* (20 June 2020). https://fssai.gov.in/upload/media/FSSAI_News_Covid_TOI_23_06_2020.pdf (accessed 27 July 2020).

Wu, S.Y., Silverberg, J.I., Joks, R. et al. (2012). Green tea (*Camelia sinensis*) mediated suppression of IgE production by peripheral blood mononuclear cells of allergic asthmatic humans. *Scand. J. Immunol.* 76 (3): 306–310.

Xing, L., Santhi, D., Shar, A. et al. (2017). Psyllium husk (*Plantago ovata*) as a potent hypocholesterolemic agent in animal, human and poultry. *Int. J. Pharmacol.* 13: 690–697.

Yadav, S.S., Singh, M.K., Singh, P.K., and Kumar, V. (2017). Traditional knowledge to clinical trials: a review on therapeutic actions of *Emblica officinalis*. *Biomed. Pharmacother.* 93: 1292–1302. https://doi.org/10.1016/j.biopha.2017.07.065.

Yang, Y. (2008). Scientific substantiation of functional food health claims in China. *J. Nutr.* 138: 1199–1205.

Zheng, Y., Hou, S.X., Chen, T., and Lu, Y. (2006). Preparation and characterization of transfersomes of three drugs in vitro. *Zhongguo Zhongyao Zazhi.* 31 (9): 728–731.

Zink, A. and Traidl-Hoffmann, C. (2015). Green tea in dermatology – myths and facts. *J. der Dtsch. Dermatologischen Gesellschaft.* 13 (8): 768–775.

11

Lycopene as Nutraceuticals

Debasmita Dutta and Debjani Dutta

Department of Biotechnology, National Institute of Technology Durgapur, Durgapur, West Bengal, India

11.1   Introduction

Lycopene belongs to the carotenoid family of phytochemicals, an acyclic isomer of β-carotene (Nguyen and Schwartz 1998; Paiva and Russell 1999). This natural pigment has drawn colossal attention globally. Both lycopene and β-carotene are hydrocarbon carotenoids (Rodriguez-Amaya and Kimura 2004). Unlike β-carotene, it has no provitamin A activity due to the absence of a β-ionone ring structure (Tapiero et al. 2004). Millardet first discover the ruby-red carotenoid in 1876 and the name "lycopene" was coined by Schunck (Vogele 1937). The red pigment is hidden under the chlorophyll. Chlorophyll disappears when the plant matures and makes lycopene and other pigments responsible for most fruits and vegetables' bright colors. The conjugated double bonds present in the structure of lycopene (Figure 11.1) form light-absorbing chromophore, which is responsible for the distinctive red color of it. The bright red color is used as natural food color or a food additive (Rodriguez-Amaya 2001). Only plants and microorganisms can synthesize it. It also protects the plants from photosensitization caused by the light absorbed during photosynthesis. Humans or animals are unable to produce it. So, they are dependent on the food sources of lycopene (Rao and Rao 2007). Generally, it is profusely found in fruits and vegetables with red color (tomato, papaya, pink grapefruit, rosehip, pink guava, and watermelon) (Vogele 1937). Lycopene degradation (trans to cis form) occurs due to isomerization and oxidation during tomato processing as lycopene is heat-, light- and oxygen-sensitive (Shi and Le Maguer 2000). Lycopene is supposed to be the freest and the highest radical scavenger among all carotenoids (Goula and Adamopoulos 2005). Several in vitro and in vivo studies showed lycopene plays a role in regulating apoptosis, cell cycle, and DNA repair mechanism, thus possessing chemopreventive properties against prostate, breast, lungs, bladder, cervix, and skin cancers and also has hypocholesterolemic and antidiabetic properties (Fuhrman et al. 1997; Okajima et al. 1997; Rao et al. 1998; Guttenplan et al. 2001; Imaida et al. 2001; Offord et al. 2002; Chalabi et al. 2006; Stahl et al. 2006; Neyestani et al. 2007; Wertz 2009; Ried and Fakler 2011).

In recent times, the world is trending toward discovering the best process to increase the nutritional quality of food, which has led to encouraging fortification practices. Food fortification is a commercial choice to provide additional nutrients in the food or health policy to improve the nutrient deficiencies for both poor and wealthy societies. Nearly about 4000 BCE, Persian physician Melampus reported that fortified sweet wine with iron fillings enhances the sailors' resistance to spears and arrows (Richardson 1990; Panda et al. 2011). Later in 1833, the French chemist

Handbook of Nutraceuticals and Natural Products: Biological, Medicinal, and Nutritional Properties and Applications, Volume 1, First Edition. Edited by Sreerag Gopi and Preetha Balakrishnan.

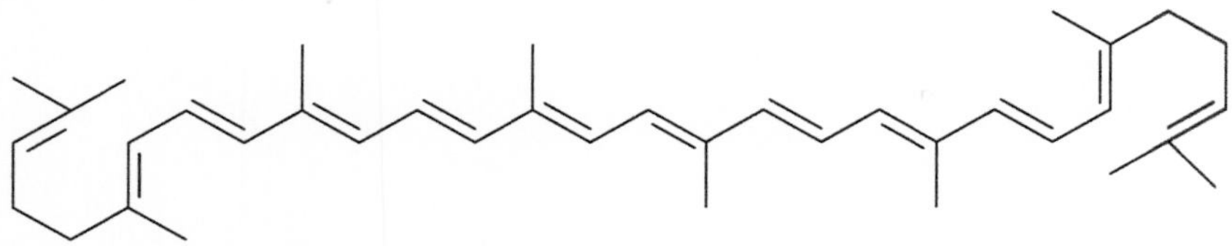

Figure 11.1   Structure of lycopene (Camara et al. 2013).

Boussingault suggested iodine fortification in salt to combat goiter in South Africa (Cowgill 1887). The antioxidant property and functional activity of lycopene increased its use as an active component in food fortification (Rao and Rao 2007). Lycopene intake has been increased from 5000 tons in 1995 to 15 000 tons in 2004 (Focus on Pigments 2007). The absorption of lycopene from fresh tomato is more inadequate than the processed one (tomato juice and paste) (Richelle et al. 2002). It is evident from the study that bioavailability of trans and cis lycopene is enhanced in processed tomato products compared to fresh tomatoes (Gartner et al. 1997). Considering all the flaws like sensitivity toward oxidation, lights and heat, low availability through dietary sources 10–30%, different strategies are being applied to enhance this bioactive in the food sector (Rao and Rao 2007).

This review paper will discuss the various ongoing practices to enhance lycopene intake through fortification and different extraction methods adopted to obtain the maximum quantity of lycopene.

11.2   Sources of Lycopene

Lycopene obtained from plant sources exists predominantly in the all-trans geometrical configuration, which is the most stable form of lycopene. In contrast, in the human body (in serum and prostate tissues), it exists as a cis isomeric form comprising 55–88% of total lycopene content (Nguyen and Schwartz 1998). Tomato skin contains three times (12 mg/100 g on a wet basis) higher concentration of lycopene than whole mature tomato (3.4 mg/100 g) (Al-Wandawi et al. 1985). Tomato skin is rich in lycopene; almost five times (53.9 mg/100 g) of the lycopene content was present in whole tomato pulp (11 mg/100 g) (Sharma and Le Maguer 1996a). Different sources of lycopene from the various components in the tables dependent on sources like natural sources (Table 11.1), processed foods

Table 11.1   Sources of lycopene from natural sources (Collins et al. 2006; Mohamadin et al. 2012).

Fruits and vegetables	Amount of lycopene (mg/100 g)
Raw tomatoes	3.7–4.4
Fresh apricots	0.0005
Fresh watermelon	2.3–7.2
Fresh papaya	2.0–5.3
Grapefruit (pink/red)	0.2–3.4
Raw guava	5.3–5.5
Vegetable juice	7.3–9.7
Bitter melon aril	41.1
Rosehips	2.182
Gac fruit aril	34.8–190.2

Table 11.2 Sources of lycopene from processed foods.

Processed foods	Lycopene (mg/100 g wet basis)	References
Tomato juice (in Israel)	5.8–9.0	Lindner et al. (1984)
Tomato ketchup (in Finland)	9.9	Heinonen et al. (1989)
Tomato puree	19.37–8.93	Tavares and Rodriguez-Amaya (1994)
Tomato paste	18.27–6.07	
Tomato ketchup	10.29–41.4	
Tomato juice (in Campinas, Brazil)	61.6	
Tomato soup	8.0–13.84	Tonucci et al. (1995)
Tomato juice	9.70–11.84	
Tomato paste	51.12–59.78	
Tomato puree	16.67	
Tomato sauce (in the USA)	6.51–19.45	
Tomato pulp	12.09–12.83	
Pulp thick fraction	41.91–42.82	
Pulp thin fraction (in Canada)	3.98–4.08	
Sauce from pizza	328.90 mg/kg	Nguyen and Schwartz (1998)
Prepared spaghetti sauce	159.90 mg/kg	
Tomato paste	287.64 mg/kg	
Canned tomato sauce	151.52 mg/kg	
Canned pizza sauce	127.10 mg/kg	
Vegetable juice cocktail	96.60 mg/kg	
Tomato juice (canned)	90.37 mg/kg	
Tomato soup	54.60 mg/kg	

(Table 11.2), microbial sources like microbial fermentation influenced by enzyme inhibitors and metabolically engineered microbial strains (Table 11.3) and synthetic sources (Table 11.4) have been given.

11.3 Disease-Preventive Nature of Lycopene

11.3.1 Antioxidant Properties

The ability to trap peroxyl radicals and the highest singlet oxygen quenching rate of lycopene defines its antioxidant activity and prevents cancers and chronic diseases (Foote and Denny 1968; Burton and Ingold 1984; Pool-Zobel et al. 1997; Agarwal and Rao 1998; Rao and Agarwal 1998; Rissanen et al. 2002). The order of quenching abilities given as: lycopene > α-tocopherol > α- carotene > β- cryptobanthin > zeaxanthin-β-carotene > lutein (Table 11.5) (Di Mascio et al. 1989; Conn et al. 1991; Di Mascio et al. 1991; Conn et al. 1992; Miller et al. 1996). Lycopene reactivity depends upon their physical properties, molecular structure, action site

Table 11.3 Sources of lycopene from microbial fermentation in the presence of enzyme inhibitors and metabolically engineered microbes.

Microbes	Fermentation type	Enzyme inhibitors	Applied metabolic engineering	Lycopene yield	Sources
Blakeslea trispora F-816(+) and F-744(−)	Mated	Imidazole and pyridine (0.2–0.8 g/l)	—	100% Lycopene of total carotenoids	López-Nieto et al. (2004)
Blakeslea trispora NRRL 2895 and 2896	Submerged	Piperidine (500 ppm)	—	Up to 269.66 mg/l	Choudhari and Singhal (2008)
Blakeslea trispora NRRL 2895 and 2896	Mated	Creatinine	—	270.3 mg/l	Liu et al. (2012)
Blakeslea trispora NRRL 2895 and 2896	Mated	Creatinine	—	98.1 mg/l	Wang et al. (2012)
Blakeslea trispora NRRL 2895 and 2896	Batch	2-Methylimidazole	—	26.4 mg/g dry biomass	Qiang et al. (2014)
Blakeslea trispora NRRL 2895 and 2896	Submerged	2-Methylimidazole	—	40.5 mg/g dry biomass	Wang et al. (2015)
Blakeslea trispora ATCC 14271 and 14272	Submerged	Ketoconazole	—	286.2 g/l	Sun et al. (2007)
Blakeslea trispora ATCC 14271 and 14272	Submerged	Nicotine	—	533 mg/l	Xu et al. (2007)
Blakeslea trispora ATCC 14271 and 14272	Mated	Nicotine	—	578 mg/l	Shi et al. (2012)
Blakeslea trispora T (+) and T (−)	Submerged	2-Amin-6 methyl pyridine 0.005% and 5% (w/v) plant oil	—	1.17 mg/l	Vereschagina et al. (2010)
Blakeslea trispora ATCC 14059 and 14060	Submerged	2-Isopropylimidazole (300 mg/l)	—	96% lycopene of total carotenoid	Wang et al. (2014)
Bacterium *Dietzia natronolimnaea* HS-1 (beet molasses)	Fed-batch	Imidazole, nicotinic acid, pyridine, piperidine, and triethylamine (0–50 ppm)	—	8.26 mg/l	Nasri Nasrabadi and Razavi (2010)
Microalga *Dunaliella salina* CCAP 19/18	—	Nicotine (20 μm)	—	0.68 mg/l	Fazeli et al. (2009)

Organism	Fermentation	Treatment	Gene/strategy	Yield	Reference
Rhodotorula glutinis and R. rubra (yeast)	Fermentation	Nicotine (20 nmol) and diphenylamine	—	77% lycopene of total carotenoids	Squina and Mercadante (2005)
Rhodotorula glutinis YB-252 (yeast)	Solid-state fermentation	Imidazole 250 ppm at 24 hours fermentation	—	6.82 mg/l	Hernández-Almanza et al. (2014)
Candida utilis	—	—	Combination of ERG gene disruption and overexpression of HMG catalytic domain	7.8 mg/g	Shimada et al. (2014)
Pichia pastoris	—	—	Plasmid pGAPZB-EbI* and pGAPZB-EpBpi*p	73.9 mg/l	Bhataya et al. (2009)
Mucor circinelloides	—	—	Disruption of negative regulator gene crgA	54 mg/l	Nicolás-Molina et al. (2008)
Escherichia coli	—	—	Identification of multiple gene targets	16 mg/g	Jin and Stephanopoulos (2007)
Escherichia coli	—	—	Genes crtE, crtB and CrtI of Pantoea ananatis, plasmid pMH1, and T7 promoter	1.234 g/l	Zhu et al. (2015)
Escherichia coli	—	—	Synthetic crt operon	260 mg/l	Kim et al. (2009)
Escherichia coli	—	—	Genes of Bacillus licheniformis is the host	198 mg/g	Rad et al. (2012)
Escherichia coli	—	—	Triclosan-induced chromosomal evolution	33.43 mg/g	Chen et al. (2013)
Escherichia coli	—	—	Engineering of global regulator cAM Preceptor protein	18.48 mg/l	Huang et al. (2015)
Escherichia coli	—	—	Deleting genes crtX and crtY from the crtEXYIB operon	10.5 mg/g	Sun et al. (2014)
Escherichia coli	—	—	pACLYCipi plasmid with genes of crtE, crtB, and crtI from Pantoea agglomerans	1.050 g/l	Zhang et al. (2015)
Saccharomyces cerevisiae	—	—	Synthetic genes derived from crtE, crtB, and crtI genes of Erwinia uredovora. Gene expression regulated by ADH2 promoter	3.3 mg lycopene/g dry cell weight	Bahieldin et al. (2014)

Table 11.4 Synthetic sources of lycopene (Ernst 2002; Olempska-Beer 2006).

Synthetic lycopene	All-trans lycopene	5 cis lycopene	9 cis lycopene	13 and 15 cis lycopene	Other cis isomers of lycopene
DSM nutritional products LTD	>70%	<23%	<1%	<1%	<3%
BASF AG	>70%	<23%	—	—	—

Table 11.5 Antioxidant activity of carotenoids (Di Mascio et al. 1989; Conn et al. 1991; Di Mascio et al. 1991; Conn et al. 1992; Miller et al. 1996).

Carotenoids	Singlet oxygen quenching activity $10^9 \times k_q$ (m^{-1}/s^{-1}) (k_q = quenching rate constant)
Lycopene	31
γ Carotene	25
α Carotene	19
β Carotene	14
Lutein	8
Astaxanthin	24
Bixin	14
Canthaxanthin	21
Zeaxanthin	10

inside cells, the potentiality to interact with other antioxidants (Britton 1995; Young and Lowe 2001); Quenching rate of lycopene is two times higher than β-carotene and ten times higher than α-tocopherol (Cantrell et al. 2003). Three mechanisms are followed by lycopene for its radical scavenging actions: Adducts formation (Figure 11.2), electron transfer to the radical, and allylic hydrogen abstraction (Burton and Ingold 1984; Conn et al. 1992; Mortensen et al. 2001; Krinsky and Yeum 2003; El-Agamey et al. 2004; Krinsky and Johnson 2005). During electron transfer reaction (Figure 11.3) of lycopene, cation radicals, anion radicals, or alkyl radicals are formed (Figure 11.4) (Krinsky and Yeum 2003). This property reduces the rate of LDL oxidation, leading to a decrease in the risk of cardiovascular disease (CVD) and atherosclerotic development (Rissanen et al. 2002). Lycopene reduces prostate, lung, and digestive tract cancer risks, as all-trans isomer reduces alcohol-induced apoptosis in 2E1 cells (Tapiero et al. 2004). After all these studies came to light, the demands of lycopene have increased.

11.3.2 Anticarcinogenic Effect

Research on lycopene has been increased due to its chemopreventive properties (Figure 11.5). It has been reported that 1–4 µM lycopene lowered the risk of prostate, lung, and digestive tract cancer (Xu et al. 2003; Salman et al. 2007) and also, 10–50 µM lycopene decreased the risk of liver and ovarian cancer (Scolastici et al. 2007; Scolastici et al. 2008). The antioxidant property of lycopene prevents DNA damage in prostate tissues (Stacewicz-Sapuntzakis and Bowen 2005). Increased intakes of lycopene or tomatoes prevent prostate cancer (Giovannucci et al. 2002). Lycopene

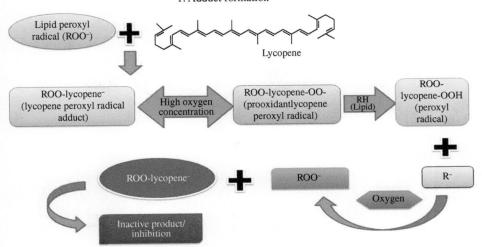

Figure 11.2 Adduct formation. The free radical will bind to the conjugated double bonds of the lycopene and form a lycopene peroxyl radical adduct. In the presence of oxygen, it will form a new intermediate pro-oxidant for lipid peroxidation. The peroxyl radical-lycopene adduct can be inhibited by another peroxyl radical.

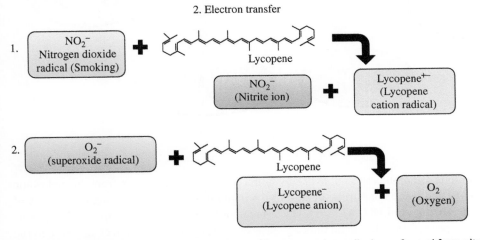

Figure 11.3 Electron transfer. Lycopene cation and lycopene anion radicals are formed from nitrogen dioxide radical and superoxide radical, respectively.

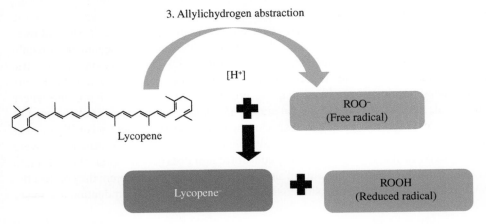

Figure 11.4 Allylic H abstraction. Lycopene acts as a hydrogen donor to reduce the free radical.

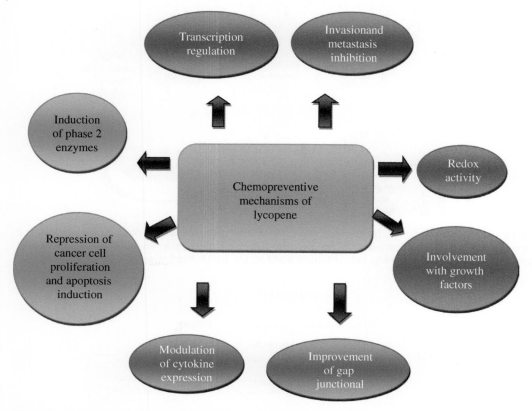

Figure 11.5 The potential mechanism of cancer prevention by lycopene.

(1–10 µM) inhibits cell proliferation of liver carcinoma cells and protects them from the metastatic process (Hwang and Lee 2006; Burgess et al. 2008). A high intake of lycopene decreases the risk of breast cancer (Huang et al. 2007a). A biological metabolite of lycopene, i.e. apo-10'-lycopenoic inhibits lung cancer and subduing the tumor genesis of the lungs in mice (Lian et al. 2007). In the lungs, mainly lycopene has been found among other carotenoids (Schmitz et al. 1991). Smoking produces nitric oxide free radicals, which may cause lung cancer after prolonged exposure (Halliwell and Gutteridge 1989). Lycopene quenches singlet oxygen and prevents the risk of lung cancer (Böhm et al. 1995). Consumption of lycopene is related to a reduced risk of cancer of the digestive tract, pancreas, and bladder (Gerster 1997). Studies on in vitro breast cells showed lycopene plays a role in regulating apoptosis, cell cycle, and DNA repair mechanism (Chalabi et al. 2006). Lycopene prevents oxidative stress by inhibiting iNOS expression (inducing Nitric Oxidative Stress) (Rafi et al. 2007) and reduces nitric oxide production. A lycopene-rich diet lowers the level of Prostate-Specific Antigen (PSA) in the serum of people diagnosed with prostate cancer (Giovannucci et al. 1995; Klein 2005).The population which intakes a minimum of one serving of tomato byproducts each day had a 50% less chance of the risk of digestive tract cancer (Franceschi et al. 1994). Harvard University conducted a study where they found old-age Americans were dying less from all types of cancer who regularly consumed tomatoes (Colditz et al. 1985). Tomato oleoresin can be considered as a cosmeceutical alone or combined with sunscreen; they protect the skin from UV radiation. Prolonged exposure to UV radiation increases ROS production leading to skin cancer. Administration of lycopene as it has antioxidant properties can give photo-protection. In this study, the consumption of lycopene for 10–12 weeks leads to decreased sensitivity toward UV-induced erythema. With vitamin C or vitamin E or both, lycopene showed photo-protection when human dermal fibroblasts were exposed to UV light (Rittié and Fisher 2002; González et al. 2008; Andreassi 2011).

The possible mechanisms by which cancer is prevented by lycopene are given below:

11.3.2.1 Redox Activity

Oxidative stress is one of the significant factors behind the increased risk of cancer. The conjugated double bonds in lycopene quench the energy from singlet oxygen and also scavenge the free radicals. In vitro lycopene deactivates free radicals like H_2O_2, Nitrogen dioxide, thyl and sulfonyl (Böhm et al. 1995; Lu et al. 1995; Mortensen et al. 1997). Oxidative DNA damage caused by Xanthine oxidase was prevented by the 1–3 μM concentration of lycopene but enhanced DNA damage at a higher concentration of 4–10 μM (Lowe et al. 1999). Carotenoids regulate redox-sensitive molecular targets that participate in cell growth signaling, such as antioxidant response elements, mitogen-activated protein kinases (MAPKs), and transcription factors (nuclear factors kappa B [NF-κB] and activators protein 1 [AP-1]). In various ways, different oxidative stress-inducing stimuli (γ irradiation, UV light, H_2O_2, and IL-1) activate AP-1 (Stein et al. 1989; Angel and Karin 1991; Devary et al. 1991; Meyer et al. 1993; Janssen et al. 1997). It has been reported lycopene inhibits AP-1 signaling in mammary malignant cells, though there is no direct evidence for the role of lycopene in cells of inflammation (Karas et al. 2000). Recent studies (in vitro and in vivo) showed lycopene and other neutraceuticals modulate cellular signaling pathways like MAPK and/or NF-κB (Agarwal and Shishodia 2006; Chalabi et al. 2007; Sarkar et al. 2009). Lycopene regulates the MAPK-signaling pathway by disturbing phosphorylation. Recent studies showed lycopene extract blocked NF-κB signaling (Kim et al. 2004; Joo et al. 2009). Some antioxidants α-tocopheryl succinate (Neuzil et al. 2001) and astaxanthin (Lee et al. 2003) inhibit NF-κB activity and block proinflammatory gene expression (Heiss et al. 2001). These postulated that ROS plays an essential role in the activation of NF-κB and inflammatory gene expression. NF-κB participates in the induced expression of the IL-2 gene (Bauerle and Henkel 1994; Bauerle and Baltimore 1996). It is the first eukaryotic transcription factor that reacts directly to oxidative stress in a particular kind of cells (Schrek and Bauerle 1991). Two mechanisms are there – one increases IκB degradation via ROS and the second enhances the upstream signal cascade via oxidation. Recent studies showed that lycopene hindered the binding abilities of NF-κB and SP1 and reduced insulin-like growth factor 1 receptor (IGF-1R) expression (Huang et al. 2007b). Also, lycopene impedes LPS-induced proinflammatory gene expression by blocking NF-κB signaling (Joo et al. 2009) (Figure 11.6). The interactivity between PPARγ and NF-κB is well known where PPARγ activators have anti-inflammatory effects (Touyz and Schiffrin 2006). PPARγ block the activation and translocation of NF-κB and their lycopene modulates these PPARγ levels to remold inflammatory response (Zaripheh et al. 2006; Campbell et al. 2006).

11.3.2.2 Repression of Cancer Cell Proliferation and Apoptosis Induction

Lycopene represses cancerous cell proliferation and cell cycle progression from the G_0/G_1 to the S phase (Nahum et al. 2001). Several studies showed lycopene decreases the level of H_2O_2, stops cell cycle progression, and represses KU DNA-binding activity with cellular and nuclear levels of KU-70 in pancreatic Acinar AR42J cells (Seo et al. 2009). These are evidence of the role of lycopene in the treatment of oxidative stress-induced cell death by protecting DNA repair protein KU-70 from loss.

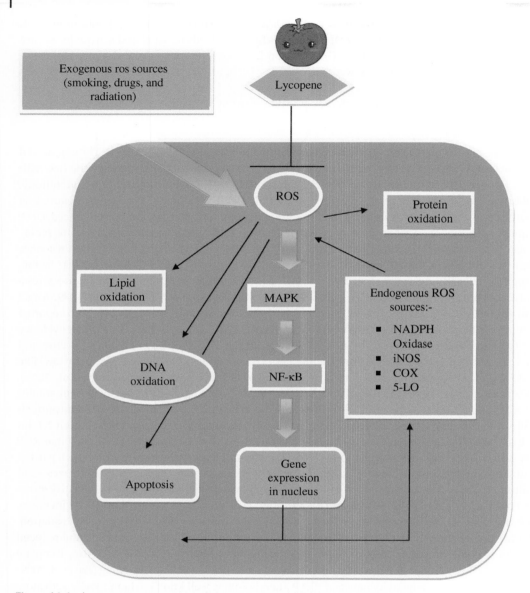

Figure 11.6 Lycopene acts as a secondary messenger and inhibits exogenous and endogenous ROS produced during the inflammatory process. That leads to reducing lipid, protein, and DNA oxidation and induction of apoptosis. That also results in decreased MAPK activation and DNA-binding activity of AP-1 and NF-κB transcription factor, which causes changes in functional proteins, some ROS-producing enzymes and apoptosis induction. (iNOS = *Inducible nitric oxide synthase,* COX = *Cyclooxygenase,* 5-LO = *5-Lipoxygenase*).

11.3.2.3 Involvement with Growth Factors' Stimulation of Cancer Cell Proliferation

Lycopene is involved with IGF-1 and enhanced cell growth. Lycopene decreases the IGF-1 stimulated cell growth and DNA-binding activity of the AP-1 transcription factors in endometrial, mammary, and lung cancer cell lines. Smoke-induced changes were protected by lycopene in a dose-dependent manner. It prevents smoke-induced squamous metaplasia by decreasing Bad phosphorylation at both Ser[136] and Ser[112] and decreasing cleaved Caspase-3 (Karas et al. 1997; Liu et al. 2003; Sarkar et al. 2009).

11.3.2.4 Induction of Phase 2 Enzymes

Administration of lycopene decreased the incidence of DMBA-induced hamster buccal pouch tumors and increased the levels of GSH (reduced glutathione) and phase 2 enzyme GST (glutathione *S*-transferase). GSH regulates cell proliferation and GST acts as an indirect antioxidant and conjugates electrophilic carcinogens that are less toxic and easily excretable (Bhuvaneswari et al. 2001).

11.3.2.5 Transcription Regulation

Lycopene affects different cellular pathways by participating in the modulation of transcription via direct interaction of their derivatives with transcriptional factors (Sharoni et al. 2004).

11.3.2.6 Modulation of Cytokine Expression

Proinflammatory (go signals) cytokine-like interleukins, TNF-α have been involved in tumorigenesis for tumor promotion. The lycopene can control cytokine levels either partially explained by lycopene localization in or within the cell membrane, modulating surface molecules for primary immune response, ROS production, MAPKs function, and transcription factors (NF-κB) (Bertram et al. 1991).

11.3.2.7 Invasion and Metastasis Inhibition

It is evident from the study that lycopene at 5 and 10 μM concentration could lower the level of the gelatinolytic activities of the matrix metalloproteinases MMP-2 and MMP-9 and also prevent adhesion, invasion, and migration of SK-Hep1 cells (Burgess et al. 2008). The same concentration of lycopene-subdued MMP9 expression in SK-Hep-1 cells and as a result, the metastasis suppressor gene nm23-H1 was induced. Hence, it can be concluded that lycopene inhibits metastasis and invasion by hepatocarcinoma cells, though at high lycopene concentration, it might not be physiologically achievable (Touyz and Schiffrin 2006).

11.3.2.8 Improvement of Gap Junctional Communication

Both carotenoids and retinoids induce intracellular communication via gap junctional communication (GJC) by stabilizing connexin 43 mRNA (Stahl et al. 2000; Aust et al. 2003) (a gene encoding major gap junction protein and upregulated GJC and acting as a chemopreventive component) (Zhang et al. 1991; Trosko and Chang 2001; Krinsky and Yeum 2003). Non-cancer cells communicate through GJC, but GJC is lost in cancer cells. Most of them have dysfunctional homologous or heterologous GJC (Krutovskikh et al. 1997). In a cell culture study, the oxidation of lycopene produces dialdehyde 2,7,11 trimethyl tetradecahexane-1,14-dialdehyde, which triggers GJC in WBF344 cells (rat liver epithelial cells) (Krutovskikh et al. 1997). The risk of tumor cell formation increases with the loss of GJC and can be prevented by restoring it (Hotz-Wagenblatt and Shalloway 1993; Trosko and Chang 2001).

11.3.3 Antidiabetic Effect

The concentration of plasma glucose and fasting insulin decreased with the increase of serum lycopene (Coyne et al. 2005). A study was conducted to determine the effects of lycopene on plasma glucose and insulin levels of streptozotocin-induced diabetic rats. The result showed that an increased blood glucose level due to diabetes was decreased by lycopene intake over eight weeks' periods (Aydin and Celik 2012). Three weeks of lycopene supplementation reduced blood glucose levels in diabetic rats (Duzguner et al. 2008). Diabetes leads to a decrease in plasma insulin level because of the damage caused by the cytotoxic effect of streptozotocin (STZ) in β cells of the pancreas. Consumption of lycopene can retrieve back to normal as free radicals are responsible for the dysfunctioning of pancreatic β cells and reduce insulin secretion. So, lycopene prevents oxidative stress and reduces lipid, protein and DNA damage, and free radicals (Dixon et al. 1998; Evans et al. 2003). The study finds out the preventive effect of lycopene on diabetic nephropathy via lessening the inflammatory response and oxidation stress. Results demonstrated that lycopene diminished the lesion occurred by STZ in DN (diabetic nephropathy) mice and increased body weight and HDL-C and decreased blood sugar levels, LDL-C, and urine protein content. Other than these, the kidney of DN mice was improved, and lycopene impaired the expression of NF-κB and TNF-α in kidney tissues for anti-inflammation (Guo et al. 2015).

11.3.4 Antihypertensive Effect

Intake of 15 mg/day of lycopene supplementation significantly decreases the systolic blood pressure from 144 to 134 mmHg in the mildly hypertensive subject. Antioxidants have an essential role in the management of hypertension. A DASH (Dietary Approach to Stop Hypertension) diet is suggested, containing a higher amount of lycopene with other carotenoids, polyphenols, and flavanols to combat hypertension (Paran and Engelhard 2001; Moriel et al. 2002; Most 2004; Paran 2006).

11.3.5 Effect on Cardiovascular Disease

A study on dietary lycopene supplementation (once in a week followed by seven days gap) through tomato juice content 50.4 mg, spaghetti sauce content 39.2 mg, and tomato oleoresin content 75.0 mg lycopene significantly increased serum lycopene (Agarwal and Rao 1998). Low plasma lycopene concentration is related to atherosclerosis onset and increases intima-media thickness of the common carotid artery wall (CCA-IMT) (Rissanen et al. 2002). This study postulated that the preventive action of lycopene against CVD is associated with an increased intake of tomato-based products like tomato sauce and pizza (Sesso et al. 2003). Atherogenesis occurs when LDL oxidation takes place by free radicals causing cell proliferation (Khachik et al. 1995). As β-carotene and lycopene are initially transported into LDL, they protect LDL from oxidation (Salonen et al. 1992). An epidemiological study exhibited that a higher intake of lycopene may prevent CVD. In their experiment, 39 876 middle-aged and older women were chosen, who were free from CVD. During seven years of follow-up, women who took two servings of oil-based tomato products (tomato sauce and pizza) per week had a 34% lower risk of CVD. In contrast, women who took 7–10 servings of lycopene per week showed a 29% lowered risk of CVD than women consuming 1.5 servings of tomato products weekly (Goulinet and Chapman 1997). It was reported that a group of 12 healthy women obtained 8 mg of lycopene per day for three weeks by consuming tomato products. The lipophilic compounds in lycopene modulate the atherogenic processes in vascular endothelium, mediated by LDL oxidation and prevent CVD (Khachik et al. 1995). From a meta-analysis, it is evident that lycopene uptake in doses of ≥25 mg daily helps decrease LDL-C by about 10%, which can be comparable to the action of low doses of statins in people with little upraised cholesterol level (Ried and Fakler 2011). An epidemiological study among ten European countries exhibited a relation between lycopene and lipid levels. Reduced risk of myocardial infarction (MI) had been observed from the content of lycopene was taken from human tissue after MI. The effect of lycopene decreased with an increasing level of PUFA and significant among individuals whose fat tissue content >16.1% polyunsaturates (Visioli et al. 2003). LDL oxidation reduced significantly among individuals who consumed lycopene in the diet of 19 healthy people and were not on drugs. In some in vitro studies, in J774A, cell line macrophages have been utilized to check cellular cholesterol synthesis, exhibiting its down gradation of 73% by 10 µmol of lycopene (Fuhrman et al. 1997). It has a preventive effect against intimal wall thickness and myocardial infarction (Kohlmeier et al. 1997; Arab and Steck 2000). In this experiment, 18 healthy men and women consumed a soy tomato beverage daily for eight weeks leading to decreased susceptibility of the LDL and VLDL blood plasma to oxidative damage and total cholesterol and HDL-C ratio and increased HDL-C level significantly (Bohn et al. 2013). The early onset of atherosclerosis is due to the oxidation of LDL in the vascular endothelium. In the study, the effect of fat-soluble vitamins and carotenoids, in the concentration of conjugated dienes in LDL as an indicator, has been found out. Lycopene and Lutein were the significant indicators of "LDL-conjugated diene formation" inhibition in women. So, it can be concluded that the antioxidant property of lycopene in vivo plays a role in the inhibition of LDL oxidation (Karppi et al. 2010).

11.3.6 Effect on Oxidative Stress

Ingestion of foods rich in lycopene showed protective effects against DNA damage in lymphocytes (Riso et al. 1999; Porrini et al. 2005; Zhao et al. 2006). By binding to the surfaces of the cells, lycopene shielded lymphoid cells from singlet oxygen (Tinkler et al. 1994). Lipid and protein oxidation are reduced by consuming ketchup or oleoresin capsules as a lycopene source (Rao and Shen 2002; Rao et al. 2007). Supplementation of lycopene about 4 mg/day for 180 days can alter the hormone replacement therapy in postmenopausal women to reduce oxidative stress and atherosclerosis (Misra et al. 2006). Fortification of tomato juice with vitamin C decreased thiobarbituric acid reactive substances (TBARS) in plasma and urine (Jacob et al. 2008).

11.3.7 Other Diseases

Lycopene supplementation significantly delayed the onset of cataract among rats (Gupta et al. 2003). Supplementation of lycopene (2 mg twice daily) to the primigravida women group showed decreased chances of preeclampsia and intrauterine growth retardation (Sharma et al. 2003). The study showed that the consumption of tomatoes plays a role against neurodegenerative diseases like Parkinsons' (Suganuma et al. 2002).

11.4 Lycopene Extraction Method

Byproducts obtained from the tomato processing industries (Table 11.6) are further utilized to produce lycopene-fortified food products. Tomato skin is the richest source of lycopene (Camara et al. 2013). Tomato skins are considered an industrial waste used for livestock feed. As it contains a higher amount of lycopene, it has been utilized as a source of functional components (Schieber et al. 2001). Various techniques are applied to extract lycopene. Heating or processing increased the bioavailability of lycopene by converting trans to cis isomers (Figure 11.7) possessing higher bioavailability (Agarwal et al. 2001). Heating or processing loosened the bond between lycopene and tissue matrix and at the same time breaks the cell walls and releases the lycopene. But the temperature should be maintained at 70 °C, otherwise too much heat could degrade the lycopene (Stahl and Sies 1992; Maulida and Zulkarnaen 2010). An experiment was done on the effect of the external condition of lycopene from watermelon by SFE (Supercritical Fluid Extraction) using 15% ethanol

Table 11.6 Byproducts from the tomato processing plant.

Sources	Byproducts	References
Algeria	Tomato skin	Benakmoum et al. (2008)
Argentina	Tomato skin	Naviglio et al. (2008)
Canada	Tomato skin	Kassama et al. (2008)
China, Canada	Tomato paste waste	Yang et al. (2004)
China	Tomato paste waste	Xi (2006) and Jun (2006)
	Mace (*Myristica fragrans*)	Dhas et al. (2004)
India	Tomato peels and seeds, tomato industrial waste	Choudhari and Ananthanarayan(2007)
	Tomato skin	Kaur et al. (2004)
Iraq	Tomato skin	Al-Wandawi et al. (1985)
Italy	Tomato peels and seeds, tomato peels	Sandei and Leoni (2004) and Lavecchia and Zuorro (2008)
Hungary	Tomato pomace	Vági et al. (2007)
Japan	Tomato skin	Topal et al. (2006)
Portugal, Brazil	Tomato skin and seeds	Nobre et al. (2006)
Spain	Tomato peels	Calvo et al. (2008)
Taiwan	Tomato pulp waste	Chiu et al. (2007)
Turkey, Netherland	Tomato paste waste	Baysal et al. (2000)
USA	Tomato pomace	Altan et al. (2008)

as an organic solvent. It showed that the leading role in lycopene yield is 14% greater at 60 °C and 20.7 MPa pressure than at 70 °C temperature (Katherine et al. 2008). It is evident from this study, response surface methodology used Central Composite Rotatable Design (CCRD) model to optimize the parameters for the extraction of all-trans lycopene from tomato peel that 62 °C temperature, 45 MPa pressure and 14% modifier concentration are adequate to obtain a higher amount of lycopene (Kassama et al. 2008). Operational pressure and temperature and extraction time are the influencing factors for lycopene yield. The optimum condition for the yield of lycopene, where 93% lycopene was recovered from 100 g of dried tomato pomace at the temperature of 57 °C, 40 MPa pressure and 1.8 hours of time (Huang et al. 2008). This study also optimized the parameters for the extraction of carotenoids (mainly content lycopene and β-carotene and significantly less amount of lutein) from rosehip fruit. It is evident from the study that all variables, i.e. temperature, pressure and CO_2 flow rate, have an influential role in lycopene extraction, but no interaction takes place among variables (Machmudah et al. 2008). Two different types of hot air-dried tomatoes possessing a higher amount of lycopene compared to freeze-dried tomatoes. As lycopene has antioxidant activity, so the drying process enhances the nutritional quality of tomatoes (Chang et al. 2006). Tomato juice was treated with high-intensity pulse electric fields (HIPEF) and evaluated its effect on antioxidant property and health-related compounds. The electric field strength and treatment time are directly proportional to vitamin C content. The lycopene kinetics was correctly described by the Peleg model (Odriozola-Serrano et al. 2008). In this study, the production of β-carotene was inhibited by adding inhibitors' piperidine to obtain a higher amount of lycopene from carotenoids producing microorganism *Blackeslea trispora*. These inhibitors inhibit lycopene cyclase and this further

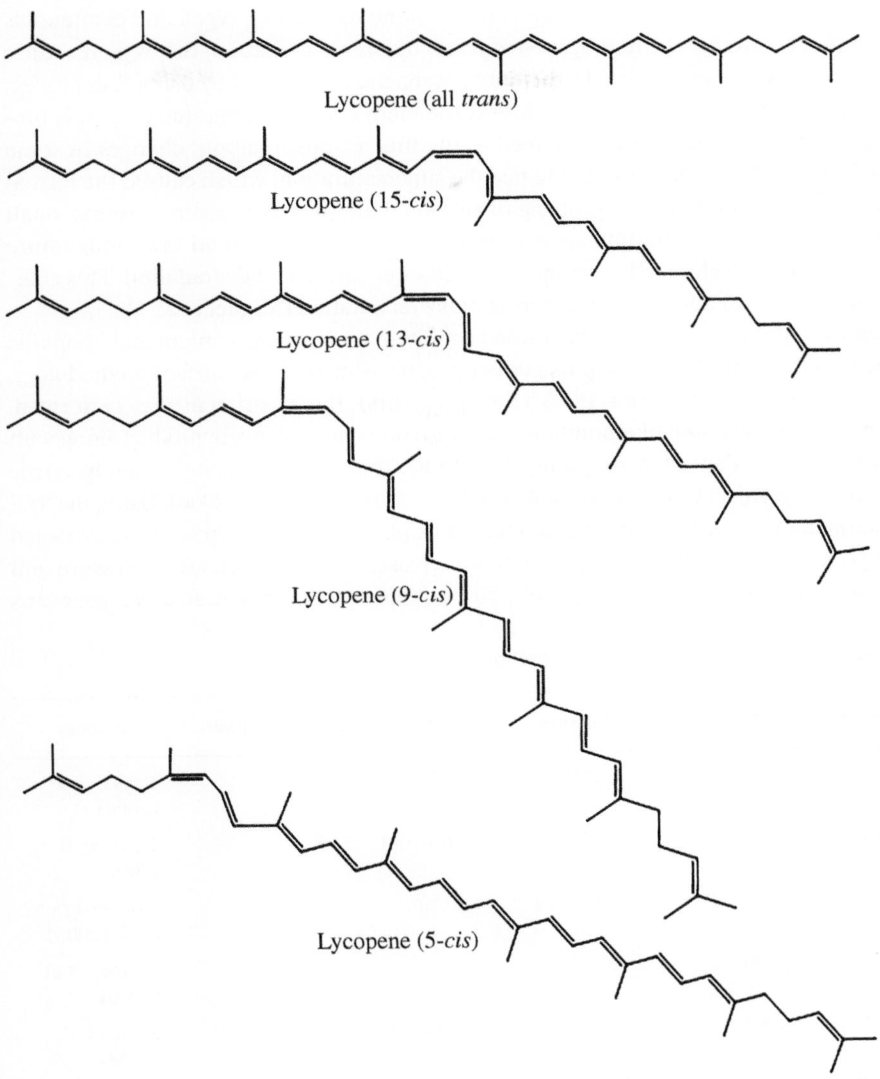

Figure 11.7 Isomeric forms of lycopene (Camara et al. 2013).

prevents the cyclization of lycopene. A significant drop in β-carotene concentration and a considerable rise in lycopene have been observed (Choudhari and Ananthanarayan 2007). Microencapsulation of lycopene has been done by spray-drying technique. Gelatine and sucrose have been used as a wall system. The optimal condition of the microencapsulation may cause little isomerization but improve storage stability. The result from SEM and XRD analysis demonstrated that the microencapsulation formed a regular spherical shape with bee net interior structure and smooth center surface along with the lycopene perfectly embedded in the wall system made of gelatine and sucrose (Shu et al. 2006). Supercritical CO_2 extraction is one of the most popular techniques used in the food processing industry as CO_2 is nontoxic with low critical temperature, but a drawback of CO_2 has been observed. As carotenoids are degraded in the presence of oxygen, there is a possibility of degradation of carotenoids when they react with the oxygen present in CO_2. But this problem can be avoided by using supercritical antioxidant solvent (SAS) process because CO_2 and carotenoids ratio is significantly less followed by the ratio of oxygen and carotenoids. As the oxygen and carotenoids stay together for a short period at the homogeneous phase before precipitation, the oxygen cannot get enough time to react with carotenoids. In this study, lycopene micronized by using SAS process showed that the equilibrium solubility of the solute is the main conclusive parameter in this process, which identified the supersaturation obtained at the time of precipitation; changes in some parameter led to decrease the solubility and enhance the supersaturation, which caused the formation of small particles. The solubility of lycopene decreased with the low pressure forming small particles along with increased maximum supersaturation. The method required low temperature and an inert environment, therefore reducing the possibilities of carotenoid degradation. This characteristic makes the process an alternative for carotenoids precipitation (Miguel et al. 2006).

This experiment was optimized under an oven-dried condition for lycopene content and lipophilic antioxidant capacity of the byproduct of the pink guava puree by using response surface methodology. At the recommended optimum condition (43.8 °C for six hours), the experiment was performed, which was proven to be the most suitable condition to dry a decanted guava pink byproduct along with high lycopene content antioxidant capacity (Kong et al. 2010). This experiment shows that lycopene was more soluble in supercritical CO_2 at 313 K and 10 MPa pressure (Juan et al. 2006). Using the SFE CO_2 technique, carotenoids, mainly lycopene and others (tocopherols and sitosterols), were extracted from the tomato pomace sample. Lycopene production increased with the increasing pressure and temperature, i.e. 460 bar and 80 °C and as a result, 90.1% (Table 11.7) concentrated lycopene was

Table 11.7 Lycopene extraction by using SFE-CO_2 method.

Food	Modifier	Temperature	Pressure	Flow rate	Lycopene obtain	References
Tomato paste waste	CO_2/5% ethanol	55 °C	30 MPa	4 kg/h	54%	Baysal et al. (2000)
Tomato seeds and skin	CO_2	86 °C	34.5 MPa	2.5 ml/min	61%	Rozzi et al. (2002)
Tomato skin and pulp	CO_2	40 °C	28.1 MPa	4 ml/min	42%	Gomez-Prieto et al. (2003)
Tomato pulp and skin	CO_2	80 °C	27.5 MPa	500 cm^3/min	65%	Cadoni et al. (2000)
Tomato seeds and skin	CO_2	80 °C	30 MPa	0.792 kg/h	80%	Sabio et al. (2003)
Sun-dried tomato	CO_2/10% hazel oil	66 °C	45 MPa	20 kg/h	60%	Vasapollo et al. (2004)
Watermelon	CO_2/15% ethanol	60 °C	20.7 MPa	1.5 ml/min	14% greater yield than obtaining in 70 °C	Katherine et al. (2008)
Tomato skin	CO_2/14% ethanol	62 °C	45 MPa	3.5 LPM	33% all-trans lycopene	Kassama et al. (2008)
Tomato pomace	CO_2/16% ethanol	57 °C	40 MPa	—	93%	Huang et al. (2008)
Rosehip	CO_2	40–80 °C	15–45 Mpa	2–4 ml/min	1.180–14.37 mg/g feed	Machmudah et al. (2008)
Dried milled tomato	CO_2	110 °C	39.5 MPa	1.5 ml/min	100%	Ollanketo et al. (2001)
Dried tomato pomace	CO_2	80 °C	460 bar	—	90.1%	Vági et al. (2007)

obtained without degradation. If the storage of the sample is done in deep-frozen conditions instead of air-dried, this increases the concentration of carotenoids ten times (Vági et al. 2007). Conventional thermal processing inactivated all the microorganisms but degraded carotenoids (lycopene) color and tomato juice viscosity. So, an alternative way was postulated to increase lycopene content during a long period of storage and the stable microbial product. With high pressure, 500 MPa gave the best result to obtain a microbial stable and high lycopene content tomato juice (Hsu et al. 2008). A study was conducted to increase lycopene production by treating the biomass with lysozyme and EDTA into organic solvents. This organic two-phase system enhanced recombinant *E. coli* to produce 40% greater amounts of lycopene than that in a conventional aqueous single-phase system (Yoon et al. 2008).

11.5 Effect of Lycopene During Processing

Lycopene degradation occurs due to exposure to light, heat, oxygen and metallic ions of copper, iron that carry out oxidation, and acids. Heating and drying tomato and tomato byproducts under different conditions during the production of tomato juice, pulp, powder, etc., lead to lycopene degradation. The oxidative degradation of lycopene was first reported in the year 1954 (Shi and Le Maguer 2000). The heating of lycopene at high temperature (130 °C) for seven minutes showed a 17% loss in lycopene content, whereas at low temperature (90 °C), the percentage of lycopene loss was less (Miki and Akatsu 1970) (Figure 11.8). Oxygen is mainly responsible for degradation. Almost 33% of the lycopene was destroyed in the presence of oxygen, whereas 5% loss was observed in the presence of CO_2 (Cole and Kapur 1957) (Figure 11.9). Time and temperature are directly proportional to the percentages of lycopene loss, indicating high temperature and heating time affect the lycopene content. In this study, a mathematical model was proposed to stimulate lycopene loss during drying processes (concentration process and spray-drying technique) of tomato pulp. The rate constant of lycopene degradation is a function of material temperature, and moisture content is obtained from the changes that occur in lycopene concentration in an equal time interval. The minimum reaction rate constant of degradation is when the moisture content of the pulp is between 50 and 55%. In the spray-drying process, the

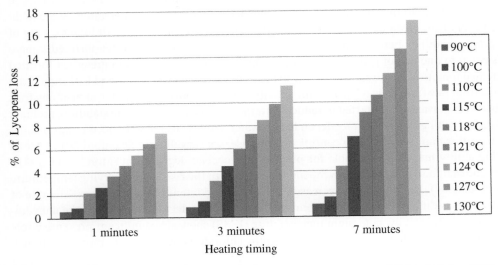

Figure 11.8 Loss of lycopene by heat treatment with different temperatures (Miki and Akatsu 1970).

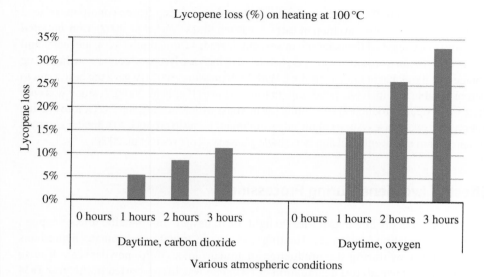

Figure 11.9   Lycopene loss from tomato pulp on heating at 100 °C temperature in the presence of oxygen (Cole and Kapur 1957).

product was in droplet form. Due to the large area, lycopene degradation was quicker than the concentration process (Goula and Adamopoulos 2005). According to an experiment, the reaction rate constant values of lycopene degradation are decreased under vacuum and dark conditions and increased under oxygen and light at each temperature. It was also reported, a freeze-dried tomato sample showed a higher amount of lycopene loss (97%) than overdried samples (73–79%) stored over four months. As the freeze-dried sample has a fluffy texture, they are more prone to air and light exposure than oven-dried as they have a texture like thin crust sheets (Sharma and Le Maguer 1996b). In the presence of oxygen, the percentage of lycopene retention decreased after a long storage period (Table 11.8). Almost 21.8% of lycopene was retained in 385 days of the storage period, whereas 65.8% of lycopene retained in the absence of oxygen under the same condition (Lovrić et al. 1970). The degradation can be decelerated by the addition of flavonols of green tea extract in dehydrated tomatoes. From 200 g fresh tomato, 140 g of dried product can be obtained and flavanol content in 10 g of dried green-tea-fortified tomato skin is equal to one cup of green tea. Flavanol content remains unaltered in green-tea-fortified heat-treated tomato skin stored at the a_w (water activity) levels between 0.17 and 0.32 than those obtained from raw fruit. This is because the activity of polyphenol oxidase in the skin of raw fruit was observed. Flavanols are started to reduce with the increased a_w level. The stability of tomato skin fortified with green tea extract depended on water activity (a_w). It enhanced antiglycoxidative and antioxidant properties to control various diseases (Lavelli and Scarafoni 2012). Metal chelating ability may be responsible for preventing lycopene degradation (Morel et al. 1993). A study showed the degradation of lycopene increased with the rise of spray-drying temperature (Quek et al. 2007). Hot air drying decreased the lycopene content of tomato slices. The rate of degradation was different and pretreatment had an impact on degradation during the dehydration process. In this study, potassium metabisulfite (KMS) showed a significant preventive role in degradation, but when combined with calcium chloride ($CaCl_2$), it was more functional.

Table 11.8 Retention of total lycopene from tomato powder in several atmospheric conditions (Lovrić et al. 1970).

Fresh tomato powder = 100%

Storage time (days)	Temperature (°C)	Atmospheric conditions	Percentage of total lycopene retention
30	2	N_2	85.5
	20		90.0
	2	Air	37
	20		46.3
80	2	N_2	66.3
	20		78.5
	2	Air	11.3
	20		28.7
160	2	N_2	54.2
	20		76.5
	2	Air	9.3
	20		25.5
210	2	N_2	53.3
	20		69.8
	2	Air	8.5
	20		23
385	2	N_2	53
	20		65.8
385	2	Air	8.2
	20		21.8

The combined effect of KMS and $CaCl_2$ prevented non-enzymatic browning (NEB) due to dehydration and prevented carotenoid discoloration. The chelating property of calcium may be the reason behind NEB prevention. Lycopene degradation was lower in tunnel drying (65 °C temperature for six hours) than solar drying (between February and May for 10 h/day). Combined treatment of $CaCl_2$ with KMS showed lower lycopene degradation in both sun- and tunnel-drying techniques. But the browning index was lower in tunnel drying with the combined pretreatment. Lycopene degradation was less observed in metalized polyester (MP) film pouches at room temperature for six months, 20% of degradation had been observed and 50–60% of the color retention was also observed. Less permeability of MP films prevented the entry of light and oxygen led to the higher retention of lycopene (Davoodi et al. 2007). In this study, researchers experimented on encapsulated watermelon-extracted lycopene by inverse gelation to prevent lycopene degradation. The watermelon puree was mixed with sunflower oil followed by heating to extract the lycopene. This extracted lycopene was further added to the oil in water emulsion containing $CaCl_2$. This emulsion was finally added to the alginate solution followed by stirring and drying respectively to obtain encapsulated lycopene. The optimum condition of low-viscosity alginate was 1.5% (w/v) alginate, 240 g/l $CaCl_2$ with 30 minutes' gelation time, and this was found to have higher encapsulated efficiency and loading capacity (Celli et al. 2016).

11.6 Daily Intake of Lycopene

Despite having lots of information about the disease-preventive effect of lycopene, still it is not accepted as an essential nutrient. Due to this, there are no recommended dietary allowances for lycopene by health care workers and government regulatory agencies. Based on the studies, daily consumption of 5–7 mg for a healthy person can be suggested to maintain lycopene levels. So, it can prevent oxidative stress and chronic diseases (Rao and Shen 2002). During disease conditions like cancer or CVD, higher lycopene (35–75 mg/day) can be suggested (Heath et al. 2006).

11.7 The Importance of Fortification

The World Health Organization defined it as a method through which food items are added with nutrients in an adequate amount to enhance the dietary quality of a targeted group or a large population (Dary and Hurrell 2006).

There are three types of fortification.

11.7.1 Mass Fortification

It is usually targeted in staple foods (rice, wheat, cereals, etc.) generally consumed by people. It is the best way of fortification when a large number of populations become deficient or become beneficial for those who are not yet suffering from any deficiency according to the biochemical criteria, e.g. fortification of wheat flour with folic acid in the USA (Dary and Hurrell 2006; Gupta 2014).

11.7.2 Targeted Fortification

The fortification is done for a specific group of a population to ensure the increased intake of deficient nutrients for the targeted group instead of the whole, e.g. school feeding programs for school children (Dary and Hurrell 2006; Gupta 2014).

11.7.3 Market-Driven fortification

It is a business-oriented initiative where one or more micronutrients are added to the food, also known as voluntary fortification and fortification levels regulated by the government (Dary and Hurrell 2006; Gupta 2014).

Lycopene is one of 600 carotenoids in nature, having lots of beneficial properties. Lycopene has been used as a natural food colorant for many years. The consumption of lycopene from natural origins and as a food color would be expected to persist within acceptable daily intake (ADI) of 0.5 mg/kg BW/day (EFSA 2010). European Food Safety Authority (EFSA) has given a guideline to use lycopene as a natural color in foods and drinks (Table 11.9). The European Economic Commission (EEC) allows using lycopene oleoresin (natural lycopene) as a novel food component, which is given in (Table 11.10). Lycopene manufactured from *B. trispora* had a GRAS limit up to 50 ppm (Table 11.11)

Table 11.9 Maximum levels of lycopene use as a natural color in foods and drinks (EFSA 2010).

Foods	Recommended maximum levels of use	Typical use levels as reported by NATCOL
Nonalcoholic flavored drinks	12 mg/l	5 mg/l
Candied fruits and vegetables, Mostarda di frutta	30 mg/kg	20 mg/kg
Confectionery	30 mg/kg	10 mg/kg
Decorations and coatings	30 mg/kg	30 mg/kg
Fine bakery wares (e.g. Viennoiserie, biscuits, cakes, and wafers)	25 mg/kg	10 mg/kg
Edible ices	40 mg/kg	10 mg/kg
Flavored processed cheese	5 mg/kg	5 mg/kg
Desserts including flavored milk products	30 mg/kg	10 mg/kg
Sauces, seasonings (for example curry powder, tandoori), pickles, relishes, chutney and piccalilli	50 mg/kg	15 mg/kg
Jams, jellies and marmalades as mentioned in Council Directive 2001/113/EC7 and similar fruit preparations	10 mg/kg	10 mg/kg
Fish paste and crustacean paste	30 mg/kg	20 mg/kg
Precooked crustaceans	30 mg/kg	20 mg/kg
Salmon substitutes	10 mg/kg	7 mg/kg
Surimi	30 mg/kg	15 mg/kg
Fish roe	30 mg/kg	20 mg/kg
Smoked fish	50 mg/kg	20 mg/kg
Snacks: extruded or expanded savory snack products	30 mg/kg	15 mg/kg
Snacks: other savory snack products and savory-coated nuts	30 mg/kg	15 mg/kg
Edible cheese and edible casings	30 mg/kg	20 mg/kg
Complete formulae for weight control intended to replace total daily intake or an individual meal	30 mg/kg	20 mg/kg
Complete formulae and nutritional supplements for use under medical supervision	30 mg/kg	20 mg/kg
Liquid food supplements/dietary integrators	30 mg/kg	20 mg/kg
Solid food supplements/dietary integrators	30 mg/kg	20 mg/kg
Soups	20 mg/kg	10 mg/kg
Meat and fish analogues based on vegetable proteins	30 mg/kg	20 mg/kg
Spirituous beverages (excluding products <15% alcohol by volume) except those mentioned in Annex II or III	30 mg/l	10 mg/l
Aromatized wines, aromatized wine-based drinks, and aromatized wine product cocktails as mentioned in Regulation (EEC) No. 1601/918 except those mentioned in Annex II or III	10 mg/l	10 mg/kg
Fruit wine (still or sparkling); Cider (except cidre bouche) and perry; Aromatized fruit wines, cider, and perry	10 mg/l	10 mg/kg

Table 11.10 Lycopene-enriched foods to which lycopene added as a novel food component (European Economic Commission (EEC) council regulation EC No. 258/97, 2009).

Food category	The maximum content of lycopene
Fruit/vegetable juice-based drinks (including concentrates)	2.5 mg/100 g
Drinks intended to meet the expenditure of intense muscular effort, especially for sportsmen	2.5 mg/100 g
Foods intended for use in energy-restricted diets for weight reduction	8 mg/meal replacement
Breakfast cereals	5 mg/100 g
Soups other than tomato soups	1 mg/100 g
Bread (including crispy bread)	3 mg/100 g
Dietary foods for special medical purposes	Following the particular nutritional requirements

Table 11.11 GRAS uses of lycopene produced by *B. trispora* in foods and beverages (FDA (U.S. Food and Drug Administration) 2005b).

Food category	Maximum use levels (ppm)
Baked goods and baking mixes	50
Beverages and beverage bases	25
Breakfast cereals	50
Cheeses	5.0
Condiments and relishes	50
Confections and frostings	25
Fats and oils	20
Frozen dairy desserts and mixes	25
Gelatins, puddings and fillings	25
Gravies and sauces	50
Hard candy	25
Milk products	50
Plant protein products	50
Processed fruits and fruit juices	25
Snack foods	30

when used as an ingredient in large varieties of foods (FDA (U.S. Food and Drug Administration) 2005b). BASF Corporation (manufacturer of synthetic crystalline lycopene) revealed that synthetic lycopene that fulfilled its established food-grade specifications is GRAS under the conditions of its intended application as a direct food component in various food levels varying from 5 to 70 mg/kg of food (Table 11.12) (FDA (U.S. Food and Drug Administration) 2005a).

Table 11.12 GRAS uses of synthetic lycopene in various foods (FDA (U.S. Food and Drug Administration) 2005a).

Food category	Maximum[a] use levels (mg synthetic lycopene[b] per 100 g food as prepared)
Breakfast cereals (ready-to-eat and cooked)	0.5, 2.0, 3.5, or 7.0[c]
Drinks (energy drinks, juice drinks, and dairy fruit drinks)	2.5
Instant soup	2.0
Low-fat dressings	2.0
Meal replacements	2.5
Meatless meat products	5.0
Nutrient bars	5.0
Salty snacks and crackers	3.0
Yogurt	2.0

[a] The maximum use level of synthetic lycopene per 100 g food may be provided by any of the three synthetic lycopene-containing products (LycoVit®10%, Lycopene 10 CWD, or lycopene Dispersion 20).
[b] Total synthetic lycopene (cis + trans isomers)
[c] 7.0 mg synthetic lycopene per 100 g Ready-to-eat (RTE) for cereals weighing <20 g per cup, 3.5 mg synthetic lycopene per 100 g RTE for high fiber cereals containing ≥28 g of fiber per 100 g; 2.0 mg synthetic lycopene per 100 g RTE for cereals weighing ≥43 g per cup; 0.5 mg synthetic Lycopene per 100 g cooked cereals.

11.8 Ongoing Fortification Process with Lycopene

There are several experiments of lycopene fortification; however, the number is significantly less compared to the other nutrient fortifications.

In this study, an experiment was done by fortifying tomato juice with lycopene powder, followed by its effect on lycopene status, antioxidants, and other nutritional changes. Fortification with 30 mg lycopene/100 g tomato juice showed the highest antioxidant activity, i.e. 30.23 mg ascorbic acid equivalence (AAE)/100 g at day 60 of storage. The maximum amount of lycopene content was 22.16 mg/100 g on day zero, but after that, the amount gradually decreased; at day 60, the content was 19.339 mg/100 g. Enzymatic and nonenzymatic oxidation taking place during storage. By inactivating oxidative enzymes, the carotenoid loss can be prevented. The organoleptic score was also decreased nonsignificantly from day 0 to day 60 (Prathibha and Narayana 2016). The result of this study exhibited the enhanced level of lutein and lycopene in the blood and liver of mice that were fed with egg yolk powder fortified with lutein, lycopene, and vitamin C (Kiss et al. 2019). In this study, tomato juice was blended with other fruit juices (apple, sweet corn, and carrot juice) in various proportions and fortified with isomerized lycopene extract and β-carotene. This significantly increased the amount of cis-lycopene at the end. The total level of lycopene content in various tomato juice blends ranged from 16.21 mg/100 g to 25.65 mg/100 g and cis-lycopene was 9.16 mg/100 g to 14.46 mg/100 g. From the organoleptic study, tomato juice content, 35% apple juice and 40% carrot juice were the most acceptable in taste. Tomato–carrot juice blend contains the highest amount of β carotene among all juice blends (Urbonavičienė et al. 2015). Refined sunflower oil was fortified with lycopene, along with other antioxidants. In the study, sunflower oil is fortified with 1000 ppm of lycopene and rosemary extract and other natural antioxidants. Lycopene reduced the Oxidative Stability Index (OSI) compared to the other antioxidant system, where lycopene was absent because the test was performed under high temperature and in the presence of light. This reduces the antioxidant property of lycopene by enhancing the reactivity of carotene resonance stabilized radical adducts. Sunflower oil containing 0.1% rosemary extract, 0.01% of ascorbyl palmitate retained the highest amount of lycopene (63.53%) (Omer et al. 2014). A similar study was done on edible oils. Lycopene and other carotenoids were added from tomato peel (industrial waste). This enhances the thermostability of refined olive oil and improved the phenol, lycopene, and β-carotene content (Benakmoum et al. 2008). In this experiment, an extruded product made of barley and tomato blends in a different ratio was produced. Tomato pomace at 2 and 10% level were incorporated at 160° C temperature and 200 rpm into the blends of barley flour to produce extruded barley tomato pomace snacks. Tomato pomace consists of the skin and seeds of the fruit. A diet rich in lycopene has several health benefits. It had a high acceptance level (Altan et al. 2008). Dry fermented sausages fortified with lycopene by adding dry tomato peel to the meat mixture utilized in sausage manufacturing. A very less amount of lycopene loss has been observed during the 21-day ripening period though the overall acceptability of the sausage along with the lycopene level (0.326–0.58 mg/100 g of sausage) was satisfactory (Calvo et al. 2008). Lycopene was extracted and added to the ice cream as a natural color source to avoid chemical colors. 0.1% addition of lycopene to the ice cream enhanced organoleptic analysis score compared to commercially available mango-flavored ice cream with sunset yellow color (Jadav et al. 2016). Yogurt is fortified with curcumin, lycopene, and bixin, as a combined effect of these three decreased glycemia, TG, total cholesterol, oxidized LDL, and enhanced the activity of antioxidant enzymes. Lycopene also lowered both paraoxonase and HDL levels. These antiatherogenic properties reduced CVD risk, which is one of the major complications for a diabetic person (Assis et al. 2017). In another study, yogurt was fortified with tomato juice, which enhanced the nutritional quality of the food, also can meet the daily intake of lycopene. Still, the fortification can decrease the viscosity of yogurt (Ademosun et al. 2019). The amount of lycopene in the wine prepared from tomatoes was enriched by the addition of tomato puree. It showed an antiobesity effect, increased HDL-C, and decreased the mass of liver and adipose tissues by inhibiting lipid biosynthesis among rats on a high-fat diet. But advanced experiments are required to establish the combined effect of alcohol and lycopene in combating weight gain (Kim et al. 2012). A beverage was prepared from pink flesh guava; the pink color of the guava flesh indicates the presence of lycopene to improve the nutritional quality and acceptability of the beverage; tomato puree with various amounts had been added to it. As a result, the lycopene content increased from 760 µg/100 g to 2010 µg/100 g with an increased tomato puree level. Among all concentrations of the puree-added beverages, the most acceptable one was 6%, stored up to six months at room temperature (Pasupuleti and Kulkarni 2014). An experiment was done for food preservation by fortifying fresh-cut apples with lycopene. Lycopene had cis-isomers' antioxidant capacity. Tomato skin is very cheap and easily available. So, lycopene was extracted from it and used as an anti-browning dipping treatment. Lycopene was encapsulated to form microspheres by adding cis-isomerized lycopene-rich oil (after extraction, resuspended in sunflower oil) dropwise into the gelatine, then gum arabic solution followed by stirring and heating. As a result, it was found that physiochemical quality and microbial quality remain unchanged. Improved bioactive quality and increased chlorogenic acid in the fresh-cut apples, which is a predominant phenolic acid and delayed browning. The fortification enhanced cis lycopene content from 33 to 52 mg/kg and all-trans lycopene from 3.4 to 5.6 mg/kg. Cis lycopene isomer remains unaltered after nine days of storage 20 mg/kg lycopene content was found. Two grams of lycopene microsphere per liter showing the lowest browning index after nine days of storage, i.e. 43.8 (Martínez-Hernández et al. 2019). Tomato-processing industries produced an excessive amount of waste material consisting mainly of peels and seeds, which are also known as tomato pomace. Tomato pomaces were utilized to produce tomato seed oil using press extractors instead of solvents for better retention of polar compounds and tomato oleoresin. Later, the seed oil is fortified with tomato oleoresin extracted by using enzymes (polygalacturonase, pectin methylesterase, cellulase, and hemicellulase) to prepare lycopene-enriched seed oil. It has a wide range of applications in food-processing industries, cosmetics and nutraceuticals' production. For these purposes, the lycopene content of seed oil was maintained between 50 and 500 mg/kg by the addition of lycopene from 0.73 to 7.3 g/kg oil. About 53% of the oil was extracted from seeds by pressing (Zuorro et al. 2013). The solvent extraction method had many problems like the solvent residuals and can also prevent the extraction of some polar compounds, thus decreasing the nutritional quality. The amount of phytosterol content in SC-CO_2-treated tomato seed oil was higher than the conventional organic solvents' treatment, but the endogenous antioxidant content was less (Eller et al. 2010). The tomato seed oil contains almost 84% unsaturated fatty acids. These fatty acids can undergo partial oxidative degradation under supercritical conditions (Demirbas 2010). Unfavorable extraction conditions can enhance the isomerization of lycopene and alter the stability of oil (Longo et al. 2012). From this data, it can be concluded that though the yield of lycopene is lower in pressing method than others, it has no adverse effect on the health and the environment and protects the functional properties of the oil. Some different techniques were applied for lycopene fortification to overcome these disadvantages due to direct lycopene fortification. Orange juice was fortified with lycopene-loaded nanoparticles (nanoencapsulation), which eliminated some drawbacks, those are undesirable after taste and less solubility of lycopene, but it significantly lowers the orange odor (Zardini et al. 2018). Soy-fortified lycopene-rich tomato juice was prepared to make available the phytochemical constituents possessing chemopreventive effect and affect biomarkers of blood lipid. Eighteen people, including men and women, consumed 300 ml soy-fortified juice containing 66 mg isoflavones and 22 mg lycopene for eight weeks. As a result, 3.1% lycopene was absorbed and 49.3% isoflavones ingested were recovered after 24 hours in urine. Also enhanced resistance of LDL and VLDL to Cu^+-mediated oxidation and increased the level of HDL-C. This juice showed no adverse effect after ingestion, so safe to intake (Bohn et al. 2013). In another study, lycopene was extracted from the edible part of papaya fruit by various solvent extraction methods. The highest yield of lycopene was 1.02 mg/100 g of fresh weight. Later, the extracted lycopene was used to enrich fruit drinks with two different compositions. The acceptability of the lycopene-added papaya drink (tomato and papaya at 1 : 2 ratio) is more acceptable than the lycopene-added mixed fruit drink (tomato, papaya, and watermelon at 1 : 1 : 1 ratio). But the mixed fruit drink showed the highest lycopene content, i.e. 3.9 mg/100 ml. The organoleptic and microbiological quality assessment results ensured that the fruit drinks can be stored for up to three months at room temperature (Rayhan et al. 2019). In this experiment, lycopene, fortified noodles, and functional grits are coated with maltodextrin. Degradation of lycopene microencapsulated by maltodextrin in functional grit is less than the instant noodle. Warming and drying do not affect this loss as the preparation of the grit required long heating and drying time than noodles. The concentration of maltodextrin-coated lycopene is 2000 and 250 ppm in the batter to prepare noodles, and grit is mostly acceptable with 8.17 and 8.11 months of the expiration period, respectively, when stored at room temperature (Sumarni and Ibrahim 2019). This experiment was done to determine the effect of lemon juice added in the tomato jelly beverage products to improve antioxidant activity to enhance the lycopene bioavailability in the body. The addition of 8.4% of lemon juice in tomato jelly was the most acceptable one in the experiment. Young tomatoes contain vitamin C of 30 mg/100 g and ripe tomatoes contain vitamin C of 34 mg/100 g. Lemon juice is rich in vitamin C (50 mg/100 g) and also contains vitamins B and E, sodium and some micronutrients, which boost up the immune system and have antiviral properties against influenza. Also, the fiber content in the form of pectin and antioxidant properties are useful in lowering cholesterol and triglycerides. The lycopene concentration in tomato jelly became double (18.70 mg/100 g of each ingredient) than fresh tomatoes (9.00 mg/100 g of each ingredient) due to the heating at the optimum temperature (70 °C). But excessive heating will decrease lycopene concentration (Nazir and Adrian 2016). Beef hamburgers were fortified with lycopene by direct addition of dry tomato peel to obtain lycopene-enriched products with minimal changes in physicochemical properties (García et al. 2009). As the peel is rich in lycopene (2.5 times higher lycopene content than pulp) and fiber, it enhanced the nutritional quality of beef hamburgers. Tomato peel powder was added to ground meat and homogenized. Hamburger containing 4.5% tomato peel was mostly accepted among all others and enhanced the lycopene content in hamburger 4.9 mg/100 g (Knoblich et al. 2005). In the experiment, tomato pulp powder was used as a thickening agent in tomato ketchup production. The addition of 1 and 2% of the powder in the ketchup enhanced the viscosity by about 50 and 100%, respectively (Farahnaky et al. 2008). Nitrite is a reactive chemical used in the curing of meat, but there are chances of the formation of n-nitrosamines and nitrite residue in the meat, which is harmful for health (Cassens et al. 1979). Fortifications of lycopene from natural sources to minced meat enhanced the organoleptic quality of the food, as well as improve health benefits. The acidic property of tomato decreases the pH in meat farces and thus, the growth of microorganisms was decreased. The red-colored lycopene crystals without nitrite had the most reddish hue and were quite stable during storage. Thus, it can be concluded that tomato products can partially or wholly replace nitrite use (Østerlie and Lerfall 2005). Another study also supported this result. In their study, frankfurters were fortified with tomato paste (12%) and showed a positive effect on color and helped in the reduction of nitrite level from 150 to 100 mg/kg without altering the desirable quality of the food. It has health benefits as it contains lycopene (Deda et al. 2007). Low-fat cooked sausage (beef and chicken meat) made with tomato juice showed the lowest pH value, as well as low total aerobic count and nitrite content (Yılmaz et al. 2002). Beef patties were fortified with tomato paste and kept in a refrigerator at 4 °C for nine days. Due to the antioxidant activity of lycopene, it increases the TBA (thiobarbituric acid) value of the fortified patties along with the pH value, and the result from the sensory evaluation score was satisfactory (Candogan 2002). A similar result was found when the cooked pork patties were fortified with tomato powder stored at 10 °C (Kim et al. 2013).

11.9 Conclusion

Lycopene is a lipophilic red-colored pigment (carotenoids) with no provitamin A activity. Various studies provide information about the preventive effect of lycopene on diseases, which encouraged the demand for lycopene intake. This led to enhance the production of lycopene-rich food. Various food products have been developed, which are fortified with lycopene. Different extraction and purification methods are evolved to reduce the loss of lycopene. Despite health benefits, no recommendation has been given for lycopene consumption. More research is required on serum lycopene levels, dietary effects, prolonged dietary interventions, disease-prevention mechanisms, and the development of different fortification techniques to produce more lycopene-fortified foods.

References

Ademosun, O.T., Ajanaku, K.O., Adebayo, A.H. et al. (2019). Physico-chemical, microbial and organoleptic properties of yogurt fortified with tomato juice. *J. Food Nutr. Res.* 7 (11): 810–814.

Agarwal, S. and Rao, A.V. (1998). Tomato lycopene and low density lipoprotein oxidation: a human dietary intervention study. *Lipids* 33: 981–984.

Agarwal, B.B. and Shishodia, S. (2006). Molecular targets of dietary agents for prevention and therapy of cancer. *Biochem. Pharmacol.* 71: 1397–1421.

Agarwal, A., Shen, H., and Rao, A.V. (2001). Lycopene content of tomato products: its stability, bioavailability and in vivo antioxidant properties. *J. Med. Food* 4: 9–15.

Altan, A., McCarthy, K.L., and Maskan, M. (2008). Evaluation of snack foods from barley–tomato pomace blends by extrusion processing. *J. Food Eng.* 84 (2): 231–242.

Al-Wandawi, H., Abdul-Rahman, M., and Al-Shaikhly, K. (1985). Tomato processing wastes as essential raw materials source. *J. Agric. Food Chem.* 33 (5): 804–807.

Andreassi, L. (2011). UV exposure as a risk factor for skin cancer. *Expert. Rev. Dermatol.* 6: 445–454.

Angel, P. and Karin, M. (1991). The role of jun, fos and the AP-1 complex in cell proliferation and transformation. *Biochim. Biophys. Acta.* 1072: 129–157.

Arab, L. and Steck, S. (2000). Lycopene and cardiovascular disease. *Am. J. Clin. Nutr.* 71 (6): 1691S–1695S.

Assis, R.P., Arcaro, C.A., Gutierres, V.O. et al. (2017). Combined effects of curcumin and lycopene or bixin in yogurt on inhibition of LDL oxidation and increases in HDL and paraoxonase levels in streptozotocin-diabetic rats. *Int. J. Mol. Sci.* 18 (4): 332.

Aust, O., Ale-Agha, N., Zhang, L. et al. (2003). Lycopene oxidation product enhances gap junctional communication. *Food Chem. Toxicol.* 41: 1399–1407.

Aydin, M. and Celik, S. (2012). Effects of lycopene on plasma glucose, insulin levels, oxidative stress, and body weights of streptozotocin-induced diabetic rats. *Turk. J. Med. Sci.* 42 (Sup. 2): 1406–1413.

Bahieldin, A., Gadalla, N.O., Al-Garni, S.M. et al. (2014). Efficient production of lycopene in *Saccharomyces cerevisiae* by expression of synthetic crt genes from a plasmid harboring the ADH2 promoter. *Plasmid* 72: 18–28.

Bauerle, P.A. and Baltimore, D. (1996). NF-kB ten years after. *Cell* 87: 13–20.

Bauerle, P.A. and Henkel, T. (1994). Function and activation of NF-kB in the immune system. *Annu. Rev. Immunol.* 12: 141–179.

Baysal, T.A., Ersus, S.E., and Starmans, D.A. (2000). Supercritical CO_2 extraction of β-carotene and lycopene from tomato paste waste. *J. Agric. Food Chem.* 48 (11): 5507–5511.

Benakmoum, A., Abbeddou, S., Ammouche, A. et al. (2008). Valorisation of low quality edible oil with tomato peel waste. *Food Chem.* 110 (3): 684–690.

Bertram, J.S., Pung, A., Churley, M. et al. (1991). Diverse carotenoids protect against chemically induced neoplastic transformation. *Carcinogenesis* 12: 671–678.

Bhataya, A., Schmidt-Dannert, C., and Lee, P.C. (2009). Metabolic engineering of Pichia pastoris X-33 for lycopene production. *Process Biochem.* 44 (10): 1095–1102.

Bhuvaneswari, V., Velmurugan, B., Balasenthil, S. et al. (2001). Chemopreventive efficacy of lycopene on 7,12-dimethylbenz[a]anthracene-induced hamster buccal pouch carcinogenesis. *Fitoterapia* 8: 865–874.

Böhm, F., Tinkler, J.H., and Truscott, T.G. (1995). Carotenoids protect against cell membrane damage by the nitrogen dioxide radical. *Nat. Med.* 1 (2): 98–99.

Bohn, T., Blackwood, M., Francis, D. et al. (2013). Bioavailability of phytochemical constituents from a novel soy fortified lycopene rich tomato juice developed for targeted cancer prevention trials. *Nutr. Cancer* 65 (6): 919–929.

Britton, G. (1995). Structure and properties of carotenoids in relation to function. *FASEB J.* 9: 1551–1558.

Burgess, L.C., Rice, E., Fischer, T. et al. (2008). Lycopene has limited effect on cell proliferation in only two of seven human cell lines (both cancerous and noncancerous) in an in vitro system with doses across the physiological range. *Toxicol. In Vitro* 22: 1297–1300.

Burton, G.W. and Ingold, K.U. (1984). β-carotene: an unusual type of lipidantioxidant. *Science* 224: 569–573.

Cadoni, E., DeGiorgi, M.R., Medda, E., and Poma, G. (2000). Supercritical CO_2 extraction of lycopene and β-carotene from ripe tomatoes. *Dyes Pigm.* 44: 27–32.

Calvo, M.M., Garcia, M.L., and Selgas, M.D. (2008). Dry fermented sausages enriched with lycopene from tomato peel. *Meat Sci.* 80 (2): 167–172.

Camara, M., de Cortes, S.-M.M., Fernández-Ruiz, V. et al. (2013). Lycopene: A review of chemical and biological activity related to beneficial health effects. In: *Studies in Natural Products Chemistry*, vol. 40, 383–426. Elsevier.

Campbell, J.K., Stroud, C.K., Nakamura, M.T. et al. (2006). Serum testosterone is reduced following shorttermphytofluene, lycopene, or tomato powder consumption in F344 rats. *J. Nutr.* 136: 2813–2819.

Candogan, K. (2002). The effect of tomato paste on some quality characteristics of beef patties during refrigerated storage. *Eur. Food Res. Technol.* 215 (4): 305–309.

Cantrell, A., McGarvey, D.J., Truscott, T.G. et al. (2003). Singletoxygen quenching by dietary carotenoids in a model membrane environment. *Arch. Biochem. Biophys.* 412 (1): 47–54.

Cassens, R.G., Greaser, M.L., Ito, T., and Lee, M. (1979). Reactions of nitrite in meat. *Food Technol.* 33: 46–57.

Celli, G.B., Teixeira, A.G., Duke, T.G., and Brooks, M.S. (2016). Encapsulationof lycopene from watermelon in calcium-alginate microparticles using an optimised inverse-gelation method by response surface methodology. *Int. J. Food Sci. Technol.* 51 (6): 1523–1529.

Chalabi, N., Delort, L., LeCorre, L. et al. (2006). Gene signature of breast cancer cell lines treated with lycopene. *Pharmacogenomics* 7: 663–672.

Chalabi, N., Satih, S., Delort, L. et al. (2007). Expression profiling by whole-genome microarray hybridization reveals differential gene expression in breast cancer cell lines after lycopene exposure. *Biochim. Biophys. Acta.* 1769: 124–130.

Chang, C.H., Lin, H.Y., Chang, C.Y., and Liu, Y.C. (2006). Comparisons on the antioxidant properties of fresh, freeze-dried and hot-air-dried tomatoes. *J. Food Eng.* 77 (3): 478–485.

Chen, Y., Shen, H., Cui, Y. et al. (2013). Chromosomal evolution of *Escherichia coli* for the efficient production of lycopene. *BMC Biotechnol.* 13: 6.

Chiu, Y.T., Chiu, C.P., Chien, J.T. et al. (2007). Encapsulation of lycopene extract from tomato pulp waste with gelatin and poly (γ-glutamic acid) as carrier. *J. Agric. Food Chem.* 55 (13): 5123–5130.

Choudhari, S.M. and Ananthanarayan, L. (2007). Enzyme aided extraction of lycopene from tomato tissues. *Food Chem.* 102 (1): 77–81.

Choudhari, S.M. and Singhal, R.S. (2008). Supercritical carbon dioxide extraction of lycopene from mated cultures of *Blakeslea trispora* NRRL 2895 and 2896. *J. Food Eng.* 89 (3): 349–354.

Colditz, G.A., Branch, L.G., Lipnick, R.J. et al. (1985). Increased green and yellow vegetable intake and lowered cancer deaths in an elderly population. *Am. J. Clin. Nutr.* 41 (1): 32–36.

Cole, E.R. and Kapur, N.S. (1957). The stability of lycopene. II.—oxidation during heating of tomato pulps. *J. Sci. Food Agric.* 8 (6): 366–368.

Collins, J.K., Perkins-Veazie, P., and Roberts, W. (2006). Lycopene: from plants to humans. *Hort. Sci. Hort. Sci.* 41 (5): 1135–1144.

Conn, P.F., Schalch, W., and Truscott, T.G. (1991). The singlet oxygen and carotenoid interaction. *J. Photochem. Photobiol. B Biol.* 11 (1): 41–47.

Conn, P.F., Lambert, C., Land, E.J. et al. (1992). *Rad. Res. Commun.* 16: 401–408.

Cowgill, G.R. (1887). Jean Baptiste Boussingault — a biographical sketch. *J. Nutr.* 84 (1): 1–9.

Coyne, T., Ibiebele, T.I., Baade, P.D. et al. (2005). Diabetes mellitus and serum carotenoids: findings of a population-based study in Queensland, Australia. *Am. J. Clin. Nutr.* 82 (3): 685–693.

Dary, O. and Hurrell, R. (2006). *Guidelines on Food Fortification with Micronutrients*. Geneva: World Health Organization, Food and Agricultural Organization of the United Nations.

Davoodi, M., Vijayanand, P., Kulkarni, S.G., and Ramana, K.V.R. (2007). Effect of different pre-treatments and dehydration methods on quality characteristics and storage stability of tomato powder. *LWT Food Sci. Technol.* 40: 1832–1840. https://doi.org/10.1016/j.lwt.2006.12.004.

Deda, M.S., Bloukas, J.G., and Fista, G.A. (2007). Effect of tomato paste and nitrite level on processing and quality characteristics of frankfurters. *Meat Sci.* 76 (3): 501–508.

Demirbas, A. (2010). Oil, micronutrient and heavy metal contents of tomatoes. *Food Chem.* 118: 504–507.

Devary, Y., Gottlieb, R.A., Laus, L.F., and Karin, M. (1991). Rapid and preferential activation of the c-jun gene during the mammalian UV response. *Mol. Cell. Biol.* 11: 2804–2811.

Dhas, P.H., Zachariah, T.J., Rajesh, P.N., and Subramannian, S. (2004). Effect of blanching and drying on quality of mace (*Myristica fragrans*). *J. Food Sci. Technol. Mysore* 41 (3): 306–308.

Di Mascio, P., Kaiser, S., and Sies, H. (1989). Lycopene as the most efficient biological carotenoid singlet oxygen quencher. *Arch. Biochem. Biophys.* 274: 532–538.

Di Mascio, P., Kaiser, S.P., Devasagayam, T.P., and Sies, H. (1991). Biological significance of active oxygen species: in vitro studies on singlet oxygen-induced DNA damage and on the singlet oxygen quenching ability of carotenoids, tocopherols and thiols. In: *Biological Reactive Intermediates IV*, 71–77. Boston, MA: Springer.

Dixon, Z.R., Shie, F.S., Warden, B.A. et al. (1998). The effect of a low carotenoid diet on malondialdehydethiobarbituric acid (MDA-TBA) concentrations in women: a placebo-controlled double-blind study. *J. Am. Coll. Nutr.* 17: 54–58.

Duzguner, V., Kucukgul, A., Erdogan, S. et al. (2008). Effect of lycopene administration on plasma glucose, oxidative stress and body weight in streptozotocin diabetic rats. *J. Appl. Anim. Res.* 33: 17–20.

EFSA (2010). Revised exposure assessment for lycopene as a food colour1 European Food Safety Authority 2, 3 European Food Safety Authority (EFSA), Parma, Italy. *EFSA J.* 8 (1): 1444. https://doi.org/10.2903/j.efsa.2010.1444.

El-Agamey, A., Lowe, G.M., McGarvey, D.J. et al. (2004). Carotenoid radical chemistry andantioxidant or pro-oxidant properties. *Arch. Biochem. Biophys.* 430: 37–48.

Eller, F.J., Moser, J.K., Kenar, J.A., and Taylor, S.L. (2010). Extraction and analysis of tomato seed oil. *J. Am. Oil Chem. Soc.* 87: 755–762.

Ernst, H. (2002). Recent advances in industrial carotenoid synthesis. *Pure Appl.Chem.* 74 (8): 1369–1382.

European Economic Community (EEC) (2009). Council Regulation EC No. 258/97. http://eurlex.europa.eu/LexUriServ/LexUriServ.do?uri=OJ:L:2009:110:0054:0057:EN:PDF. http://eurlex.europa.eu/LexUriServ/LexUriServ.do?uri=OJ:L:2009:109:0047:0051:EN:PDF (accessed 9 December 2011).

Evans, J.L., Goldfine, I.D., Maddux, B.A., and Grodsky, G.M. (2003). Are oxidative stress-activated signaling pathways mediatorsofinsulin resistance and β-cell dysfunction? *Diabetes* 52: 1–8.

Farahnaky, A., Abbasi, A., Jamalian, J., and Mesbahi, G. (2008). The use of tomato pulp powder as a thickening agent in the formulation of tomato ketchup. *J. Text. stud.* 39 (2): 169–182.

Fazeli, M.R., Tofighi, H., Madadkar-Sobhani, A. et al. (2009). Nicotine inhibition of lycopene cyclase enhances accumulation of carotenoid intermediates by *Dunaliella salina* CCAP 19/18. *Eur. J. Phycol.* 44 (2): 215–220.

FDA (U.S. Food and Drug Administration) (2005a). Agency response letter GRAS notice no. GRN 000119: synthetic lycopene. http://www.fda.gov/Food/FoodIngredientsPackaging/ GenerallyRecognizedasSafeGRAS/GRASListings/ucm153934.htm (accessed 7 November 2011).

FDA (U.S. Food and Drug Administration) (2005b). Agency response letter GRAS notice no. GRN 000173: lycopene from *B. trispora*. http://www.fda.gov/Food/FoodIngredientsPackaging/ GenerallyRecognizedasSafeGRAS/GRASListings/ucm154597.htm (accessed 7 November 2011).

Focus on Pigments (2007). World spends more than $50 M on lycopene red. *Focus. Pigment.* 4: 3–4.

Foote, C.S. and Denny, R.W. (1968). Chemistry of singlet oxygen. VII. Quenching by β-caotene. *J. Am. Chem. Soc.* 90: 6233–6235.

Franceschi, S., Bidoli, E., Vecchia, C.L. et al. (1994). Tomatoes and risk of digestive? Tract cancers. *Int. J.Cancer.* 59 (2): 181–184.

Fuhrman, B., Elis, A., and Aviram, M. (1997). Hypocholesterolemic effect of lycopene and beta-carotene is related to suppression of cholesterol synthesis and augmentation of LDL receptor activity in macrophages. *Biochem. Biophys. Res. Commun.* 233 (3): 658–662.

García, M.L., Calvo, M.M., and Selgas, M.D. (2009). Beef hamburgers enriched in lycopene using dry tomato peel as an ingredient. *Meat Sci.* 83 (1): 45–49.

Gartner, C., Stahl, W., and Sies, H. (1997). Lycopene is more bioavailable from tomato paste than from fresh tomatoes. *Am. J. Clin. Nutr.* 66 (1): 116–122.

Gerster, H. (1997). The potential role of lycopene for human health. *J. Am. Coll. Nutr.* 16 (2): 109–126.

Giovannucci, E., Ascherio, A., Rimm, E.B. et al. (1995). Intake of carotenoids and retinol in relation to risk of prostate cancer. *J. Natl. Cancer Inst.* 87: 1767–1776.

Giovannucci, E., Rimm, E.B., Liu, Y. et al. (2002). A prospective study of tomato products, lycopene, and prostate cancer risk. *J. Nat. Cancer Inst.* 94: 391–398.

Gomez-Prieto, M.S., Caja, M.M., Herraiz, M., and Santa-Maria, G. (2003). Supercritical fluid ex-traction of all-trans-lycopene from tomato. *J. Agric. Food Chem.* 51: 3–7.

González, S., Fernandez-Lorente, M., and Gilaberte-Calzada, Y. (2008). The latest on skin photoprotection. *Clin. Dermatol.* 26: 614–616.

Goula, A.M. and Adamopoulos, K.G. (2005). Stability of lycopene during spray drying of tomato pulp. *LWT Food Sci. Technol.* 38 (5): 479–487.

Goulinet, S. and Chapman, M.J. (1997). Plasma LDL and HDL subspecies heterogenous in particle content of tocopherols and oxygenated hydrocarbon carotenoids. Relevance to oxidative resistance therogenesis. *Arterioscler. Thromb. Vasc. Biol.* 17: 786–796.

Guo, Y., Liu, Y., and Wang, Y. (2015). Beneficial effect of lycopene on anti-diabetic nephropathy through diminishing inflammatory response and oxidative stress. *Food Funct.* 6 (4): 1150–1156.

Gupta, A. (2014). Fortification of foods with vitamin D in India. *Nutrients* 6 (9): 3601–3623.

Gupta, S.K., Trivedi, D., Srivastava, S. et al. (2003). Lycopene attenuates oxidative stress induced experimental cataract development: an in vitro and in vivo study. *Nutrition* 19 (9): 794–799.

Guttenplan, J.B., Chen, M., Kosinska, W. et al. (2001). Effects of a lycopene-rich diet on spontaneous and benzo[a]pyrene-induced mutagenesis in prostate, colon and lungs of the lacZ mouse. *Cancer Lett.* 164: 1–6.

Halliwell, B. and Gutteridge, J.M. (1989). *Free Radicals in Biology and Medicine*, vol. 2. New York: Oxford University Press.

Heath, E., Seren, S., Sahin, K., and Kucuk, O. (2006). The role of tomato lycopene in the treatment of prostate cancer. In: *Tomatoes, Lycopene and Human Health*, 127–140. Caledonian Science Press.

Heinonen, M.I., Ollilainen, V., Linkola, E.K. et al. (1989). Carotenoids in finnish foods, vegetables, fruits, and berries. *J. Agric. Food Chem.* 37: 655–659.

Heiss, E., Herhaus, C., Klimo, K. et al. (2001). Nuclear factor B is a molecular target for sulforaphane mediated antiinflammatory mechanisms. *J. Biol. Chem.* 276: 32008–32015.

Hernández-Almanza, A., Montañez-Sáenz, J., Martínez-Ávila, C. et al. (2014). Carotenoid production by *Rhodotorula glutinis* YB-252 in solid-state fermentation. *Food Biosci.* 7 (0): 31–36.

Hotz-Wagenblatt, A. and Shalloway, D. (1993). Gap junctional communication and neoplastic transformation. *Crit. Rev. Oncog.* 4: 541–558.

Hsu, K.C., Tan, F.J., and Chi, H.Y. (2008). Evaluation of microbial inactivation and physicochemical properties of pressurized tomato juice during refrigerated storage. *LWT Food Sci. Technol.* 41 (3): 367–375.

Huang, J.P., Zhang, M., Holman, C.D.J., and Xie, X. (2007a). Dietary carotenoids and risk of breast cancer in Chinese women. *Asia-Pac. J. Clin. Nutr.* 16: 437–442.

Huang, C.S., Fan, Y.E., Lin, C.Y., and Hu, M.L. (2007b). Lycopene inhibits matrix metalloproteinase-9 expression and down-regulates the binding activity of nuclear factor-kappa B and stimulatory protein-1. *J. Nutr. Biochem.* 18: 449–456.

Huang, W., Li, Z., Niu, H. et al. (2008). Optimization of operating parameters for supercritical carbon dioxide extraction of lycopene by response surface methodology. *J. Food Eng.* 89 (3): 298–302.

Huang, L., Pu, Y., Yang, X. et al. (2015). Engineering of global regulator cAMP receptor protein (CRP) in *Escherichia coli* for improved lycopene production. *J. Biotechnol.* 199 (0): 55–61.

Hwang, E.-S. and Lee, H.J. (2006). Inhibitory effects of lycopene on the adhesion, invasion, and migration of SK-Hep1 human hepatoma cells. *Exp. Biol. Med.* 231: 322–327.

Imaida, K., Tamano, S., Kato, K. et al. (2001). Lack of chemopreventive effects of lycopene and curcumin on experimental rat prostate carcinogenesis. *Carcinogenesis* 22: 467–472.

Jacob, K., Periago, M.J., Böhm, V., and Berruezo, G.R. (2008). Influence of lycopene and vitamin C from tomato juice on biomarkers of oxidative stress and inflammation. *Br. J. Nutr.* 99 (1): 137–146.

Jadav, P., Akbari, S., and Bhatt, H. (2016). Studies on lycopene fortified ice cream. *Advances* 5: 108–112.

Janssen, Y.M., Matalon, S., and Mossman, B.T. (1997). Differential induction of c-fos, c-jun, and apoptosis in lung epithelial cells exposed to ROS or RNS. *Am. J. Phys. Lung Cell. Mol. Phys.* 273: 789–796.

Jin, Y.-S. and Stephanopoulos, G. (2007). Multi-dimensional gene target search for improving lycopene biosynthesis in *Escherichia coli*. *Metab. Eng.* 9 (4): 337–347.

Joo, Y.E., Karrasch, T., Mühlbauer, M. et al. (2009). Tomato lycopene extract prevents lipopolysaccharide-induced NF-kappa B signaling but worsens dextran sulfate sodium-induced colitis in NF-kappa B EGFP mice. *PLoS ONE* 4: 4562.

Juan, C., Oyarzún, B., Quezada, N., and del Valle, J.M. (2006). Solubility of carotenoid pigments (lycopene and astaxanthin) in supercritical carbon dioxide. *Fluid Phase Equilib.* 247 (1-2): 90–95.

Jun, X. (2006). Application of high hydrostatic pressure processing of food to extracting lycopene from tomato paste waste. *High Press. Res.* 26 (1): 33–41.

Karas, M., Danilenko, M., Fishman, D. et al. (1997). Membrane-associated insulin-like growth factorbinding protein-3 inhibits insulin-like growth factor-Iinduced insulin-like growth factor-I receptor signaling in ishikawa endometrial cancer cells. *J. Biol. Chem.* 26: 16514–16520.

Karas, M., Amir, H., Fishman, D. et al. (2000). Lycopene interferes with cell cycle progression and insulin-like growth factor I signaling in mammary cancer cells. *Nutr. Cancer* 36: 101–111.

Karppi, J., Nurmi, T., Kurl, S. et al. (2010). Lycopene, lutein and β-carotene as determinants of LDL conjugated dienes in serum. *Atherosclerosis* 209 (2): 565–572.

Kassama, L.S., Shi, J., and Mittal, G.S. (2008). Optimization of supercritical fluid extraction of lycopene from tomato skin with central composite rotatable design model. *Sep. Purif. Technol.* 60 (3): 278–284.

Katherine, L.V., Edgar, C.C., Jerry, W.K. et al. (2008). Extraction conditions affecting supercritical fluid extraction (SFE) of lycopene from watermelon. *Bioresour. Technol.* 99 (16): 7835–7841.

Kaur, C., George, B., Deepa, N. et al. (2004). Antioxidant status of fresh and processed tomato a review. *J. Food Sci. Technol. Mysore* 41 (5): 479–486.

Khachik, F., Beecher, G.R., and Smith, J.C. Jr. (1995). Lutein, lycopene, and their oxidative metabolites in chemoprevention of cancer. *J. Cell. Biochem.* 22 (4): 236–246.

Kim, G.Y., Kim, J.H., Ahn, S.C. et al. (2004). Lycopene suppresses the lipopolysaccharide induced phenotypic and functional maturation of murine dendritic cells through inhibition of mitogen-activated protein kinases and nuclear factor-kappa B. *Immunology* 113: 203–211.

Kim, S., Kim, J., Ryu, J. et al. (2009). High-level production of lycopene in metabolically engineered *E. coli. Process Biochem.* 44 (8): 899–905.

Kim, A.Y., Jeong, Y.J., Park, Y.B. et al. (2012). Dose dependent effects of lycopene enriched tomato-wine on liver and adipose tissue in high-fat diet fed rats. *Food Chem.* 130 (1): 42–48.

Kim, I.S., Jin, S.K., Yang, M.R. et al. (2013). Efficacy of tomato powder as antioxidant in cooked pork patties. *Asian Australas. J. Anim. Sci.* 26 (9): 1339.

Kiss, Z., Kert, A., Szabó, C., and Bordán, J. (2019). Experiments of fortified egg yolk powder in mice. *J. Microbiol. Biotechnol. Food Sci.* 2019: 556–563.

Klein, E.A. (2005). Chemoprevention of prostate cancer. *Crit. Rev. Oncol. Hematol.* 54 (1): 1–10.

Knoblich, M., Anderson, B., and Latshaw, D. (2005). Analysis of tomato peel and seed byproducts and their use as a source of carotenoids. *J. Sci. Food Agric.* 85: 1166–1170.

Kohlmeier, L., Kark, J.D., Gomez-Gracia, E. et al. (1997). Lycopene and myocardial infarction risk in the EURAMIC Study. *Am. J. Epidemiol.* 146 (8): 618–626.

Kong, K.W., Ismail, A., Tan, C.P., and Rajab, N.F. (2010). Optimization of oven drying conditions for lycopene content and lipophilic antioxidant capacity in a by-product of the pink guava puree industry using response surface methodology. *LWT Food Sci. Technol.* 43 (5): 729–735.

Krinsky, N.I. and Johnson, E.J. (2005). Carotenoid actions and their relation tohealth and disease. *Mol. Asp. Med.* 26: 459–516.

Krinsky, N.I. and Yeum, K.J. (2003). Carotenoid–radical interactions. *Biochem. Biophys. Res. Commun.* 305: 754–760.

Krutovskikh, V., Asamoto, M., Takasuka, N., and Murakoshi, M. (1997). Differential dose-dependent effects of alpha-carotene and lycopene on gap juctional intercellular communication in rat liver in vivo. *Jpn. J. Cancer Res.* 88: 1121–1124.

Lavecchia, R. and Zuorro, A. (2008). Improved lycopene extraction from tomato peels using cell-wall degrading enzymes. *Eur. Food Res. Technol.* 228: 153–158.

Lavelli, V. and Scarafoni, A. (2012). Effect of water activity on lycopene and flavonoid degradation in dehydrated tomato skins fortified with green tea extract. *J. Food Eng.* 110 (2): 225–231.

Lee, S.J., Bai, S.K., Lee, K.S. et al. (2003). Astaxanthin inhibits nitric oxide production and inflammatory gene expression by suppressing IB kinase-dependent NF-B activation. *Mol. Cell.* 16: 97–105.

Lian, F., Smith, D.E., Ernst, H. et al. (2007). Apo-10?-lycopenoic acid inhibits lung cancer cell growth in vitro, and suppresses lung tumorigenesis in the A/J mouse model in vivo. *Carcinogenesis* 28: 1567–1574.

Lindner, P., Shomer, I., and Vasiliver, R. (1984). Distribution of protein, lycopene and the elements Ca Mg, P and N among various fractions of tomato juice. *J. Food Sci.* 49: 1214–1215.

Liu, C., Lian, F., Smith, D.E. et al. (2003). Lycopene supplementation inhibits lung squamous metaplasia and induces apoptosis via up-regulating insulin-like growth factor-binding protein 3 in cigarette smoke-exposed ferrets. *Cancer Res.* 63: 3138–3144.

Liu, X.J., Liu, R.S., Li, H.M., and Tang, Y.J. (2012). Lycopene production from synthetic medium by *Blakeslea trispora* NRRL 2895 (+) and 2896 (−) in a stirred-tank fermenter. *Bioproc. Biosyst. Eng.* 35 (5): 739–749.

Longo, C., Leo, L., and Leone, A. (2012). Carotenoids, fatty acid composition and heat stability of supercritical carbon dioxide extracted oleoresins. *Int. J. Mol. Sci.* 13: 4233–4254.

López-Nieto, M.J., Costa, J., Peiro, E. et al. (2004). Biotechnological lycopene production by mated fermentation of *Blakeslea trispora*. *Appl. Microbiol. Biotechnol.* 66 (2): 153–159.

Lovrić, T., Sablek, Z., and Bošković, M. (1970). Cis–trans isomerisation of lycopene and colour stability of foam—mat dried tomato powder during storage. *J. Sci. Food Agric.* 21 (12): 641–647.

Lowe, G.M., Bilton, R.F., Davies, I.G. et al. (1999). Carotenoid composition and antioxidant potential in subfractions of human low-density lipoprotein. *Ann. Clin. Biochem.* 36: 323–332.

Lu, Y., Etoh, H., and Watanaba, N. (1995). A new carotenoid, hydrogen peroxide oxidation products from lycopene. *Biosci. Biotechnol. Biochem.* 59: 2153–2155.

Machmudah, S., Kawahito, Y., Sasaki, M., and Goto, M. (2008). Process optimization and extraction rate analysis of carotenoids extraction from rosehip fruit using supercritical CO_2. *J. Supercrit. Fluids.* 44 (3): 308–314.

Martínez-Hernández, G.B., Castillejo, N., and Artés-Hernández, F. (2019). Effect of fresh-cut apples fortification with lycopene microspheres, revalorized from tomato by-products, during shelf life. *Postharvest Biol. Technol.* 156: 110925.

Maulida, D. and Zulkarnaen, N. (2010). Ekstraksi antioksidan (likopen) dari buah tomat dengan menggunakan solven campuran, n-heksana, aseton, dan etanol. (Extraction of antioxidants (lycopene) from tomatoes using mixed solvents, n-hexane, acetone, and ethanol). In: *Final Assignment Seminar for Bachelor Degree in Chemical Engineering UNDIP 2010*, 1–8. Indonesia: Department of Chemical Engineering.

Meyer, M., Schreck, R., and Baeuerle, P.A. (1993). H_2O_2 and antioxidants have opposite effects on activation of NF-kB and AP-1 in intact cells. AP-1 as secondary antioxidant response factor. *EMBO J.* 12: 2005–2015.

Miguel, F., Martin, A., Gamse, T., and Cocero, M.J. (2006). Supercritical anti solvent precipitation of lycopene: Effect of the operating parameters. *J. Supercrit. Fluids.* 36 (3): 225–235.

Miki, N. and Akatsu, K. (1970). Effect of heating sterilization on color of tomato juice. *J. Jpn. Food Ind.* 17 (5): 175–181.

Miller, N.J., Sampson, J., Candeias, L.P. et al. (1996). Antioxidant activities of carotenes and xanthophylls. *FEBS Lett.* 384 (3): 240–242.

Misra, R., Mangi, S., Joshi, S. et al. (2006). LycoRed as an alternative to hormone replacement therapy in lowering serum lipids and oxidative stress markers: a randomized controlled clinical trial. *J. Obstet. Gynaecol. Res.* 32 (3): 299–304.

Mohamadin, A.M., Elberry, A.A., Mariee, A.D. et al. (2012). Lycopene attenuates oxidative stress and heart lysosomal damage in isoproterenol induced cardiotoxicity in rats: a biochemical study. *Pathophysiology* 19 (2): 121–130.

Morel, I., Lescoat, G., Cogrel, P. et al. (1993). Antioxidant and iron-chelating activities of the flavonoids catechin, quercetin and diosmetin on iron-loaded rat hepatocyte cultures. *Biochem. Pharmacol.* 45 (1): 13–19.

Moriel, P., Sevanian, A., Ajzen, S. et al. (2002). Nitric oxide, cholesterol oxides and endotheliumdependent vasodilation in plasma of patients with essential hypertension. *Braz. J. Med. Biol. Res.* 35: 1301–1309.

Mortensen, A., Skibsted, L.H., Sampson, J. et al. (1997). Comparative mechanisms and rates of free radical scavenging by carotenoid antioxidants. *FEBS Lett.* 418: 91–97.

Mortensen, A., Skibsted, L.H., and Truscott, T.G. (2001). The interaction of dietarycarotenoids with radical species. *Arch. Biochem. Biophys.* 385: 13–19.

Most, M.M. (2004). Estimated phytochemical content of the dietary approaches to stop hypertension (DASH) diet is higher than in the control study diet. *Am. Diet Assoc.* 104: 1725–1727.

Nahum, A., Hirsch, K., and Danilenko, M. (2001). Lycopene inhibition of cell cycle progression in breast and endometrial cancer cells is associated with reduction in cyclin D levels and retention of p27(Kip1) in the cyclin E-cdk2 complexes. *Oncogene* 26: 3428–3436.

Nasri Nasrabadi, M. and Razavi, S. (2010). High levels lycopene accumulation by *Dietzia natronolimnaea* HS-1 using lycopene cyclase inhibitors in a fed-batch process. *Food Sci. Biotechnol.* 19 (4): 899–906.

Naviglio, D., Caruso, T., Iannece, P. et al. (2008). Characterization of high purity lycopene from tomato wastes using a new pressurized extraction approach. *J. Agric. Food chem.* 56 (15): 6227–6231.

Nazir, N. and Adrian, M.R. (2016). The improvement lycopene availability and antioxidant activities of tomato (*Lycopersicum esculentum*, Mill) Jelly drink. *Agric. Agric. Sci. Proc.* 9: 328–334.

Neuzil, J., Weber, C., and Kontush, A. (2001). The role of vitamin E in atherogenesis. Linking the chemical, biological and clinical aspects of the disease. *Atherosclerosis* 157: 257–283.

Neyestani, T.R., Shariatzadeh, N., Gharavi, A. et al. (2007). Physiological dose of lycopene suppressed oxidative stress and enhanced serum levels of immunoglobulin M in patients with Type 2 diabetes mellitus: a possible role in the prevention of long-term complications. *J. Endocrinol. Investig.* 30 (10): 833–838.

Nguyen, M.L. and Schwartz, S.J. (1998). Lycopene stability during food processing. *Proc. Soc. Exp. Biol. Med.* 218 (2): 101–105.

Nicolás-Molina, F., Navarro, E., and Ruiz-Vázquez, R. (2008). Lycopene over-accumulation by disruption of the negative regulator gene crgA in *Mucor circinelloides*. *Appl. Microbiol. Biotechnol.* 78 (1): 131–137.

Nobre BP, Pessoa FL, Palavra AF, Mendes RL.(2006). Supercritical CO_2 extraction of lycopene from tomato industrial waste. CHISA 2006—17th International Congress of Chemical and Process Engineering, Prague – Czech Republic (27–31 August).

Odriozola-Serrano, I., Soliva-Fortuny, R., Gimeno-Añó, V., and Martín-Belloso, O. (2008). Modeling changes in health-related compounds of tomato juice treated by high-intensity pulsed electric fields. *J. Food Eng.* 89 (2): 210–216.

Offord, E.A., Gautier, J.C., Avanti, O. et al. (2002). Photoprotective potential of lycopene, β-carotene, vitamin E, vitamin C and carnosic acid in UVAirradiated human skin fibroblasts. *Free Radic. Biol. Med.* 32: 1293–1303.

Okajima, E., Ozono, S., Endo, T. et al. (1997). Chemopreventive efficacy of piroxicam administered alone or in combination with lycopene and beta-carotene on the development of rat urinary bladder carcinoma after *N*-butyl-*N*-(4-hydroxybutyl)nitrosamine treatment. *Jpn. J. Cancer Res. Gann.* 88 (6): 543–552.

Olempska-Beer, Z. (2006). Lycopene (Synthetic) Chemical and Technical Assessment (CTA). Submitted to the Joint Expert Committee on Food Additives (JECFA), Rome.

Ollanketo, M., Hartonen, K., Riekkola, M.-L. et al. (2001). Supercritical carbon dioxide extraction of lycopene in tomato skins. *Eur. Food Res. Technol.* 212: 561–565.

Omer, E., Thapa, M., Hong, L., and Lianfu, Z. (2014). The influence of lycopene and other natural antioxidants on refined sunflower oil stability. *Int. J. Eng. Res. Technol.* 3 (3): 86–91.

Østerlie, M. and Lerfall, J. (2005). Lycopene from tomato products added minced meat: effect on storage quality and colour. *Food Res. Int.* 38 (8–9): 925–929.

Paiva, S.A.R. and Russell, R.M. (1999). β-Carotene and other carotenoids as antioxidants. *J. Am. Coll. Nutr.* 18 (5): 426–433.

Panda, A.K., Mishra, S., and Mohapatra, S.K. (2011). Iron in ayurvedic medicine. *J. Adv. Dev. Res.* 2: 287–293.

Paran, E. (2006). Reducing hypertension with tomato lycopene. In: *Tomatoes, Lycopene and Human Health* (ed. A.V. Rao), 169–182. Scotland: Caledonian Science Press.

Paran, E. and Engelhard, Y. (2001). Effect of Lyc-O-Mato, standardized tomato extract on blood pressure, serum lipoproteins plasma homocysteine and oxidative stress markers in grade 1 hypertensive patients. *Am. J. Hypertens* 14: 141A. Abstract P-333.

Pasupuleti, V. and Kulkarni, S.G. (2014). Lycopene fortification on the quality characteristics of beverage formulations developed from pink flesh guava (*Psidiumguajava L.*). *J. Food Sci. Technol.* 51 (12): 4126–4131.

Pool-Zobel, B., Bub, A., Müller, H. et al. (1997). Consumption of vegetables reduces genetic damage in humans: first results of a human intervention trial with carotenoid-rich foods. *Carcinogenesis* 18: 1847–1850.

Porrini, M., Riso, P., Brusamolino, A. et al. (2005). Daily intake of a formulated tomato drink affects carotenoid plasma and lymphocyte concentrations and improves cellular antioxidant protection. *Br. J. Nutr.* 93 (1): 93–99.

Prathibha, G. and Narayana, C.K. (2016). Influence of level of lycopene, antioxidants and other nutritional changes on fortification of lycopene powder in tomato juice. *Bioscan* 11 (3): 1437–1440.

Qiang, W., Ling-ran, F., Luo, W. et al. (2014). Mutation breeding of lycopene-producing strain *Blakeslea trispora* by a novel atmospheric and room temperature plasma (ARTP). *Appl. Biochem. Biotechnol.* 174 (1): 452–460.

Quek, S.Y., Chok, N.K., and Swedlund, P. (2007). The physicochemical properties of spray-dried watermelon powders. *Chem. Eng. Process. Process Intensif.* 46 (5): 386–392.

Rad, S., Zahiri, H., Noghabi, K. et al. (2012). Type 2 IDI performs better than type 1 for improving lycopene production in metabolically engineered *E. coli* strains. *World J. Microbiol. Biotechnol.* 28 (1): 313–321.

Rafi, M.M., Yadav, P.N., and Reyes, M. (2007). Lycopene inhibits LPS? Induced proinflammatory mediator inducible nitric oxide synthase in mouse macrophage cells. *J. Food Sci.* 72 (1): S069–S074.

Rao, A. and Agarwal, S. (1998). Bioavailability and in vivo antioxidant properties of lycopene from tomato products and their possible role in the prevention of cancer. *Nutr. Cancer.* 31: 199–203.

Rao, A.V. and Rao, L.G. (2007). Carotenoids and human health. *Pharmacol. Res.* 55: 207–216.

Rao, A.V. and Shen, H. (2002). Effect of low dose lycopene intake on lycopene bioavailability and oxidative stress. *Nutr. Res.* 22: 1125–1131.

Rao, A.V., Waseem, Z., and Agarwal, S. (1998). Lycopene content of tomatoes and tomato products and their contribution to dietary lycopene. *Food Res. Int.* 31: 737–741.

Rao, L.G., Mackinnon, E.S., Josse, R.G. et al. (2007). Lycopene consumption decreases oxidative stress and bone resorption markers in postmenopausal women. *Osteoporos. Int.* 18 (1): 109–115.

Rayhan, M., Mumtaz, B., Motalab, M. et al. (2019). Extraction and quantification of lycopene, β-carotene and total phenolic contents from papaya (*carica papaya*) and formulation of lycopene enriched fruit drinks. *Am. J. Food Nutr.* 7 (2): 55–63.

Richardson, D.P. (1990). Food fortification. *Proc. Nutr. Soc.* 49 (1): 39–50.

Richelle, M., Bortlik, K., Liardet, S. et al. (2002). A food-based formulation provides lycopene with the same bioavailability to humans as that from tomato paste. *J. Nutr.* 132 (3): 404–408.

Ried, K. and Fakler, P. (2011). Protective effect of lycopene on serum cholesterol and blood pressure: meta-analyses of intervention trials. *Maturitas* 68 (4): 299–310.

Riso, P., Pinder, A., Santangelo, A., and Porrini, M. (1999). Does tomato consumption effectively increase the resistance of lymphocyte DNA to oxidative damage? *Am. J. Clin. Nutr.* 69 (4): 712–718.

Rissanen, T., Voutilainen, S., Nyyssönen, K., and Salonen, J.T. (2002). Lycopene, atherosclerosis, and coronary heart disease. *Exp. Biol. Med.* 227 (10): 900–907.

Rittié, L. and Fisher, G.J. (2002). UV-light-induced signal cascades and skin aging. *Ageing Res. Rev.* 1: 705–720.

Rodriguez-Amaya, D.B. (2001). *A Guide to Carotenoid Analysis in Foods*, 1–45. Washington, D.C.: ILSI Press.

Rodriguez-Amaya, D.B. and Kimura, M. (2004). Carotenoids in foods. In: *Harvestplus Handbook for Carotenoid Analysis*, 2–7. Washington, DC: IFPRI and CIAT.

Rozzi, N.L., Singh, R.K., Vierling, R.A., and Watkins, B.A. (2002). Supercritical fluid extraction oflycopene from tomato processing byproducts. *J. Agric. Food Chem.* 50: 2638–2643.

Sabio, E., Lozano, M., Montero de Espinosa, V. et al. (2003). Lycopene and β-carotene extraction from tomato processing waste using supercritical CO_2. *Ind. Eng. Chem. Res.* 42 (25): 6641–6646.

Salman, H., Bergman, M., Djaldetti, M., and Bessler, H. (2007). Lycopene affects proliferation and apoptosis of four malignant cell lines. *Biomed. Pharmacother.* 61: 366–369.

Salonen, J.T., Korpela, H., Salonen, R. et al. (1992). Autoantibody against oxidized LDL and progression of carotid atherosclerosis. *Lancet* 339: 883–887.

Sandei, L. and Leoni, C. (2004). Exploitation of by-products (solid wastes) from tomato processing to obtain high value antioxidants. *IX Int. Symp. Process. Tomato* 724: 249–257.

Sarkar, F.H., Li, Y., Wang, Z., and Kong, D. (2009). Cellular signalling perturbation by natural products. *Cell Signal.* 21: 1541–1547.

Schieber, A., Stintzing, F.C., and Carle, R. (2001). By-products of plant food processing as a source of functional compounds—recent developments. *Trends Food Sci. Technol.* 12: 401–413.

Schmitz, H.H., Poor, C.L., Wellman, R., and Erdman, J.W. Jr. (1991). Concentrations of selected carotenoids and vitamin A in human liver, kidney and lung tissue. *J. Nutr.* 121: 1613–1621.

Schrek, R. and Bauerle, P.A. (1991). Reactive oxygen intermediates as apparently widely used messengers in the activation of NF-kB transcription factor and HIV-1. *Trends Cell Biol.* 1: 39–42.

Scolastici, C., Alves de Lima, R.O., Barbisan, L.F. et al. (2007). Lycopene activity against chemically induced DNA damage in Chinese hamster ovary cells. *Toxicol. In Vitro* 21: 840–845.

Scolastici, C., Alves de Lima, R.O., Barbisan, L.F. et al. (2008). Antigenotoxicity and antimutagenicity of lycopene in HepG2 cell line evaluated by the comet assay and micronucleus test. *Toxicol. In Vitro* 22: 510–514.

Seo, Y., Masamune, A., Shimosegawa, T., and Kim, H. (2009). Protective effect of lycopene on oxidative stress-induced cell death of pancreatic acinar cells Jeong. *Ann. N.Y. Acad. Sci.* 1171: 570–575.

Sesso, H.D., Liu, S., Gaziano, J.M., and Buring, J.E. (2003). Dietary lycopene, tomato-based food products and cardiovascular disease in women. *J. Nutr.* 133 (7): 2336–2341.

Sharma, S.K. and Le Maguer, M. (1996a). Lycopene in tomatoes and tomato pulp fractions. *Ital. J. Food Sci.* 2: 107–113.

Sharma, S.K. and Le Maguer, M. (1996b). Kinetics of lycopene degradation in tomato pulp solids under different processing and storage conditions. *Food Res. Int.* 29 (3–4): 309–315.

Sharma, J.B., Kumar, A., Kumar, A. et al. (2003). Effect of lycopene on pre-eclampsia and intra-uterine growth retardation in primigravidas. *Int. J. Gynecol. Obstet.* 81 (3): 257–262.

Sharoni, Y., Danilenko, M., Dubi, N. et al. (2004). Carotenoids and transcription. *Arc. Biochem. Biophys.* 430 (1): 89–96.

Shi, J. and Le Maguer, M. (2000). Lycopene in tomatoes: Chemical and physical properties affected by food processing. *Crit. Rev. Food Sci. Nutr.* 40: 1–42.

Shi, Y.Q., Xin, X.L., and Yuan, Q.P. (2012). Improved lycopene production by *Blakeslea trispora* with isopentenyl compounds and metabolic precursors. *Biotechnol. Lett.* 34 (5): 849–852.

Shimada, H., Kondo, K., Fraser, P.D. et al. (2014). Increased carotenoid production by the food yeast *Candida utilis* through metabolic engineering of the isoprenoid pathway. *Appl. Environ. Microbiol.* 64 (7): 2676–2680.

Shu, B., Yu, W., Zhao, Y., and Liu, X. (2006). Study on microencapsulation of lycopene by spray-drying. *J. Food Eng.* 76 (4): 664–669.

Squina, F.M. and Mercadante, A.Z. (2005). Influence of nicotine and diphenylamine on the carotenoid composition of rhodotorula strains. *J. Food Biochem.* 29 (6): 638–652.

Stacewicz-Sapuntzakis, M. and Bowen, P.E. (2005). Role of lycopene and tomato products in prostate health. *Biochim. Biophys. Acta-Mol. Basis Dis.* 1740: 202–205.

Stahl, W. and Sies, H. (1992). Uptake of lycopene and its geometrical isomers is greater from heat-processed than from unprocessed tomato juice in humans. *J. Nutr.* 122: 2161–2166.

Stahl, W., von Laar, J., Martin, H.D. et al. (2000). Stimulation of gap junctional communication: comparison of acyclo-retinoic acid and lycopene. *Arch. Biochem. Biophys.* 1: 271–274.

Stahl, W., Heinrich, U., Aust, O. et al. (2006). Lycopene-rich products and dietary photoprotection. *Phytochem. Photobiol. Sci.* 5: 238–242.

Stein, B., Rahmsdorf, H.J., Steffen, A. et al. (1989). UVinduced DNA damage is an intermediate step in UV-induced expression of human immunodeficiency virus type 1, collagenase, cfos, and metallothionein. *Mol. Cell. Biol.* 9: 5169–5181.

Suganuma, H., Hirano, T., Arimoto, Y., and Inakuma, T. (2002). Effect of tomato intake on striatal monoamine level in a mouse model of experimental parkimson's disease. *J Nutr. Sci. Vitiminol.* 48: 251–254.

Sumarni, N.K. and Ibrahim, N. (2019). The organoleptic quality of noodles and functional grits with fortified lycopene coated bymaltodextrin during storage. *J. Phys. Conf. Ser.* 1242 (1): 012006. IOP Publishing.

Sun, Y., Yuan, Q.-P., and Vriesekoop, F. (2007). Effect of two ergosterol biosynthesis inhibitors on lycopene production by *Blakeslea trispora*. *Process Biochem.* 42: 1460–1464.

Sun, T., Miao, L., Li, Q. et al. (2014). Production of lycopene by metabolically-engineered *Escherichia coli*. *Biotechnol. Lett.* 36 (7): 1515–1522.

Tapiero, H., Townsend, D.M., and Tew, K.D. (2004). The role of carotenoids in the prevention of human pathologies. *Biomed. Pharmacother.* 58: 100–110.

Tavares, C.A. and Rodriguez-Amaya, D.B. (1994). Carotenoid composition of Brazilian tomatoes and tomato products. *Lebensm. Wiss. U. Technol.* 27: 219–224.

Tinkler, J.H., Böhm, F., Schalch, W., and Truscott, T.G. (1994). Dietary carotenoids protect human cells from damage. *J. Photochem. Photobiol. B: Biol.* 26 (3): 283–285.

Tonucci, L.H., Holden, J.M., Beecher, G.R. et al. (1995). Carotenoid content of thermally processed tomato-based food products. *J. Agric. Food Chem.* 43: 579–586.

Topal, U., Sasaki, M., Goto, M., and Hayakawa, K. (2006). Extraction of lycopene from tomato skin with supercritical carbon dioxide: effect of operating conditions and solubility analysis. *J. Agric. Food Chem.* 54 (15): 5604–5610.

Touyz, R.M. and Schiffrin, E.L. (2006). Peroxisome proliferator-activated receptors in vascular biology-molecular mechanisms and clinical implications. *Vasc. Pharmacol.* 45: 19–28.

Trosko, J.E. and Chang, C.C. (2001). Mechanism of up-regulated gap junctional intercellular communication during chemoprevention and chemotherapy of cancer. *Mutat. Res.* 480/481: 219–229.

Urbonavičienė D, Bobinaitė R, Viškelis J, et al. (2015). Characterisation of tomato juice and different tomato-based juice blends fortified with isomerised lycopene extract. *Proceedings of the 7th International Scientific Conference Rural Development*, Lithuania. doi:10.15544/RD.2015.029.

Vági, E., Simándi, B., Vásárhelyiné, K.P. et al. (2007). Supercritical carbon dioxide extraction of carotenoids, tocopherols and sitosterols from industrial tomato by-products. *J. Supercrit. Fluids.* 40 (2): 218–226.

Vasapollo, G., Longo, L., Rescio, L., and Ciurlia, L. (2004). Innovative supercritical CO_2 extraction of lycopene from tomato in the presence of vegetable oil as co-solvent. *J. Supercrit. Fluids.* 29 (1–2): 87–96.

Vereschagina, O.A., Memorskaya, A.S., and Tereshina, V.M. (2010). The role of exogenous lipids in lycopene synthesis in the mucoraceous fungus *Blakeslea trispora*. *Microbiology* 79 (5): 593–601.

Visioli, F., Riso, P., Grande, S. et al. (2003). Protective activity of tomato products on in vivo markers of lipid oxidation. *Eur. J. Nutr.* 42 (1): 201–206.

Vogele, A.C. (1937). Effect of environmental factors upon the color of the tomato and the watermelon. *Plant Physiol. 12*: 929–955.

Wang, J., Liu, X., Liu, R. et al. (2012). Optimization of the mated fermentation process for the production of lycopene by Blakeslea trispora NRRL 2895 (+) and NRRL 2896 (−). *Bioprocess Biosyst. Eng.* 35 (4): 553–564.

Wang, H.-B., He, F., Lu, M.-B. et al. (2014). High-quality lycopene overaccumulation via inhibition of γ-carotene and ergosterolbiosyntheses in *Blakeslea trispora*. *J. Funct. Foods.* 7 (0): 435–442.

Wang, Q., Feng, L.R., Luo, W. et al. (2015). Effect of inoculation process on lycopene production by *Blakeslea trispora* in a stirred-tank reactor. *Appl. Biochem. Biotechnol.* 175 (2): 770–779.

Wertz, K. (2009). Lycopene effects contributing to prostate health. *Nutr. Cancer* 61 (6): 775–783.

Xi, J. (2006). Effect of high pressure processing on the extraction of lycopene in tomato paste waste. *Chem. Eng. Technol. Ind. Chem. Plant Equip. Process Eng. Biotechnol.* 29 (6): 736–739.

Xu, Y., Leo, M.A., and Lieber, C.S. (2003). Lycopene attenuates alcoholic apoptosis in HepG2 cells expressing CYP2E1. *Biochem. Biophys. Res. Commun.* 308: 614–618.

Xu, F., Yuan, Q., and Zhu, Y. (2007). Improved production of lycopene and β-carotene by *Blakesle trispora* with oxygen-vectors. *Process Biochem.* 42 (2): 289–293.

Yang, S.X., Shi, W., and Zeng, J. (2004). Modelling the supercritical fluid extraction of lycopene from tomato paste waste using neuro-fuzzy approaches. In: *International Symposium on Neural Networks*, 880–885. Berlin, Heidelberg: Springer.

Yılmaz, I., Şimşek, O., and Işıklı, M. (2002). Fatty acid composition and quality characteristics of low-fat cooked sausages made with beef and chicken meat, tomato juice and sunflower oil. *Meat Sci.* 62 (2): 253–258.

Yoon, K.W., Doo, E.H., Kim, S.W., and Park, J.B. (2008). In situ recovery of lycopene during biosynthesis with recombinant *Escherichia coli*. *J. Biotechnol.* 135 (3): 291–294.

Young, A.J. and Lowe, G.M. (2001). Antioxidant and prooxidant properties of carotenoids. *Arch. Biochem. Biophys.* 385: 20–27.

Zardini, A.A., Mohebbi, M., Farhoosh, R., and Bolurian, S. (2018). Production and characterization of nanostructured lipid carriers and solid lipid nanoparticles containing lycopene for food fortification. *J. Food Sci. Technol.* 55 (1): 287–298.

Zaripheh, S., Nara, T.Y., Nakamura, M.T., and Erdman, J.W. Jr. (2006). Dietary lycopene downregulates carotenoid 15,159-monooxygenase and PPAR – in selected rat tissues. *J. Nutr.* 136: 932–938.

Zhang, L.X., Cooney, R.V., and Bertram, J. (1991). carotenoids enhance gap junctional communication and inhibit lipid peroxidation in C3H/10T1/2 cells: relationship to their cancer preventive action. *Carcinogenesis* 12: 2109–2114.

Zhang, T.-C., Li, W., Luo, X.-G. et al. (2015). Increase of the lycopene production in the recombinant strains of *Escherichia coli* by supplementing with fructose. *Lect. Notes Electr. Eng.* 332: 29–35.

Zhao, X., Aldini, G., Johnson, E.J. et al. (2006). Modification of lymphocyte DNA damage by carotenoid supplementation in postmenopausal women. *Am. J. Clin. Nutr.* 83 (1): 163–169.

Zhu, F., Lu, L., Fu, S. et al. (2015). Targeted engineering and scale up of lycopene overproduction in *Escherichia coli*. *Process Biochem.* 50 (3): 341–346.

Zuorro, A., Lavecchia, R., Medici, F., and Piga, L. (2013). Enzyme-assisted production of tomato seed oil enriched with lycopene from tomato pomace. *Food Bioprocess Technol.* 6 (12): 3499–3509.

12

Nutraceutical Compounds from Marine Microalgae

K. Renugadevi[1], C. Valli Nachiyar[1], Jayshree Nellore[1], Swetha Sunkar[2], and S. Karthick Raja Namasivayam[1]

[1] *Department of Biotechnology, Sathyabama Institute of Science and Technology, Chennai, Tamil Nadu, India*
[2] *Department of Bioinformatics, Sathyabama Institute of Science and Technology, Chennai, Tamil Nadu, India*

12.1   Introduction

With an increase in industrialization, the lifestyle of human beings has drastically changed. Food habits, poor food quality, contaminated food, increased work pressure, and pollution have deteriorated human health. This has also caused oxidative stress-related diseases like cancers, vascular diseases, physiological disorders, etc. (Sanjukta 2017). To overcome these issues, the recent research interests mainly focus on the exploration of nutraceutical compounds from microbes, especially microalgae due to their significant therapeutic properties, which can help in improving human health. Nutraceuticals are also called medical foods that have the property to improve health or prevent diseases. It includes compounds like vitamins, minerals, antioxidant supplements, medicinal foods etc. They are used to treat diseases like Parkinson's disease, Alzheimer's disease, obesity, diabetes, cancer, and coronary heart disease. It involves an array of biological processes like activation of endogenous antioxidant defences, cell survival-associated gene expression, signal transduction pathways, mitochondrial integrity preservation, etc., which help in fighting the various age-related diseases (Mandel et al. 2005).

12.2   Marine Environment

Marine or ocean is a resource of ample variety of organisms due to its diversified environment with different oceanic zones. Out of the known 33 animal phyla, 32 phyla exist in the marine environment, out of which 15 wholly exist in the marine environment (Margulis and Schwartz 1998). Since ancient times, mankind has exploited numerous marine resources for their nutritional value, pharmaceutical property as well as economic uses. One of the major resources which are exploited is food resources from marine animals like fish and algae. The marine environment is an excellent warehouse for the exploration of novel potential metabolites with varied structural and chemical features distinct from the terrestrial metabolites. In recent decades, researchers are focusing on the exploration of new metabolites with potential pharmaceutical activity from marine organisms. Most of these molecules are secondary metabolites that are not produced by regular metabolic

Handbook of Nutraceuticals and Natural Products: Biological, Medicinal, and Nutritional Properties and Applications,
Volume 1, First Edition. Edited by Sreerag Gopi and Preetha Balakrishnan.

pathways and are not vital for their growth and development processes. Marine organisms like sponges, fish, tunicates, molluscs, corals, worms, bryozoa, algae, fungi, and bacteria are adventured for their metabolites (Malve 2016). The metabolites from these organisms were found to have activities like antibacterial, anti-inflammatory, neuroprotective, antiparasitic, antiviral agents, anticancer, analgesic, and antimalarial activities. Nearly, 13000 molecules have been discovered and out of these, 3000 were found to have potential activities (Vignesh et al. 2011). The recent focus of marine pharmacology is on marine microbes like microalgae, bacteria, and fungi.

12.3 Algae

Algae are simple, a vast group of photosynthetic unicellular or multicellular organisms that can exist in a diverse ecosystem like soil, freshwater, marine water, and wastewater. They are the major producers of water ecosystem (Renugadevi et al. 2014). Based on their size, algae can be classified as microalgae or macroalgae. Macroalgae or seaweeds are multicellular and possess plant-like characteristics, whereas microalgae or phytoplankton are unicellular. Many microalgae are autotrophs that use photosynthesis. Some are heterotrophs that can grow in dark by consuming sugars. Few are mixotrophs that grow by combining both autotrophic and heterotrophic modes of nutrition.

12.4 Cyanobacteria

Cyanobacteria, blue-green algae, are classified under gram-negative bacteria, considered as the primitive form of life on earth that originated approximately 2.6–3.5 billion years ago (Hedges et al. 2001, Devendra et al. 2014). They can exist as unicellular, filamentous, colonial, and planktonic. They can thrive in marine, freshwater, and terrestrial environments. Various value-added products like vitamins, carbohydrates, enzymes, proteins, amino acids, and fatty acids are produced by heterotrophic methods from cyanobacteria.

12.5 Microalgae

Microalgae are one of the most primitive forms of life on earth over 3 billion years ago. Microalgae include prokaryotic cyanobacteria and eukaryotic microalgae. More than 50000 different microalgal species exist in marine and freshwater (Ramaraj et al. 2019). The most commonly explored microalgal species are Cyanophyceae (blue-green algae), Bacillariophyceae (diatoms), Chlorophyceae (green algae), and Chryophyceae (brown algae) (Valli and Renugadevi 2015). Some of the nutraceutical compounds from microalgae are polyols, polyunsaturated fatty acids, phycobiliproteins, carotenoids, polysaccharides, antioxidants, etc., and they are found to have antioxidant, antimicrobial, antiviral, antifungal activities, anti-inflammatory, anticancer, and act as immune modulators (Table 12.1).

The commonly exploited microalgae for their nutraceutical compounds are species of cyanobacteria used are *Spirulina maxima* and *Spirulina platensis* (Guedes et al. 2011), and eukaryotic microalgae are *Chlorella vulgaris*, *Chlorella pyrenoidosa*, *Chlamydomonas reinhardtii*, *Crypthecodinium*, *Dunaliella salina* (Plaza et al. 2009), *Dunaliella primolecta* (Ohta et al. 1998), *Diacronema*, *Euglenaviridis*, *Gonyostomium semen*, *Haematococcus pluvialis* (Plaza et al. 2009), *Isochrysis*, *Tribonemaaequala*, *Acuolariavirescens*, *Pleurochloris meiringensis* (Oono et al. 1995), *Porphyridium*

Table 12.1 List of valuable microalgal metabolites and their uses.

Type of metabolite	Metabolite name	Uses
Pigments	Phycocyanin	Colorant for health food and cosmetics (lipsticks and eyeliners) Chu (2012), antioxidant property (Renugadevi et al. 2018), anti-inflammation (Romay et al. 1998), hepatoprotectant (Vadiraja et al. 1998; Gonzalez et al. 2003; Sathyasaikumar et al. 2007; Ou et al. 2010), nephroprotectant (Fernandez et al. 2014; Rodríguez et al. 2012; Farooq et al. 2006), neuroprotectant (Pentón et al. 2011), oxidative stress protectant (Riss et al. 2007), brain mitochondria protection (Marín et al. 2012), lung protection (Sun et al. 2011, Leung et al. 2013), cardioprotection (Khan et al. 2006), and eyes' protection (Kumari and Anbarasu 2014)
	Phycoerythrin	Food colorant, fluorescent probes, tool for biomedical research, diagnostic (Chu 2012; Ramaraj et al. 2019)
	Allophycocyanin	Food colorant, used in cosmetics, antioxidant
	α-Carotene	Lowers premature death risk (Matsukawa et al. 2000; Ramaraj et al. 2019)
	Astaxanthin	Potent antioxidant, prevents age-related macular degeneration, photoprotective effect, anti-inflammatory activity, anticancer activity, prevents cardiovascular diseases, detoxificant, neuroprotectant, feed for salmon fish, ornamental fish, hen, shrimp, protects skin from UV radiation (Todd Lorenz and Cysewski 2000)
	β-Carotene	Food colorant, antioxidant activity, anticancer property, prevents night blindness, prevents liver fibrosis (Chu 2012, Ramaraj et al. 2019)
	Canthaxanthin	Tanning pills, food colorant, antioxidant (Leya et al. 2009)
	Fucoxanthin	Antioxidant, antiobese, anticancer, anti-inflammatory effect, antimalarial activity, antiangiogenic property (Kim et al. 2012a, b; Eilers et al. 2016; Crupi et al. 2013)
	Lutein	Reduces the risks of cataract and age-related macular degeneration, potent antioxidant, anticancer property, anti-inflammatory effect, prevents cardiovascular diseases (Matsukawa et al. 2000; Ramaraj et al. 2019)
	Zeaxanthin	Prevents age-related macular degeneration, antioxidant activity, neutralizes free radicals, and prevents both nonalcoholic fatty liver disease and alcoholic fatty liver disease (Leya et al. 2009)
Fatty acids	α-Linolenic acid	Preventative effect against cardiovascular diseases (Martinez-Fernandez et al. 2006)
	Arachidonic acid (AA)	Nutritional supplements (Zhang et al. 2002)
	Docosahexenoic acid (DHA)	Infant formula and baby food, nutritional supplements, aquaculture feed (Chu 2012)
	Eicosapentaenoic acid (EPA)	Prevents heart attacks, reduces blood clots, prevents vision loss due to age-related macular degeneration, anticancer property, Nutritional supplements, aquaculture feed (Chu 2012)
	γ-Linolenic acid (GLA)	Nutritional supplements, medicine for skin diseases like psoriasis, eczema, systemic sclerosis, and anticancer property (Chu 2012)
	Linolenic acid	Anti-inflammatory, acne reductive, moisture-retentive properties (Day et al. 2009)
	Stearidonic acid	To treat acne, skin diseases, inflammation, rheumatoid arthritis, increasing tissue EPA concentrations in tissues (Martinez-Fernandez et al. 2006)

(Continued)

Table 12.1   (Continued)

Type of metabolite	Metabolite name	Uses
Vitamins	Vitamin B	Reduces fatigue, reduces depression, prevents heart disease, protects the skin, and anticancer property (Becker 2004)
	Vitamin C	Prevents cardiovascular disease, protects prenatal health issues, prevents eye disease, and reduces skin wrinkling (Becker 2004)
	Vitamin E	Protects against free radicals, prevents eye disorders, anti-Alzheimer's disease, and antidiabetic properties (Becker 2004; Matsukawa et al. 2000)
Poly-saccharides	Sulfated polysaccharides	Anticoagulant, antiviral, antioxidative, anticancer activities (Mohamed 2008)
	Extracellular polysaccharides	Antioxidants and used in cosmetics
Sterols	Sterols	Antidiabetic, anticancer, anti-inflammatory, anti-photoaging, anti-obesity, anti-inflammatory, and antioxidant activity (Cardozo et al. 2007)
Glutathione	Glutathione	Prevents heart attack, antioxidant property, anticancer activity, prevents Parkinson's disease, detoxifies the metals, and controls blood pressure (Li et al. 2004)
Glycerol	Glycerol	Controls skin drying and acts as a moisturizer (Hadi et al. 2008)

species, *Nannochloropsis*, *Nitzschia*, *Phaedactylum*, and *Schizochytrim* (Simopoulos 2002). They have been exploited for their value-added products like protein, vitamins, polysaccharides, fatty acids, phycotoxins, polysaccharides, etc. (Table 12.1).

Microalgae are found to contain approximately 40% of lipids, 50% of proteins, and 10% of carbohydrates. Due to their value-dded products, they are cultivated on a large scale. Some of the microalgae and their potential metabolites are listed in Table 12.2. Asia is the major commercial microalgal producer and most of the producers are in China, India, and Taiwan.

12.6   Cultivation Strategies of Microalgae

Mass cultivation of microalgae or cyanobacteria can be carried out by photoautotrophic, photoheterotrophic, heterotrophic, and mixotrophic processes. The most common mass cultivation process is a photoautotrophic method which utilizes sunlight as an energy source and atmospheric CO_2 as a carbon source. Open system or outdoor cultivation is one of the photoautotrophic methods. Advantages of this process are (i) can utilize abundant sunlight and CO_2 from nature, (ii) easy to install and operate, (iii) cheaper, (iv) less consumption of energy source like electrical and mechanical for agitation of culture during the process (Brennan and Owende 2010). The major disadvantages of this process are (i) limited to certain species which do not get easily contaminated, (ii) depth of the system limited to 20 cm, biomass yield is less than 10 g/l in outdoor open pond or raceway pond cultivation, whereas, in photobioreactor process, maximum yield is around 40 g/l (Jianjun et al. 2018; Xianhai et al. 2011). *Spirulina*, *Dunaliela* and *Chlorella* are grown for single cell protein (SCP) and pigment production by open system method. Closed cultivation in photobioreactors is used for the production of pharmaceutical compounds, which requires the maintenance of axenic cultures. This requires the designing, installation, and operating of photobioreactors which are costly.

Table 12.2 List of microalgae and their valuable metabolites (Ramaraj et al. 2019).

Genus	Microalgae	Valuable metabolites
Aphanizomenon	*Aphanizomenon flosaquae*	Mycosporine-like amino acids (MAAs)
Anabaena	*Anabaena flos-aquae*	Anatoxin, Saxitoxin
Ankistrodesmus	*Ankistrodesmus braunii*	Astaxanthin
	Ankitrodesmus spp.	α-Linolenic acid, Hexadecatetraenoic acid
	Ankitrodesmus spiralis	MAAs
Aurora	*Aurora* sp.	EPA
Botryococcus	*Botryococcus braunii*	Lutein, Triglycerides and hydrocarbons, Linolenic acid, β-carotene
Chaetoceros	*Chaetoceros calcitrans*	Fucoxanthin, Triglycerides and hydrocarbons
	Chaetoceros gracilis	Fucoxanthin
	Chaetoceros muelleri	Triglycerides and hydrocarbons
Characium	*Characium californicum*	Triglycerides and hydrocarbons
	Characium oviforme	Triglycerides and hydrocarbons
Chlamydomonas	*Chlamydomonas acidophila*	β-Carotene, Lutein
	Chlamydomonas eugametos,	Vitamin B
	Chlamydomonas moewusii	α-Linolenic acid, Hexadecatetraenoic acid, Linolenic acid
	Chlamydomonas nivalis,	MAAs, Phenolic antioxidant, Astaxanthin, β-carotene, Canthaxanthin, Lutein, Zeaxanthin
	Chlamydomonas pulsatilla	Glycerol
	Chlamydomonas reinhardtii	Glycerol, Vitamin C, Vitamin E
Chlorella	*Chlorella emersonii*	Canthaxanthin, Triglycerides and hydrocarbons
	Chlorella fusa	Astaxanthin, Canthaxanthin, Lutein
	Chlorella homosphaera	γ-Linolenic acid (GLA)
	Chlorella luteo-viridis	MAAs, Triglycerides and hydrocarbons
	Chlorella minutissima	MAAs, EPA
	Chlorella protothecoides	Lutein, Triglycerides and hydrocarbons, Linolenic acid, Vitamin C
	Chlorella pyrenoidosa	Lutein, Polysaccharides, Vitamin B, Vitamin E,
	Chlorella sorokiniana	Vitamin E, MAAs, a-carotene, b-carotene, Lutein, Triglycerides and hydrocarbons
	Chlorella sphaerica	MAAs
	Chlorella stigmatophora	Polysaccharides
	Chlorella vulgaris	Vitamin C, Vitamin E, Astaxanthin, Canthaxanthin, Lutein, Triglycerides and hydrocarbons, Sulfonated polysaccharides, α-linolenic acid, EPA, Linolenic acid, Glycoprotein, Vitamin C, Vitamin E
	Chlorella zofingiensis	Astaxanthin, Canthaxanthin, Lutein
Chloridella	*Chloridella neglecta*	Triglycerides and hydrocarbons
	Chloridella simplex	Triglycerides and hydrocarbons

(Continued)

Table 12.2 (Continued)

Genus	Microalgae	Valuable metabolites
Chlorococcum	*Chlorococcum citriforme*	Lutein
	Chlorococcum costazygoticum	Triglycerides and hydrocarbons
	Chlorococcum infusionum	Triglycerides and hydrocarbons
	Chlorococcum submarinum	Glycerol
Chloromonas	*Chloromonas nivalis*	MAAs
Chromulina	*Chromulina ochromonoides*	Fucoxanthin
Coccomyxa	*Coccomyxa chodati*	Triglycerides and hydrocarbons
Coelastrella	*Coelastrella striolata*	Astaxanthin, β-carotene, Canthaxanthin, Triglycerides and hydrocarbons
Coelastrum	*Coelastrum proboscideum*	Lutein
Crypthecodinium	*Crypthecodinium cohnii*	Essential fatty acids-40–50% DHA, Triglycerides and hydrocarbons
Cylindrotheca	*Cylindrotheca closterium*	Fucoxanthin
Dunaliella	*Dunaliella bardawil*	β-Carotene, α-linolenic acid, Hexadecatetraenoic acid, Linolenic acid
	Dunaliella primolecta	γ-Linolenic acid (GLA), Linolenic acid
	Dunaliella salina	β-Carotene, lutein, Zeaxanthin, Glycerol, Triglycerides and hydrocarbons, α-linolenic acid
	Dunaliella tertiolecta	Vitamin C, Vitamin E, β-carotene, lutein, α-linolenic acid, Hexadecatetraenoic acid, Linolenic acid
Euglena	*Euglena gracillis*	Triglycerides and hydrocarbons
Geitlerinema	*Geitlerinema* sp.	Phycocyanin (Renugadevi et al. 2018), Anticancer activity (Srivastava et al. 2015)
Haematococcus	*Haematococcus lacustris*	Astaxanthin, Canthaxanthin
	Haematococcus pluvalis	Astaxanthin
Isochrysis	*Isochrysis aff. galbana*	Fucoxanthin
	Isochrysis galbana	Fucoxanthin, Triglycerides and hydrocarbons
Lobochlamys	*Lobochlamys culleus*	Triglycerides and hydrocarbons
	Lobochlamys segnis	Triglycerides and hydrocarbons
Microcystis	*Microcystis aeruginosa*	Microcystins
Micromonas	*Micromonas pusilla*	α-Linolenic acid, Linolenic acid
Monallanthus	*Monallanthus salina*	Triglycerides and hydrocarbons
Monodus	*Monodus subterraneus*	Triglycerides and hydrocarbons
Monoraphidium	*Monoraphidium arcuatum*	Triglycerides and hydrocarbons
	Monoraphidium contortum	Triglycerides and hydrocarbons
	Monoraphidium dybowskii	Triglycerides and hydrocarbons
	Monoraphidium griffithii	Triglycerides and hydrocarbons
	Monoraphidium neglectum	Triglycerides and hydrocarbons
	Monoraphidium terrestre	Triglycerides and hydrocarbons
	Monoraphidium tortile	Triglycerides and hydrocarbons

Table 12.2 (Continued)

Genus	Microalgae	Valuable metabolites
Nannochloris	*Nannochloris atomus*	α-Linolenic acid, Arachidonic acid (AA), EPA, Linolenic acid
	Nannochloris eucaryotum	EPA, Triglycerides and hydrocarbons
Nannochloropsis	*Nannochloropsis oculata*	EPA, Triglycerides and hydrocarbons
Muriella	*Muriella aurantiaca*	Lutein, Triglycerides and hydrocarbons
Navicula	*Navicula salinicola*	Triglycerides and hydrocarbons
Neochloris	*Neochloris oleaobundans*	Linolenic acid
Neospongiococcum	*Neospongiococcum gelatinosum*	Lutein
Nitzschia	*Nitzschia* sp.	EPA
Nostoc	*Nostoc* sp.	γ-Linolenic acid (GLA)
Ochromonas	*Ochromonas danica*	Fucoxanthin
Odontella	*Odontella aurita*	Fucoxanthin
Parachlorella	*Parachlorella kessleri*	Triglycerides and hydrocarbons
Pavlova	*Pavlova lutheri*	Triglycerides and hydrocarbons
	Pavlova salina	Triglycerides and hydrocarbons
Pediastrum	*Pediastrum boryanum*	Arachidonic acid (AA)
Phaeodactylum	*Phaeodactylum tricornutum*	Fucoxanthin, Triglycerides and hydrocarbons
Pleurastrum	*Pleurastrum insigne*	Triglycerides and hydrocarbons
Porphyridium	*Porphyridium cruentum*	Phycoerythrin
Prototheca	*Prototheca moriformis*	Vitamin C
Prymnesium	*Prymnesium parvum*	Fucoxanthin
Pseudokirchneriella	*Pseudokirchneriella subcapitata*	α-Linolenic acid, Linolenic acid
Pyramimonas	*Pyramimonas amylifera*	β-Carotene
	Pyramimonas cf. cordata	Sterols
	Pyramimonas obovata	β-Carotene
	Pyramimonas urceolata	Lutein
Sarcinochrysis	*Sarcinochrysis marina*	Fucoxanthin
Scenedesmus	*Scenedesmus acutus*	Vitamin B, Vitamin C, Vitamin E, α-linolenic acid
	Scenedesmus almeriensis	Lutein
	Scenedesmus armatus	Lutein
	Scenedesmus obliquus	Astaxanthin, α-linolenic acid, Linolenic acid, Vitamin B, Vitamin C, Vitamin E
	Scenedesmus quadricauda	Vitamin B, Vitamin C, Vitamin E, Sulfonated polysaccharides, α-linolenic acid
Spirulina	*Spirulina platensis*	Phycocyanin, γ-linolenic acid (GLA), linolenic and γ-linolenic acid, and ω-3 and ω-6 polyunsaturated fatty acids, Gamma-linolenic acid, Docohexaenoic acid (DHA),

(Continued)

Table 12.2 (Continued)

Genus	Microalgae	Valuable metabolites
Tetracystis	*Tetracystis intermedium*	Lutein
	Tetracystis tetrasporum	Lutein
Tetraselmis	*Tetraselmis suecica*	α-Linolenic acid, EPA, Hexadecatetraenoic acid, Linolenic acid, Sterols, Vitamin E
	Tetraselmis wettsteinii	β-Carotene, lutein

Growing microalgae in the absence of light, using organic carbon sources in a conventional bioreactor is heterotrophic cultivation, which is used for the economic cultivation of microalgae. Several obligate heterotrophs like thraustochytrids are cultivated by the heterotrophic method for the production of polyunsaturated fatty acids (Jianjun et al. 2018). Several microalgal species like *Chorella vulgaris*, *Chlorella zofingensis*, *Tetraselmis*, and *Neochloris* are capable of both autotrophic and heterotrophic cultivation. The advantages of heterotrophic cultivations are (i) can grow under dark conditions, in the absence of light, using carbon source as energy source, (ii) yield is 100 g/l more when compared to the phototrophic method (Scaife et al. 2015), (iii) can be carried out in conventional reactors which operate under control conditions like pH, Temperature, oxygen level, etc. (Perez et al. 2010), (iv) can be operated under fed-batch and continuous fermentation.

12.7 Conclusion

Eukaryotic microalgae and prokaryotic cyanobacteria have been exploited from the ancient periods due to their value-added products. These value-added products were found to have pharmaceutical and nutraceutical applications. The most commonly exploited nutraceuticals are pigments, fatty acids which were found to have antioxidant activity, neuroprotective activity, nephroprotectant, photoprotectant, prevent age-related diseases etc.,. ... These compounds will neutralize free radicals and protect the biomolecules from oxidative degradation, thus further protecting the cell and preventing the onset of age-related diseases.

Acknowledgments

The authors are thankful to the management and staff of Sathyabama Institute of Science and Technology for their constant support.

Conflict of Interest

The authors have declared that no conflict of interest exists. All authors have equally contributed.

References

Becker, W. (2004). Microalgae in human and animal nutrition. In: *Microalgal Culture Handbook* (ed. A. Richmond), 312–351. Oxford: Blackwell.

Brennan, L. and Owende, P. (2010). Biofuels from microalgae—a review of technologies for production, processing, and extractions of biofuels and co-products. *Renew. Sust. Energ. Rev.* 14: 557–577.

Cardozo, K.H., Guaratini, T., Barros, M.P. et al. (2007). Metabolites from algae with economical impact. *Comput. Biochem. Physiol. C Toxicol. Pharmacol.* 146: 60–78.

Chu, W.L. (2012). Biotechnological applications of microalgae. *Int. E-J. Sci. Med. Edu.* 6: 24–37.

Crupi, P., Toci, A.T., Mangini, S. et al. (2013). Determination of fucoxanthin isomers in microalgae (*Isochrysis* sp.) by high-performance liquid chromatography coupled with diode-array detector multistage mass spectrometry coupled with positive electrospray ionization. *Rapid Commun. Mass Spectrom.* 27: 1027–1035.

Day, A.G., Brinkmann, D., Franklin, S. et al. (2009). Safety evaluation of a high-lipid algal biomass from *Chlorella protothecoides*. *Regul. Toxicol. Pharmacol.* 55: 166–180.

Devendra, K., Dolly, W.D., Sunil, P. et al. (2014). Extraction and purification of C-phycocyanin from *Spirulina platensis* (CCC540). *Ind. J. Plant Physiol.* 19 (2): 184–188.

Eilers, U., Bikoulis, A., Breitenbach, J. et al. (2016). Limitations in the biosynthesis of fucoxanthin as targets for genetic engineering in *Phaeodactylum tricornutum*. *J. Appl. Phycol.* 28: 123–129.

Farooq, S.M., Ebrahim, A.S., Subramhanya, K.H. et al. (2006). Oxalate mediated nephronal impairment and its inhibition by c-phycocyanin: a study on urolithic rats. *Mol. Cell. Biochem.* 284: 95–101.

Fernandez, R.B., Medina, C.O.N., Hernandez, P.R. et al. (2014). C-Phycocyanin prevents cisplatin-induced nephrotoxicity through inhibition of oxidative stress. *Food Funct.* 5: 480–490.

Gonzalez, R., Gonzalez, A., Remirez, D. et al. (2003). Protective effects of phycocyanin on galactosamine-induced hepatitis in rats. *Biotecnol. Apl.* 20: 107–110.

Guedes, A.C., Amaro, H.M., and Malcata, F.X. (2011). Microalgae as source of high added value compounds – a brief review of recent work. *Biotechnol. Prog.* 27 (3): 597–613.

Hadi, M.R., Shariati, M., and Afsharzadeh, S. (2008). Microalgal biotechnology: carotenoid and glycerol production by the green algae *Dunaliella* isolated from the Gave-Khooni salt marsh, Iran. *Biotechnol. Bioprocess Eng.* 13: 540–544.

Hedges, S.B., Chen, H., Kumar, S. et al. (2001). A genomic timescale for the origin of eukaryotes. *BMC Evol. Biol.* 1 (4): 10.

Jianjun, H., Dillirani, N., Quanguo, Z. et al. (2018). Heterotrophic cultivation of microalgae for pigment production: a review. *Biotechnol. Adv.* 36: 54–67.

Khan, M., Varadharaj, S., Ganesan, L.P. et al. (2006). C-Phycocyanin protects against ischemia-reperfusion injury of heart through involvement of p38 MAPK and ERK signaling. *Am. J. Physiol. Heart Circul. Physiol.* 290 (5): H2136–H2145.

Kim, S.M., Jung, Y.J., Kwon, O.N. et al. (2012a). A potential commercial source of fucoxanthin extracted from the microalga *Phaeodactylum tricornutum*. *Appl. Biochem. Biotechnol.* 166: 1843–1855.

Kim, S.M., Kang, S.W., Kwon, O.N. et al. (2012b). Fucoxanthin as a major carotenoid in *Isochrysis aff. galbana*: characterization of extraction for commercial application. *J. Korean Soc. Appl. Biol. Chem.* 55: 477–483.

Kumari, R.P. and Anbarasu, K. (2014). Protective role of C-phycocyanin against secondary changes during sodium selenite mediated cataractogenesis. *Nat. Prod. Bioprospect.* 4: 81–89.

Leung, P.O., Lee, H.H., Kung, Y.C. et al. (2013). Therapeutic effect of C-phycocyanin extracted from blue green algae in a rat model of acute lung injury induced by lipopolysaccharide. *Evid. Based Compl. Alternat. Med.* 91: 65–90.

Leya, T., Rahn, A., Lütz, C., and Remias, D. (2009). Response of arctic snow and permafrost algae to high light and nitrogen stress by changes in pigment composition and applied aspects for biotechnology. *FEMS Microbiol. Ecol.* 67: 432–443.

Li, Y., Wei, G., and Chen, J. (2004). Glutathione: a review on biotechnological production. *Appl. Microbiol. Biotechnol.* 66: 233–242.

Malve, H. (2016). Exploring the ocean for new drug developments: Marine pharmacology. *J. Pharm. Bioall. Sci.* 8: 83–91.

Mandel, S., Packer, L., Youdim, M.B. et al. (2005). Proceedings from the third international conference on mechanism of action of nutraceuticals. *J. Nutr. Biochem.* 16 (9): 513–520.

Margulis, L. and Schwartz, K.V. (1998). *Five Kingdoms – An Illustrated Guide to the Phyla of Life on Earth*, 3e. New York, USA: W.H. Freeman and Company.

Marín, P.J., Pentón, R.G., Rodrigues, F.P. et al. (2012). C-Phycocyanin protects SH-SY5Y cells from oxidative injury, rat retina from transient ischemia and rat brain mitochondria from Ca^{2+}/phosphate-induced impairment. *Brain Res. Bull.* 89: 159–167.

Martinez-Fernandez, E., Acosta-Salmon, H., and Southgate, P.C. (2006). The nutritional value of seven species of tropical microalgae for blacklip pearl oyster (*Pinctada margaritifera*, L.) larvae. *Aquaculture* 257: 491–503.

Matsukawa, R., Hotta, M., Masuda, Y. et al. (2000). Antioxidants from carbon dioxide fixing *Chlorella sorokiniana*. *J. Appl. Phycol.* 12: 263–267.

Mohamed, Z.A. (2008). Polysaccharides as a protective response against microcystininduced oxidative stress in *Chlorella vulgaris* and *Scenedesmus quadricauda* and their possible significance in the aquatic ecosystem. *Ecotoxicology* 17: 504–516.

Ohta, S., Ono, F., Shiomi, Y. et al. (1998). Anti-herpes simplex virus substances produced by the marine green alga, *Dunaliella primolecta*. *J. Appl. Phys.* 10 (4): 349–356.

Oono, M., Kikuchi, K., Oonishi, S. et al. (1995). *Anticancer Agents Containing Carotenoids*, 5. Japan, Kokai: TokkyoKoho.

Ou, Y., Zheng, S., Lin, L. et al. (2010). Protective effect of C-phycocyanin against carbon tetrachloride-induced hepatocyte damage in vitro and in vivo. *Chem. Biol. Interact.* 185 (2): 94–100.

Pentón, R.G., Martínez, S.G., Cervantes, L.M. et al. (2011). C-Phycocyanin ameliorates experimental autoimmune encephalomyelitis and induces regulatory T cells. *Int. Immunopharmacol.* 11: 29–38.

Perez, A., Casas, A., Fernández, C.M. et al. (2010). Winterization of peanut biodiesel to improve the cold flow properties. *Bioresour. Technol.* 101 (19): 7375–7381.

Plaza, M., Herrero, M., Cifuentes, A. et al. (2009). Innovative natural functional ingredients from microalgae. *J. Agric. Food. Chem.* 57 (16): 7159–7170.

Ramaraj, S., Ramalingam, R., Abeer, H., and sayed, F.A.A. (2019). Microalgae metabolites: a rich source for food and medicine. *Saudi. J. Biol. Sci.* 26: 709–722.

Renugadevi, K., Valli, N.C., Sandeep, P., and Nishant, K. (2014). Biopotential activity of marine microalgae extracts. *Int. J. Chem. Tech. Res.* 62 (2): 5101–5106.

Renugadevi, K., Valli, N.C., Sowmiya, P., and Swetha, S. (2018). Antioxidant activity of phycocyanin pigment extracted from marine filamentous cyanobacteria *Geitlerinema* sp. TRV57. *Biocatal. Agric. Biotechnol.* 16: 237–242.

Riss, J., Décordé, K., Sutra, T. et al. (2007). Phycobiliprotein C-phycocyanin from *Spirulina platensis* is powerfully responsible for reducing oxidative stress and NADPH oxidase expression induced by an atherogenic diet in hamsters. *J. Agric. Food Chem.* 55 (19): 7962–7967.

Rodríguez, S.R., Ortiz, B.R., Blas, V.V. et al. (2012). Phycobiliproteins or C-phycocyanin of *Arthrospira* (Spirulina) *maxima* protect against HgCl₂-caused oxidative stress and renal damage. *Food Chem.* 135: 2359–2365.

Romay, C., Armesto, J., Remirez, D. et al. (1998). Antioxidant and anti-inflammatory properties of C-phycocyanin from blue-green algae. *Inflamm. Res.* 47: 36–41.

Sanjukta, S. (2017). Bioprospecting for algal based nutraceuticals and high value added compounds. *J. Pharm. Pharmaceut.* 4 (2): 145–150.

Sathyasaikumar, K.V., Swapna, I., Reddy, P.V.B. et al. (2007). Co-administration of C-phycocyanin ameliorates thioacetamide-induced hepatic encephalopathy in Wistar rats. *J. Neurol. Sci.* 252 (1): 67–75.

Scaife, M.A., Merkx, J.A., Woodhall, D.L., and Armenta, R.E. (2015). Algal biofuels in Canada: status and potential. *Renew. Sust. Energ. Rev.* 44: 620–642.

Simopoulos, A.P. (2002). The importance of the ratio of omega-6/omega-3 essential fatty acids. *Biomed. Pharmacother.* 56 (8): 365–379.

Srivastava, A., Tiwari, R., Srivastava, V. et al. (2015). Fresh water cyanobacteria *Geitlerinema* sp. CCC728 and *Arthrospira* sp. CCC729 as an anticancer drug resource. *PLoS ONE* 10 (9): e0136838.

Sun, Y., Zhang, J., Yan, Y. et al. (2011). The protective effect of C-phycocyanin onparaquat-induced acute lung injury in rats. *Environ. Toxicol. Pharmacol.* 32: 168–174.

Todd Lorenz, R. and Cysewski, G.R. (2000). Commercial potential for Haematococcus microalgae as a natural source of astaxanthin. *Tibtech. April* 18: 160–167.

Vadiraja, B.B., Gaikwad, N.W., and Madyastha, K.M. (1998). Hepatoprotective effect of C-phycocyanin: protection for carbon tetrachloride and R-(+)-pulegone-mediated hepatotoxicity in rats. *Biochem. Biophys. Res Commun.* 249 (2): 428–431.

Valli, N.V. and Renugadevi, K. (2015). Bio-prospecting microalgae for value added products. *Res. J. Pharm. Biol. Chem. Sci.* 6 (3): 893–900.

Vignesh, S., Raja, A., and James, R.A. (2011). Marine drugs: Implication and future studies. *Int. J. Pharmacol.* 7: 22–30.

Xianhai, Z., Michael, K.D., Xiao, D.C., and Yinghua, L. (2011). Microalgae bioengineering: from CO₂ fixation to biofuel production. *Renew. Sust. Energ. Rev.* 15: 3252–3260.

Zhang, C.W., Cohen, Z., Khozin-Goldberg, I., and Richmond, A. (2002). Characterization of growth and arachidonic acid production of *Parietochloris incisa* comb. Nov (Trebouxiophyceae, Chlorophyta). *J. Appl. Phycol.* 14: 453–460.

13

Polylysine: Natural Peptides as Antimicrobial Agents.
A Recent Scenario in Food Preservation

*Iffath Badsha[1], S. Karthick Raja Namasivayam[2], C. Jayaprakash[3], C. Valli Nachiyar[2],
and R. S. Arvind Bharani[2]*

[1] Department of Nanotechnology, Anna University, Chennai, Tamil Nadu, India
[2] Department of Biotechnology, Sathyabama Institute of Science and Technology, Chennai, Tamil Nadu, India
[3] Defense Food Research Laboratories (DFRL), Mysore, Karnataka, India

The issue of food losses is of great importance to combat hunger raise income and improve food security in the developing countries. Food losses have an impact on food security, food quality, and safety economic development and environment. The rationale behind food losses vary globally and are dependent on the specific conditions and local situation in a given country. Regardless of the extent of economic development and maturity of systems in a country, food losses must be kept to a minimum. Food losses portray an array of wastage of resources (land water energy and inputs) used in its production. Producing food which will not be consumed leads to unnecessary CO_2 emissions in addition to loss of economic value of the food produced. Economically, evitable food losses have a direct and negative impact on the income of both farmers and consumers. As most of the farmers live on the margins of food insecurity, an alleviation in food losses could have a significant and remarkable impact on their livelihoods. For consumers, the priority is mainly to have access to food products that are nutritious safe and affordable. Improving the efficiency of the food supply chain could also help to reduce the cost of food to the consumers and thus increase access to healthy food.

Many food products are perishable by nature itself and demand protection from being spoiled during their preparation, storage, and distribution to give them desired shelf life. Since food products are often sold in areas of the world far distant from their production sites, the need for extended safe shelf life for these products has also expanded. The development of food preservation processes has been driven by the necessity to extend the shelf life of foods. Food preservation is a continuous war against microorganisms spoiling the food or making it unsafe. Several traditional food preservation systems such as heating, refrigeration, and addition of antimicrobial compounds can be used to reduce the risk of outbreaks of food poisoning. However, these techniques have frequently been associated with adverse changes in organoleptic characteristics and loss of nutrients in food. Within the disposable arsenal of preservation techniques, the food industry explores the replacement of traditional food preservation techniques by new preservation techniques owing to the consumer's preference for minimally processed foods prepared without chemical preservatives and also increased consumer demands for taste, nutrition, natural, and easy-to-handle food products. Against this background, and relying on improved understanding and knowledge of the

Handbook of Nutraceuticals and Natural Products: Biological, Medicinal, and Nutritional Properties and Applications,
Volume 1, First Edition. Edited by Sreerag Gopi and Preetha Balakrishnan.
© 2022 John Wiley & Sons, Inc. Published 2022 by John Wiley & Sons, Inc.

complexity of microbial interactions, recent approaches are increasingly directed toward possibilities offered by biological preservation (Arneborg et al. 2000).

13.1 Scenario of Food Spoilage Worldwide

Worldwide losses of postharvest fruit and vegetables are around 30–40% and even much higher in some developing countries. Reducing postharvest losses is very crucial to ensure the availability of sufficient food in terms of both quantity and quality to every inhabitant in our planet. The prospects are also that the world population will grow from 5.7 billion inhabitants in 1995 to 8.3 billion in 2025. Global production of vegetables amounted to 486 million ton, while that of fruits approached 392 million ton. Minimizing the postharvest losses curtails the cost of production, trade, and distribution, thereby lowering the price for the consumer and elevating the farmer's income.

Fresh fruits and vegetables are perishable and highly prone to the decay than cereals due to their nature and composition, as they are composed of living tissues comprising thousands of living cells that must be kept alive and healthy throughout the process of marketing. Proper management in conserving the vital nutrients of processed foods could reduce the cost of production of processed foods, besides minimizing pollution hazards. The decline of postharvest loss of fruit and vegetables is a complementary means for inflating production. Conceptualization of postharvest food loss reduction as a significant means to escalate food availability was given by the World Food Conference held in Rome in 1974. The global dairy industry is impressive by large. In 2005, world milk production was estimated to be 644 million tons, of which 541 million tons was cows' milk. The leading producers of milk were the European Union at 142 million tons, India at 88 million tons, the United States at 80 million tons (20.9 billion gallons), and Russia at 31 million tons. Cheese production amounted to 8.6 million tons in Western Europe and 4.8 million tons in the United States (Kutzemeier 2006). The vast array of products made from milk worldwide leads to an equally impressive array of spoilage microorganisms. A survey of dairy product consumption revealed that 6% of US consumers would eat more dairy products if they stayed fresher longer (Lempert 2004). Products range from those that are readily spoiled by microorganisms to those that are shelf stable for many months, and the spoilage rate can be influenced by other factors such as moisture content, pH, processing parameters, and temperature of storage (Rawat 2015).

13.2 Scenario of Food Spoilage in India

In India, there is a huge scope for cultivating crops, fruits, and vegetables throughout the year in one or other part of the country because the climatic conditions are highly suitable for farming. Fruits and vegetables are available in surplus only in certain seasons and regions. In peak season, due to food spoilage, around 20–25% fruits and vegetables are spoilt in various stages. A variety of fresh fruit and vegetable in India can be made available in plenty due to favorable agro-climatic situations, thereby improving the national picture significantly.

Fruits and vegetables are very essential food commodities not only in India but all over the world, with specific importance providing a balance and healthy diet to the people. India, being the second most populated country in the world, is still struggling to achieve self-sufficiency to feed about 800 million people. India is the second largest producer of vegetables and fourth largest producer of fruits in the world contributing 10% of world fruit production and 14% of world vegetable production. Nevertheless, India is producing adequate quantities of fruits and vegetables, yet on account of losses in the field, as well as in storage, they become insufficient. Approximately, 30% fruits and vegetables are rendered unfit for consumption due to spoilage after harvesting. India annually produces fruits and vegetables of the value of about Rs. 7000 crores and wastage may be of the order of Rs. 2100 crores, which is an enormous loss of valuable food despite the minimum food requirement of the population is not met. Therefore, it is of immense importance to not only cultivate more but also to save what is grown.

According to India Agricultural Research Data Book (2004), the losses in fruits and vegetables are to the tune of 30% (Rawat 2015). Taking estimated production of fruits and vegetables in India at 150 million tons, the total waste generated comes to 50 million tons per annum. Like all other foods, fruits and vegetables are susceptible to microbial spoilage caused by fungi, bacteria, yeast, and molds. A major portion of losses during postharvest period is attributed to diseases caused by fungi and bacteria. The succulent nature of fruits and vegetables makes them easily invaded by these organisms. Besides affecting fresh fruits and vegetables, these organisms also cause damage to canned and processed products.

13.3   The Global Need for Food Preservation

The food industry has developed along with globalization, resulting in an increased risk of foodstuffs being contaminated with pathogens and toxins. The demand for minimally processed and ready-to-eat fresh food products, globalization of food trade, and distribution from centralized processing present major challenges for food safety and quality. Recent food-borne microbial outbreaks are driving a hunt to explore innovative ways to inhibit microbial growth in the foods while maintaining quality, freshness, and safety. The proliferation of pathogenic and spoilage bacteria should be controlled to guarantee food safety. One option is to use packaging of food to provide an increased margin of safety and quality.

The risk of contracting foodborne illnesses is reduced by various food preservation methods such as thermal processing, drying, freezing, refrigeration, irradiation, modified atmosphere packaging and the addition of antimicrobial agents, salts, or other chemical preservatives. Unfortunately, these techniques cannot be applied to all food products because of undesired effects (texture, color, etc.) depending on food type, such as ready-to-eat foods and fresh foods. Especially, preserving meat products is more complex, which requires higher pH and mild pasteurization temperatures.

Conventional preservatives are a group of synthetic chemical substances including nitrates/nitrites, sulfites, sodium benzoate, propyl gallate, and potassium sorbate. These conventional preservatives in food have various side effects. Nitrites and nitrates have been linked to leukemia, colon, bladder, and stomach cancer. Sorbate and sorbic acid are rare; however, they are related to urticaria and contact dermatitis. Benzoates have been suspected to cause allergies, asthma, and skin rashes. During recent decades, investigation on food preservation has enthralled on more natural and healthier food (Caminiti et al. 2011; Fangio and Fritz 2014).

Natural preservatives are the chemical agents derived from plants, animals, and microorganisms and are usually related to the host defense system (Singh et al. 2010; Tiwari et al. 2009). The requirements of natural preservatives are safety, stability during food processing (pH, heat, pressure, etc.), and antimicrobial efficacy. The representative food pathogens are *Escherichia coli*, *Salmonella* spp., *Listeria monocytogenes*, *Staphylococcus aureus*, *Bacillus cereus*, *Yersinia enterocolitica*, *Clostridium perfringens*, *Clostridium botulinum*, and *Campylobacter jejuni*. The pathogenic fungi often related to food-borne diseases are toxin-producing *Aspergillus flavus* and *Aspergillus parasiticus* (Prange et al. 2005).

Biopreservation has dealt with extending food shelf life and enhancing food safety using plants, animals, microorganisms, and their metabolites (Settanni and Corsetti 2008). Particularly, meat and meat products are perishable materials and are controlled by the Hazard Analysis Critical Control Point (HACCP) approach. As the demand for biopreservation in food systems has increased, the next generation of food packaging may include materials with antimicrobial properties. New natural antimicrobial compounds of various origin are being developed, including animal-derived systems (lysozyme, lactoferrin, and magainins), plant-derived products (phytoalexins, herbs, and spices), and microbial metabolites (bacteriocins, hydrogen peroxide, and organic acids) (Lavermicocca et al. 2003). Packaging technology is one of the possible ways that could play a significant role in extending the shelf life of foods by minimizing the risk from pathogens and providing an increased margin of safety and quality.

13.4 Antimicrobial Packaging in Food Preservation

Antimicrobial packaging is a next-generation packaging that interacts with the product to obtain a desired outcome (Brody et al. 2001; Labuza and Breene 1989; Rooney 1995). It is a rapidly emerging technology that has an important role in enhancing the shelf life of packaged foods and inhibiting the growth rate of microorganism through direct contact with food, thereby reducing the risk of pathogens (Appendini and Hotchkiss 2002). The basic idea behind this technology is the usage of antimicrobial substances (such as actively functional polymers), which help to control the microbial population and target-specific microorganisms in food products, thereby extending the shelf life of food (Espitia et al. 2013; Han and Rooney 2002). Antimicrobial packaging system prevents microbial growth by eliminating their essential growth requirements from the products (Singh and Shalini 2016) or by extending the lag period and declining the growth rate or decreasing the live counts of microorganisms (Han 2000). The primary goals of an antimicrobial packaging system are safety assurance, quality maintenance, and shelf life extension, which is the reversed order of the primary goals of conventional packaging systems (Han 2000). Antimicrobial packaging besides packaging has many applications and attractive innovation of active packaging to increase food safety and food security (Floros et al. 1997) and also has sanitizing and self-sterilizing properties (Appendini and Hotchkiss 2002).

Meat, dairy, fruits, vegetables, bakery, and confectionery are the common food products that are easily attacked by microorganism and have to be protected from spoilage by antimicrobial packaging (Leister 1994). All antimicrobial agents have different activities on microorganisms due to the characteristic antimicrobial mechanisms and various physiologies of the microorganisms. Besides the microbial characteristics, the characteristic antimicrobial function of the antimicrobial agent is also important to understand the efficacy, as well as the limits of the activity. Some antimicrobial agents inhibit essential metabolic or reproductive genetic pathways of microorganisms while some others alter cell membrane or cell wall structure. The basic principle of antimicrobial packaging is based on the hurdle technology. Hurdle technology employs hurdles like water activity, pH, redox potential, heat treatment, etc. to achieve a maximum lethality of microorganisms at an optimum level by a combination of two or more such hurdles so that minimum damage to the nutritional and sensory properties of food (Singh and Shalini 2016). The combination of various parameters (such as water activity reduction, low and high temperature, pH reduction, addition of competitive microorganisms, and preservatives agents) to inhibit the microorganisms in food products is called "hurdle effect" (Leister 1994). Intelligent use of hurdles in food product design ensures that products have an adequate shelf life and remain safe (Leister 1994). Antimicrobial packaging system is a hurdle to prevent degradation of the total quality of processed food, thus providing protection against microorganisms. The extra antimicrobial function of the packaging system is another hurdle to prevent the degradation of total quality of packaged foods while satisfying the conventional functions of moisture and oxygen barriers, as well as physical protection. Release, absorption, and immobilization are three types of modes for antimicrobial functions in antimicrobial polymeric materials (Ahvenainen 2003). The first one is the release type mode of antimicrobial functions that allows the migration of antimicrobial agents into foods or headspace inside packages and inhibits the growth of microorganisms. The second one is the absorption mode of antimicrobial system, which eliminates all essential factors (moisture, oxygen, carbon dioxide, and pH) of microbial growth from the food systems, thereby inhibiting the growth of microorganisms (like CO_2 and O_2 scavengers, moisture absorbers, ethanol emitters, etc.) and preventing the growth of bacteria, fungi, and molds inside food packages. Immobilization system does not release antimicrobial agents but suppresses the growth of microorganisms at the contact surface such as immobilized lysozyme and glucose oxidase enzyme on polymer package for cheese, beef, and culture media. Immobilization system is more effective in liquid foods, because of direct contact between the antimicrobial package and the whole food products. Package/food and package/headspace/food packaging are two types of antimicrobial packaging system (Han 2000). In the former, diffusion involves the main migration phenomena between the packaging material and the food and partitioning at the interface; hence, diffusion and partitioning processes through which antimicrobial agents embedded into the packaging materials migrate into the food (Quintavalla and Vicini 2002). In the later, the evaporation of a substance to the headspace is the main migration phenomena in this system; therefore, a volatile active substance should be used. Then, the active substances that are equilibrated may diffuse into the food (Quintavalla and Vicini 2002). Diffusional mass transfer does not occur in immobilization situation of non-food-grade antimicrobial for inhibiting surface microbial growth (Appendini and Hotchkiss 1997; Quintavalla and Vicini 2002).

13.5 Antimicrobial Packaging with Bacteriocin

Over the recent couple of years, bacteriocins have acquired significant attention owing to their potential applications in the food industry as natural preservatives and more recently in the health industry as antimicrobial agents (El-Gendy et al. 2013; Zacharof and Lovitt 2012). Bacteriocin is metabolic by-product generated by bacteria as their defense system to withstand elevated temperatures and acidic environment (Sofi et al. 2018). Bacteriocins are a member of a group of antimicrobial polypeptides produced by a diverse group of Gram-negative and Gram-positive bacteria exhibiting bactericidal or bacteriostatic activity (Castellano et al. 2012; El-Gendy et al. 2013; Tagg et al. 1976). Bacteriocins are ribosomally synthesized proteinaceous molecules produced during the primary phase of growth of bacteria. They are unique in their mechanism of action exhibiting a relatively narrow spectrum of antibacterial activity against pathogenic bacteria (Riley and Wertz 2002) and are inactivated by digestive enzymes, which makes them nontoxic to human cells if used as biopreservatives (Balciunas et al. 2013; Perez et al. 2014; Tagg et al. 1976; Zacharof and Lovitt 2012). In food preservation, these compounds are often incorporated either directly as purified or partially purified agents to food or through cultivation of the bacteriocin-producer strain in the food substrate (Deegan et al. 2006). Bacteriocins have exhibited activity against Gram-positive pathogens of human and animal origin and most resistant strains of bacteria including

Table 13.1 Advantages and limitations of chemical free preservatives.

Advantages	Limitations
Chemical-free preservation (Deegan et al. 2006)	High cost of commercial production of bacteriocins (Bradshaw 2003)
Shelf-life extension (Deegan et al. 2006)	Low yield due to ineffective purification methods (Carolissen-Mackay et al. 1997)
Inhibition of food-borne pathogenic bacteria during food-processing stages (Deegan et al. 2006)	Loss of activity and degradation by proteolytic enzymes (Bradshaw 2003)
Non-toxic to human cells (Perez et al. 2014)	Unfavorable interactions with the constituents of food decreases the availability and necessitates a huge amount of these compounds to be added (Jung et al. 1992; Schillinger et al. 1996)
Antibacterial against many resistant strains of bacteria (Millette et al. 2008)	Alterations of the chemical and physical properties of these compounds during the various food-processing stages (Davidson et al. 2005)

methicillin-resistant *S. aureus* (MRSA), and two vancomycin-resistant *Enterococcus faecalis* strains (Kruszewska et al. 2004; Millette et al. 2008). These antibacterial activities of bacteriocins make them a synergistic substitute to antibiotics to overcome bacterial resistance. Advantages and limitations of chemical-free preservatives is as follows (Table 13.1).

13.6 Polylysine as Antimicrobial Peptides in Food Preservation

Polylysine (ε-poly-L-lysine) is one such food-grade antimicrobial cationic homopolymer, which is used as a natural preservative in food products. Since the late 1980s, Polylysine has been approved by the Japanese Ministry of Health, Labour and Welfare as a preservative in food. In January 2004, The US Food and Drug Administration (FDA) conferred generally regarded as safe (GRAS) status on ε-polylysine to be incorporated into various food items at levels of 10–500 ppm (Chheda and Vernekar 2015; Lopez-Pena et al. 2015).

13.6.1 Polylysine

Polylysine is a homo polypeptide of essential amino acid lysine and belongs to the group of cationic polymers containing a positively charged hydrophilic amino group at pH 7. The precursor lysine contains two amino groups, one at the α-carbon and one at the ε-carbon; of these, either can be the position of polymerization, forming α-polylysine or ε-polylysine. There are several types of polylysine (Figure 13.1) differing from each other in terms of stereochemistry and link position.

α-Polylysine is a synthetic polymer produced by a basic polycondensation reaction. It is composed of either L-lysine or D-lysine residues where "L" and "D" refer to the chirality at lysine's central carbon, resulting in poly-L-lysine (PLL) and poly-D-lysine (PDL), respectively (Sitterley 2008). α-Polylysine is commonly used to coat tissue culture-ware as an attachment factor, which improves cell adherence. This phenomenon is predicated on the interaction between the positively charged polymer and negatively charged cells (or proteins). While the precursor amino acid of poly-L-lysine (PLL) occurs naturally, the poly-D-lysine (PDL) precursor is an artificial product. The latter is

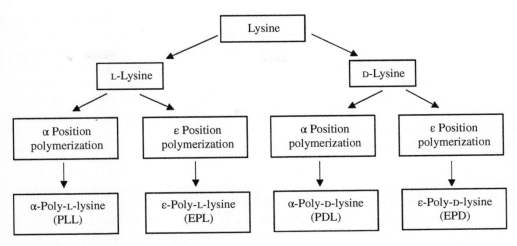

Figure 13.1 Several types of polylysine.

therefore thought to be resistant to enzymatic degradation and so may prolong cell adherence (Mazia et al. 1975).

ε-Polylysine (ε-poly-L-lysine, EPL) is typically produced as a homopolypeptide of approximately 25–30 L-lysine residues linked by isopeptide bonds between ε-amino and α-carboxyl groups (Dodd et al. 2018; Shima and Sakai 1977), with molecular weight of approximately 5000. It is produced by bacterial fermentation, and it has an antimicrobial effect against bacteria, yeast, fungi, virus, Gram-positive, and Gram-negative bacteria making it suitable for versatile applications in the food, feed, nutraceutical, and cosmetic industry. ε-Polylysine is employed commercially as a food preservative in Japan, Korea, and United States. Processed food products containing polylysine are predominantly found in Japan. The use of polylysine is common in food applications such as boiled rice, cooked vegetables, soups, noodles, and sliced fish called sushi (Hiraki et al. 2003). Literature studies have reported an antimicrobial effect of ε-polylysine against yeast, fungi, Gram-positive bacteria and Gram-negative bacteria (Hiraki 1995).

Structure of ε-polylysine.

13.6.2 Origin and Distribution of Polylysine

The production of ε-polylysine by natural fermentation was first described by researchers Shoji Shima and Heiichi Sakai in 1977 (Shima and Sakai 1977). ε-Polylysine was identified as an extracellular material produced by filamentous actinomycetes such as *Streptomyces albulus* and Lysinopolymerus strain 346 more than 25 years ago. It was discovered that polylysine-producing organisms belong to two major groups named Streptomycetaceae and Ergot fungi. The most common organism producing ε-polylysine commercially is a filamentous bacterium known as

S. albulus. But the main concern with respect to *S. albulus* is the enzymatic and pH-induced degradation of secreted ε-polylysine in the culture medium. Hence, different organisms like *Streptomyces diastatochromogenes* CGMCC 3145, *Streptomyces aureofaciens*, *Streptomyces noursei* NRRL 5126, *Streptomyces griseofuscus*, *Kitasatospora* sp. MY 5-36, *Kitasatospora kifunensine*, *Kitasatospora* sp. PL6, etc. have been explored to substitute *S. albulus* for the industrial production of ε-PL. The first ε-PL producer reported for eukaryotes is an ergot fungus *Epichloe* sp. MN-9, which produces ε-PL with 24–29 residues. Recently, ε-PL was detected and produced using a novel marine bacteria *Bacillus subtilis* species.

Properties of ε-Polylysine (EPL)

- ε-Polylysine is a natural biological product of metabolism, with strong bactericidal ability, broad antibacterial spectrum, good water solubility, thermal stability, biodegradability, nontoxicity, edibility, innocuousness, and will not affect food flavor. Therefore, ε-PL has been widely used as a preservative in many foods such as meat, rice, fruits, cooked vegetables, etc. (Chheda and Vernekar 2015) and also has great interest to the food and pharmaceutical industry.
- Polylysine has a light-yellowish appearance and is slightly bitter in taste whether in powder or liquid form.
- It is basic in nature, highly soluble in water and slightly soluble in ethanol, insoluble in organic solvents such as ethyl acetate and ether. ε-PL has been reported to display high water solubility and thermal stability.
- ε-Polylysine does not decompose or lose antibacterial activity even if treated for 20 minutes in an aqueous solution of 120 °C. It was found that on boiling a solution of ε-PL at 100 °C for 30 minutes or autoclaving it for 20 minutes at 72 °C, no degradation is observed and the polymer length is maintained. No structural change is reported upon heat treatment at pH 3.0. Therefore, ε-polylysine can go through the general heat process in food processing with raw materials, thereby preventing secondary food pollution.
- It is effective over a wide range of pH values from 3 to 9 and suitable for most foods. The isoelectric point (pI) for 25–35 L-lysine residues is around 9.
- The food safety level of ε-PL as an additive was demonstrated by experiments using rats. In Japan, ε-PL has entered the commercial market producing it industrially by fermentation using a mutant derived from *S. albulus*.
- Apart from being used as a preservative in food industry, derivatives of ε-PL offer a wide range of applications such as emulsifying agent, dietary agent, biodegradable fibers, hydrogels, drug carriers, anticancer agent enhancer, biochip coatings, etc.

13.7 Antimicrobial Activity of Polylysine

The antimicrobial activities of ε-PL have been reported during the past few years (Geornaras et al. 2007; Liu et al. 2017). ε-Polylysine exhibits broad inhibitory activity against several microorganisms, including fungi, such as *Aspergillus niger*, *Trichophyton mentagrophytes*, *Candida* spp., and *Phaffia rhodozyma*. In addition, ε-polylysine restricts a broad range of Gram-positive and Gram-negative bacterial taxa, such as *Bacillus coagulans*, *S. aureus*, *E. coli*, and *Salmonella typhimurium* (Geornaras et al. 2007; Lopez-Pena et al. 2016; Yoshida and Nagasawa 2003).

Several studies suggest that ε-polylysine is adsorbed electrostatically to the cell surface of the bacteria, which is followed by a stripping of the outer membrane. This eventually leads to the abnormal distribution of the cytoplasm causing damage to the bacterial cell that is produced by bacterial fermentation (Shima et al. 1984).

It was reported that the antimicrobial activity of ε-polylysine has been largely attributed to its cationic charge, as this allows it to adsorb onto negatively charged microbial surfaces and disrupt the cell envelope (Hyldgaard et al. 2014). The cationic nature of ε-polylysine curtails its application in some foods as it could interact with anionic mucins in the mouth or spontaneously complex with negatively charged molecules to impact food integrity (Chang et al. 2011, 2012; Lopez-Pena and McClements 2014). However, its antibacterial mechanism has not been absolutely elucidated (Bo et al. 2015; Hyldgaard et al. 2014; Wei et al. 2018).

Lin et al. (2018) found that addition of ε-PL could induce the marked change on the morphology of *L. monocytogenes* cells and further illustrated the destructive effect of ε-PL on cell structure (Lin et al. 2018). Similarly, Ye et al. found that *E. coli* O157:H7 cells exposed to ε-PL showed collapsed, lysis, and rough membranes (Ye et al. 2013). Besides mycelial growth, spore germination rate and germ-tube length of *Penicillium digitatum* were markedly inhibited by ε-PL. Meanwhile, ε-PL caused serious damages on mycelial morphology and plasma membrane (Liu et al. 2017). Studies have demonstrated that ε-PL could significantly change the cell wall composition of *Saccharomyces cerevisiae* (*S. cerevisiae*) and result in cell wall more fragile, thus increasing the cell wall permeability (Tan et al. 2018). In general, researchers concur that the antimicrobial effect of ε-PL is to destroy cell membranes or cell walls (Li et al. 2014; Melo et al. 2009; Zhang et al. 2018). Up to now, its antimicrobial mechanism at the metabolomics has not been yet thoroughly described.

13.8 Preservation Mechanism of ε-Polylysine

The main preservation mechanism of ε-polylysine is described as the following steps:

- ε-Polylysine is a highly polymerized polyvalent cation (positively charged), which interacts and binds with negatively charged microbial cell membranes of microorganisms and form holes in the membrane. It destroys the cell membrane structure of microorganisms and causes the leakage of intracellular substances.
- ε-Polylysine enters the cell through the holes in the membrane, which affects the structure and function of the cell membrane, and interferes the normal physiological metabolism of microorganisms, destroys the transmission of materials and energy in the cell, induces the cell to autolysis, and finally causes the death of the bacterial cell.

13.9 Polylysine on Major Food-Borne Pathogens

Staphylococcus aureus (*S. aureus*) is considered as one of the major food-borne pathogens that causes diverse symptoms of food poisoning. Therefore, *S. aureus* poses a serious threat to food safety owing to its high tolerance to salt and the stability of its toxins at high temperature. Furthermore, in recent years, *S. aureus* has also been used as a model strain of Gram-positive bacteria in the research of antibacterial mechanism.

13.10 Global Market of ε-Poly-L-Lysine

Globally, Japan is the largest consumption region, consumed 820.9 MT (metric ton) ε-polylysine in 2017. South Korea is the second largest consumption region with consumption share of 21.89%, followed by China and Europe, they separately consumed 297.3 and 201.3 MT in 2017. The ε-polylysine market was valued at US $420 million in 2017 and is projected to reach US $740 million by 2025, at a CAGR of 7.3% during the forecast period. The year 2017 is considered as the base year and the years 2018–2025 as the forecast period to estimate the market size for ε-polylysine (https://www.radiantinsights.com).

Geographically, the global ε-polylysine market is segmented into North America (United States, Canada, Mexico, etc.), Asia-Pacific (China, Japan, India, Korea, Australia, Indonesia, Taiwan, Thailand, etc.), Europe (Germany, United Kingdom, France, Italy, Russia, Spain, etc.), Middle East and Africa (Turkey, Saudi Arabia, Iran, Egypt, Nigeria, UAE, Israel, South Africa, etc.), and South America (Brazil, Argentina, Colombia, Chile, Venezuela, Peru, etc.) (https://reports.valuates.com).

Some of the leading vendors in the global ε-polylysine market are Chisso Corporation, Zhejiang Silver Elephant Bioengineering Co., Ltd., Nanjing Shineking Biotech Co., Ltd., Chengdu Jin Kai Biological Engineering Co., Ltd., Zhangshu City Lion Biotechnology Co., Ltd., Nanjing Sai Taisi Biotechnology Co., Ltd., Siveele B.V. (https://www.regalintelligence.com).

ε-Polylysine is used in many sectors such as food grade, medical grade, industry grade, and many other sectors. It is used as a preservative in many products such as processed meat, poultry, fish, dairy products, bakery products, grain mill products, snack foods, etc. (https://www.regalintelligence.com).

13.11 Approval, Safety, and Regulations

ε-Polylysine is food grade and meets FAO/WHO specifications. It is certified as GRAS (Generally Recognized As Safe) at levels up to 50 mg/kg in food by the U.S. Food and Drug Administration (US FDA) with US GRAS No.: GRN000135, CAS No.: 28211-04-3 (Ye et al. 2013). Currently, ε-polylysine has approval as a food additive in Korea, Japan, USA, and some more countries.

Acute oral toxicity assays showed that ε-PL is nontoxic at high dose levels of 5 g/kg in rats (Hiraki et al. 2003). Absorption, distribution, metabolism, and excretion studies demonstrated that ε-PL has low absorption in rat gastrointestinal tract (Hiraki et al. 2003). Based on its strong antibacterial activity and low toxicity, ε-PL is utilized in Japan as food additive for meat or fish sushi (1–5 mg/g), rice, cooked vegetables (0.01–0.5 mg/g), and other food (Chang et al. 2010).

Its safety has been approved by the Japan Ministry of Health, Labor and Welfare, U.S. Food and Drug Administration in 2003 and afterward, National Health Commission of the People's Republic of China (NHC) approved it in 2014. It is also authorized in some other countries. It is considered safer than chemical preservatives as it is natural and it is partly hydrolyzed to L-lysine (an essential amino acid) after ingested by the human body. It has the function of both preservation and nutrition fortification. Chemical synthetic preservatives (e.g. sodium benzoate, potassium sorbate) are widely used in food to extend shelf life in today's food industry. However, the health concerns surrounding them are always coming up, which makes consumers afraid of the safety of their food and seeks safe preservatives, and thus biological preservatives stand out (https://foodadditives.net).

ε-Poly-L-lysine is regarded as vegetarian diet as it does not contain any animal-derived product and also meets the demands of natural food preservatives of vegetarians. It is gluten-free as complied with the FDA's definition of gluten-free (it does not contain wheat, rye, barley, or crossbreeds of these grains), and it is generally considered safe for people with celiac disease (https://foodadditives.net/).

13.12   Food and Drug Administration (FDA)

- In 2004, FDA had no questions regarding the conclusion of Japan manufacturer Chisso Corporation that polylysine was generally recognized as safe (GRAS) for use as an antimicrobial agent in cooked rice or sushi rice at the maximum use levels 50 mg/kg. (Agency Response Letter GRAS Notice No. GRN 000135, FDA).
- In 2011, FDA also had no questions regarding the conclusion of the supplier Purac Biochem b.v. that polylysine was GRAS under the intended uses as an antimicrobial agent in several food categories except for meat and poultry products at levels up to 0.025%. (Agency Response Letter GRAS Notice No. GRN 000336, FDA).

13.13   China National Health Commission (NHC)

ε-Polylysine is approved to be used in baked goods, cooked meat products, fruit and vegetable juices, and their beverages. ε-Polylysine hydrochloride can be used in the following food list:

- Fruits, vegetables (including roots), beans, edible fungi, algae, nuts, and seeds
- Rice and products
- Wheat flour and its products
- Cereal products
- Meat and meat products
- Condiment
- drink
- Spiced corned egg

13.14   Global Application of ε-Polylysine in Food Preservation

ε-Polylysine is suitable for versatile applications in food, feed, cosmeceutical, and pharmaceutical industries. ε-Polylysine is commercially used as a food preservative in Japan, the republic of Korea, and in the United States. Food products containing polylysine are mainly found in Japan. The use of polylysine is common in food applications like boiled rice, cooked vegetables, soups, noodles, and sliced fish (sushi). (http://www.siveele.com).

13.15   Key Benefits (https://foodadditives.net)

- Natural and non-animal source
- Broad range of antibacterial spectrum
- Extends shelf life
- Effective over a wide range of pH values (4–10)
- Could be used before or after heat treatment owing to its high range of thermal stability
- Secures desired food flavor
- Improved cost efficiency due to the low dosage rate
- Meets consumer demands for food preserved with natural additives by fully or partially replacing synthetic additives.

It has the antibacterial effects on following microorganisms list (https://foodadditives.net):

- *Escherichia coli*
- *Staphylococcus aureus*
- *Bacillus subtilis*
- *Streptococcus thermophilus*
- *Lactobacillus bulgaricus*
- *Lactobacillus plantarum*
- *Saccharomyces cerevisiae*
- *Pichia*
- *Candida*
- *Rhizopus niger*
- *Mucor tall*

The following food may contain it (https://foodadditives.net):

- Meat and poultry
- Fish and shellfish-based foods
- Processed fruits and vegetables
- Soft drinks
- Rice
- Processed cheese and cheese spreads
- Pickles
- Salad dressings
- Yogurt
- Soups
- Tomato-based sauces
- Fruit-flavored drinks

13.16   Synergy with Other Additives or Preservatives

ε-Poly-L-lysine can not only be used alone but also can be mixed with other food additives to improve its antimicrobial effects. It has synergistic effects with hydrochloric acid, acetic acid, malic acid, citric acid, glycine, and senior fatty glycerides. It has significant synergistic effects against *L. mono-cytogenes* and *B. cereus* when used with another natural preservative Nisin. ε-PL has antibacterial effects on *Escherichia coli* and yeasts, which Nisin cannot inhibit (https://foodadditives.net).

13.17   Possible Side Effects

According to the information from the supplier Purac and FDA, that ε-poly-L-lysine is safe under the intended conditions of use after the studies on acute, subchronic, chronic oral toxicity, carcinogenicity, reproduction, teratogenicity, and mutagenicity. No allergenic reactions or other adverse effects were reported. Synergy with glycine to exhibit an antibacterial effect on *B. subtilis* and *A. flavus*. The combined use of ε-PL and acetic acid can effectively inhibit the growth of *Bacillus subtilis* (https://foodadditives.net).

References

Ahvenainen, R. (2003). *Noval Food Packaging Technique*, 50–65. Cambridge, England: Wood Head Publishing Limited.

Appendini, P. and Hotchkiss, J. (1997). Immobilization of lysozyme on food contact polymers as potential antimicrobial films. *Packag. Technol. Sci.* 10: 271–279.

Appendini, P. and Hotchkiss, J.H. (2002). Review of antimicrobial food packaging. *Innov. Food. Sci. Emerg.* 3 (2): 113–126.

Arneborg, N., Jespersen, L., and Jakobsen, M. (2000). Individual cells of *Saccharomyces cerevisiae* and *Zygosaccharomyces bailii* exhibit different short-term intracellular pH responses to acetic acid. *Arch. Microbiol.* 174: 125–128.

Balciunas, E.M., Martinez, F.A.C., Todorov, S.D. et al. (2013). Novel biotechnological applications of bacteriocins: a review. *Food Control.* 32: 134–142. https://doi.org/10.1016/j.foodcont.2012.11.025.

Bo, T., Han, P., Su, Q. et al. (2015). Antimicrobial ε-poly-l-lysine induced changes in cell membrane compositions and properties of *Saccharomyces cerevisiae*. *Food Cont.* 61: 123–134.

Bradshaw, J.P. (2003). Cationic antimicrobial peptides. *BioDrugs* 17: 233–240. https://doi.org/10.2165/00063030-200317040-00002.

Brody, A., Strupinsky, E., and Kline, L. (2001). *Active Packaging for Food Applications*. Lancaster, PA: Technomic Publishing Co.

Caminiti, I.M., Noci, F., Muñoz, A. et al. (2011). Impact of selected combinations of non-thermal processing technologies on the quality of an apple and cranberry juice blend. *Food Chem.* 124: 1387–1892.

Carolissen-Mackay, V., Arendse, G., and Hastings, J.W. (1997). Purification of bacteriocins of lactic acid bacteria: problems and pointers. *Int. J. Food Microbiol.* 34: 1–16. https://doi.org/10.1016/S0168-1605(96)01167-1.

Castellano, P., Aristoy, M.C., Sentandreu, M.A. et al. (2012). *Lactobacillus sakei* CRL1862 improves safety and protein hydrolysis in meat systems. *J. Appl. Microbiol.* 113: 1407–1416. https://doi.org/10.1111/jam.12005.

Chang, S.S., Lu, W.Y., Park, S.H., and Kang, D.H. (2010). Control of foodborne pathogens on ready-to-eat roast beef slurry by epsilon-polylysine. *Int. J. Food Microbiol.* 141: 236–241.

Chang, Y., McLandsborough, L., and McClements, D.J. (2011). Physicochemical properties and antimicrobial efficacy of electrostatic complexes based on cationic epsilon-polylysine and anionic pectin. *J. Agric. Food Chem.* 59: 6776–6782.

Chang, Y., McLandsborough, L., and McClements, D.J. (2012). Cationic antimicrobial (epsilon-polylysine)–anionic polysaccharide (pectin) interactions: influence of polymer charge on physical stability and antimicrobial efficacy. *J. Agric. Food Chem.* 60: 1837–1844.

Chheda, A.H. and Vernekar, M.R. (2015). A natural preservative ε-poly-l-lysine: fermentative production and applications in food industry. *Int. Food Res. J.* 22: 23–30.

Davidson, P.M., Sofos, J.N., and Branen, A.L. (2005). *Antimicrobials in Food*. Florida, FL: CRC Press.

Deegan, L.H., Cotter, P.D., Hill, C., and Ross, P. (2006). Bacteriocins: biological tools for bio-preservation and shelf-life extension. *Int. Dairy J.* 16: 1058–1071. https://doi.org/10.1016/j.idairyj.2005.10.026.

Dodd, A., Swanevelder, D., Zhou, N. et al. (2018). *Streptomyces albulus* yields ε-poly-l-lysine and other products from salt contaminated glycerol waste. *J. Ind. Microbiol. Biot.* 45: 1083–1090.

El-Gendy, A.O., Essam, T.M., Amin, M.A. et al. (2013). Clinical screening for bacteriocinogenic Enterococcus faecalis isolated from intensive care unit inpatient in Egypt. *J. Microb. Biochem. Technol.* 4: 161–167. https://doi.org/10.4172/1948-5948.1000089.

Espitia, P.J.P., Soares, N.D.F., Teofilo, R.F. et al. (2013). Physical–mechanical and antimicrobial properties of nanocomposite films with pediocin and ZnO nanoparticles. *Carbohydr. Polym.* 94 (1): 199–208.

Fangio, M.F. and Fritz, R. (2014). Potential use of a bacteriocin-like substance in meat and vegetable food biopreservation. *Int. Food Res. J.* 21: 677–683.

Floros, J.D., Dock, L.L., and Han, J.H. (1997). Active packaging technologies and applications. *Food Cosmet. Drug Packag.* 20: 10–17.

Geornaras, I., Yoon, Y., Belk, K.E. et al. (2007). Antimicrobial activity of epsilon–polylysine against *Escherichia coli* O157:H7, *Salmonella typhimurium*, and *Listeria monocytogenes* in various food extracts. *J. Food Sci.* 72: M330–M334.

Han, J.H. (2000). Antimicrobial food packaging. *Food Technol.* 54 (3): 56–65.

Han, J.H. and Rooney, M.L. (2002). Active food packaging workshop. *Annual Conference of the Canadian Institute of Food Science and Technology (CIFST)*, Canada.

Hiraki, J. (1995). Basic and applied studies on ε-polylysine. *J. Antibact. Antifung. Agents* 23: 349–354.

Hiraki, J., Ichikawa, T., Ninomiya, S. et al. (2003). Use of ADME studies to confirm the safety of ε-polylysine as a preservative in food. *Regul. Toxicol. Pharmacol.* 37 (2): 328–340. https://doi.org/10.1016/S0273-2300(03)00029-1. PMID 12726761.

Hyldgaard, M., Mygind, T., Vad, B.S. et al. (2014). The antimicrobial mechanism of action of epsilon-poly-l-lysine. *Appl. Environ. Microbiol.* 80: 7758–7770.

Jung, D.-S., Bodyfelt, F.W., and Daeschel, M.A. (1992). Influence of fat and emulsifiers on the efficacy of nisin in inhibiting *Listeria monocytogenes* in fluid milk. *J. Dairy Sci.* 75: 387–393. https://doi.org/10.3168/jds.S0022-0302(92)77773-X.

Kruszewska, D., Sahl, H.-G., Bierbaum, G. et al. (2004). Mersacidin eradicates methicillin-resistant *Staphylococcus aureus* (MRSA) in a mouse rhinitis model. *J. Antimicrob. Chemother.* 54: 648–653. https://doi.org/10.1093/jac/dkh387.

Kutzemeier, T. (2006). Milk and dairy products in human nutrition. *Europ. Dairy Magzin.* 7: 34–36.

Labuza, T. and Breene, W. (1989). Applications of active packaging for improvement of shelf-life and nutritional quality of fresh and extended shelf-life foods. *J. Food Process. Preserv.* 13: 1–89.

Lavermicocca, P., Valerio, F., and Visconti, A. (2003). Antifungal activity of phenyllactic acid against molds isolated from bakery products. *Appl. Environ. Microbiol.* 69: 634–640.

Leister, L. (1994). Further developments in the utilization of hurdle technology for food preservation. *J. Food Engg.* 22: 421–432.

Lempert, P. (2004). Waste not, want not. *Progress. Grocer.* 83 18 p.

Li, Y.Q., Han, Q., Feng, J.L. et al. (2014). Antibacterial characteristics and mechanisms of ε-poly-lysine against *Escherichia coli*, and *Staphylococcus aureus*. *Food Cont.* 43: 22–27.

Lin, L., Gu, Y.L., Li, C.Z. et al. (2018). Antibacterial mechanism of ε-poly-lysine against *Listeria monocytogenes* and its application on cheese. *Food Cont.* 91: 76–84.

Liu, K., Zhou, X., and Fu, M. (2017). Inhibiting effects of ε-poly-lysine (PL) on *Penicillium digitatum* and its involved mechanism. *Postharvest. Biol. Technol.* 123: 94–101.

Lopez-Pena, C.L. and McClements, D.J. (2014). Optimizing delivery systems for cationic biopolymers: competitive interactions of cationic polylysine with anionic kappa-carrageenan and pectin. *Food Chem.* 153: 9–14.

Lopez-Pena, C.L., Song, M., Xiao, H. et al. (2015). Potential impact of biopolymers (ε-polylysine and/or pectin) on gastrointestinal fate of foods: in vitro study. *Food Res. Int.* 76: 769–776.

Lopez-Pena, C.L., Zheng, B., Sela, D.A. et al. (2016). Impact of epsilon-polylysine and pectin on the potential gastrointestinal fate of emulsified lipids: in vitro mouth, stomach and small intestine model. *Food Chem.* 192: 857–864.

Mazia, D., Schatten, G., and Sale, W. (1975). Adhesion of cells to surfaces coated with polylysine. Applications to electron microscopy. *J. Cell Biol.* 66 (1): 198–200. https://doi.org/10.1083/jcb.66.1.198. PMC 2109515 PMID 1095595.

Melo, M.N., Ferre, R., and Castanho, M.A.R.B. (2009). Antimicrobial peptides: linking partition, activity, and high membrane-bound concentrations. *Nat. Rev. Microbiol.* 7: 245–250.

Millette, M., Cornut, G., Dupont, C. et al. (2008). Capacity of human nisin-and pediocin-producing lactic acid bacteria to reduce intestinal colonization by vancomycin-resistant enterococci. *Appl. Environ. Microbiol.* 74: 1997–2003. https://doi.org/10.1128/AEM.02150-07.

Perez, R.H., Zendo, T., and Sonomoto, K. (2014). Novel bacteriocins from lactic acid bacteria (LAB): various structures and applications. *Microb. Cell Fact.* 13 (Suppl. 1): S3. https://doi.org/10.1186/1475-2859-13-s1-s3.

Prange, A., Birzele, B., Hormes, J., and Modrow, H. (2005). Investigation of different human pathogenic and food contaminating bacteria and mould grown on selenite/selenate and tellurite/tellurate by X-ray absorption spectroscopy. *Food Control* 16: 713–728.

Quintavalla, S. and Vicini, L. (2002). Antimicrobial food packaging in meat industry. *Meat Sci.* 62 (3): 373–380.

Rawat, S. (2015). Food spoilage: microorganisms and their prevention. *Asian J. Plant Sci. Res.* 5 (4): 47–56.

Riley, M.A. and Wertz, J.E. (2002). Bacteriocins: evolution, ecology, and application. *Annu. Rev. Microbiol.* 56: 117–137. https://doi.org/10.1146/annurev.micro.56.012302.161024.

Rooney, M. (1995). *Active Food Packaging*. Glasgow, UK: Blackie Academic and Professional.

Schillinger, U., Geisen, R., and Holzapfel, W. (1996). Potential of antagonistic microorganisms and bacteriocins for the biological preservation of foods. *Trends Food Sci. Technol.* 7: 158–164. https://doi.org/10.1016/0924-2244(96)81256-8.

Settanni, L. and Corsetti, A. (2008). Application of bacteriocins in vegetable food biopreservation. *Int. J. Food Microbiol.* 121: 123–138.

Shima, S. and Sakai, H. (1977). Polylysine produced by *Streptomyces*. *Agric. Biol. Chem.* 41 (9): 1807–1809. https://doi.org/10.1271/bbb1961.41.1807.

Shima, S., Matsuoka, H., Iwamoto, T., and Sakai, H. (1984). Antimicrobial action of ε-poly-l-lysine. *J. Antibiot.* 37 (11): 1449–1455. https://doi.org/10.7164/antibiotics.37.1449. PMID 6392269.

Singh, S. and Shalini, R. (2016). Effect of hurdle technology in food preservation: a review. *Crit. Rev. Food Sci. Nutr.* 56 (4): 641–649.

Singh, A., Sharma, P.K., and Garg, G. (2010). Natural products as preservatives. *Int. J. Pharm. Bio Sci.* 1: 101–612.

Sitterley, G. (2008). Poly-l-lysine cell attachment protocol. *BioFiles* 3 (8): 12.

Sofi, S.A., Singh, J., Rafiq, S. et al. (2018). A comprehensive review on antimicrobial packaging and its use in food packaging. *Curr. Nutr. Food Sci.* 14 (4): 305–312. https://doi.org/10.2174/1573401313666170609095732.

Tagg, J.R., Dajani, A.S., and Wannamaker, L.W. (1976). Bacteriocins of grampositive bacteria. *Bacteriol. Rev.* 40: 722.

Tan, Z.L., Bo, T., Guo, F.Z. et al. (2018). Efects of ε-poly-l-lysine on the cell wall of *Saccharomyces cerevisiae* and its involved antimicrobial mechanism. *Int. J. Biol. Macromol.* 118: 2230–2236.

Tiwari, B.K., Valdramidis, V.P., O'Donnell, C.P. et al. (2009). Application of natural antimicrobials for food preservation. *J. Agric. Food Chem.* 57: 5987–6000.

Wei, M.L., Ge, Y.H., Li, C.Y. et al. (2018). Antifungal activity of ε-poly-l-lysine on Trichothecium roseum in vitro and its mechanisms. *Physiol. Mol. Plant P* 103: 23–27.

Ye, R.S., Xu, H.Y., Wan, C.X. et al. (2013). Antibacterial activity and mechanism of action of ε-poly-l-lysine. *Biochem. Biopharm. Res. Co.* 439: 148–153. https://doi.org/10.1016/j.bbrc.2013.08.001.

Yoshida, T. and Nagasawa, T. (2003). Epsilon-poly-l-lysine: microbial production, biodegradation and application potential. *Appl. Microbiol. Biotechnol.* 62: 21–26.

Zacharof, M. and Lovitt, R. (2012). Bacteriocins produced by lactic acid bacteria a review article. *APCBEE Proc.* 2: 50–56. https://doi.org/10.1016/j.apcbee.2012.06.010.

Zhang, X.W., Shi, C., Liu, Z.J. et al. (2018). Antibacterial activity and mode of action of ε-polylysine against *Escherichia coli* O157:H7. *J. Med. Microbiol.* 67: 838–845.

14

Nutraceuticals Approach as a Treatment for Cancer Cachexia

Gabriela de Matuoka e Chiocchetti, Laís Rosa Viana, Leisa Lopes-Aguiar, Natalia Angelo da Silva Miyaguti, and Maria Cristina Cintra Gomes-Marcondes

Laboratory of Cancer and Nutrition, Department of Structural and Functional Biology, Institute of Biology, University of Campinas – UNICAMP, Campinas, São Paulo, Brazil

14.1 Cancer-Induced Cachexia

14.1.1 Definition and Main Metabolic Changes

Cachexia is characterized as a multifactorial syndrome, with severe lean body mass loss, reduced food intake, decreased physical activity, and accelerated proteolysis due to underlying illness (Langstein and Norton 1991; Blum et al. 2010; Fearon et al. 2011; Johns et al. 2013; Baracos et al. 2018). Typically, it is associated with increased catabolism, which can be partially, but not totally, reversed by merely nutritional support. This metabolic dysfunction occurs in response to pathologic influence by many chronic diseases such as acquired immunodeficiency syndrome, chronic heart and lung failure, liver cirrhosis, kidney failure, rheumatoid arthritis, sepsis, and cancer, which we outline more specifically about cancer-induced cachexia. Although cachexia always includes a component of reduced food intake – anorexia, as unlike "semi-starvation," there are metabolic changes that differ from the normal response to reduced food intake (Inui 1999; Holecek and Kovarik 2011). Cachexia represents the clinical consequence of a chronic systemic inflammatory response, intense body weight reduction, comorbidity, with functional limitation, whether or not accompanied by a decrease in fat mass, a significant increase in protein degradation, mainly of skeletal muscle mass, and increased resting energy expenditure. According to Fearon et al. (2011), a variety of criteria has been used to characterize cancer cachexia to facilitate a standard of clinical trial and development of treatment. In this way, the authors reported a framework that included a continuum of three diagnostic stages: precachexia, cachexia, and refractory cachexia, which not all patients go through these three stages (Fearon et al. 2011; Fearon et al. 2012; Baracos et al. 2018). According to Fearon, precachexia is defined as an earlier clinical and metabolic abnormalities, such as anorexia or impaired glucose control, preceding less than 5% involuntary weight loss, with progression depending on some factors as cancer type and stage, systemic inflammation, low food intake, and less response to anticancer therapy. Cachexia is defined in patients who have more than 5% involuntary weight loss over the preceding six months or a body mass

---

All authors have equal contribution to write, research, and develop data from experimental procedures for this work.

Handbook of Nutraceuticals and Natural Products: Biological, Medicinal, and Nutritional Properties and Applications, Volume 1, First Edition. Edited by Sreerag Gopi and Preetha Balakrishnan.
© 2022 John Wiley & Sons, Inc. Published 2022 by John Wiley & Sons, Inc.

index lower than 20 kg/m^2 and ongoing weight loss over 2% or signs of sarcopenia and ongoing weight loss more than 2%, and nonassociated with a refractory stage. Refractory cachexia is defined by the clinical presentation of the patient with advanced cancer (preterminal stage) or the presence of fast progression and unresponsive cancer to the treatment, also associated with active catabolism, and presence of factors, that make body weight loss no longer possible to manage, low-performance status, and lower expectance of life (<three months) (Fearon et al. 2011; Fearon et al. 2012). This severe syndrome occurs in most patients with terminal cancer and is responsible for 22% of cancer deaths (Argilés et al. 2005). The conventional therapies for cancer, including surgery, chemotherapy, radiotherapy and immunotherapy, also lead to anorexia and weight loss, which can aggravate the cachexia process. Depending on the type of tumor, weight loss occurs in 30–80% of cancer patients and is severe (with 10% loss of initial body weight) in 15% of these patients (Tisdale 2009, 2010). Patients with pancreatic or gastric cancer have the highest incidence of cachexia, while patients with non-Hodgkin's lymphoma, breast cancer, acute nonlymphocytic leukemia, and sarcomas have the lowest frequency of cachexia (Tisdale 2010; Prado et al. 2013; Del Fabbro 2015; Baracos et al. 2018).

The changes observed in cancer cachexia and the mechanisms of this syndrome are outlined here pointing some of the critical metabolic changes that occur in cachexia include deviations from the homeostatic pattern of carbohydrate metabolism, lipids, and especially proteins. Depletion of muscle protein is an aspect of high relevance, as it involves not only skeletal muscle tissue but also cardiac proteins, which results in important changes in patients' cardiac performance (Argilés et al. 2005; Sandri 2015). Currently, cachexia is considered to have an epidemic potential for the coming decades.

The tumor growth modifies the harmony of metabolic processes through profound changes, leading to unintentional body weight loss that occurs, in the presence of cancer, depending on a lower intake of nutrients with an increased expenditure of basal energy substrate, obtained by the mobilization of glycogen, and fat and spoliation of muscle mass (Ventrucci et al. 2001; Gomes-Marcondes et al. 2003; Salomão et al. 2012; Oliveira and Gomes-Marcondes 2016; Viana et al. 2018). In the presence of cancer cachexia, the patient loses the ability to adapt carbohydrate metabolism, since cancer affects host tissues changing the characteristics of the enzymes, tissue hormone sensitivity and disturbing the negative feedback responses. Cachectic patients have an increased level of catabolic hormones such as glucagon, catecholamines, and glucocorticoids, associated with insulin resistance. In this state, many studies have shown that tumor cells, mainly solid tumors such as pancreas, colon, gastric, use glucose as a primary energy source, causing hypoglycemia. Therefore, in the cachectic host, the alteration of glycemia homeostasis increases the liver demand. Thus, the glycemia disturbance is weakly supported by hepatic glycogenolysis and by new glucose synthesis via gluconeogenesis, mainly from muscle catabolism amino acids, from glycerol of lipolysis and also from lactate, in this case, from the anaerobic glycolysis of tumor cell (Pisters and Brennan 1990). Thus, gluconeogenesis remains higher in the cachectic host leading to greater excretion of nitrogen as a result of intense protein catabolism, with a general hypercatabolic state, reducing lean body mass and consequently increasing the body weight loss (Costelli and Baccino 2003). In these cases, the whole-body energy expenditure, especially the resting energy, is related to a higher negative energy balance, further aggravating the body weight loss. Most of the energy expenditure is mainly related to tumor metabolism. Glucose requirement increased in tumor cells due to the targeting of glucose-6-phosphate and fructose-6-phosphate for the synthesis of purines, pyrimidines, DNA, and tumor RNA. In parallel, the pentose cycle increases, which supports the tumor cell proliferation. Besides, these cells are unable to maintain an adequate level of intracellular ATP in the absence of glucose. Thus the anaerobic glycolytic rate in tumor cells is extremely high, even under normal or higher levels of O_2, and provides lactate and non-pyruvate and CO_2, resulting in energy deficit per cell (Denko 2008). Therefore, in tumor cells, the lactate produced, in some areas of solid tumors, is converted into glucose by hepatic gluconeogenesis, corresponding to the Cori cycle under an inefficiency way to the host (Tisdale 2003; McLean et al. 2014). Moreover, the higher disruption of some mitochondrial enzymes activity is the major cause of massive lactate production. This point together with the increased cytosolic NADH/NAD+ ratio favor the action of lactate dehydrogenase, which is also associated with failing of electron transfer chain and jeopardizing the Na/K ATPase pump, limiting the mitochondria membrane potential. Besides, in other host tissues also occurs mitochondrial dysfunction, especially in skeletal muscles, which enhances the cachexia state (Vitorino et al. 2015; Carson et al. 2016; Cruz et al. 2020). Since the oxidative stress leads to lipid peroxidation and also protein carbonylation, this fail accounts for this partial uncoupling of respiration and phosphorylation in mitochondria (Gomes-Marcondes and Tisdale 2002; Vitorino et al. 2015; Carson et al. 2016; Fukawa et al. 2016). Also, the disrupted balance of antioxidant enzymes increases the microenvironment of tumor cells spreading and jeopardizes the normal function of the other host cells/tissue. Thus, the changes in carbohydrate metabolism due to the consequences of metabolic demands of tumor tissue lead to a worsening development of the cachectic state.

The factors postulated as mediators of cancer cachexia are also related to a complex tumor secretome directly related to host catabolism and by the pro-inflammatory factors that affect host metabolism direct or indirectly (Barbosa et al. 2012; Fukawa et al. 2016; Cruz et al. 2017). Compounds with hormone-like characteristics secreted by tumor cells can exert their effects directly on host catabolism. Small peptides such as 24 kDa proteoglycan isolated from the urine of cachectic patients or in tumor tissue in experimental models, named proteolysis-inducing factor (PIF), promote skeletal muscle degradation. The main effect is related to increasing proteolysis, specifically through the ubiquitin-proteasome pathway, and inhibiting the incorporation of amino acids in muscle, which is prevalent in cachexia state (Todorov et al. 1996; Yano et al. 2008; Gonçalves et al. 2013; Cruz et al. 2017; Cruz et al. 2019). Another 43 kDa glycoprotein isolated from colon adenocarcinoma (MAC16) and also found in the urine of cancer patients, and characterized as lipid mobilization factor (LMF) is capable of increasing lipolysis leading to adipose tissue loss as verified in cachectic patients (Mulligan et al. 1992; Russell and Tisdale 2005). Pro-inflammatory cytokines also include a long list that leads to a generation of catabolic process modulating the homeostatic control in the central nervous system, triggering the sympathetic nervous system, which as mentioned above releases or stimulates the increased levels of catabolic hormones (Tisdale 2009, 2010). The most important cytokines that mediating cachexia include tumor necrosis factor-alpha (TNF-α), interleukin-1 and -6 (IL-1 and IL-6), interferon-gamma (INF-γ), leukemia inhibitory factor (LIF), TNF-related weak inducer of apoptosis (TWEAK or TNFSF12), growth/differentiation factor 15 (GDF15), and transforming growth factor-β (TGFβ) superfamily – including activins, myostatin, adrenomedullin, and others (Langstein and Norton 1991; Tisdale 2009, 2010; Cruz et al. 2017). All these mediators act over host tissues promoting the catabolic state of cachexia (Langstein and Norton 1991; Tisdale 2009, 2010; Cruz et al. 2017). These humoral factors are released mainly by the immune system or tumor cells and exert effects on numerous cells of the body, such as bone marrow cells, myocytes, cardiomyocytes, hepatocytes, adipocytes, endothelial cells, and neurons, producing a complex cascade of biological responses such as activating proteolysis and lipolysis, responsible for most of the metabolic alterations associated with cachexia.

Body fat, which represents the large stock of body energy, is depleted to supply the increase in metabolic demand of the host, caused by the tumor evolution. Fat depletion in cancer is related to direct growth of tumor mass (Gomes-Marcondes et al. 2003; Salomão et al. 2012; Argiles et al. 2013).

The mobilization of fatty acids of adipose tissue can occur even before the perception of weight loss. In this case, as mentioned above, the LMF factor acts directly on adipose tissue releasing free fatty acids and glycerol, through the elevation of intracellular adenosine monophosphate cyclic, as in the same way as lipolytic hormones acting. Besides, this LMF and others cytokines such as TNFα inhibit lipoprotein lipase, preventing adipocytes from removing fatty acids from plasma lipoprotein stock, resulting in increased circulating lipids in these cancer patients (Tisdale 2009, 2010). Adipocytes of cancer patients respond two to three times more to the lipolysis effects of catecholamine or natriuretic peptide than healthy organism (Tisdale 2009). These adipocytes present a 50% increase in mRNA expression for the sensitive hormone lipase, which in turn can be activated by LMF (Tisdale 2009). Increased levels of pro-inflammatory cytokines in cachectic patients show the inflammatory state, which conducts to lipid metabolic alteration and also leading the skeletal muscle waste (Tisdale 2009; Salomão et al. 2010; Cruz et al. 2017). In this way, cancer cachexia is considered a chronic inflammatory disease. In adipocyte of a cachectic host, the activation of apoptosis induced by DNA fragmentation is correlated to a higher release of free fatty acids in serum, up to two to four times more than in healthy organism (Tisdale 2009; Salomão et al. 2010; Cruz et al. 2017). Thus, associated with this fact, there is a diminished insulin secretion and resistance enhancing the lipid mobilization, increased by the lipolytic factors, such as glucocorticoids, which contribute to hypertriglyceridemia. Indeed, as mentioned before, cachectic patients have an intense weight loss caused by depletion of adipose tissue, driven by many pro-inflammatory cytokines, such as TNF, and also by the crosstalk among host tissues. Thus, some findings of the crosstalk between the peritumoral adipose tissue and tumor can show that the release of adipokines and angiogenic, apoptotic, and growth factors predict the modulation of proliferative environment closely linked to the tumor (Neto et al. 2018; Lengyel et al. 2018). In addition, considering the decreased glucose oxidation by peripheral tissues by up to 40% associated with increased expression of pyruvate dehydrogenase kinase, phosphorylation (inactivation) of pyruvate dehydrogenase complex, there is a favoring way to fatty acid oxidation. Indeed, the liver has a higher energy demand by the gluconeogenesis process, which can be provided by beta-oxidation of fatty acids by the Krebs cycle producing not only ATP but also ketone bodies (Viana et al. 2016). This explains the high oxidation of fatty acids by peripheral tissues and high oxidation of glucose by tumor tissue. Together with the high activity of lipolysis, the increased thermogenesis process in adipose tissue also happens to enhance the browning of white adipose cells. Mitochondria regulate the thermogenesis process by the uncoupling protein 1, in which the gene expression increases in both animal models of cancer cachexia and white adipose tissue in cachectic patients (Petruzzelli and Wagner 2016; Porporato 2016). The researchers are raising to understand better how the adipose tissue loss leads to muscle mass loss, and how this crosstalk between adipose and muscle tissue can be one of the most important driven to cachexia definition.

Indeed, the depletion of lean body mass in cancer is the principal responsible for reducing the survival time of cancer patients. The increase in catabolism associated with reduced protein synthesis is present in the skeletal muscle of patients and experimental animals with cancer, which is the main factor for the establishment of cachexia (Gomes-Marcondes et al. 2003; Tisdale 2009, 2010; Cruz et al. 2019). The protein synthesis process during cachexia corresponds to about 8% of the total body compared to healthy individuals who have 53% of total body protein synthesis. On the other hand, in cancer-induced cachexia, there may be an increased protein synthesis by specific tissues or organs, as acute-phase proteins secreted by the liver. Most of the pro-inflammatory cytokines and tumoral factors associated with reduced insulin and insulin-like growth factor 1 (IGF-1) levels disrupt the central core of protein synthesis – the mechanistic target of rapamycin (mTOR). In the host tissues, the upstream proteins such as protein kinase B (AKT) and phosphoinositide 3-kinase (PI3K) are inhibited impairing the phosphorylation of mTOR, which would phosphorylate the downstream proteins – S6K, protein ribosomal S6 kinase-β1 (S6K), and eukaryotic translation initiation factor 4E-binding protein 1 (4EBP1), which are part of the assembling of the ribosomal unit and activating the cap-dependent mRNA translation for protein synthesis. In this way, most of the host tissues are impaired protein synthesis and also cellular activity due to the inhibited mTOR pathway (Gordon et al. 2013; Sharples et al. 2015; Viana et al. 2016; Cruz et al. 2017, 2019). The main pathway of protein degradation, especially in muscle, that is upregulated in cachexia is related to the ATP-dependent ubiquitin-proteasome system, where the E3 ubiquitin-protein ligase (MuRF-1) and F-box only protein 32 (Fbxo32, or atrogin1) play a key role in this system, which is regulated by the transcription factor forkhead box protein O1 (FoxO1) and O3 (FoxO3). These activities are posttranslationally regulated, managing a regulatory intersection between the anabolic and catabolic process. In a cachectic state, many factors as PIF, proinflammatory cytokines and other reduce the AKT activity, allowing the translocation of FoxO to nucleus consequently the transcription of MuRF-1 and atrogin1, which increase the muscle myofibrillar protein degradation (Dutt et al. 2015; Cruz et al. 2017). Together with others such as TNF-α and TWEAK activating factor nuclear kappa B (NFkB), IL6 and LIF activating signal transducer and activator of transcription (STAT3) increase the transcription of E3 ubiquitin ligase genes. Thus, activins, TGFβ, and myostatin increasing the activation of SMAD family member 2 and 3 (SMAD2/SMAD3) also enhanced the transcription of E3 ubiquitin ligases, autophagy, and lead to muscle atrophy and contractile dysfunction (de Oliveira et al. 2020). Furthermore, protein catabolism provides amino acids which offer gluconeogenic substrate would further stimulate the gluconeogenesis process, further increasing the energy needs of the host and neoplastic cells. Some amino acids are preferably used by neoplastic cells because these cells are unable to synthesize certain amino acids, which implies an increased demand for host amino acids. Glutamine, for example, is not synthesized by various types of cancer; it is a precursor of proteins and nucleotides in neoplastic cells. There is evidence that neoplastic protein synthesis is accelerated due to the increase of enzymes responsible for the biosynthesis of DNA, pyrimidines, and purines in neoplastic cells. As a result of the high neoplastic cellular activity and host demand, the protein ingested in adequate quantity for the nitrogen balance of a healthy organism is insufficient for cachectic patients. Thus, the lower intake of nutrients due to anorexia and consequently lower protein and caloric intake associated with high energy expenditure increase the weight loss and functional impairment in cachexia state. Again, healthy individuals adapt to lower nutrient intake by increasing fatty acid mobilization and reducing protein catabolism, a condition where there would be lower glucose production from amino acids. The lack of nutrients, imposed by anorexia and the progression of cancer, promotes the non-adaptation of cachectic patients to the metabolism of body proteins, reducing protein synthesis and increasing the proteolysis.

The best management to treat cachexia includes an appropriate antitumor treatment, nutrition intervention, exercise or physical activity plan, and supportive pharmacologic intervention. According to the literature, the most important treatments are linked to experimental approaches and also applied in patients, but still under empirical procedures. These methods are related to the nutrients intake improvement including orexigenic substances to increase the food intake/appetite, such as cannabinoids (Dronabinol), progesterone analogues (megestrol acetate, medroxyprogesterone), ghrelin, melatonin and corticosteroids (dexamethasone), and drugs which minimize nausea/vomiting (thalidomide) or delay of gastric emptying, approved by Food and Drug Administration (FDA). These substances can also inhibit some cytokines that are related to the inflammatory process (such as IL1α, IL6, TNFα), stimulating the anti-inflammatory process (increasing IL10), or in other cases can stimulate the release of neuropeptide Y (NPY), which modulates directly the ventromedial hypothalamic nucleus related to satiety. Moreover, the inhibitors of the ubiquitin-proteasome pathway and PI3K pathway minimize the muscle proteolysis and improve the lean body mass to recover or to improve the quality of life (QOL). Despite the advances, there is still a gap between studies in cachectic patients and animal models of cachexia, which could lead to a specific medication or a set of drugs to act in important points for the management of cancer-related cachexia.

Given all metabolic abnormalities, leading to an elevated proteolysis process and inflammatory state, as described above, the treatment of cancer cachexia is usually recognized not as a single treatment plan, but a multimodal approach, especially because of the multifactorial characteristics of this syndrome. Considering that cachexia occurs in approximately 80% of severe cancer cases and is responsible for up to 22% of all cancer-related deaths, as mentioned before, it is important to investigate non-pharmacological strategies to mitigate the severe changes in host metabolism. Strategies such as nutritional supplementation, especially as pointed here as a nutraceutical approach, have been considered as a coadjutant treatment in cancer cachexia.

14.2   Probiotics and Prebiotics

In general, probiotics are defined as live microorganisms that, when administered in adequate quantities, provide a benefit to the health of the host (Hill et al. 2014). Traditional probiotics are isolated from sources as the gut and traditional fermented foods, which have been listed as Generally Regarded as Safe (GRAS) at the strain level by the FDA (Martín and Langella 2019). The extensive application of probiotics and their status as GRAS organisms make them suitable for use as dietary supplementation strategies to enhance the effects of muscle preservation and improvement (Jäger et al. 2016; Chen et al. 2016). Additionally, probiotics also present an anti-inflammatory profile, which can modulate cancer development (Jeong et al. 2015; Gamallat et al. 2016; Jacouton et al. 2017), showing possible beneficial effects in cancer-associated cachexia.

Kimchi, a traditional fermented food highly consumed in Korea, with an additional of *Leuconostoc mesenteroides* CJ LM119 and *Lactobacillus plantarum* CJ LP133 was studied by An and colleagues to assess the possible contribution to ameliorate cancer cachexia in colon carcinoma C26-bearing mice. The animals that consumed kimchi daily had lesser weight loss, higher muscle preservation, as well as higher survival, compared with mice that consumed a standard diet. Through the significant reduction of the IL-6 signaling pathway, kimchi afforded significant downregulation of muscle-specific ubiquitin-proteasome system, including inhibition of atrogin-1 and MuRF-1. The NF-kB activation, known as a pivotal inflammatory mechanism, also reduced under kimchi consumption, with a decreased phosphorylation of NF-kB 65 and NF-kB p50. On the other hand, kimchi significantly decreased AMP-activated protein kinase (AMPK) activation, which could improve muscle regeneration. Also, regarding the changes of mitogen-activated protein kinases (MAPKs), extracellular signal-regulated kinase 1 and 2 (ERK1/2), p38, and c-Jun N-terminal kinase (JNK) activations were all noted in the tumor-bearing group, and these MAPKs were all significantly inactivated by kimchi treatment. Moreover, signals of AKT, mTOR, and PI3K were significantly improved in those C26 tumor-bearing mice subjected to kimchi administration, restoring the atrophied muscle in cancer cachexia (An et al. 2019).

Varian and colleagues showed that *Lactobacillus reuteri,* originally isolated from human mother's milk, was able to lower systemic indices of inflammation (IL-6, IL-1β, and TNFα) and inhibit cachexia (improving the gastrocnemius muscle mass and muscle fiber cross-sectional area compared to controls mice) when administered to ApcMIN mice, a murine model of cachexia.

Lactobacillus reuteri administration improved the life span and was also associated with increased thymus and decreased forkhead box N1 (FoxN1) expression, a transcription factor involved in systemic inflammation. Nevertheless, the authors point out that *L. reuteri* treatment in ApcMIN mice also reduced the intestinal tumor burden, which was difficult to assess if the extent of the reduced tumor burden contributed in the prevention of cancer-associated cachexia itself or by the modulation of the inflammatory process (Varian et al. 2016).

In another study, the supplementation with *L. reuteri* 100-23 reduced the expression of atrophy markers (Atrogin-1, MuRF-1, microtubule-associated protein 1A/1B-light chain 3 (LC3), Cathepsin L) in the gastrocnemius and the tibialis muscles, and decreased inflammatory cytokines (IL-6, IL- 4, monocyte chemoattractant protein-1 (MCP-1) and granulocyte colony-stimulating factor (G- CSF)) in a murine model of cachexia, but had no change in cachexia parameters, as body and muscle weight, food intake, and serum parameters. Also, in this study, a similar result was seen with the supplementation with *Lactobacillus gasseri* 311476 (Bindels et al. 2012). Although these results show a beneficial effect of *Lactobacillus* ssp. supplementation on the skeletal muscle, it is important to stress that these positive effects are strain- and species-specific and cannot extrapolate to all *Lactobacillus* ssp., as found by Bindels and colleagues, who verified that *Lactobacillus acidophilus* NCFM supplementation had no impact on muscle atrophy markers and systemic inflammation (Bindels et al. 2012).

Emerging research has pointed out that the microbiota can play a role in cancer cachexia (Bindels and Thissen 2016; Herremans et al. 2019; Genton et al. 2019). Nevertheless, just a few studies have reported effectively how cancer cachexia affects the microbiota. Bindels and colleagues have been the pioneer group investigating this topic, and they found a dysbiosis and a selective modulation of *Lactobacillus* spp. (decrease of *L. reuteri* and *Lactobacillus johnsonii/gasseri* in favor of *Lactobacillus murinus/Lactobacillus animalis*), an increase of *Enterobacteriaceae*, specifically *Klebsiella oxytoca*, and *Parabacteroides goldsteinii*/ASF 519, in two different experimental models of cachexia (Bindels et al. 2012, 2016, 2018; Pötgens et al. 2018). The authors also reported that these alterations in microbiota were not related to food intake reduction and partially counteracted by the anti-IL-6 treatment, suggesting that cancer cells and associated increased IL-6 levels contribute to the gut microbial dysbiosis (Bindels et al. 2018). Despite there is some evidence that microbiota and inflammation are linked in cancer (Roy and Trinchieri 2017; Lucas et al. 2017), the association of microbiota and inflammation in cancer cachexia remains unclear.

Probiotics can be used as a supplementation way to restore the normal balance of the intestinal ecosystem by modulating the microbiota (Bindels et al. 2012). However, not just probiotics can modulate the microbiota to benefit the host health; prebiotics could also present a similar effect. The term prebiotics is defined as "a nondigestible food ingredient that beneficially affects the host by selectively stimulating the growth and the activity of a limited number of bacteria in the colon, and thus improves host health" (Gibson and Roberfroid 1995). However, with the advances in the understanding of the interactions among the diet, the microbiota, and the host (Bindels et al. 2015; Martín and Langella 2019), this traditional concept has been updated as "a substrate that is selectively utilised by host/commensal microorganisms conferring a health benefit" (Gibson et al. 2017).

Bindels and colleagues found the supplementation of two prebiotics (pectic oligosaccharides – POS and inulin – INU) in a mouse model, which mimics acute leukemia and cause cachexia to decrease the microbial diversity and richness of cecal microbiota, whereas the population of *Bifidobacterium* spp., *Roseburia* spp., and *Bacteroides* spp. increased. In addition, POS reduced the metabolic alterations associated with cachexia and delayed anorexia linked to cancer progression (Bindels et al. 2015). Huang and colleagues assessed the prebiotic ginsenoside-Rb3 and ginsenoside-Rd in an ApcMin/+ mice model, showing the effectively reinstated the dysbiotic-gut microbial composition and intestinal microenvironment, by promoting the growth of beneficial bacteria such as *Bifidobacterium* spp., *Lactobacillus* spp., *Bacteroides acidifaciens*, and *Bacteroides xylanisolvens*. Rb3/Rd supplementation also showed anti-inflammatory activity by suppressing pro-inflammatory cytokines and enhancing anti-inflammatory cytokines (Huang et al. 2017).

Also, at the intestinal level, a profound change in intestinal functions (gut permeability, impaired barrier function, and gut immunity) is observed in experimental models of cachexia (Puppa et al. 2011; Klein et al. 2013; Bindels et al. 2018) and also verified in clinical studies (Jiang et al. 2014a, b). Despite clinical evidence that gut functions can be modulate by probiotics (Bron et al. 2017; Wang et al. 2018), the treatment with *Faecalibacterium prausnitzii* (a principal member of the human microbiota, which is reduced upon chemotherapy in cancer patients) was not able to modulate the gut dysfunction (did not modify gut permeability and intestinal markers of the gut barrier function) in C26 tumor-bearing mice (Bindels et al. 2018).

Nevertheless, Bindels and colleagues showed that a symbiotic approach – a mixture of probiotics and prebiotics that beneficially affect the host (Martín and Langella 2019) – can restore intestinal homeostasis in cachectic mice (Bindels et al. 2016). In two different models of cancer cachexia, mice fed the prebiotic inulin-type fructans and *L. reuteri* showed restoration of the expression of antimicrobial proteins controlling intestinal barrier function and gut immunity markers. It was also associated with the improvement of some cachectic features such as muscle mass loss and the expression of atrophy markers in tibialis and gastrocnemius muscles (cathepsin L and LC3) (Bindels et al. 2016).

From our knowledge, there is no clinical study demonstrating that solely supplementation with probiotics is beneficial in cancer cachexia. Besides, Hassan and colleagues performed a systematic review and meta-analysis investigation on the efficacy and safety of probiotics in cancer patients. The authors concluded that there remain insufficient studies to assess the exact effect of probiotics in people with cancer, and the reporting of adverse events was variable and inconsistent (Hassan et al. 2018). Based on that, the safety of probiotics in cancer patients needs to be better examined before their clinical implementation as a coadjutant in cancer cachexia treatment.

14.3 Amino Acids

14.3.1 Leucine

Leucine is the most important essential branched-chain amino acid (BCAA) among the other two valine, and isoleucine. These three BCAAs have a similar lateral radical chain, and they exert an essential role in many metabolic pathways in skeletal muscle, acting as an energy source, anti-inflammatory, and stimulatory agents for protein synthesis (Shimomura et al. 2006; Nicastro et al. 2011; de Campos-Ferraz et al. 2014). Although all three BCAAs have these important roles, leucine is the most powerful, among valine and isoleucine, in stimulating muscle protein synthesis (Garlick 2005). Leucine can attenuate proteolysis and enhance protein synthesis in skeletal muscle, mainly through activation of the mTOR pathway (Kimball et al. 1999; Kimball and Jefferson 2006; Columbus et al. 2015a, b). Knowing that skeletal muscle protein synthesis decreased and the proteolysis is extremely increased in cancer cachexia, leucine supplementation may exert a therapeutic effect for cancer cachexia. Besides having a key role in muscle protein metabolism, leucine also plays an essential role in oxidative phosphorylation, activating peroxisome proliferator-activated receptor gamma PPARγ activity and increasing mitochondrial biogenesis and elevated substrate oxidation (Liang et al. 2014; Schnuck et al. 2016). Despite having a significant anabolic effect in skeletal muscle tissue, few clinical studies investigated the effects of leucine supplementation in patients suffering from cancer cachexia.

Engelen and colleagues performed a nutritional intervention comparing a mixture of the essential amino acid (EAA) with high leucine levels (EAA/leucine) versus a balanced amino acid mixture (containing both EAA and non-EAA) in patients with advanced non-small-cell lung cancer (stages III and IV) and in healthy age-matched subjects (Engelen et al. 2015). The authors found that protein synthesis and net protein anabolism were higher after intake of the EAA/leucine than the balanced amino acid mixture. The high anabolic potential of dietary EAA/leucine in cancer patients was independent of their nutritional status, systemic inflammatory response, or disease trajectory. Therefore, the authors suggested a key role of EAA/leucine as a nutritional approach to preventing muscle loss, thereby improving the outcome of patients with advanced cancer (Engelen et al. 2015). Deutz and colleagues presented a randomized controlled study in patients with radiographic evidence of cancer (Deutz et al. 2011). The authors evaluated the fractional rate of muscle protein synthesis in the experimental group that received a medical food containing 40 g protein + 10% of leucine and the control group that received the standard medical food containing 24 g of protein. The plasma leucine concentration and muscle protein synthesis were significantly increased in the experimental group. On the other hand, standard food failed to increase muscle protein synthesis. Despite the interesting result, it is not possible to conclude to a specific effect of leucine, as both medical foods were not isonitrogenous (Deutz et al. 2011). This study brings a very important aspect that cancer patients require a special diet, with high protein and amino acid (especially leucine) content to stimulate muscle protein synthesis, since these patients often suffer from cachexia.

Since clinical studies evaluating the effects of a leucine-rich diet are rare, outcomes from preclinical models of cancer cachexia studies have brought significant progress in the knowledge of how leucine protects skeletal muscle tissue under cancer cachexia. Peters et al. (2011) demonstrated that muscle wasting, associated with high skeletal muscle protein breakdown was attenuated after leucine supplementation (8 g leucine per kilogram feed, containing 14.8% leucine per gram protein) in a murine colon adenocarcinoma (C26) tumor-bearing cachectic mouse model (Peters et al. 2011). In our previous study, we found that the association of leucine supplementation (18% protein + 3% leucine) with aerobic exercise training in Walker 256 tumor-bearing rats was effective in increasing protein synthesis in gastrocnemius muscle, leading to higher total net protein content (Salomão et al. 2010). Also, we showed that pregnant Walker 256 tumor-bearing rats fed with a leucine-rich diet (18% protein + 3% leucine) conferred protection for the fetal muscle tissue, which resulted from the maintenance of muscle protein synthesis and decreased proteolysis due to the lower activity of the proteasomal and lysosomal pathways (Cruz and Gomes-Marcondes 2014). Another study found that adult Walker 256 tumor-bearing rats fed with a leucine-rich diet presented better heart functional parameters and lower sudden death risk when compared to tumor-bearing rats fed with the standard diet. Leucine was effective in modulating heart damage, cardiomyocyte proteolysis, and apoptosis induced by cancer cachexia (Toneto et al. 2016). Furthermore, we demonstrated that the role of dietary leucine supplementation in decreased muscle protein degradation in adult Walker 256 tumor-bearing rats was related to an increase in anti-inflammatory cytokines that diminished the inflammation, relieving muscle catabolism (Cruz et al. 2017). Moreover, as a prevention approach, we also verified that a leucine-rich diet, when administered to the dams rats, during pregnancy and lactation, showed improvements related to muscle wasting. The tumor-bearing offspring maternally supplemented with this amino acid had lesser muscle mass loss. This study reported an improved protein balance, with differences in the mTOR pathway and modified proteasome and calpain protein breakdown systems provided by the maternal diet (Miyaguti et al. 2019). Additionally, we have recently shown, in a skeletal muscle proteomic and metabolomic study, that the beneficial effects of a leucine-rich diet in Walker 256 tumor-bearing rats are also due to a significant improvement in muscle mitochondria function and biogenesis (Cruz et al. 2020). Whereas understanding the effects of a leucine-rich diet in tumor tissue is as important as the effects in muscles, we have recently evaluated the effects of the administration of the leucine-rich diet on the Walker 256 tumor metabolism (Viana et al. 2019). We found similar tumor weight between tumor-bearing rats and tumor-bearing rats fed with leucine-rich diet. Despite the similar tumor weights, leucine diet led to a tumor metabolic shifting from glycolytic toward oxidative phosphorylation, reducing glucose consumption and metastasis formation, suggesting that the leucine nutritional supplementation does not benefit this type of tumor. Further studies must be done to evaluate the effects of a leucine diet in other experimental models of cancer cachexia.

14.3.2 β-Hydroxy-β-Methylbutyrate

Approximately 80% of leucine is generally used for protein synthesis while the remainder is converted to α-ketoisocaproate (α-KIC) and only a small proportion of leucine (5%) is converted into β-hydroxy-β-methylbutyrate (HMB) in skeletal muscle (Van Koevering and Nissen 1992). Several studies revealed the effects of HMB as a skeletal muscle protector, attenuating muscle damage (Rossi et al. 2017), enhancing muscle protein synthesis and decreasing muscle protein breakdown, and consequently increasing muscle strength (Aversa et al. 2011; Park et al. 2013; Silva et al. 2017). Kovarik and colleagues proposed that HMB might affect muscle protein metabolism through changes in proteasome-dependent proteolysis and protein synthesis in experimental models (Kovarik et al. 2010). As mentioned above, the skeletal muscle protein synthesis decreased, and the proteolysis enhanced in cancer cachexia; thus, the HMB supplementation could be considered as a potential target for cancer cachexia treatment. Aversa and colleagues showed that a 4% HMB supplemented diet attenuated muscle and body weight loss in AH-130 tumor-bearing rats, improving protein anabolism in muscle, through the increasing of the phosphorylation of ribosomal p70 S6 kinase (p70S6K) and mTOR, without changing the phosphorylation of 4EBP1 (Aversa et al. 2011). Besides activating muscle protein synthesis through mTOR pathway, HMB administration (320 mg/kg body weight) seems to stimulate GH/IGF-1 axis activity, and this axis may mediate some of the effects on skeletal muscle exerted by HMB (Gerlinger-Romero et al. 2011). Giron and colleagues performed an in vitro study using rat L6 myotubes comparing the anabolic effects of leucine and HMB in the absence of any catabolic stimuli (Girón et al. 2016). The authors observed that HMB was significantly more effective than leucine in exerting stimulatory effects through mTOR pathway, activating the downstream elements such as S6K, 4EBP1, and eIF4E (Girón et al. 2016). The ineffectiveness of leucine could be related to the fact that L6 myotubes lack the ability to convert leucine into HMB, once L6 myotubes were transfected with a plasmid that codes for α-KIC dioxygenase, the key enzyme involved in the catabolic conversion of α-KIC into HMB leucine was able to promote protein synthesis and mTOR pathway activation equally to HMB. The study proposes that HMB may be very useful to stimulate protein synthesis in wasting conditions, such as cancer cachexia. Likewise, Mirza et al. (2014) suggested that HMB could be more effective than leucine in attenuating body weight loss in an experimental model of cancer cachexia (Mirza et al. 2014). In this study, MAC16 tumor-bearing mice were administrated with leucine (1 g/kg) or HMB (0.25 g/kg), and then, at the endpoint criteria, the muscle protein degradation and synthesis were measured. The authors found that a low dose of HMB was 60% more effective than leucine in attenuating loss of body weight in cachectic animals (Mirza et al. 2014). For this reason, the authors proposed that HMB might be a more clinically feasible approach in the treatment of cancer cachexia. It is also important to emphasize that tumor weight and tumor cell proliferation reduced in Walker 256 tumor-bearing rats treated with HMB (Kuczera et al. 2012). Further studies must be done to evaluate the effects of HMB treatment in other cancer cachexia experimental models.

Unfortunately, the lack of randomized, blinded placebo-controlled clinical trials limits any extrapolation to patients (Molfino et al. 2013). Likewise, Bear and colleagues recently performed a systematic review and meta-analysis investigating the efficacy of HMB alone, or supplements containing HMB, on skeletal muscle mass and function in a variety of clinical conditions mainly characterized by loss of skeletal mass and weakness (Bear et al. 2019). The authors concluded that the effect size of the studies was small and due to the bias associated with the studies, they suggested that further high-quality studies should be undertaken to enable interpretation and translation into clinical practice.

14.3.3 Glycine

Glycine is a nonessential amino acid and considered biologically neutral. Some studies indicate that glycine could be an effective anti-inflammatory agent that could preserve muscle function during wasting conditions. Since increased inflammation plays a key role in the loss of skeletal muscle and adipose tissue in cancer cachexia, glycine supplementation could represent a simple, safe, and promising treatment option (Ham et al. 2014; Koopman et al. 2017).

Based on this knowledge, Ham and colleagues performed the first study testing the hypothesis that glycine treatment would reduce systemic inflammation and attenuate the loss of skeletal muscle and function in a C26 murine model of cancer cachexia (Ham et al. 2014). The authors treaded C26 tumor-bearing and healthy mice with 1 g/kg/day of glycine for 21 days (which represented an increase in amino acid intake of only 3.7%). Glycine treatment attenuated the loss of body mass, the reduction on food intake, provided some protection from the loss of fat, and significantly reduced tumor mass by approximately 32%. Also, the authors observed that in glycine-treated animals, the reductions in mass of the quadriceps, gastrocnemius and tibialis muscles were significantly less than in PBS-treated C26 tumor-bearing mice (Ham et al. 2014). In line with muscle mass results, glycine treatment attenuated the reduction of the muscle cross-sectional area. Moreover, in order to evaluate if glycine treatment would reduce inflammation, authors measured some markers of inflammation (IL-6) and macrophage infiltration (F4/80) and found that both markers reduced significantly and not differed from the non-tumor control group. Additionally, glycine treatment prevented the tumor-induced increase in MuRF and atrogin-1, the two major effector proteins of muscle degradation (Reed et al. 2012). Taken together, the results show that glycine treatment could be considered a potential therapeutic agent for cancer cachexia since it reduces tumor growth and attenuates cancer-induced cachexia (Koopman et al. 2017).

Among the described pathways involved in cancer cachexia, such as upregulation of degradation ubiquitin-proteasome pathway and downregulation of mTOR pathway, Zhang and colleagues recently proposed that tumor induces muscle wasting through releasing extracellular heat shock proteins (Hsp), Hsp70 and Hsp90 (Zhang et al. 2017). Thus, the authors observed that Hsp70 and Hsp90 induced muscle catabolism by activating Toll-like receptor 4 (TLR4) signaling and were responsible for elevating circulating cytokines. In parallel, glycine suppressed the TLR4 signaling, although it is not known whether skeletal muscle fibers express glycine receptors, this could be partially responsible for beneficial effects found by Ham and colleagues (Ham et al. 2014). While the mechanism of glycine action may be somewhat obscure, the impact of glycine supplementation on cancer cachexia merits more study once it has great potential as a therapeutic agent for cancer cachexia. From our knowledge, there is no clinical study if glycine administration in cancer cachexia context.

14.3.4 Carnitine

Carnitine is an amino acid derivative that can be synthesized through endogenous conversion from lysine and methionine, but 75% of the required levels come from the diet. Carnitine plays a significant role as blocking inflammatory state, which is known to play an essential role in cancer cachexia (Liu et al. 2011). Moreover, carnitine has a fundamental role in fatty acids β-oxidation for energy generation via mitochondria. Despite having these important roles, acting as anti-inflammatory and energy agent, low-carnitine serum levels have been shown in advanced cancer patients, and this carnitine deficiency seems to be one of the causes of cancer cachexia (Malaguarnera et al. 2006). Additionally, chemotherapy leads to further depletion of carnitine (Mancinelli et al. 2007). On the other hand, oral carnitine supplementation is effective in normalizing this deficiency (Cruciani et al. 2009) and minimize chemotherapy-related side effects (Pisano et al. 2010).

Based on the exposed above, a study performed a randomizing multicenter trial with advanced cancer pancreatic patients, receiving carnitine supplementation (4 g/day) or placebo for 6 and 12 weeks (Kraft et al. 2012). The authors found that carnitine treatment reduced malnutrition, increased body weight, and improved both body composition and quality of life, and also suggested that carnitine supplementation is an inexpensive and very well tolerated supplementation with significant improvement for advanced cancer patients. On the other hand, another clinical trial with cancer cachexia patients also evaluated the effects of 4 g carnitine supplementation per day during four months, but the authors had no changes or improvements on the lean body mass, resting energy expenditure and fatigue (Mantovani 2010).

As the other amino acids described above, the mechanism of action and better knowledge on how they act come from preclinical studies. Liu and colleagues evaluated the effect of two doses of oral administration of carnitine (4.5 and 18 mg/kg/day) for seven days in C26 tumor-bearing mice (Liu et al. 2011). Both doses of carnitine treatment were effective in increasing food intake, gastrocnemius muscle weight, and fat mass compared to saline-treated C26 group. Also, carnitine administration reduced pro-inflammatory cytokines, recuperates serum carnitine levels, and recovers the expression and activity of liver carnitine palmitoyltransferase. The beneficial effects of carnitine supplementation could be associated with PPAR-γ signaling pathway (Jiang et al. 2015). In a study conducted by Busquets and colleague, the AH-130 Yoshida ascites hepatoma cells were implanted in rats that were treated with a daily dose of carnitine (1 g/kg) for seven days (Busquets et al. 2012). Carnitine administration increased food intake, muscle weights (gastrocnemius, extensor digitalis lateral, and soleus), improved physical activity, and tended to increase muscle strength. Treatment with carnitine resulted in a significant decrease in proteasome activity in skeletal muscle, associated with decreases in mRNA content for ubiquitin and MuRF-1. No effects of carnitine were found on other proteolytic pathways such as calcium-dependent or lysosomal. More recently, the same research group found that daily dose of carnitine 1 g/kg for seven days ameliorated the atrophy of both slow- and fast-twitch fibers, minimized the structural muscle alterations, and attenuated oxidative stress, proteolytic and signaling markers in AH-130 Yoshida ascites hepatoma tumor-bearing rats (Busquets et al. 2020).

Although clinical studies are inconclusive, studies in animal models clearly show that carnitine administration ameliorates muscle mass and function in cancer cachexia models, mainly by decreasing oxidative stress and improving mitochondrial function. More clinical trials are necessary to establish carnitine as a therapeutic strategy for cachexia associated with cancer.

14.4 Antioxidants

14.4.1 Curcumin

Curcumin, a natural phenolic compound extracted from *Curcuma longa* L., is the major component of turmeric, commonly used as a spice and food-coloring material and exhibits anti-inflammatory, antitumor, and antioxidant properties (Menon and Sudheer 2007; Sahebkar et al. 2017). in vivo and in vitro studies have explored the role of curcumin, alone or in combination with chemotherapy or other nutraceuticals, in reducing tumor weight and, mainly, in conserving of body weight and muscle mass.

Quan-Jun and colleagues observed that curcumin treatment in C26 tumor-bearing mice resulted in 13% less body weight loss and conserved 91% of epididymal fat, and minimized the gastrocnemius and tibialis anterior muscles waste (Quan-Jun et al. 2015). Moreover, the pathway analysis showed that the main metabolic regulation of curcumin involved the metabolism of valine, leucine, and phenylalanine, and the synthesis and degradation of ketone bodies (Quan-Jun et al. 2015). Also, Archer-Lahlou and colleagues identified C_2C_{12} myotube muscle cells atrophy after exposure with a combination of doxorubicin and dexamethasone under the modified culture conditions, which was partially prevented by coadministration of curcumin (Archer-Lahlou et al. 2018). Busquets and colleagues found that Lewis lung carcinoma-bearing mice subjected to curcumin plus omega-3-enriched fruit juices had a reduction of 18% in tumor weight. Besides, this juice, when combined with the chemotherapeutic drug sorafenib, had a significant effect reversing the body weight loss, and tibialis muscle mass was increased as a result of juice treatment (Busquets et al. 2018). The combination of curcumin with eicosapentaenoic acid induced a significant increase in protein synthesis in C_2C_{12} myotube muscle cells minimizing the effects of TNF-α and PIF. Moreover, this combination of nutraceuticals produced complete inhibition in protein degradation caused only by PIF (Mirza et al. 2016).

14.4.2 Resveratrol

Resveratrol, a polyphenolic compound naturally found mainly in grape skin and seeds, berries, peanuts, and other plant sources, reveals a wide range of biological properties including anti-glycation, antioxidant, anti-inflammatory, neuroprotective, anticancer and antiageing activity (Galiniak et al. 2019). Currently, resveratrol is a subject of considerable scientific investigations, particularly, about the effects on preventing protein degradation induced by PIF, angiotensin I and II, dexamethasone, and others. Besides, resveratrol has shown a protective effect on muscle wasting under diverse catabolic conditions, including cachexia (Dutt et al. 2015).

Shadfar and colleagues demonstrate that daily resveratrol intake inhibits skeletal muscle and cardiac atrophy in C26 tumor-bearing mice, throughout inhibition of NFκB (p65 subunit) activity in the muscle and heart tissues (Shadfar et al. 2011). Furthermore, in vitro administration of resveratrol led to an inhibition of muscle proteolysis, and muscle wasting, by downregulating the atrogin-1, MuRF1, and FoxO1, counteracting with upregulation of AKT, mTOR, p70S6K, 4E-BP1 in C_2C_{12} myotube in response to hyperthermia (Olivan et al. 2011), and TNF-α (Wang et al. 2014) and in L6 myotube exposed to dexamethasone (Alamdari et al. 2012).

14.4.3 Selenium

Selenium, an essential mineral naturally found in soil, water, and some of the food, fulfils essential functions in the organism, mainly connected with antioxidant properties, as this micronutrient acts as essential cofactor of important antioxidant enzymes (Kielczykowska et al. 2018). Therefore, the importance of selenium supplementation in boosting up the internal antioxidative defense has been highlighted in recent years (Wang et al. 2017).

Wang and colleagues observed that consumption of selenium supplementation combined with fish oil by lung carcinoma (Line-1)-bearing mice showed a synergistic effect: the population of regulatory T cells and myeloid-derived suppressor cells decreased as opposed to an increase of antitumor immunity. Also, the selenium and fish oil -supplemented group had a significant improvement in body weight and muscle/fat mass (Wang et al. 2013). Subsequently, these researchers evaluated the mechanisms of tumor and chemotherapy on skeletal muscle proteolysis, demonstrating that the lung carcinoma (Line-1)-bearing mice under docetaxel, cisplatin, or 5-FU, supplementation associated with selenium, and fish oil had no rise in IL-6, TNF-α, and myostatin and muscle atrophy (Wang et al. 2015). Moreover, the combined effect of aerobic interval training and selenium nanoparticles prevented cachexia and muscle wasting and, additionally, decreased tumor volume in the breast (4T1) cancer-bearing mice (Molanouri Shamsi et al. 2017).

14.4.4 Vitamin D

Vitamin D, found as two isoforms cholecalciferol (D3) and ergocalciferol (D2), is a fat-soluble vitamin obtainable about 80% by ultraviolet B (290–320 nm) sunlight-induced production of a seco-steroidal prohormone in the skin, whereas dietary intake accounts for the minor role (Jeon and Shin 2018). The classical role of vitamin D is to regulate the metabolism of calcium and phosphate, in addition to the regulation of cell proliferation and differentiation (Penna et al. 2017; Jeon and Shin 2018). Serum vitamin D levels have been correlated to muscle cell contractility, muscle strength, and postural stability (Polly and Tan 2014). For these reasons, the possibility of using vitamin D supplementation to improve muscle mass loss, with a special focus on cancer cachexia, has been discussed (Penna et al. 2017).

Camperi and colleagues demonstrated in rats bearing hepatoma (AH130) that both circulating vitamin D and muscle vitamin D receptor expression increased after vitamin D administration, without exerting appreciable effects on body weight and gastrocnemius and tibialis muscle mass. Furthermore, vitamin D treatment resulted in vitamin D receptor overexpression and myogenin downregulation in C_2C_{12} myocyte muscle cells (Camperi et al. 2017).

The supplementation of 1α,25-dihydroxy vitamin D_3 reversed the tumor cell-mediated changes in mitochondrial oxygen consumption and proteasomal activity in CC-2561 myoblast muscle cells exposed to Lewis lung carcinoma cell-conditioned medium (Ryan et al. 2018). On the other hand, 1α,25-dihydroxy vitamin D_3 had an atrophic activity, increasing FoxO3 levels, inducing the expression of atrogenes and blocking the autophagic flux in C_2C_{12} myotube muscle cells were exposed to Lewis lung carcinoma cell-conditioned medium. At the same time, 25-hydroxy vitamin D_3 was able to protect from muscle atrophy by activating AKT signaling, inducing protein synthesis and stimulating the autophagic flux (Sustova et al. 2019).

14.4.5 Polyunsaturated Fatty Acids

Polyunsaturated fatty acids (PUFAs) comprise mainly two groups of essential fatty acids: omega-3 (*n*-3) and omega-6 (*n*-6) groups. The main types of *n*-3 PUFAs are α-linolenic acid (ALA), mainly found in several plants, seeds, and nuts, is a precursor to the synthesis of eicosapentaenoic acid (EPA) and docosahexaenoic acid (DHA), found in large quantities in deep-sea fish

(Wiktorowska-Owczarek et al. 2015; Burdge and Calder 2015), which are mostly related to cell signaling pathways and gene expression modifying the host responses, especially as anti-inflammatory responses (Burdge and Calder 2015; Baker et al. 2016; Calder 2017). The characteristics of n-3 PUFAs have being explored in in vitro and in vivo studies and, nowadays, in clinical trials, being the most studied nutraceuticals in cancer cachexia interventions (Malta et al. 2019).

The n-3 fatty acids action was already pointed in relation to modulate the balance between protein synthesis and degradation pathways (Malta et al. 2019). An in vitro study with C_2C_{12} myotube cells showed the effects of DHA supplementation in counteracting the catabolic effects of palmitate treatment restoring the AKT/FoxO signaling and limiting the autophagy (Woodworth-Hobbs et al. 2014). Other works showed the relation of fish oil supplementation and cancer cachexia outcomes in experimental models. A study showed the protective effects of fish oil rich in EPA and DHA supplementation on reducing tumor growth and improving renal function in Walker-256 tumor-bearing rats (Coelho et al. 2012). Also, a study in tumor-bearing animals subjected to a fish oil and Oro Inca Oil (derived from an Andean plant, which is rich in ALA) supplementation, showed a positive effect of both oils, diminishing tumor size and cell proliferation, as well, improving glycemia, triacylglycerolemia, and minimizing the plasma pro-inflammatory markers, such as IL-6 and TNF-α (Schiessel et al. 2015). Plas and colleagues combined a fish oil and leucine supplementation, showing improvement in hypercalcemia in C26 tumor-bearing mice. The authors correlated this effect to the DHA treatment, as the in vitro experiment corroborated the DHA effects in C26 cells, on reducing the parathyroid hormone-related protein (PTHrP) secretion by these tumor cells (Plas et al. 2019).

Besides fish oil supplementation studies in cancer cachexia, other marine sources were already evaluated, such as EPA-enriched phospholipids (EPA-PL) derived from a starfish. An intragastric of EPA-PL administration in ascitic tumor-bearing mice ameliorated cachexia by preventing white adipose tissue loss. The anti-inflammatory effects of this administration were reported by a reduced IL-6 and TNF-α serum levels. Moreover, this supplementation prevented the adipose tissue browning in cachectic mice, and an inhibited TNF-α-stimulated lipolysis corroborated all these data in adipocytes cells (Du et al. 2015). As a multimodal therapy, a study from Penna and colleagues showed the effects of a combined endurance exercise and EPA supplementation in Lewis tumor-bearing mice (Penna et al. 2011). The grip strength loss was not prevented by the EPA administration alone, even though the combined therapy showed a limited recovery. Also, the exercise plus EPA slightly inhibited gastrocnemius depletion and decreased the Pax7 protein levels, which was related to the inhibition of myogenesis process.

Also, in order to maximize the translational capacity of these findings, it is important to considerate the effects of n-3 supplementation during a chemotherapy situation, making the experimental study more closely to the human condition. In this way, Wang and colleagues showed the effects of a fish oil and selenium supplementation in tumor-bearing rats under chemotherapy. This study revealed a positive effect of this treatment in preventing the increase of inflammatory cytokines, downregulated myostatin, and prevented muscle atrophy (Wang et al. 2015). A study with a cachexia model induced by chemotherapy showed the effects of the DHA supplementation in minimizing the body weight loss in induced mammary tumor-bearing rats. However, some concerning in the use of this tumor model, dose, and time of the DHA administration was raised by the authors, who suggested the need of more investigations on the effects of the DHA supplementation benefits when administered alone (Hajjaji et al. 2012).

Studies using nutraceuticals as a preventive approach in cachexia studies recently started to be reported in the literature. In our previous study, concerning a preventive supplementation approach in cancer cachexia studies, maternal nutritional supplementation with fish oil, rich in EPA and DHA, in combination or not to leucine enrichment was evaluated. These nutrients, when administered to pregnant dams rats until the weaning period, affected the responses of the tumor-bearing offspring to cachexia spoliation. Miyaguti and colleagues reported improved survival, cachexia indexes, liver function antioxidant responses in the offspring supplemented with fish oil and fish oil plus leucine (Miyaguti et al. 2018). Therefore, further epigenetics studies should be done to provide more information about the use of nutraceuticals as nutritional supplementation in cancer cachexia prevention, as a new and important investigation area.

In accordance with the experimental studies, positive effects were also found in the literature review. A randomized clinical trial showed the effects of a combined *n*-3 PUFAs, micronutrient, and probiotic nutritional supplement in ameliorating the cachexia parameters with an improvement of body weight, as well as serum albumin and pre-albumin in head and neck cachectic patients under chemotherapy or radiotherapy (Yeh et al. 2013). Moreover, van der Meji and colleagues investigated the effects of an oral protein and energy-dense supplementation rich in EPA and DHA in lung cancer patients. In the first clinical trial, the authors found an improvement in the nutritional status of these cancer patients with the maintenance of body weight and free fat mass, but no improvements on inflammatory markers (van der Meij et al. 2010). In another study, the authors assessed the QOL and physical parameters of these patients. The supplementation was efficient in improving the QOL, physical and cognitive function, global health status, which tended to a higher physical activity after five weeks of intervention and chemotherapy, showing a significant number of positive effects of the *n*-3 supplementation (Van Der Meij et al. 2012).

More recent studies also showed the *n*-3 supplementation improvements in cancer patients with different tumor types. Werner and colleagues tested fish oil and a low dose of marine phospholipids supplementation, which contained the same *n*-3 amount, in pancreatic cancer patients. Both interventions showed positives effects related to weight and appetite stabilization. Interestingly, oral marine phospholipids were better tolerated, and with fewer side effects, an essential fact to considerate in cancer patients undergoing other treatments options, such as chemotherapy (Werner et al. 2017). An increased body weight, lean body mass and CRP levels were found in a study with gastrointestinal cachectic patients (Shirai et al. 2017) supplemented with fish oil supplementation during chemotherapy. Associated with these improvements, also were related to improved tolerance to chemotherapy and prognosis in those patients, showing another positive effect of the *n*-3 supplementation in the management of cancer cachexia syndrome. In head and neck cancer patients, an EPA supplementation for six weeks before antineoplastic treatment also showed beneficial effects in ameliorating the serum levels of inflammatory cytokines and preserve lean and fat body mass and improved QOL (Solís-Martínez et al. 2018).

Although the experimental studies with different sources of *n*-3, in a combination of EPA plus DHA, or each PUFAs alone, showed some benefits in cancer cachexia, the clinical studies are still controversial (Malta et al. 2019). In our searching, the literature review showed studies with none improved effect in related cachexia parameters. In patients with head and neck cancer, a double-blind, randomized controlled trial with Echium oil, rich in *n*-3 α-linolenic acid (ALA), stearidonic acid, and in *n*-6 γ-linoleic acid, showed no effects on improving the nutritional status and body weight in patients undergoing (chemo)radiotherapy (Pottel et al. 2014). Also, a prospective randomized study reported no positive effect of a high-blend supplementation rich in

EPA, administered during the perioperative period, in minimizing the head and neck patients weight loss and inflammatory markers (Hanai et al. 2018). Moreover, negative effects were reported, and in a randomized study comprising gastrointestinal and lung cancer patients, an EPA enriched supplementation, administered 72 hours before chemotherapy and continued for 4 weeks, had no efficient effect in reducing the C-reactive protein (CRP) in those patients. Besides that, a high number of patients interrupted the treatment, especially in EPA intervention group. This is possibly related to the gastrointestinal intolerance provided by the combination of the treatments when an optimal time to initiate the supplementation was not adopted (Pastore et al. 2014).

Some concerning should be taken into consideration to the clinical studies. There is still a lack of standardization among the works, and this fact does not allow extracting the real effects of the *n*-3 supplementation in these clinical studies (Malta et al. 2019; Freitas and Campos 2019). Besides the cancer type, stage, concurrent therapies adopted and gold standard physical and physiological analysis employed, further studies should carefully be designed. There is a need to considering which *n*-3 type should be administered (EPA alone, DHA alone, fish oil, marine or plants *n*-3 sources), dosage, the administration route (in capsules or oral formulas), in combination or not with others nutraceuticals (Lavriv et al. 2018). Also, the time of administration is extremely important so that this supplementation can affect the composition of the cell membrane and change the lipid content of muscles and other tissues (McGlory et al. 2019). With more homogeneous studies, it would be possible to obtain more information, which could assess the mechanisms underlying the effects of *n*-3 supplementation.

14.5 Conclusions

Nutraceuticals as an approach to the treatment of the cancer-induced cachexia mean that the main metabolic alterations imposed by this syndrome could be minimized and improved the host responses and the QOL. Concerning the whole host tissues and organs that suffer by the damage effects of cancer evolution, important synergistic, and potentially effect of one nutraceutical or acting together to other nutraceuticals should be considered. Indeed, in view of the raising epigenetics studies, as mentioned here, the use of nutraceuticals as a nutritional approach in cancer prevention should be very important to minimize the cachexia damages. From the minimizing or perhaps reversing the state of anorexia, to the amelioration of the microbiota, the enhancement of the anti-inflammatory process, in addition to minimizing liver disorders associated with muscle mass gain (Figure 14.1), all these points should provide some improved response to conventional treatment and better quality of life in the cachectic patient.

Acknowledgments

The authors are thankful for the financial support of Coordenação de Aperfeiçoamento de Pessoal de Nível Superior (CAPES), Conselho Nacional de Desenvolvimento Cientifico e Tecnológico (CNPq #301771/2019-7), and Fundação de Amparo à Pesquisa do Estado de São Paulo (FAPESP #2015/21890-0; #2017/02739-4; #2019/13937-7; #2019/14803-4; #2019/20558-2). The authors gratefully thank Biol. R.W. Santos for technical support and Designer A.C. Gomes Marcondes for the graphical art.

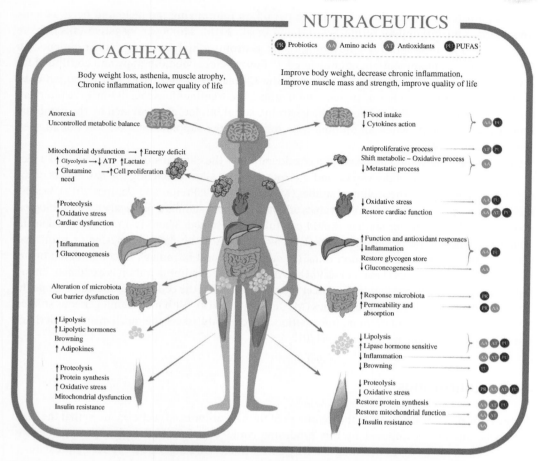

Figure 14.1 Schematic representation of cancer-induced cachexia and positive effects of nutraceuticals approach. Most of the aspects presented here were taken from preclinical (experimental models of cancer-induced cachexia), including in vitro assay, and from clinical trials studies from the last 10 years. The cachectic state leads to intense loss of body weight and chronic inflammatory state, imposed by severe catabolic process, where the most cellular catabolic pathway is upregulated, inducing substantial skeletal muscle proteolysis added or not to increased lipolysis. In addition, aggravating the entire process, the energy supply is deficient by the anorexia, with an enormous energetic deficit, associated with downregulated anabolic processes, which lead to atrophy, asthenia, and reduced quality of life. The nutraceuticals described here – probiotics (PR), amino acids (AA), antioxidants (AT) and PUFAS (PU) – demonstrated positive effects, mainly in anabolic process, and minimizing catabolic points such as inflammatory and oxidative stress and, more importantly, reducing the proteolytic pathways, which can improve the whole-body responses, increasing quality of life. More specific details are found in the main text.

References

Alamdari, N., Aversa, Z., Castillero, E. et al. (2012). Resveratrol prevents dexamethasone-induced expression of the muscle atrophy-related ubiquitin ligases atrogin-1 and MuRF1 in cultured myotubes through a SIRT1-dependent mechanism. *Biochem. Biophys. Res. Commun.* 417: 528–533. https://doi.org/10.1016/j.bbrc.2011.11.154.

An, J.M., Kang, E.A., Han, Y. et al. (2019). Dietary intake of probiotic kimchi ameliorated I6 driven cancer cachexia. *J. Clin. Biochem. Nutr.* 65: 109–117. https://doi.org/10.3164/jcbn.19910.

Archer-Lahlou, E., Lan, C., and Jagoe, R.T. (2018). Physiological culture conditions alter myotube morphology and responses to atrophy treatments: implications for in vitro research on muscle wasting. *Physiol. Rep.* 6: 1–14. https://doi.org/10.14814/phy2.13726.

Argilés, J.M., Busquets, S., Felipe, A., and López-Soriano, F.J. (2005). Molecular mechanisms involved in muscle wasting in cancer and ageing: cachexia versus sarcopenia. *Int. J. Biochem. Cell Biol.* 37: 1084–1104.

Argiles, J.M., Lopez-Soriano, F.J., and Busquets, S. (2013). Mechanisms and treatment of cancer cachexia. *Nutr. Metab. Cardiovasc. Dis.* 23 (Suppl 1): S19–S24. https://doi.org/10.1016/j.numecd.2012.04.011.

Aversa, Z., Bonetto, A., Costelli, P. et al. (2011). β-Hydroxy-β-methylbutyrate (HMB) attenuates muscle and body weight loss in experimental cancer cachexia. *Int. J. Oncol.* 38: 713–720. https://doi.org/10.3892/ijo.2010.885.

Baker, E.J., Miles, E.A., Burdge, G.C. et al. (2016). Metabolism and functional effects of plant-derived omega-3 fatty acids in humans. *Prog. Lipid Res.* 64: 30–56. https://doi.org/10.1016/j.plipres.2016.07.002.

Baracos, V.E., Martin, L., Korc, M. et al. (2018). Cancer-associated cachexia. *Nat. Publ. Gr.* 4: 1–18. https://doi.org/10.1038/nrdp.2017.105.

Barbosa, A.W.C., Benevides, G.P., Alferes, L.M.T. et al. (2012). A leucine-rich diet and exercise affect the biomechanical characteristics of the digital flexor tendon in rats after nutritional recovery. *Amino Acids* 42: 329–336. https://doi.org/10.1007/s00726-010-0810-1.

Bear, D.E., Langan, A., Dimidi, E. et al. (2019). β-Hydroxy-β-methylbutyrate and its impact on skeletal muscle mass and physical function in clinical practice: a systematic review and meta-analysis. *Am. J. Clin. Nutr.* 109: 1119–1132. https://doi.org/10.1093/ajcn/nqy373.

Bindels, L.B. and Thissen, J.P. (2016). Nutrition in cancer patients with cachexia: a role for the gut microbiota? *Clin. Nutr. Exp.* 6: 74–82. https://doi.org/10.1016/j.yclnex.2015.11.001.

Bindels, L.B., Beck, R., Schakman, O. et al. (2012). Restoring specific lactobacilli levels decreases inflammation and muscle atrophy markers in an acute leukemia mouse model. *PLoS One* 7: e37971. https://doi.org/10.1371/journal.pone.0037971.

Bindels, L.B., Delzenne, N.M., Cani, P.D., and Walter, J. (2015). Towards a more comprehensive concept for prebiotics. *Nat. Rev. Gastroenterol. Hepatol.* 12: 303–310. https://doi.org/10.1038/nrgastro.2015.47.

Bindels, L.B., Neyrinck, A.M., Salazar, N. et al. (2015). Non digestible oligosaccharides modulate the gut microbiota to control the development of leukemia and associated cachexia in mice. *PLoS One* 10: e0131009. https://doi.org/10.1371/journal.pone.0131009.

Bindels, L.B., Neyrinck, A.M., Claus, S.P. et al. (2016). Synbiotic approach restores intestinal homeostasis and prolongs survival in leukaemic mice with cachexia. *ISME J.* 10: 1456–1470. https://doi.org/10.1038/ismej.2015.209.

Bindels, L.B., Neyrinck, A.M., Loumaye, A. et al. (2018). Increased gut permeability in cancer cachexia: mechanisms and clinical relevance. *Oncotarget* 9: 18224–18238.

Blum, D., Omlin, A., Fearon, K. et al. (2010). Evolving classification systems for cancer cachexia: ready for clinical practice? *Support. Care Cancer* 18: 273–279.

Bron, P.A., Kleerebezem, M., Brummer, R.J. et al. (2017). Can probiotics modulate human disease by impacting intestinal barrier function? *Br. J. Nutr.* 117: 93–107.

Burdge, G.C. and Calder, P.C. (2015). Introduction to fatty acids and lipids. *World Rev. Nutr. Diet.* 112: 1–16. https://doi.org/10.1159/000365423.

Busquets, S., Serpe, R., Toledo, M. et al. (2012). l-Carnitine: an adequate supplement for a multi-targeted anti-wasting therapy in cancer. *Clin. Nutr.* 31: 889–895. https://doi.org/10.1016/j.clnu.2012.03.005.

Busquets, S., Marmonti, E., Oliva, F. et al. (2018). Omega-3 and omega-3/curcumin – enriched fruit juices decrease tumour growth and reduce muscle wasting in tumour – bearing mice. *J. Cachexia Sarcopenia Muscle – Rapid Commun.* 1: 1–10.

Busquets, S., Pérez-Peiró, M., Salazar-Degracia, A. et al. (2020). Differential structural features in soleus and gastrocnemius of carnitine-treated cancer cachectic rats. *J. Cell. Physiol.* 235: 526–537. https://doi.org/10.1002/jcp.28992.

Calder, P.C. (2017). Omega-3 fatty acids and inflammatory processes: From molecules to man. *Biochem. Soc. Trans.* 45: 1105–1115. https://doi.org/10.1042/BST20160474.

Camperi, A., Pin, F., Costamagna, D. et al. (2017). Vitamin D and VDR in cancer cachexia and muscle regeneration. *Oncotarget* 8: 21778–21793. https://doi.org/10.18632/oncotarget.15583.

de Campos-Ferraz, P.L., Andrade, I., das Neves, W. et al. (2014). An overview of amines as nutritional supplements to counteract cancer cachexia. *J. Cachexia. Sarcopenia Muscle* 5: 105–110.

Carson, J.A., Hardee, J.P., and VanderVeen, B.N. (2016). The emerging role of skeletal muscle oxidative metabolism as a biological target and cellular regulator of cancer-induced muscle wasting. *Semin. Cell Dev. Biol.* 54: 53–67. https://doi.org/10.1016/j.semcdb.2015.11.005.

Chen, Y.M., Wei, L., Chiu, Y.S. et al. (2016). Lactobacillus plantarum TWK10 supplementation improves exercise performance and increases muscle mass in mice. *Nutrients* 8: 205. https://doi.org/10.3390/nu8040205.

Coelho, I., Casare, F., Pequito, D.C.T. et al. (2012). Fish oil supplementation reduces cachexia and tumor growth while improving renal function in tumor-bearing rats. *Lipids* 47: 1031–1041. https://doi.org/10.1007/s11745-012-3715-9.

Columbus, D.A., Fiorotto, M.L., and Davis, T.A. (2015a). Leucine is a major regulator of muscle protein synthesis in neonates. *Amino Acids* 47: 259–270.

Columbus, D.A., Steinhoff-Wagner, J., Suryawan, A. et al. (2015b). Impact of prolonged leucine supplementation on protein synthesis and lean growth in neonatal pigs. *Am. J. Physiol. – Endocrinol. Metab.* 309: E601–E610. https://doi.org/10.1152/ajpendo.00089.2015.

Costelli, P. and Baccino, F.M. (2003). Mechanisms of skeletal muscle depletion in wasting syndromes: role of ATP-ubiquitin-dependent proteolysis. *Curr. Opin. Clin. Nutr. Metab. Care* 6: 407–412. https://doi.org/10.1097/01.mco.0000078984.18774.02.

Cruciani, R.A., Dvorkin, E., Homel, P. et al. (2009). L-Carnitine supplementation in patients with advanced cancer and carnitine deficiency: a double-blind, placebo-controlled study. *J. Pain Symptom Manage.* 37: 622–631. https://doi.org/10.1016/j.jpainsymman.2008.03.021.

Cruz, B. and Gomes-Marcondes, M.C.C. (2014). Leucine-rich diet supplementation modulates foetal muscle protein metabolism impaired by Walker-256 tumour. *Reprod. Biol. Endocrinol.* 12: 2. https://doi.org/10.1186/1477-7827-12-2.

Cruz, B., Oliveira, A., and Gomes-Marcondes, M.C.C. (2017). l-Leucine dietary supplementation modulates muscle protein degradation and increases pro-inflammatory cytokines in tumour-bearing rats. *Cytokine* 96: 253–260. https://doi.org/10.1016/j.cyto.2017.04.019.

Cruz, B., Oliveira, A., Ventrucci, G., and Gomes-Marcondes, M.C.C. (2019). A leucine-rich diet modulates the mTOR cell signalling pathway in the gastrocnemius muscle under different Walker-256 tumour growth conditions. *BMC Cancer* 19: 349. https://doi.org/10.1186/s12885-019-5448-0.

Cruz, B., Oliveira, A., Viana, L.R. et al. (2020). Leucine-rich diet modulates the metabolomic and proteomic profile of skeletal muscle during cancer cachexia. *Cancers (Basel).* 12: 1880–1905.

Del Fabbro, E. (2015). Current and future care of patients with the cancer anorexia–cachexia syndrome. *Am. Soc. Clin. Oncol. Educ. Book. Am. Soc. Clin. Oncol. Meet.* 35: e229–e237. https://doi.org/10.14694/EdBook_AM.2015.35.e229.

Denko, N.C. (2008). Hypoxia, HIF1 and glucose metabolism in the solid tumour. *Nat. Rev. Cancer* 8: 705–713. https://doi.org/10.1038/nrc2468.

Deutz, N.E.P., Safar, A., Schutzler, S. et al. (2011). Muscle protein synthesis in cancer patients can be stimulated with a specially formulated medical food. *Clin. Nutr.* 30: 759–768. https://doi.org/10.1016/j.clnu.2011.05.008.

Du, L., Yang, Y.H., Wang, Y.M. et al. (2015). EPA-enriched phospholipids ameliorate cancer-associated cachexia mainly via inhibiting lipolysis. *Food Funct.* 6: 3652–3662. https://doi.org/10.1039/c5fo00478k.

Dutt, V., Gupta, S., Dabur, R. et al. (2015). Skeletal muscle atrophy: potential therapeutic agents and their mechanisms of action. *Pharmacol. Res.* 99: 86–100. https://doi.org/10.1016/j.phrs.2015.05.010.

Engelen, M.P.K.J., Safar, A.M., Bartter, T. et al. (2015). High anabolic potential of essential amino acid mixtures in advanced nonsmall cell lung cancer. *Ann. Oncol.* 26: 1960–1966. https://doi.org/10.1093/annonc/mdv271.

Fearon, K., Strasser, F., Anker, S.D. et al. (2011). Definition and classification of cancer cachexia: an international consensus. *Lancet Oncol.* 12: 489–495.

Fearon, K.C.H., Glass, D.J., and Guttridge, D.C. (2012). Cancer cachexia: mediators, signaling, and metabolic pathways. *Cell Metab.* 16: 153–166. https://doi.org/10.1016/j.cmet.2012.06.011.

Freitas, R. and Campos, M.M. (2019). Protective effects of omega-3 fatty acids in cancer-related complications. *Nutrients* 11: 945. https://doi.org/10.3390/nu11050945.

Fukawa, T., Yan-Jiang, B.C., Min-Wen, J.C. et al. (2016). Excessive fatty acid oxidation induces muscle atrophy in cancer cachexia. *Nat. Med.* 22: 666–671. https://doi.org/10.1038/nm.4093.

Galiniak, S., Aebisher, D., and Bartusik-Aebisher, D. (2019). Health benefits of resveratrol administration. *Acta Biochim. Pol.* 66: 13–21.

Gamallat, Y., Meyiah, A., Kuugbee, E.D. et al. (2016). Lactobacillus rhamnosus induced epithelial cell apoptosis, ameliorates inflammation and prevents colon cancer development in an animal model. *Biomed. Pharmacother.* 83: 536–541. https://doi.org/10.1016/j.biopha.2016.07.001.

Garlick, P.J. (2005). The role of leucine in the regulation of protein metabolism. *J. Nutr.* 135: 1553S–1556S.

Genton, L., Mareschal, J., Charretier, Y. et al. (2019). Targeting the gut microbiota to treat cachexia. *Front. Cell. Infect. Microbiol.* 9: 1–8. https://doi.org/10.3389/fcimb.2019.00305.

Gerlinger-Romero, F., Guimarães-Ferreira, L., Giannocco, G., and Nunes, M.T. (2011). Chronic supplementation of beta-hydroxy-beta methylbutyrate (HMβ) increases the activity of the GH/IGF-I axis and induces hyperinsulinemia in rats. *Growth Horm. IGF Res.* 21: 57–62. https://doi.org/10.1016/j.ghir.2010.12.006.

Gibson, G.R. and Roberfroid, M.B. (1995). Dietary modulation of the human colonic microbiota: introducing the concept of prebiotics. *J. Nutr.* 125: 1401–1412. https://doi.org/10.1093/jn/125.6.1401.

Gibson, G.R., Hutkins, R., Ellen Sanders, M. et al. (2017). Expert consensus document: the International Scientific Association for Probiotics and Prebiotics (ISAPP) consensus statement on the definition and scope of prebiotics. *Nat. Rev. Gastroenterol. Hepatol.* 14: 491–502. https://doi.org/10.1038/nrgastro.2017.75.

Girón, M.D., Vílchez, J.D., Salto, R. et al. (2016). Conversion of leucine to β-hydroxy-β-methylbutyrate by α-keto isocaproate dioxygenase is required for a potent stimulation of protein synthesis in L6 rat myotubes. *J. Cachexia. Sarcopenia Muscle* 7: 68–78. https://doi.org/10.1002/jcsm.12032.

Gomes-Marcondes, M.C.C. and Tisdale, M.J. (2002). Induction of protein catabolism and the ubiquitin-proteasome pathway by mild oxidative stress. *Cancer Lett.* 180: 69–74.

Gomes-Marcondes, M.C.C., Ventrucci, G., Toledo, M.T. et al. (2003). A leucine-supplemented diet improved protein content of skeletal muscle in young tumor-bearing rats. *Braz. J. Med. Biol. Res.* 36: 1589–1594. https://doi.org/10.1590/S0100-879X2003001100017.

Gonçalves, E.M., Salomão, E.M., Gomes-Marcondes, M.C.C. et al. (2013). Leucine modulates the effect of Walker factor, a proteolysis-inducing factor-like protein from Walker tumours, on gene expression and cellular activity in C_2C_{12} myotubes. *Cytokine* 64: 343–350. https://doi.org/10.1016/j.cyto.2013.05.018.

Gordon, B.S., Kelleher, A.R., and Kimball, S.R. (2013). Regulation of muscle protein synthesis and the effects of catabolic states. *Int. J. Biochem. Cell Biol.* 45: 2147–2157. https://doi.org/10.1016/j.biocel.2013.05.039.

Hajjaji, N., Couet, C., Besson, P., and Bougnoux, P. (2012). DHA effect on chemotherapy-induced body weight loss: an exploratory study in a rodent model of mammary tumors. *Nutr. Cancer* 64: 1000–1007. https://doi.org/10.1080/01635581.2012.714832.

Ham, D.J., Murphy, K.T., Chee, A. et al. (2014). Glycine administration attenuates skeletal muscle wasting in a mouse model of cancer cachexia. *Clin. Nutr.* 33: 448–458. https://doi.org/10.1016/j.clnu.2013.06.013.

Hanai, N., Terada, H., Hirakawa, H. et al. (2018). Prospective randomized investigation implementing immunonutritional therapy using a nutritional supplement with a high blend ratio of ω-3 fatty acids during the perioperative period for head and neck carcinomas. *Jpn. J. Clin. Oncol.* 48: 356–361. https://doi.org/10.1093/jjco/hyy008.

Hassan, H., Rompola, M., Glaser, A.W. et al. (2018). Systematic review and meta-analysis investigating the efficacy and safety of probiotics in people with cancer. *Support. Care Cancer* 26: 2503–2509.

Herremans, K.M., Riner, A.N., Cameron, M.E., and Trevino, J.G. (2019). The microbiota and cancer cachexia. *Int. J. Mol. Sci.* 20: 6267. https://doi.org/10.3390/ijms20246267.

Hill, C., Guarner, F., Reid, G. et al. (2014). The International Scientific Association for Probiotics and Prebiotics consensus statement on the scope and appropriate use of the term probiotic. *Nat. Rev. Gastroenterol. Hepatol.* 11: 506–514. https://doi.org/10.1038/nrgastro.2014.66.

Holecek, M. and Kovarik, M. (2011). Alterations in protein metabolism and amino acid concentrations in rats fed by a high-protein (casein-enriched) diet – effect of starvation. *Food Chem. Toxicol.* 49: 3336–3342. https://doi.org/10.1016/j.fct.2011.09.016.

Huang, G., Khan, I., Li, X. et al. (2017). Ginsenosides Rb3 and Rd reduce polyps formation while reinstate the dysbiotic gut microbiota and the intestinal microenvironment in ApcMin/+ mice. *Sci. Rep.* 7: 1–14. https://doi.org/10.1038/s41598-017-12644-5.

Inui, A. (1999). Cancer anorexia-cachexia syndrome: are neuropeptides the key? *Cancer Res.* 59: 4493–4501.

Jacouton, E., Chain, F., Sokol, H. et al. (2017). Probiotic strain *Lactobacillus casei* BL23 prevents colitis-associated colorectal cancer. *Front. Immunol.* 8: 17. https://doi.org/10.3389/fimmu.2017.01553.

Jäger, R., Shields, K.A., Lowery, R.P. et al. (2016). Probiotic *Bacillus coagulans* GBI-30, 6086 reduces exercise-induced muscle damage and increases recovery. *PeerJ* 4: e2276. https://doi.org/10.7717/peerj.2276.

Jeon, S.M. and Shin, E.A. (2018). Exploring vitamin D metabolism and function in cancer. *Exp. Mol. Med.* 50: 1–4. https://doi.org/10.1038/s12276-018-0038-9.

Jeong, M., Park, J.M., Han, Y.M. et al. (2015). Dietary prevention of *Helicobacter pylori*-associated gastric cancer with kimchi. *Oncotarget* 6: 29513–29526. https://doi.org/10.18632/oncotarget.4897.

Jiang, Y., Lin, J., Zhang, D. et al. (2014a). Bacterial translocation contributes to cachexia and its possible pathway in patients with colon cancer. *J. Clin. Gastroenterol.* 48: 131–137. https://doi.org/10.1097/01.mcg.0000436437.83015.17.

Jiang, Y., Guo, C., Zhang, D. et al. (2014b). The altered tight junctions: an important gateway of bacterial translocation in cachexia patients with advanced gastric cancer. *J. Interf. Cytokine Res.* 34: 518–525. https://doi.org/10.1089/jir.2013.0020.

Jiang, F., Zhang, Z., Zhang, Y. et al. (2015). L-Carnitine ameliorates cancer cachexia in mice partly via the carnitine palmitoyltransferase-associated PPAR-γ signaling pathway. *Oncol. Res. Treat.* 38: 511–516. https://doi.org/10.1159/000439550.

Johns, N., Stephens, N.A., and Fearon, K.C.H. (2013). Muscle wasting in cancer. *Int. J. Biochem. Cell Biol.* 45: 2215–2229. https://doi.org/10.1016/j.biocel.2013.05.032.

Kielczykowska, M., Kocot, J., Pazdzior, M., and Musik, I. (2018). Selenium – a fascinating antioxidant of protective properties. *Adv. Clin. Exp. Med.* 27: 245–255. https://doi.org/10.17219/acem/67222.

Kimball, S.R. and Jefferson, L.S. (2006). Signaling pathways and molecular mechanisms through which branched-chain amino acids mediate translational control of protein synthesis. *J. Nutr.* 136: 227S–231S. https://doi.org/10.1093/jn/136.1.227S.

Kimball, S.R., Shantz, L.M., Horetsky, R.L., and Jefferson, L.S. (1999). Leucine regulates translation of specific mRNAs in L6 myoblasts through mTOR-mediated changes in availability of eIF4E and phosphorylation of ribosomal protein S6. *J. Biol. Chem.* 274: 11647–11652. https://doi.org/10.1074/jbc.274.17.11647.

Klein, G.L., Petschow, B.W., Shaw, A.L., and Weaver, E. (2013). Gut barrier dysfunction and microbial translocation in cancer cachexia: a new therapeutic target. *Curr. Opin. Support. Palliat. Care* 7: 361–367. https://doi.org/10.1097/SPC.0000000000000017.

Koopman, R., Caldow, M.K., Ham, D.J., and Lynch, G.S. (2017). Glycine metabolism in skeletal muscle: implications for metabolic homeostasis. *Curr. Opin. Clin. Nutr. Metab. Care* 20: 237–242.

Kovarik, M., Muthny, T., Sispera, L., and Holecek, M. (2010). Effects of β-hydroxy-β-methylbutyrate treatment in different types of skeletal muscle of intact and septic rats. *J. Physiol. Biochem.* 66: 311–319. https://doi.org/10.1007/s13105-010-0037-3.

Kraft, M., Kraft, K., Gärtner, S. et al. (2012). l-Carnitine-supplementation in advanced pancreatic cancer (CARPAN) – a randomized multicentre trial. *Nutr. J.* 11: 52. https://doi.org/10.1186/1475-2891-11-52.

Kuczera, D., Paro de Oliveira, H.H., de Fonseca Guimarães, F.S. et al. (2012). Bax/Bcl-2 protein expression ratio and leukocyte function are related to reduction of Walker-256 tumor growth after β-hydroxy-β-methylbutyrate (HMB) administration in Wistar rats. *Nutr. Cancer* 64: 286–293. https://doi.org/10.1080/01635581.2012.647229.

Langstein, H.N. and Norton, J.A. (1991). Mechanisms of cancer cachexia. *Hematol Oncol. Clin. North Am.* 5: 103–123.

Lavriv, D.S., Neves, P.M., and Ravasco, P. (2018). Should omega-3 fatty acids be used for adjuvant treatment of cancer cachexia? *Clin. Nutr. ESPEN* 25: 18–25. https://doi.org/10.1016/j.clnesp.2018.02.006.

Lengyel, E., Makowski, L., DiGiovanni, J., and Kolonin, M.G. (2018). Cancer as a matter of fat: the crosstalk between adipose tissue and tumors. *Trends Cancer* 4: 374–384. https://doi.org/10.1016/j.trecan.2018.03.004.

Liang, C., Curry, B.J., Brown, P.L., and Zemel, M.B. (2014). Leucine modulates mitochondrial biogenesis and SIRT1-AMPK signaling in C_2C_{12} myotubes. *J. Nutr. Metab.* 2014: 239750. https://doi.org/10.1155/2014/239750.

Liu, S., Wu, H.J., Zhang, Z.Q. et al. (2011). L-carnitine ameliorates cancer cachexia in mice by regulating the expression and activity of carnitine palmityl transferase. *Cancer Biol. Ther.* 12: 125–130. https://doi.org/10.4161/cbt.12.2.15717.

Lucas, C., Barnich, N., and Nguyen, H.T.T. (2017). Microbiota, inflammation and colorectal cancer. *Int. J. Mol. Sci.* 18: 1310. https://doi.org/10.3390/ijms18061310.

Malaguarnera, M., Risino, C., Gargante, M.P. et al. (2006). Decrease of serum carnitine levels in patients with or without gastrointestinal cancer cachexia. *World J. Gastroenterol.* 12: 4541–4545. https://doi.org/10.3748/wjg.v12.i28.4541.

Malta, F.A.P.S., Estadella, D., and Gonçalves, D.C. (2019). The role of omega 3 fatty acids in suppressing muscle protein catabolism: A possible therapeutic strategy to reverse cancer cachexia? *J. Funct. Foods* 54: 1–12. https://doi.org/10.1016/j.jff.2018.12.033.

Mancinelli, A., D'Iddio, S., Bisonni, R. et al. (2007). Urinary excretion of l-carnitine and its short-chain acetyl-l-carnitine in patients undergoing carboplatin treatment. *Cancer Chemother. Pharmacol.* 60: 19–26. https://doi.org/10.1007/s00280-006-0341-3.

Mantovani, G. (2010). Randomised phase III clinical trial of 5 different arms of treatment on 332 patients with cancer cachexia. *Eur. Rev. Med. Pharmacol. Sci.* 15: 200–211. https://doi.org/10.1634/theoncologist.2009-0153.

Martín, R. and Langella, P. (2019). Emerging health concepts in the probiotics field: streamlining the definitions. *Front. Microbiol.* 10: 1047. https://doi.org/10.3389/fmicb.2019.01047.

McGlory, C., Calder, P.C., and Nunes, E.A. (2019). The influence of omega-3 fatty acids on skeletal muscle protein turnover in health, disuse, and disease. *Front. Nutr.* 6: 1–13. https://doi.org/10.3389/fnut.2019.00144.

McLean, J.B., Moylan, J.S., and Andrade, F.H. (2014). Mitochondria dysfunction in lung cancer-induced muscle wasting in C_2C_{12} myotubes. *Front. Physiol.* 5: 1–8. https://doi.org/10.3389/fphys.2014.00503.

van der Meij, B.S., Langius, J.A.E., Smit, E.F. et al. (2010). Oral nutritional supplements containing (*n*-3) polyunsaturated fatty acids affect the nutritional status of patients with stage III non-small cell lung cancer during multimodality treatment. *J. Nutr.* 140: 1774–1780. https://doi.org/10.3945/jn.110.121202.

Menon, V.P. and Sudheer, A.R. (2007). Antioxidant and anti-inflammatory properties of curcumin. *Adv. Exp. Med. Biol.* 595: 105–125.

Mirza, K.A., Pereira, S.L., Voss, A.C., and Tisdale, M.J. (2014). Comparison of the anticatabolic effects of leucine and Ca-β-hydroxy-β-methylbutyrate in experimental models of cancer cachexia. *Nutrition* 30: 807–813. https://doi.org/10.1016/j.nut.2013.11.012.

Mirza, K.A., Luo, M., Pereira, S. et al. (2016). in vitro assessment of the combined effect of eicosapentaenoic acid, green tea extract and curcumin C_3 on protein loss in C_2C_{12} myotubes. *Vitr. Cell. Dev. Biol. - Anim.* 52: 838–845. https://doi.org/10.1007/s11626-016-0051-z.

da Miyaguti, N.A.S., de Oliveira, S.C.P., and Gomes-Marcondes, M.C.C. (2018). Maternal nutritional supplementation with fish oil and/or leucine improves hepatic function and antioxidant defenses, and minimizes cachexia indexes in Walker-256 tumor-bearing rats offspring. *Nutr. Res 51*: 29–39. https://doi.org/10.1016/j.nutres.2017.12.003.

Miyaguti, N.A.d.S., de Oliveira, S.C.P., and Gomes-Marcondes, M.C.C. (2019). Maternal leucine-rich diet minimises muscle mass loss in tumour-bearing adult rat offspring by improving the balance of muscle protein synthesis and degradation. *Biomolecules* 9: 229. https://doi.org/10.3390/biom9060229.

Molanouri Shamsi, M., Chekachak, S., Soudi, S. et al. (2017). Combined effect of aerobic interval training and selenium nanoparticles on expression of IL-15 and IL-10/TNF-α ratio in skeletal muscle of 4T1 breast cancer mice with cachexia. *Cytokine* 90: 100–108. https://doi.org/10.1016/j.cyto.2016.11.005.

Molfino, A., Gioia, G., Rossi Fanelli, F., and Muscaritoli, M. (2013). Beta-hydroxy-beta-methylbutyrate supplementation in health and disease: a systematic review of randomized trials. *Amino Acids* 45: 1273–1292.

Mulligan, H.D., Beck, S.A., and Tisdale, M.J. (1992). Lipid metabolism in cancer cachexia. *Br. J. Cancer* 66: 57–61.

Neto, N.I.P., de Murari, A.S.P., Oyama, L.M. et al. (2018). Peritumoural adipose tis sue pro-inflammatory cytokines are associated with tumoural growth factors in cancer cachexia patients. *J. Cachexia. Sarcopenia Muscle* 9: 1101–1108. https://doi.org/10.1002/jcsm.12345.

Nicastro, H., Artioli, G.G., Dos Santos Costa, A. et al. (2011). An overview of the therapeutic effects of leucine supplementation on skeletal muscle under atrophic conditions. *Amino Acids* 40: 287–300.

Olivan, M., Busquets, S., Figueras, M. et al. (2011). Nutraceutical inhibition of muscle proteolysis: a role of diallyl sulphide in the treatment of muscle wasting. *Clin Nutr* 30: 33–37. https://doi.org/10.1016/j.clnu.2010.06.004.

Oliveira, A.G. and Gomes-Marcondes, M.C.C. (2016). Metformin treatment modulates the tumour-induced wasting effects in muscle protein metabolism minimising the cachexia in tumour-bearing rats. *BMC Cancer* 16: 418. https://doi.org/10.1186/s12885-016-2424-9.

de Oliveira, A.G., Cruz, B., Oliveira, S.C.P. et al. (2020). Leucine and its importance for cell signalling pathways in cancer cachexia-induced muscle wasting, chapter 6. In: *Muscle Cells. Recent Advances and Future Prespectives* (ed. M.T. Valarmathi), 109–129. IntechOpen.

Park, B.S., Henning, P.C., Grant, S.C. et al. (2013). HMB attenuates muscle loss during sustained energy deficit induced by calorie restriction and endurance exercise. *Metabolism* 62: 1718–1729. https://doi.org/10.1016/j.metabol.2013.06.005.

Pastore, C.A., Orlandi, S.P., and Gonzalez, M.C. (2014). Introduction of an omega-3 enriched oral supplementation for cancer patients close to the first chemotherapy: may it be a factor for poor compliance? *Nutr. Cancer* 66: 1285–1292. https://doi.org/10.1080/01635581.2014.956253.

Penna, F., Busquets, S., Pin, F. et al. (2011). Combined approach to counteract experimental cancer cachexia: Eicosapentaenoic acid and training exercise. *J. Cachexia. Sarcopenia Muscle* 2: 95–104. https://doi.org/10.1007/s13539-011-0028-4.

Penna, F., Camperi, A., Muscaritoli, M. et al. (2017). The role of vitamin D in cancer cachexia. *Curr. Opin. Support. Palliat. Care* 11: 287–292. https://doi.org/10.1097/SPC.0000000000000302.

Peters, S.J., van Helvoort, A., Kegler, D. et al. (2011). Dose-dependent effects of leucine supplementation on preservation of muscle mass in cancer cachectic mice. *Oncol. Rep.* 26: 247–254. https://doi.org/10.3892/or.2011.1269.

Petruzzelli, M. and Wagner, E.F. (2016). Mechanisms of metabolic dysfunction in cancer-associated cachexia. *Genes Dev.* 30: 489–501. https://doi.org/10.1101/gad.276733.115.

Pisano, C., Vesci, L., Milazzo, F.M. et al. (2010). Metabolic approach to the enhancement of antitumor effect of chemotherapy: a key role of acetyl-l-carnitine. *Clin. Cancer Res.* 16: 3944–3953. https://doi.org/10.1158/1078-0432.CCR-10-0964.

Pisters, P.W. and Brennan, M.F. (1990). Amino acid metabolism in human cancer cachexia. *Annu. Rev. Nutr.* 10: 107–132. https://doi.org/10.1146/annurev.nu.10.070190.000543.

Plas, R.L.C., Poland, M., Faber, J. et al. (2019). A diet rich in fish oil and leucine ameliorates hypercalcemia in tumour-induced cachectic mice. *Int. J. Mol. Sci.* 20: 4978. https://doi.org/10.3390/ijms20204978.

Polly, P. and Tan, T.C. (2014). The role of vitamin D in skeletal and cardiac muscle function. *Front. Physiol.* 5: 145. https://doi.org/10.3389/fphys.2014.00145.

Porporato, P. (2016). Understanding cachexia as a cancer metabolism syndrome. *Oncogenesis* 5: e200. https://doi.org/10.1038/oncsis.2016.3.

Pötgens, S.A., Brossel, H., Sboarina, M. et al. (2018). *Klebsiella oxytoca* expands in cancer cachexia and acts as a gut pathobiont contributing to intestinal dysfunction. *Sci. Rep.* 8: 1–12. https://doi.org/10.1038/s41598-018-30569-5.

Pottel, L., Lycke, M., Boterberg, T. et al. (2014). Echium oil is not protective against weight loss in head and neck cancer patients undergoing curative radio(chemo)therapy: a randomised-controlled trial. *BMC Complement. Altern. Med.* 14: 382. https://doi.org/10.1186/1472-6882-14-382.

Prado, C.M., Sawyer, M.B., Ghosh, S. et al. (2013). Central tenet of cancer cachexia therapy: do patients with advanced cancer have exploitable anabolic potential? *Am. J. Clin. Nutr.* 98: 1012–1019. https://doi.org/10.3945/ajcn.113.060228.

Puppa, M.J., White, J.P., Sato, S. et al. (2011). Gut barrier dysfunction in the Apc Min/+ mouse model of colon cancer cachexia. *Biochim. Biophys. Acta – Mol. Basis Dis.* 1812: 1601–1606. https://doi. org/10.1016/j.bbadis.2011.08.010.

Quan-Jun, Y., Jun, B., Li-Li, W. et al. (2015). NMR-based metabolomics reveals distinct pathways mediated by curcumin in cachexia mice bearing CT26 tumor. *RSC Adv.* 5: 11766–11775. https://doi. org/10.1039/c4ra14128h.

Reed, S.A., Sandesara, P.B., Senf, S.M., and Judge, A.R. (2012). Inhibition of FoxO transcriptional activity prevents muscle fiber atrophy during cachexia and induces hypertrophy. *FASEB J.* 26: 987–1000. https://doi.org/10.1096/fj.11-189977.

Rossi, A.P., D'Introno, A., Rubele, S. et al. (2017). The potential of β-hydroxy-β-methylbutyrate as a new strategy for the management of sarcopenia and sarcopenic obesity. *Drugs Aging* 34: 833–840.

Roy, S. and Trinchieri, G. (2017). Microbiota: a key orchestrator of cancer therapy. *Nat. Rev. Cancer* 17: 271–285.

Russell, S.T. and Tisdale, M.J. (2005). The role of glucocorticoids in the induction of zinc-alpha2-glycoprotein expression in adipose tissue in cancer cachexia. *Br. J. Cancer* 92: 876–881. https://doi. org/10.1038/sj.bjc.6602404.

Ryan, Z.C., Craig, T.A., Wang, X. et al. (2018). 1α,25-Dihydroxyvitamin D_3 mitigates cancer cell mediated mitochondrial dysfunction in human skeletal muscle cells. *Biochem. Biophys. Res. Commun.* 496: 746–752. https://doi.org/10.1016/j.bbrc.2018.01.092.

Sahebkar, A., Saboni, N., Pirro, M., and Banach, M. (2017). Curcumin: an effective adjunct in patients with statin-associated muscle symptoms? *J. Cachexia. Sarcopenia Muscle* 8: 19–24. https://doi. org/10.1002/jcsm.12140.

Salomão, E.M., Toneto, A.T., Silva, G.O., and Gomes-Marcondes, M.C.C. (2010). Physical exercise and a leucine-rich diet modulate the muscle protein metabolism in Walker tumor-bearing rats. *Nutr. Cancer* 62: 1095–1104.

Salomão, E.M., Gomes-Marcondes, M.C.C., and Salomao, E.M. (2012). Light aerobic physical exercise in combination with leucine and/or glutamine-rich diet can improve the body composition and muscle protein metabolism in young tumor-bearing rats. *J. Physiol. Biochem.* 68: 493–501. https:// doi.org/10.1007/s13105-012-0164-0.

Sandri, M. (2015). Protein breakdown in cancer cachexia. *Semin. Cell Dev. Biol.* 54: 11–19. https://doi. org/10.1016/j.semcdb.2015.11.002.

Schiessel, D.L., Yamazaki, R.K., Kryczyk, M. et al. (2015). α-Linolenic fatty acid supplementation decreases tumor growth and cachexia parameters in Walker 256 tumor-bearing rats. *Nutr. Cancer* 67: 839–846. https://doi.org/10.1080/01635581.2015.1043021.

Schnuck, J.K., Sunderland, K.L., Gannon, N.P. et al. (2016). Leucine stimulates PPARβ/δ-dependent mitochondrial biogenesis and oxidative metabolism with enhanced GLUT4 content and glucose uptake in myotubes. *Biochimie* 128–129: 1–7. https://doi.org/10.1016/j.biochi.2016.06.009.

Shadfar, S., Couch, M.E., McKinney, K.A. et al. (2011). Oral resveratrol therapy inhibits cancer-induced skeletal muscle and cardiac atrophy in vivo. *Nutr. Cancer* 63: 749–762. https://doi.org/10.1080/01635 581.2011.563032.

Sharples, A.P., Hughes, D.C., Deane, C.S. et al. (2015). Longevity and skeletal muscle mass: the role of IGF signalling, the sirtuins, dietary restriction and protein intake. *Aging Cell* 14: 511–523. https:// doi.org/10.1111/acel.12342.

Shimomura, Y., Yamamoto, Y., Bajotto, G. et al. (2006). Nutraceutical effects of branched-chain amino acids on skeletal muscle. *J. Nutr.* 136: 529S–532S. https://doi.org/10.1093/jn/136.2.529s.

Shirai, Y., Okugawa, Y., Hishida, A. et al. (2017). Fish oil-enriched nutrition combined with systemic chemotherapy for gastrointestinal cancer patients with cancer cachexia. *Sci. Rep.* 7: 1–9. https://doi. org/10.1038/s41598-017-05278-0.

Silva, V.R., Belozo, F.L., Micheletti, T.O. et al. (2017). β-Hydroxy-β-methylbutyrate free acid supplementation may improve recovery and muscle adaptations after resistance training: a systematic review. *Nutr. Res.* 45: 1–9.

Solís-Martínez, O., Plasa-Carvalho, V., Phillips-Sixtos, G. et al. (2018). Effect of eicosapentaenoic acid on body composition and inflammation markers in patients with head and neck squamous cell cancer from a public hospital in Mexico. *Nutr. Cancer* 70: 663–670. https://doi.org/10.1080/01635581.2018.1460678.

Sustova, H., De Feudis, M., Reano, S. et al. (2019). Opposing effects of 25-hydroxy- and 1α,25-dihydroxy-vitamin D_3 on pro-cachectic cytokine-and cancer conditioned medium-induced atrophy in C_2C_{12} myotubes. *Acta Physiol.* 226: 1–10. https://doi.org/10.1111/apha.13269.

Tisdale, M.J. (2003). Pathogenesis of cancer cachexia. *J. Support Oncol.* 1: 159–168.

Tisdale, M.J. (2009). Mechanisms of cancer cachexia. *Physiol. Rev.* 89: 381–410. https://doi.org/10.1152/physrev.00016.2008.

Tisdale, M.J. (2009). Zinc-alpha2-glycoprotein in cachexia and obesity. *Curr. Opin. Support Palliat. Care* 3: 288–293. https://doi.org/10.1097/SPC.0b013e328331c897.

Tisdale, M.J. (2010). Cancer cachexia. *Curr. Opin. Gastroenterol.* 26: 146–151. https://doi.org/10.1097/MOG.0b013e3283347e77.

Todorov, P., Cariuk, P., McDevitt, T. et al. (1996). Characterization of a cancer cachectic factor. *Nature* 379: 739–742. https://doi.org/10.1038/379739a0.

Toneto, A.T., Ferreira Ramos, L.A., Salomão, E.M. et al. (2016). Nutritional leucine supplementation attenuates cardiac failure in tumour-bearing cachectic animals. *J. Cachexia. Sarcopenia Muscle* 7: 577–586. https://doi.org/10.1002/jcsm.12100.

Van Der Meij, B.S., Langius, J.A.E., Spreeuwenberg, M.D. et al. (2012). Oral nutritional supplements containing n-3 polyunsaturated fatty acids affect quality of life and functional status in lung cancer patients during multimodality treatment: An RCT. *Eur. J. Clin. Nutr.* 66: 399–404. https://doi.org/10.1038/ejcn.2011.214.

Van Koevering, M. and Nissen, S. (1992). Oxidation of leucine and alpha-ketoisocaproate to beta-hydroxy-beta-methylbutyrate in vivo. *Am. J. Physiol.* 262: E27–E31.

Varian, B.J., Goureshetti, S., Poutahidis, T. et al. (2016). Beneficial bacteria inhibit cachexia. *Oncotarget* 7: 11803–11816.

Ventrucci, G., Mello, M.A.R., and Gomes-Marcondes, M.C.C. (2001). Effect of a leucine-supplemented diet on body composition changes in pregnant rats bearing Walker 256 tumor. *Braz. J. Med. Biol. Res.* 34: 333–338.

Viana, L.R., Canevarolo, R., Luiz, A.C.P. et al. (2016). Leucine-rich diet alters the (1)H-NMR based metabolomic profile without changing the Walker-256 tumour mass in rats. *BMC Cancer* 16: 764. https://doi.org/10.1186/s12885-016-2811-2.

Viana, L.R., Luiz, A.C.P., Favero-Santos, B.C. et al. (2018). Leucine-rich diet minimises liver glycogen mobilisation and modulates liver gluconeogenesis enzyme expression in tumour-bearing cachectic rats. *JCSM Rapid Commun.* 1: 1–9. https://doi.org/10.1002/j.2617-1619.2018.tb00003.x.

Viana, L.R., Tobar, N., Busanello, E.N.B. et al. (2019). Leucine-rich diet induces a shift in tumour metabolism from glycolytic towards oxidative phosphorylation, reducing glucose consumption and metastasis in Walker-256 tumour-bearing rats. *Sci. Rep.* 9: 1–11. https://doi.org/10.1038/s41598-019-52112-w.

Vitorino, R., Moreira-Gonçalves, D., and Ferreira, R. (2015). Mitochondrial plasticity in cancer-related muscle wasting: potential approaches for its management. *Curr. Opin. Clin. Nutr. Metab. Care* 18: 226–233. https://doi.org/10.1097/MCO.0000000000000161.

Wang, H., Chan, Y.L., Li, T.L. et al. (2013). Reduction of splenic immunosuppressive cells and enhancement of anti-tumor immunity by synergy of fish oil and selenium yeast. *PLoS One* 8: 1–11. https://doi.org/10.1371/journal.pone.0052912.

Wang, D.T., Yin, Y., Yang, Y.J. et al. (2014). Resveratrol prevents TNF-α-induced muscle atrophy via regulation of Akt/mTOR/FoxO1 signaling in C_2C_{12} myotubes. *Int. Immunopharmacol.* 19: 206–213. https://doi.org/10.1016/j.intimp.2014.02.002.

Wang, H., Li, T., Hsia, S. et al. (2015). Skeletal muscle atrophy is attenuated in tumor-bearing mice under chemotherapy by treatment with fish oil and selenium. *Oncotarget* 6: 7758–7773.

Wang, N., Tan, H.Y., Li, S. et al. (2017). Supplementation of micronutrient selenium in metabolic diseases: Its role as an antioxidant. *Oxid. Med. Cell. Longev.* 2017: 7478523. https://doi.org/10.1155/2017/7478523.

Wang, J., Ji, H., Wang, S. et al. (2018). Probiotic *Lactobacillus plantarum* promotes intestinal barrier function by strengthening the epithelium and modulating gut microbiota. *Front. Microbiol.* 9: 1953. https://doi.org/10.3389/fmicb.2018.01953.

Werner, K., Küllenberg de Gaudry, D., Taylor, L.A. et al. (2017). Dietary supplementation with *n*-3-fatty acids in patients with pancreatic cancer and cachexia: marine phospholipids versus fish oil - a randomized controlled double-blind trial. *Lipids Health Dis.* 16: 1–12. https://doi.org/10.1186/s12944-017-0495-5.

Wiktorowska-Owczarek, A., Berezińska, M., and Nowak, J.Z. (2015). PUFAs: structures, metabolism and functions. *Adv. Clin. Exp. Med.* 24: 931–941. https://doi.org/10.17219/acem/31243.

Woodworth-Hobbs, M.E., Hudson, M.B., Rahnert, J.A. et al. (2014). Docosahexaenoic acid prevents palmitate-induced activation of proteolytic systems in C_2C_{12} myotubes. *J. Nutr. Biochem.* 25: 868–874. https://doi.org/10.1016/j.jnutbio.2014.03.017.

Yano, C.L., Ventrucci, G., Tisadale, M.J., and Gomes-Marcondes, M.C. (2008). Metabolic and morphological alterations induced by proteolysis-inducing factor from Walker tumour in C_2C_{12} myotubes. *BMC Cancer* 8: 24.

Yeh, K.Y., Wang, H.M., Chang, J.W.C. et al. (2013). Omega-3 fatty acid-, micronutrient-, and probiotic-enriched nutrition helps body weight stabilization in head and neck cancer cachexia. *Oral Surg. Oral Med. Oral Pathol. Oral Radiol.* 116: 41–48. https://doi.org/10.1016/j.oooo.2013.01.015.

Zhang, G., Liu, Z., Ding, H. et al. (2017). Tumor induces muscle wasting in mice through releasing extracellular Hsp70 and Hsp90. *Nat. Commun.* 8: 589. https://doi.org/10.1038/s41467-017-00726-x.

15

Early Life Nutrition, Epigenetics, and Programming of Later Life

Jayshree Nellore[1], Jaya Krishna Tippabathani[1], Aparna S. Narayan[1], Swetha Sunkar[2],
C. Valli Nachiyar[1], K. Renugadevi[1], and S. Karthick Raja Namasivayam[1]

[1] Department of Biotechnology, Sathyabama Institute of Science and Technology, Chennai, Tamil Nadu, India
[2] Department of Bioinformatics, Sathyabama Institute of Science and Technology, Chennai, Tamil Nadu, India

15.1 Introduction

The current epidemic of noncommunicable diseases (NCDs), such as metabolic syndrome, cardio-vascular diseases (CVD), type-2 diabetes mellitus (T2DM), osteoporosis, obesity, hypertension, hyperlipidemia, some cancers, neurological disorders, and chronic respiratory disease presents one of our greatest-ever challenges to the global health (Islam et al. 2014). The total deaths from NCDs are projected to increase by 17% over the next 10 years. Knowing the risk factors for a chronic disease means that approximately 80% of premature heart disease and stroke, 80% of T2DM and 40% of cancers are preventable (Habib and Saha 2010). In particular, the World Health Organization has identified tobacco use, harmful use of alcohol, physical inactivity, unhealthy diet, and pollution as the main modifiable risk factors.

Evidence has shown that predisposition to these chronic diseases of adulthood arises at the earliest times of life. The developmental origins of health and disease (DOHaD) hypothesis suggested that nutrition in early life (fetal, neonatal, and infantile periods) and prenatal nutritional environments could influence or "program" the long-term health of an individual (Calkins and Devaskar 2011). Although initial studies focused on the detrimental effects of fetal undernutrition, subsequent studies on humans, and animal models have consistently reported that either deficiency (undernutrition) or excess (overnutrition) availability of nutrients, oxygen, and hormones influence tissue development, and lead to an increased risk of "NCDs" in adult progeny (Fleming et al. 2018).

The late onset of such diseases in response to earlier transient experiences has led to the suggestion that developmental programming may have an epigenetic component, as epigenetic marks such as DNA methylation or histone tail modifications could provide a persistent memory of earlier nutritional states. Recent evidence has shown that some of the epigenetic changes ensuing from early nutrition can be transgenerationally inherited (Vickers 2014).

This chapter attempts to inform readers about the causative links identified between nutrition, epigenetics, and developmental programming that can lead to different and unintended long-term consequences on health and disease. Moreover, a better understanding of the underlying mechanisms may be fundamental to improve the approach to disease prevention.

Handbook of Nutraceuticals and Natural Products: Biological, Medicinal, and Nutritional Properties and Applications,
Volume 1, First Edition. Edited by Sreerag Gopi and Preetha Balakrishnan.
© 2022 John Wiley & Sons, Inc. Published 2022 by John Wiley & Sons, Inc.

15.2   Nutritional Influence on Epigenetic Marks

Intrauterine programming happens at "critical time windows" of fetal growth- specified by a high rate of differentiation and/or proliferation, and comprise genes, cells, tissues, and even whole organs (Sferruzzi-Perri and Camm 2016). Programming is an adaptive response of the organism to the surrounding environment. This ability, named "developmental plasticity," enables the development of a variety of phenotypes from a single genotype. According to DOHaD, the organism exposed to in utero malnutrition diverts the limited nutrients to preserve the growth and function of vital organs, such as the brain, at the expense of the growth of organs, such as the liver and pancreas (Gluckman et al. 2010). This intrauterine adaptation is promising for survival in cases where the fetus is born into conditions of insufficient nutrition. However, detrimental consequences of developmental programming arise when the fetus is born in an environment with normal or even increased nutrient supply. The mismatch between pre- and postnatal environments may ultimately predispose the offspring to the development of disease in adulthood, the inheritance of risk factors, and a cycle of disease transmission across generations (Gluckman et al. 2008).

Prenatal environmental exposures may have important and permanent effects on epigenetic mechanisms. The study of food nutrients and their effects on human health through epigenetic modifications is called Nutriepigenomics (Paparo et al. 2014). Epigenetics relates to relatively stable, mitotically heritable changes in chromosomes that influence the phenotype of an organism within a generation but are not due to alterations in the DNA nucleotide sequence. Two major epigenetic mechanisms implicated in nutriepigenomics are DNA methylation and histone modification. In addition to histone modifications and DNA methylation, there are also other gene regulatory networks, including microRNAs (miRNAs), small interfering RNAs, and long noncoding RNAs, all of which serve to control gene expression. Given that these modifications are reversible and sensitive to environmental factors, they provide a mechanistic link between environmental exposures, developmental programming, and the risk for disease (Ho et al. 2012). Hence, early life nutrition may influence development through direct epigenetic mechanisms.

15.2.1   DNA Methylation and Nutrition

DNA methylation is a chemical process that adds a methyl group to DNA. It is highly specific and almost exclusively affects position five of the pyrimidine ring of cytosines in the context of the dinucleotide sequence, CpG. CpG sites are methylated by a group of enzymes called DNA methyltransferases (DNMTs), namely DNMT1, DNMT2, DNMT3a, DNMT3b, and DNMTL. DNMT1 maintains DNA methylation during cell replication while the rest of the DNMT family, mainly DNMT3a and DNMT3b, are responsible for de novo DNA methylation (Gujar et al. 2019). DNA methylation is essential for cell-specific gene expression, plays a crucial role during embryonic development, and establishes imprinting and X chromosome inactivation. DNA methylation in promoter regions is generally associated with transcriptional silencing (Jin et al. 2011).

Several studies have focused on the link between diet and DNA methylation in mammals to elucidate the lifelong consequences of dietary exposures on epigenetic marks. Various researchers (*in vitro* and *in vivo*) have reported the relationship between nutrition and DNA methylation, inclusive of prenatal and postnatal periods, showing that diets deficient in methyl donors and proteins may cause global DNA hypomethylation, or that high-fat (HF) diet consumption may result in changes in DNA methylation (Kadayifci et al. 2018). The "yellow agouti (Avy) mice" model is one of the most popular models that have studied the link between diet and DNA methylation.

The agouti gene regulates the eumelanin (brown/black) and pheomelanin (yellow) pigmentation in the mammalian coat. It has been demonstrated that the supplementation of dams with dietary methyl donors altered the coat color by correlating it with the Avy methylation status (Dolinoy 2008). However, most of these studies using the agouti mice model failed to explain the underlying epigenetic mechanisms concerning DNA methylation and whether it occurred due to the expression or inhibition of special binding sites of methylation enzymes, substrates, cofactors, etc. (Kadayifci et al. 2018). Besides this, there are too many uncertainties about the necessary nutrition doses and the exact duration of dietary exposure to DNA methylation.

There is now increasing evidence substantiating that nutrients may alter the pattern of DNA methylation, either at the global scale or at locus-specific sites. Earlier evidence has proposed that nutrition affects the epigenetic regulation of DNA methylation in several possible ways: first, by providing necessary substrates for proper DNA methylation; second, by providing cofactors that modulate the enzymatic activity of DNMT; third, by modulating the activity of enzymes regulating the one-carbon cycle. Importantly, all three mechanisms are mutually compatible and may collectively operate in time (Zhang 2015).

15.2.1.1 Methylation Cycle and Methyl Donors

Various nutrients present in the diet, including methionine, folate, choline, betaine, and vitamins B2, B6, and B12 serve as precursors and contribute to the production of S-adenosylmethionine (SAM). SAM is the principal methyl group donor for the majority of methyltransferases. Therefore, any deficits in these nutrients may result in changes in the SAM pool, which can influence the DNMTs' activity as well as DNA methylation (Qiu and Schlegel 2015).

Actually, it is the DNMTs that convert into S-adenosylhomocysteine (SAH), which strongly competes with SAM for the active site on the methyltransferase enzyme. The ratio of SAM to SAH is called "methylation index" which is a better marker for methylation status (DNA hypermethylation or hypomethylation). Furthermore, elevated levels of plasma homocysteine concentrations increase the levels of SAH, but not SAM; increased SAH levels have been associated with global DNA hypomethylation (Tehlivets et al. 2013; Zhang 2018).

The methyl- and folate-deficient diets have been reported to reduce SAM/SAH ratios in the livers of male rats and mice. Also, the changes in SAM and SAH levels demonstrated irreversible alteration in hepatic DNA methylation (Pogribny et al. 2006). Besides, zinc deficiency has resulted in global DNA hypomethylation due to reduced use of methyl groups from SAM in rat liver (Brabin et al. 2001). On the other hand, low protein or 50% global malnutrition during gestation in mice led to both hyper- and hypo-methylation at specific loci in the offspring (Van Straten et al. 2010).

Also, other studies demonstrated that high dietary methionine intake is believed to increase DNA methylation. High doses of folate supplementation are believed to induce a substantial increase of the intracellular pool of the SAM, the SAM/SAH ratio and showed an increase in methylation and normalized gene expression at specific loci (Ingrosso et al. 2003). Very few studies have examined the epigenetic mechanisms of the effects of high methionine intake on DNA methylation (Brabin et al. 2001). In an epigenetic mouse model, protracted methionine treatment in mice elicited an increase in brain SAH levels, whereas SAM was not affected. The decrease in the SAM/SAH ratio would be anticipated to hypomethylate DNA, but it has been found that specific CpG islands of the reelin (RELN) promoter were actually hypermethylated in the cortex of methionine-treated mice (Dong et al. 2005). This significant increase in CpG methylation appeared to down-regulate RELN expression (Rhizobium 2013). A follow-up study showed that protracted methionine increased the binding of methyl CpG-binding protein 2 (MeCP2) to the RELN promoter, which is believed to be the reason behind hypermethylation (Zhubi et al. 2014). However, contradictory effects were found in other control genes (Gad65 and β-globin). Another model found no significant dietary methionine effects on genome-wide DNA methylation, although methionine supplementation significantly decreased the SAM/SAH ratio in the liver and brain (Devlin et al. 2004).

The other major methyl donor is betaine which can be produced by choline or taken through diet. Upon oxidative conversion to betaine, choline can modulate methylation via the enzyme betaine homocysteine methyltransferase (BHMT), this nutrient (and its metabolite, betaine) regulates the concentrations of SAM and SAH (Coleman et al. 2019). Choline methyl-deficient diets showed reduced hepatic concentrations of SAM and increased levels of SAH in the livers of mice (Shivapurkar and Poirier 1983). Additionally, a rat study demonstrated that administration of a choline-deficient diet for seven days significantly reduced liver methionine formation by 20–25%, SAM by 60%, and increased liver SAH by 50% (Zeisel et al. 1989). Studies also demonstrated another complex scenario, folate deficiency led to reduced choline and betaine levels in the liver (Kim et al. 1994). A choline deficiency decreased hepatic folate stores and affected the methyl transfer of the one-carbon cycle in the liver. Besides, a study demonstrated that folic acid-supplemented diets to BHMT-deleted mice have produced more hepatic SAM compared to mice fed with folate-deficient diets or a control diet (Teng et al. 2011). Previous studies have shown that a diet very low in choline and methionine has resulted in decreased methylation of cytosine in the liver (Wilson et al. 1984). However, the direct interaction between choline, biotin, and DNA methylation through SAM and SAH activities or different mechanisms remains elusive.

15.2.1.2 Cofactor and Enzyme Activities in One-Carbon Cycles

Nutrients possibly modify DNA methylation by participating in a cellular process known as "one-carbon metabolism" that donates methyl groups for the biological methylation of DNA, protein, or phospholipids (Friso et al. 2017). One-carbon metabolism is a process that is involved in amino acid and nucleotide metabolism and includes a set of biochemical reactions that are catalyzed by a specific set of enzymes and coenzymes (Ducker and Rabinowitz 2017). This set of reactions is named one-carbon metabolism because they transfer one-carbon groups from donors to protein or DNA. During this process, cyclical chemical reactions take place in mammalian cells where micronutrients such as folate, vitamin B12, and vitamin B6 play a significant role as cofactors or methyl acceptors or donors (Anderson et al. 2012). This process starts with a one-carbon transfer from the amino acid serine to tetrahydrofolate. Tetrahydrofolate is a form of vitamin B9 that is essential for the nucleic acid synthesis and is naturally present in many food sources. Apart from this, it is also important for other vital biological processes in the body. This reaction is catalyzed by the enzyme serine hydroxymethyltransferase (SMHT), a vitamin B6-containing enzyme (Kandi and Vadakedath 2015; Mentch and Locasale 2016).

The outcome of this reaction is 5,10-methylenetetrahydrofolate, which, in turn, is transformed into 5-methyl tetrahydrofolate via the enzyme methylenetetrahydrofolate reductase (*MTHFR*), a vitamin B2-containing enzyme (Jiang and Huang 2015). The product 5-methyl tetrahydrofolate is the primary methyl donor for the reaction that remethylates homocysteine into methionine. The latter reaction is catalyzed by the enzyme methionine synthase (MS or MTR), which contains vitamin B12 as a cofactor (Froese et al. 2019). Methionine is then converted to SAM, the DNMT cofactor, and the universal methyl donor for all the biological methylation processes inside mammalian cells including DNA methylation (Kandi and Vadakedath 2015; Mentch and Locasale 2016; Ducker and Rabinowitz 2017).

Additionally, it is believed that supplementing diets with micronutrients such as folate, vitamins B2, B6, and B12 contributes to the maintenance of DNA methyl marks and thus regulates DNA methylation (Kulkarni et al. 2011). It is assumed that changes in the bioavailability of these nutrients alter the activity of the one-carbon cycle and the production of SAM, thereby affecting the DNA methylation (Wu et al. 2019).

Studies have also reported a common polymorphism in the gene encoding *MTHFR.MTHFR* 677TT results in thermolability and lower levels of methylated DNA in the presence of low folate concentrations (Wan et al. 2018). Another study in cultured lymphocytes has shown that vitamin B2, folic acid, and *MTHFR* C677T polymorphism affect genome instability and that high concentrations of vitamin B2 may increase the activity of *MTHFR*, which may cause folate to transfer methyl groups for the methionine synthesis enzyme. Furthermore, it has been suggested that low vitamin B2 concentration in the presence of low folate may increase the risk of genome hypomethylation. However, more studies are necessary to evaluate the link between diet-enzyme activities in the one-carbon cycle and DNA methylation (Brabin et al. 2001).

15.2.1.3 DNA Methyltransferase Activity

SAM acts as a cofactor for the full activation of DNMT. Methyl donors from the diet may play a crucial role in regulating the DNMT activity by altering the intracellular concentration of SAM. Besides an indirect regulation of DNA methylation patterns through modulation of SAM pools, several compounds can also directly affect the expression or activity of DNMT. These assumptions have been demonstrated for several bioactive food components such as epigallocatechin-3-gallate (EGCG), genistein, caffeic acid, ascorbate, etc. (Zhang 2015).

Evidence of competitive inhibition of DNMT activity has been demonstrated for each of the tea polyphenols, catechin, epicatechin, and EGCG, or the genistein present in soybean. Bioflavonoids such as quercetin, fisetin, and myricetin can also decrease DNA methylation by inhibiting SssI DNMT and DNMT1-mediated DNA methylation in a concentration-dependent manner (Won et al. 2005).

Reactivation of many methylation-silenced genes by EGCG was also demonstrated through inhibition of DNMT1in human colon cancer HT-29 cells, prostate cancer PC3 cells, and KYSE cells (Fang et al. 2003). Several other studies have also revealed that EGCG decreased global DNA methylation levels, and also showed a protective effect by inhibiting the promoter hypermethylation of specific genes. These effects were attributed to the decreased mRNA and protein expression activity of DNMT1 whose binding domain is induced by EGCG to connect to the promoter of the specific genes (Zhang et al. 2013; Remely et al. 2017).

Genistein was also found to decrease DNMT activity in a dose-dependent manner, but this activity was found to be weaker than that of EGCG. However, the mechanistic role of genistein has not been explored. While it has been shown that other dietary phenolic compounds, including hesperetin, naringin, apigenin, and luteolin, can also indirectly moderate DNMT activity by regulating the ratio of SAM and SAH, these compounds are not as efficient as EGCG in inhibiting DNMT activity (Won et al. 2005; Fang et al. 2007).

Molecular docking studies have suggested that curcumin covalently blocks the catalytic thiolate of DNMT's C1226 to exert its inhibitory effect. In addition, curcumin was found to induce global hypomethylation by inhibiting DNMT (Liu et al. 2009). In contrast, a multidocking approach has suggested that curcumin does not elicit any significant effect on DNMT inhibition and global hypomethylation (Liu et al. 2009). Thus, more studies are warranted to detect a definitive interaction between curcumin and DNA methylation.

15.2.2 Histone Modifications and Nutrition

The NH2-terminal tail of histones can be covalently modified by histone methyltransferases (HMTs), histone deacetylases (HDACs), and histone acetyltransferases (HATs) (Bannister and

Kouzarides 2011). Histone modifications alter chromatin compaction and influence the recruitment of transcriptional regulators which modulate gene expression. Multiple histone post-translational modifications (PTMs) have been described, including acetylation, methylation, phosphorylation, ubiquitination, and SUMOylation of amino acid residues (e.g. lysine or arginine). Many of these act in concert to regulate gene expression. In fact, several studies have demonstrated that histone PTMs are excellent intermediaries to connect changes between environmental input (nutritional availability) and the biological output (transcriptional regulation) (Bannister and Kouzarides 2011; MolinaSerrano et al. 2019).

15.2.2.1 Acetylation of Histones

The two dietary compounds directly involved in acetylation events are acetate and coenzyme A (CoA). Acetate can be derived from the metabolism of glucose, amino acids, fatty acids, and other compounds in intermediary metabolism (Shi and Tu 2015). Except for circumstances of prolonged total starvation, it is nearly impossible to deplete the body's pool of acetates. CoA is required for the generation of the energy-rich acetyl-CoA for subsequent acetylation reactions. The vitamin, pantothenic acid is an integral part of the CoA molecule. Excess acetyl-CoA is exported from the mitochondria to the cytoplasm and diffuses into the nucleus, where it can be used by HATs (Pietrocola et al. 2015; Sivanand et al. 2018). Therefore, the major nutrients, i.e. carbohydrates, lipids, and proteins are linked with histone acetylation.

Both in vitro and in vivo studies provide evidence that the medicinal natural product curcumin directly inhibits HAT activity (Hassan et al. 2019).

The family of HDACs is categorized into four classes depending on sequence identity and domain organization. Classes I, II, and IV are zinc-dependent enzymes whereas class III HDACs are dependent on NAD+ concentration and are also called sirtuins (Gregoretti et al. 2004). Sir2 (silent information regulator 2), which is present in simple eukaryotes, and its mammalian ortholog SIRT1 "sense" the positive effects of caloric restriction on the physiology of the cell and are key controllers of mitochondrial energy metabolism, senescence of the cell, inflammation and, most importantly, tumorigenesis (Motta et al. 2004; Brenmoehl and Hoeflich 2013). When fasting happens, the available NAD+ and activity of *SIRT1* are high (Rodgers and Puigserver 2007). In contrast, when energy resources are high, NAD+ would be converted to Nicotinamide Adenine Dinucleotide (Nad) + Hydrogen (H) (NADH) and, consequently, its concentration would decrease (Cantó et al. 2015). Another interesting possibility about links between nutrition and histone PTMs is that the ketone body β-hydroxybutyrate – a product of activation of fatty acid β oxidation – acts as an endogenous HDAC inhibitor. This would lead to increased H3 acetylation (Lys9 and Lys14) and transcription of genes that are controlled with the forkhead box O gene (*FOXO3a*) (Nakahata et al. 2008; Martins et al. 2016). Other studies confirmed that caloric restriction – mostly low-carbohydrate diets – would lead to ketogenesis and this is associated with class I HDACs (yeast, Caenorhabditis elegans, Drosophila) in the extension of life span along with protection against reactive oxygen species (ROS) (Pallos et al. 2008; Newman and Verdin 2014). It seems that this metabolite-controlled HDAC is a process that is involved in lots of cell events and not just longevity.

Resveratrol (RSV), a phenolic compound isolated from the skins of red grapes, is a caloric restriction mimetic that activates sirtuins in a dose-dependent manner. RSV also increases the life span of Saccharomyces cerevisiae, Caenorhabditis elegans, Drosophila melanogaster, and the fish – Nothobranchiusfurzeri. However, its efficacy in mammals is uncertain. A number of studies have investigated certain bioactive food components that can act as HDAC inhibitors, e.g. sulforaphane and isothiocyanate from broccoli and broccoli sprouts; diallyl sulfide, an organosulfur compound from garlic; and butyrate, a short-chain fatty acid from fiber. The extent to which these dietary compounds affect HDAC activity is still unknown (Nian et al. 2009; Stacchiotti et al. 2019).

15.2.2.2 Methylation of Histones

The effects of nutrients or bioactive components on histone methylation are less explored compared to histone acetylation. HMTs transfer methyl groups from SAM onto the lysine or arginine residues of the H3 and H4 histones. Reduction of threonine, a metabolic precursor for the genesis of SAM, results in reduced levels of H3K4me2 and H3K4me3 but not H3K4me1 (Nicolas et al. 2003; Janke et al. 2015). Different dietary interventions like HF diet, low-protein diet (LPD), and CR (caloric restrictions) showed that extreme dietary conditions affect multiple nutrient-sensing pathways and can cause global histone modification changes (Piper and Bartke 2008; Donohoe and Bultman 2012; MolinaSerrano et al. 2019).

Histone methylation is a dynamic and reversible process. Demethylases are enzymes that remove methyl groups not only from histones but from other proteins as well (Piper and Bartke 2008). They are important in epigenetic modification mechanisms. The largest class of demethylase enzymes contains a Jumonji C (JmjC) domain which can demethylate mono-, di-, and trimethylated histones by an oxidative mechanism that requires Fe (II) and alpha-ketoglutarate as cofactors. Nevertheless, it is unclear to what extent iron deficiency affects histone demethylation events (Cloos et al. 2008; Donohoe and Bultman 2012; MolinaSerrano et al. 2019). Lysine-specific demethylase 1 (LSD1) is the founding member of the second class of histone demethylases (Hou and Yu 2010). Enzymes in this class that demethylate only mono- or dimethylated H3K4me and H3K9me depend on flavin adenine dinucleotide (FAD) as a coenzyme for oxidative demethylation (Zempleni et al. 2013). FAD is one of the two coenzyme forms of the vitamin riboflavin. It is unknown whether riboflavin deficiency affects histone demethylation to a meaningful extent. Peptidylarginine deiminase 4 is the third class of histone demethylases, and it was the first to be identified. It converts methylated arginine to citrulline (as opposed to producing unmethylated arginine) in a Ca2+-dependent reaction (Dolinoy and Jirtle 2008). It is unknown whether calcium deficiency affects histone demethylation to a meaningful extent. Please note that vitamin D and biotin play important roles in calcium homeostasis and cellular compartmentalization, respectively.

15.2.2.3 Biotinylation of Histones

Holocarboxylase synthetase (HLCS) plays a pivotal role in covalently linking biotin to histones. The vitamin biotin acts as a cofactor of HLCS. Also, evidence has been provided that biotin regulates the genetic expression of HLCS at the mRNA level (Zempleni et al. 2011). Dietary supplementation of biotin is required for biotinylation and a deficiency in biotin may have profound effects on chromatin structure. However, a recent cultured cell study strongly argues that biotin is absent in native histones (Camporeale et al. 2006; Healy et al. 2009). Because there are many unanswered questions in histone biotinylation, further studies are needed to delineate the significance of histone biotinylation, a modification of the histone directly by a nutrient.

15.2.2.4 Poly(ADP-ribosylation) of Histones

Histones are ADP-ribosylated by ADP-ribosyl transferase at specific amino acid residues, in particular at the lysine's, of the histone's tails. The water-soluble vitamin niacin (as nicotinamide) is an essential building block of NAD^+ (Hassa et al. 2006). Poly (ADP-ribosylation) of histones depends on niacin supply. NAD+ can also be derived from dietary sources other than niacin (Kirkland 2009).

15.2.2.5 Ubiquitination and SUMOylation of Histones

As of today, there are no published reports linking nutrient intake to aberrant patterns of histone ubiquitination and SUMOylation.

15.2.3 miRNAs and Nutrients

MicroRNA is a new class of noncoding, endogenous, small RNA that regulates gene expression by translational repression, representing a new and important class of regulatory molecules (Felekkis et al. 2010). MicroRNA can play important roles in controlling DNA methylation and histone modifications, creating a highly controlled feedback mechanism. Interestingly, epigenetic mechanisms such as promoter methylation or histone acetylation can also modulate microRNA expression (Morales et al. 2017). Further, they can be controlled by environmental and dietary factors, particularly by isolated nutrients or bioactive compounds (Quintanilha et al. 2017).

15.3 Nutriepigenomics and Development: Windows of Vulnerability in DOHaD

The mechanisms previously described provide convincing evidence that nutrients can modify epigenetic marks and may serve as a memory of exposure to inadequate or inappropriate nutritional factors (Tiffon 2018). The period of life of the organism in which these environmental stimuli occur is very important in determining which disease-related genes will be affected. Different organs have critical developmental stages and the time point at which they are compromised will predispose individuals to specific diseases. Epigenetic modifications that occur during development may not be expressed until later in life depending on the function of the gene (Moosavi and Ardekani 2016). While the majority of studies implicate prenatal and perinatal periods as critical time windows, some research has shown that nutritional intake during adulthood can also affect the epigenome (Rothstein et al. 2009).

15.3.1 Prenatal Nutrition and Nutrition in Pregnancy: Effects on Body Composition, Obesity, and Metabolic Function

Maternal malnutrition, both undernutrition and overnutrition (obesity), may have predominant effects on the growth of the fetus. Intrauterine restricted growth (IURG) is defined as a fetus that fails to achieve its growth potential. Antenatal small for gestational age (SGA) is defined as a fetus with weight <10th percentile. IUGR and SGA are commonly used interchangeably. The identification of IUGR is important. Epidemiological studies and animal models link IUGR or SGA to risk of low birth weight (LBW), adult obesity, and metabolic syndrome, including insulin resistance (Parlee and MacDougald 2014).

15.3.1.1 Evidence from Animal Studies

Experiments in rhesus monkeys show strong evidence that maternal undernutrition exhibited IUGR in females. Additionally, the growth-restricted females were at risk for poor reproductive outcomes in adulthood. These associations were observed across five generations (Price et al. 1999; Price and Coe 2000). In rats, protein-restricted diet showed an inhibitory effect on birth size and adult size as well as organ size and this recessive effect increased in every generation (Stewart et al. 1975). To reverse the effects of maternal malnutrition in terms of size, it took three generations and still there were some observable effects with regard to lack of learning and behavior (Stewart et al. 1980). Another study assessed the effect of maternal malnutrition in index pregnancy and dietary rehabilitation for offspring and studied whether this was reversible during early childhood. Results showed that malnourished mothers gave birth to small-sized babies. However, when offspring were fed an adequate diet, the final size was the same for experimental and control groups (Rogers 2003). In summary, animal studies showed that maternal undernutrition can have intergenerational effects on growth and development and these effects can be reversed with adequate nutritional rehabilitation of mothers and offspring.

Maternal overnutrition has also been investigated in numerous experimental animal models (Nathanielsz et al. 2013) including those involving rodents, and nonhuman primates (Samuelsson et al. 2008; Gupta et al. 2009; Kirk et al. 2009; McCurdy et al. 2009; Yan et al. 2011; Nathanielsz et al. 2013). The outcome of these studies demonstrated that maternal obesity can induce several adverse effects on offspring's metabolism and may include increased adult body weight and fat mass, reduced insulin sensitivity, increased blood glucose and triglyceride levels, increased lipid deposition and defects in fatty acids metabolism in adult liver, as well as increased leptin levels, and hypothalamic alterations of appetite-regulating neuropeptides (Nathanielsz et al. 2013). However, most of these studies were observatory and further studies are warranted to establish exact mechanisms by which maternal obesity adversely affects the offspring.

15.3.1.2 Human Studies

Famine studies are quasi-experimental studies that have assessed the effect of maternal malnutrition on offspring. During the Dutch famine, adverse effects of acute maternal malnutrition resulted in maternal weight loss, which further resulted in an increased incidence of low body weight (LBW) and inflated perinatal mortality. Maternal undernutrition had the highest impact during the second and third trimesters of pregnancy. However, the infants who were conceived during the famine and whose mothers were exposed through the second trimester but then received adequate nutrition during the third trimester had normal size at birth. Intrauterine exposure was thought to be associated with increased risk of development of hypertension, obesity, and diabetes mellitus in middle age in offspring (England et al. 2004; Ross and Desai 2005; Koupil et al. 2007; Huang et al. 2010; Hult et al. 2010). Similar observations were reported from Leningrad and Germany. Chinese famine was prolonged and had exposure windows that included prenatal as well as postnatal life and negative effects were reported during adult life (Huang et al. 2010).

On the other hand, a link between maternal obesity to the development of elements of the metabolic syndrome, cardiovascular and renal diseases, hypertension, and cerebral dysfunction, as well as type 2 diabetes and obesity, later in the life of the offspring were observed in recent epidemiological studies (Howie et al. 2009; Maric-Bilkan et al. 2011). There are also studies that have showed maternal obesity can impact neurodevelopment during childhood as well. The exact mechanisms, by which maternal obesity adversely affects the health of offspring, are not clear. Several metabolic pathways are likely to influence fetal development and neonatal outcomes and may include altered placental nutrient transport, glucose metabolism, excessive fetal exposure to insulin, and state of inflammation (Poston et al. 2011). In terms of long-term effects, "programming" must include permanent changes in cellular structure or function in the offspring in response to the metabolic consequences of maternal obesity (Poston et al. 2011). This may involve hormone dysregulation, hyperinsulinemia, fat deposit during fetal life, and epigenetic modification of DNA (Symonds et al. 2009; Zhang et al. 2011; Zambrano and Nathanielsz 2013). The human data in this regard are relatively scarce; however, animal studies have helped explain some of the above-listed mechanisms (Zambrano and Nathanielsz 2013). More research is needed to discover the mechanisms in humans.

Maternal prepregnancy nutritional status also determines the pregnancy outcomes and health of offspring later in life. Women who are underweight before pregnancy have an increased risk of preterm birth and having small-for-gestational-age babies (Dean et al. 2014). Prepregnancy overweight, on the other hand, increases the risk for hypertensive disorders of pregnancy and gestational diabetes mellitus. Different studies have reported high prepregnancy body mass index increases the risk of obesity during childhood (Castillo et al. 2015); abnormal cardiometabolic profile during adolescence; (Gaillard et al. 2016) and significant problems with inattention, hyperactivity, and negative emotionality children (Rodriguez 2010). However, the mechanisms underlying these relationships are poorly understood, but modulation of the epigenome, in particular DNA methylation, is thought to be a key mechanism.

15.3.1.3 Prenatal Nutrition and Epigenetic Mechanisms

15.3.1.3.1 *Epigenetic Contribution to Prenatal Nutritional Programming of Obesity*

Obesity is attributed/impacted by an increase in fat cell number, size, or both. Prenatal and early postnatal periods are crucial windows in the development of fat mass or adipogenesis. Recent studies delineated the modulatory effects of nutritional cues on genes important to the development of adipose tissue. Animal studies have revealed that fat cells exposed to a high substrate supply during crucial windows in their development have an augmented capacity for lipid storage in postnatal life (Muhlhausler et al. 2006, 2007). This increased lipogenic capacity manifests these individuals as more likely to store excess energy in the form of fat and increases their susceptibility to weight gain and obesity and its metabolic outcome. In individuals exposed to undernutrition before birth, the development of adipocyte is primarily sacrificed in favour of "essential" organs (Padoan et al. 2004; McMillen and Robinson 2005). If an *in utero* "restricted" individual is born into a postnatal environment in which nutrient supply is no longer constrained, a period of "catchup" fat deposition ensues, mainly in the visceral adipose depot (Crescenzo et al. 2003). These individuals are at increased risk of visceral obesity (Ibáñez et al. 2006) and, consequently, to the development of insulin resistance and type 2 diabetes (Jaquet et al. 2000). But the developmental contribution to such phenotypic characteristics has remained uncertain and controversial.

In this section, we introduce the proposed mechanisms and related research that have explained the phenomena and manifestations ascribed to early nutritional programming through different mechanisms such as the involvement of the adipose tissue, the participation of different hormones and endocrine systems, enzymes, transcription factors, and signaling mediators (glucocorticoids, insulin, PPAR family, adipokines,. . .), the regulation of specific nutrient-related metabolic pathways (lipogenesis, glyconeogenesis,. . .), the control of neural networks affecting the appetite system (specific orexigenic/anorexigenic neuropeptides and the HPA axis) and the up/down feedback concerning the gene expression machinery and epigenetic marks (Brakowski et al. 2017; Ehlers and Todd 2017).

Adult men conceived during the Dutch famine in 1944–1945; whose mothers were undernourished during pregnancy were at a significantly greater risk of developing obesity than comparable subjects. This was later related to hypomethylation, on a certain region of the *insulin-like growth factor 2 (IGF2) gene* – which is important to induce adipose tissue expansion during fetal growth and development in the offspring – compared with control children (Stein et al. 1972; Lumey et al. 2011).

While the development of obesity in adult rodents born to hyperleptinemic dams due to feeding restriction during the gestation period has been partly explained by hypothalamic leptin sensitivity. Leptin is an adipose-tissue-secreted anorexic cytokine, which regulates energy homeostasis and food intake through its action in specific hypothalamic nuclei (Elmquist et al. 1998; Férézou-Viala et al. 2007). In the arcuate nucleus, leptin binds to its long form of the receptor

(*ObRb*), leading to activation of signal transducer and activator of transcription 3 (*STAT3*) by phosphorylation and nuclear translocation. Upon activation, STAT3 binds to the Specificity Protein 1 (*SP1*) – POMC promoter complex driving POMC transcription to suppress food intake (Münzberg et al. 2003). Interestingly, recent studies clearly indicate that maternal undernutrition alters the expression of POMC, maybe due to an epigenetic modification in the key regulatory elements of the POMC promoter region, which subsequently affects the appetite regulatory pathway in the hypothalamus, resulting in impaired energy homeostasis, causing obesity in adulthood (Gali Ramamoorthy et al. 2018).

In a study of two independent cohorts, Godfrey and colleagues suggested that higher methylation levels at retinoid X receptor-*α* (*RXRA*) in cord blood are associated with lower maternal carbohydrate intake in early pregnancy to child's adiposity at age nine years. *RXRA* encodes retinoid X receptor-α, which regulates the transcription of many genes involved in energy metabolism, adipocyte differentiation, and adipogenesis to a large extent via heterodimerization with the nuclear receptor Peroxisome proliferator-activated receptor gamma (*PPARG*) (Godfrey et al. 2011).

Moreover, in experimental models, IUGR-altered hepatic *IGF-1* mRNA expression due to histone H3K4 methylation pattern changes that may contribute to early epigenetic reprogramming toward obesity in the rat (Tosh et al. 2010). A recent prospective birth cohort indicates that maternal folate deficiency can increase obesity-induced child metabolic risk. This process is due to altering metabolism-related key gene expression such as *PGC1*-α through epigenetic regulation due to a decrease in SAM and genome-wide hypomethylation (Guéant et al. 2014).

On the other hand, a recent study shows that postnatal exposure to soybean genistein increased the risk of obesity development in female offspring and the mechanisms may involve activation of adipogenic genes via regulation of DNA methylation (Strakovsky et al. 2014). These results recommend the importance of exposure window of soybean genistein in maternal diets that may lead to different health sequelae in later life.

Researchers highlighted that the *agouti* gene product can also control the *melancholic 4 receptor (MC4R)* gene which is known to induce obesity when mutated. The dam's diet was supplemented with a folate diet, conferred a protective effect preventing the mutant *MC4R* from inducing obesity highlighting the importance of DNA methylation in regulating obesity (Huang et al. 2017). Furthermore, the question remains regarding the translatability of the murine model finding to humans. For example, Cone et al. 2000 highlight that the *agouti-MC4R* mechanism is quite well conserved between mice and human. However, further studies must be conducted to assess whether other epigenetic, genetic, and environmental interactions are also conserved (Butler et al. 2000).

In murine models, fetal type III histone deacetylase, sirtuin 1 (*SIRT1*) has been shown to be altered by maternal HF diets and, consequently, shown to be involved in the regulation of adipogenesis and obesity development (Suter et al. 2012). Nevertheless, in a murine model, changes to chromatin were discovered upon feeding HFDs and multiple histone marks were misregulated at the genes responsible for adipocyte differentiation and proliferation. They specifically found the accumulation of permissive histone markers such as acetylation. Although the researcher highlights that an association between acetylation and obesity is hypothesized, it remains to be established whether the histone modification is the cause for obesity or vice versa.

Liu et al. (2018) found over 1000 differentially expressed ncRNA in children with obesity. Further analysis of these ncRNA revealed them to be involved in a wide range of biological processes including lipid and fatty acid metabolism and adipogenesis. Although these results are predominately based on bioinformatic analysis, further validation of these ncRNA can reveal the molecular mechanism of obesity providing important strategies for diagnostic tools and therapeutic intervention (Liu et al. 2018) (Figure 15.1).

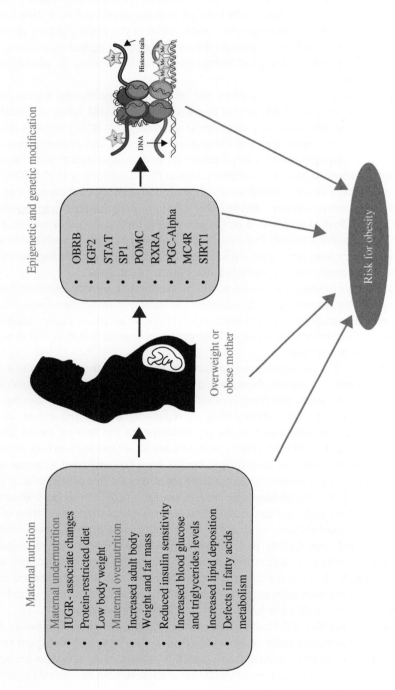

Figure 15.1 Effect of maternal health and nutritional status and altered epigenetic programming cycle during development on offspring as a risk factor for obesity.

15.3.1.3.2 Epigenetic Contribution to Prenatal Nutritional Programming of T2D

A causal link between developmental nutrition and T2D in adulthood was demonstrated in rodent models of 50% dietary restriction (DR) throughout gestation (Nakahata et al. 2008). Rat offspring exposed to intrauterine DR had decreased beta-cell mass both at birth and throughout their early postnatal development (Garofano et al. 1997; Garofano et al. 1998; Dumortier et al. 2007). In adulthood, these offspring in response to increasing metabolic demands lacked the ability to adaptively increase beta-cell mass which consequently resulted in insulin resistance. As a result, the rats developed diabetic phenotypes of β-cells' failure associated with impaired insulin secretion, insufficient expansion of beta-cell mass, glucose intolerance, and fasting hyperglycemia (Blondeau et al. 1999; Garofano et al. 1999). Along with these physiological changes, the genes involved in the development of β-cell showed strong epigenetic changes. For instance, maternal DR in rats caused a significant reduction in expression of pancreatic and duodenal homeobox 1 (*Pdx-1*), *an* important transcription factor that contributes to the beta-cell development in embryos (Pinney et al. 2011). Recently, this decrease has been reported to be due to gradual epigenetic silencing of the *Pdx1* gene locus following proximal promoter methylation. These epigenetic changes may be associated with the reduced beta-cell formation in postnatal life and the inability to expand beta-cell mass in response to metabolic stresses (Pinney et al. 2011; Pasyukova and Vaiserman 2017). Furthermore, in Zhang et al.'s study in IUGR, rat pancreas recorded lowered expression of Pdx1 and other genes encoding transcription factors involved in regulating gluconeogenesis such as *FoxO1* and *MafA* genes, and also altered expression levels of miRNAs contributed to pancreatic development (Zhang et al. 2016). Another study postulated that protein restriction in dams modulates fetal mechanistic target of rapamycin (mTOR) signaling pathway and β cell development to the susceptibility to diabetes.

An alternative mechanism suggested elucidating reduced beta-cell mass after IUDR is linked to prenatal glucocorticoid exposure. In rats, maternal undernutrition significantly increased both fetal and maternal corticosterone levels and subsequently impairs both fetal and postnatal beta-cell formation. Glucocorticoid receptors (GRs) are expressed during the embryonic development of the pancreas and glucocorticoids are known to suppress fetal endocrine differentiation by binding to *Pdx1* promoter (Blondeau et al. 2001).

It has also been demonstrated that a gestational LPD modifies the transcriptional activity of *Hnf4β*, a key transcription factor for beta-cell differentiation and glucose homeostasis, subsequently inducing glucose intolerance in pancreatic islets of rat adult offspring (Sandovici et al. 2011). The mechanistic basis for reduced *Hnf4a* expression was associated with increased DNA methylation at the active *Hnf4a* promoter (P2) and increased repression through histone methylation at the enhancer region of this gene. Furthermore, in programmed offspring islets, the repressive histone mark, histone 3 lysine 27 trimethylation (H3K27me3), was found to accumulate with age (Sandovici et al. 2011). Hypermethylation of the imprinted *Igf2/H19* loci in pancreatic islets was observed and suggested to cause impaired islet structure and function (Ding et al. 2012) and impaired glucose tolerance in offspring of gestational LPD.

Nonetheless, in the liver of offspring rats, gestational LPD effected the expression of crucial metabolic genes such as Igf2, *GR* (Glucocorticoid Receptor), Nr3c1(Nuclear Receptor Subfamily 3 Group C Member 1), *Ppara* (Peroxisome proliferator-activated receptor alpha), and *Cyp2c34* (cytochrome P450 2C34) (Lillycrop et al. 2008; Gong et al. 2010; Altmann et al. 2013), as well as genes involved in amino acid response pathway (Zhou and Pan 2011). Maternal LPD during pregnancy also caused an increased expression of *PEPCK, a* glucoregulatory gene and a reduced expression of nutrient transporters including glucose transporter, *GLUT4*. All these factors cause a predisposition to insulin resistance in adult life via persisting histone code modifications. Such histone modifications are regulated by elevated activity of HDACs *HDAC1* and *HDAC4*, increased binding of *DNMT3a* and *DNMT3b*, deacetylation of histone 3 lysine 14 (*H3K14*), increased recruitment of heterochromatin protein 1α, and demethylation of H3K9 (H3K9me2) in adult life (Raychaudhuri et al. 2008).

Human data substantiating the link between epigenetic alterations during development and risk for metabolic disorders including T2D in adulthood are still elusive due to limited access to suitable human biological samples. The information about these associations comes mainly from observational studies conducted with a quasi-experimental design. The Dutch famine (1944–1945) provided researchers with an opportunity to study the long-term health outcomes of prenatal malnutrition (Lumey et al. 2011). In subsequent investigations carried out to ascertain whether changes in DNA methylation occurred as a result of famine showed that although there was no association between prenatal famine exposure and overall DNA methylation in adulthood, whole blood samples showed a correlation between methylation levels of several genes with prenatal exposure to famine (Wang et al. 2020). In particular, genes associated with metabolic and cardiovascular development showed irregular methylation in comparison to their control counterparts. These abnormally methylated genes comprise *IGF2*, *GNASAS*, *IL10*, *LEP*, *ABCA1*, *INSIGF*, and *MEG3*. These findings are corroborated with recent genome-scale analysis of differential DNA methylation in whole blood, which has found that periconceptional exposure to famine results in differential methylation of those genomic regions which are extended along the growth and metabolism-related pathways (Heijmans et al. 2009).

Early gestation has been identified as the most crucial period for DNA methylation changes which persist into adulthood. In contrast, mid or late gestational exposure to famine has shown negligible mutuality with anomalous DNA methylation (Tobi et al. 2015). In the case of the Dutch famine cohort, a definitive link was reported between DNA methylation and impaired metabolic homeostasis in adult subjects prenatally exposed to famine (Lumey et al. 2007). In a similar study performed in rural Bangladesh, perinatal exposure to famine was associated with a distinctly higher risk of developing T2D and obesity in their adulthood. Famine studies have found the following metastable epialleles to be liable to changes in methylation: *VTRNA2-1*, *PAX8*, *PRDM-9*, near *ZFP57*, near *BOLA*, and *EXD3* (Finer et al. 2016).

T2DM susceptibility in offspring may also be established by multiple miRNAs sensitive to maternal nutrients. A recent study has shown that a maternal LPD alters microRNA and mTOR expression in the islets of offspring, influencing insulin secretion and glucose homeostasis. Blockade of these miRNAs restored mTOR and insulin secretion to normal (Alejandro et al. 2014). In another study, a maternal HF diet has been shown to alter levels of certain hepatic miRNAs concomitant with changes in gene expression including *IGF-2* which has been shown important for islet β-cell survival (Zhang et al. 2009). A specific set of miRNAs plays an important role in three crucial aspects; first, in the differentiation of pancreatic β-cell; second, in the fine-tuning of insulin secretion; and third, for compensatory β-cell mass expansion in response to insulin resistance (Guay et al. 2012; Nesca et al. 2013). It must be noted at this juncture that several independent, recent investigations have reported significant differences between the microRNA levels in the islets of diabetic animal models and the islets isolated from diabetic patients. Many of the changes in microRNA expression observed in animal models of diabetes were not detected in the islets of diabetic human patients and vice versa which may reflect fundamental differences in the experimental approaches (Guay and Regazzi 2015) (Figure 15.2).

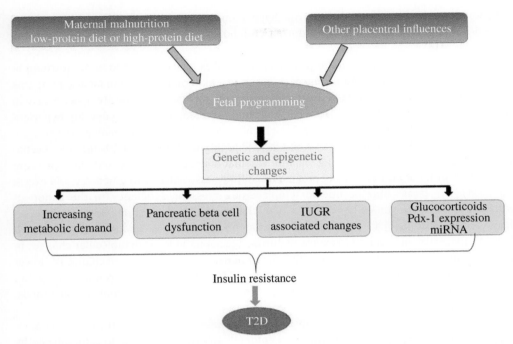

Figure 15.2 An overview of potential maternal factors impacting the fetal programming via epigenetic modifications including DNA methylation on insulin resistance and T2D.

15.3.1.3.3 *Prenatal Malnutrition-Induced Epigenetic Dysregulation as a Risk Factor for CVD*

Findings from the Dutch Famine Birth Cohort Study suggested long-term effects of prenatal deficiency on adult health of offspring, with surprising correlations between LBW and increased incidence later in the life of atherogenic lipid profile and coronary heart disease (CHD) (Stein et al. 2007; Lumey et al. 2009). Another epidemiological study also has shown that fetal exposure to famine in Biafra during the *Nigerian civil war* (1967–1970) could be associated with higher levels of systolic pressure and diastolic pressure in 40-year-old Biafrans (Hult et al. 2010). A similar risk of hypertension was demonstrated in those offspring exposed to "The Great Chinese Famine," during the first half of their mother's pregnancy (Wang et al. 2012). Taken together, the findings clearly demonstrated that there is a relevant relationship between maternal malnutrition and higher susceptibility to the development of hypertension in the offspring.

Numerous experimental models use maternal undernutrition as a means to recapitulate the mechanisms that link birth weight and blood pressure. In rats, undernutrition (70% food restriction) during gestation programs a marked increase in blood pressure associated with vascular dysfunction in the offspring in later life (Ozaki et al. 2001). Similarly, in a mouse model, global undernutrition programs an increase in blood pressure that is accompanied by cardiac enlargement and an increase in coronary perivascular fibrosis (Kawamura et al. 2009). An LPD (8% versus 18%) during gestation has been associated with long-lasting growth restriction and hypertension, even when the rat offspring is weaned on a control diet (Costa-Silva et al. 2009; Barros et al. 2015; de Brito Alves et al. 2015; Langley-Evans 2015). Previous findings relate that female offspring exposed to a nutritional insult during fetal life are resistant to the development of hypertension in young adulthood (Woods et al. 2005). This chapter is not focused to perform a comparison between gender in maternal malnutrition induced-hypertension models; hence, the evidences are not discussed.

As demonstrated by a cohort study, maternal hypovitaminosis D during pregnancy is associated with cardiovascular disease risk factors during childhood and adolescence of their offspring (Timpka et al. 2016).

Also, fetal exposure to overnutrition is just as detrimental as fetal exposure to undernutrition in regards to long-term CV health. For instance, exposure to a maternal diet rich in fat also programs a marked increase in blood pressure in the offspring. Yet, only female offspring are hypertensive in young adulthood (Khan et al. 2003). However, both male and female offspring develop hypertension following fetal exposure to dams being fed a high-sucrose diet (Samuelsson et al. 2013).

Continued research in humans and animal models has provided some insights into the mechanisms involved in *in utero* programming of cardiovascular disease. First, increased blood pressure observed in offspring of an LPD during pregnancy could be associated with glucocorticoid excess (Seckl 2004). An excess may be due to fetoplacental stress or deficiency in the action of β-hydroxysteroid dehydrogenase type 2 (*11β-HSD2*) that shields the fetus from maternal glucocorticoids. Such a deficiency can be produced experimentally in rats by undernutrition (Cottrell et al. 2014). Excessive glucocorticoid exposure during development leads to molecular changes in the myocardium that can cause a predisposition for adult heart disease. One such change is a lower adult expression of cardiac glucose transporter proteins (*GLUT-1* and *GLUT-4*) (Wadley et al. 2013), which may result in an impaired ability for energy provision from glucose during critical periods, such as ischemia.

In addition, a protein-restricted diet during pregnancy epigenetically affects the energy homeostasis gene, peroxisome proliferator-activated receptor (*PPAR*)–α, contributing to cardiomyopathy in adult rats. Such changes in the expression of the *GLUT-1*, *GLUT-4*, and of the *PPAR*–α, in the offspring of maternal LPD, were associated with significantly reduced methylation of CpGs in the promoter regions of the same genes (Laker et al. 2013).

Alternatively, there are reports suggesting the fetal programming of adult-onset hypertension associated with alterations of the renin-angiotensin system (RAS). The RAS modulates cardiovascular regulation by operating in organs such as the heart, large arteries, and kidneys (Kumar et al. 2007; De Mello and Frohlich 2014). In the RAS, renin first converts the precursor protein angiotensinogen (*AGT*) to angiotensin I (*Ang I*). Later, angiotensin-converting enzymes (ACE) hydrolyze Ang I to Ang II-IX. Ang II is a biological key hormone that mediates its function via the receptors of Ang II type 1 (*AGTR1*) or Ang II type 2 (*AGTR2*) (Muñoz-Durango et al. 2016). Excessive activation of *AGTR1* results in increased expression levels of the extracellular matrix components, such as collagen 1 (*COL1*) and collagen 3 (*COL3*) (Billet et al. 2008), which are distributed in several layers of the heart wall to provide rigidity and elasticity (Carver et al. 1993). Maternal protein deprivation reduces renal renin mRNA, angiotensin II levels, and glomerular number in the offspring, which, in turn, are associated with hypertension in the adult (Woods and Rasch 1998; Woods et al. 2001; Woods et al. 2004). Further, a study demonstrated that the hypomethylation observed in 3 CpG sites, within the *ACE* gene promoter, directly contributes to a higher ACE protein activity and could predispose LBW children to undesirable outcomes later in life, such as elevated SBP levels observed in these children (Rangel et al. 2014). Another study indicated that maternal HFD-induced vascular dysfunction and the development of a hypertensive phenotype in adulthood in a sex-dependent manner is associated with differential regulation of vascular AT_1R and AT_2R gene expression through a DNA methylation mechanism (Chen et al. 2020).

On the other hand, there are reports associating low-renin hypertension with dysfunction of the renal Na^+, K^+ ATPase (Muñoz-Durango et al. 2016). Experimental and clinical studies have reported that offspring from dams subjected to a maternal HF diet during pregnancy exhibited a reduction in nephron number and activity of renal Na^+, K^+ ATPase, which is strongly associated with hypertension. The mechanisms underpinning the reduced activity of renal activity of Na^+, K^+ ATPase remain speculative (Armitage et al. 2005; Gilbert and Nijland 2008).

In Sprague-Dawley rats, feeding the parents a vitamin-D-depleted diet resulted in increased BP in the offspring, which was accompanied by hypermethylation of the promoter region of the Pannexin-1 (*Panx1*) gene in the kidney. *Panx1* is a transmembrane protein that plays an important role in the endothelial relaxation in the large vessels and deficiency causes increased blood pressure (Meems et al. 2016).

Then again, a lab demonstrated that hypertension evidenced in rat adult offspring (90 days old) from dams exposed to protein restriction during pregnancy and lactation is associated with augmented sympathetic activity (De Brito Alves et al. 2014; Barros et al. 2015). The interface between the sympathetic fibers and the cardiovascular system is formed by the adrenergic receptors (ARs). Dysregulation of cardiac beta-AR signaling and transduction are salient features of heart failure progression. The male offspring from dams exposed to protein restriction during pregnancy exhibited a decrease in the density of β1-adrenergic receptors and also have higher levels of circulating epinephrine. It is likely that the long-term increased adrenergic stimulation observed in these animals will lead to compromised cardiac function and possibly heart failure. Studies show that hypomethylation mechanisms can lead to higher β-adrenergic receptors' expression in the hypertensive condition (Rivière et al. 2011; Friso et al. 2015; Zampieri et al. 2015).

In sheep models, 50% nutrient restriction causes substantial upregulation in the expression of various genes in the fetal heart (Dong et al. 2005). Some of the genes identified as being upregulated have been implicated in cardiac hypertrophy, while others are vital regulatory proteins. However, the effects of this alteration in gene expression have not been fully clarified, and it has not been established if the changes seen in the fetal gene expression are persistent (Gluckman et al. 2008; Edlow et al. 2019). Alterations are not confined to protein-restriction diets; a low maternal sodium diet increases the levels of atrial natriuretic peptide in the adult offspring, which is implicated in cardiac hypertrophy (Lafontan et al. 2005). A maternal LPD also changes the plasma membrane composition and the fatty acid content of the cardiomyocytes of the pups studied up to 21 days after birth (Ghosh et al. 2001). The increased levels of sphingomyelin and lysophosphatidylcholine observed may be factors in the increased level of myocardial apoptosis noticed in response to maternal protein restriction (Tappia et al. 2005).

MiRNAs also play an important role in the pathogenesis of hypertension. miRNA-130a regulates the proliferation of vascular smooth muscle cells. miRNA-155 is involved in the regulation of the activity of the renin-angiotensin-aldosterone system by affecting the expression of angiotensin II receptors. miRNA-17, 21, 145, 204, 208, etc., participate in the pathogenesis of hypertension through vascular endothelial injury, platelet damage, angiogenesis, cardiac hypertrophy, and the like (Pacurari and Tchounwou 2015).

Sheane et al. study pointed toward a positive association between miRNA-21 expression and vitamin D deficiency in coronary artery disease (Patel et al. 2017).

Taken together, these observations strongly suggest that maternal diet alters different pathways that contribute to the control of blood pressure.

15.3.1.3.4 *Epigenetic Contribution to Prenatal Nutritional, Immune Programming, and Allergies*
Early immune development is altered in children affected by asthma and allergic diseases. Alterations in the immune system lead to dysregulated immunity characterized by a reduced interferon g (*IFN- g*) production, altered innate immunity, and deficient T regulatory cell (*Treg*) networks, which leads to uncontrolled T helper (Th) 2 immune responses (Chen et al. 2016;

Martín-Orozco et al. 2017). These are notably manifested at birth, suggesting that gene-environmental interactions that lead to allergic disease are already operating in the prenatal period. Most importantly, immune development is regulated by epigenetic mechanisms (Gilles et al. 2018). These mechanisms control both Th1 and Th2 cell differentiation and are also regulating FoxP3 expression and Treg differentiation (Kaiko et al. 2008; Poojary et al. 2010). Hence, there is a growing interest in *in utero* exposures that can activate or silence these genes and alter the balance of neonatal immune responses.

During pregnancy, the bidirectional relationship of the fetal-maternal immune system is mediated by various complex immunologic mechanisms. For a healthy pregnancy, the maternal cellular immune system adapts subtly to a "Th2 state" to downregulate Th1 *IFN- g* cell-mediated immune responses to both environmental and fetal antigens (Raghupathy et al. 1999; Breckler et al. 2008; Breckler et al. 2010). The balance between Th17 cells and the regulatory T-cells (Tregs) is another important maternal immunoregulatory mechanism associated with pregnancy outcome. Tregs can inhibit both Th1and Th2 responses (O'Garra and Vieira 2004), while Th17 cells are crucial for the induction of autoimmunity and protection against infectious diseases. Thus, maintaining the Tregs/T17 cell balance is critical in immunity and has been demonstrated to play an important role in maternal immune tolerance to fetal antigens and fetal and neonatal immune development (Gustafsson et al. 2008; Prescott and Clifton 2009). Importantly, the Treg (CD4$^+$CD25$^+$FoxP3$^+$) regulatory response is reported to be initiated even before conception, subsequent to paternal antigens in seminal fluid (Robertson et al. 2009).

The suppression of fetal *IFN-g* production is achieved through hypermethylation (gene silencing) of the *IFNG* gene promoter in CD4 1 T cells at the maternofetal interface. *FOXP3* cells are also attracted to the maternofetal interface 26 by human chorionic gonadotrophin, and recent studies now provide preliminary evidence that the FOXP3 gene is expressed at lower levels in the placentas of allergic women (and allergic infants) (Martino and Prescott 2011). This has fueled speculation that factors that increase gene methylation may increase the risk of disease by silencing pathways (Th1 and Treg differentiation) that normally inhibit Th2 allergic differentiation and propensity for allergic airways disease (Prescott and Saffery 2011).

15.3.1.3.4.1 Animal and Epidemiological Evidences

Various experimental, epidemiological, and intervention studies show that nutritional exposures during this critical period of life can affect the development of the immune system and postnatal allergic susceptibilities (Prescott 2016). However, the increased risk may continue throughout childhood, adolescence, and adult life. Here we outline the current knowledge of the nutritional programming of immune health and nutritional epigenetics in the context of allergic disease.

Work in this field has primarily considered general nutritional conditions reflected by anthropometric measures (e.g. LBW) more so than micronutrient nutriture. Epidemiological evidence links LBW, a rough indicator of intrauterine growth retardation, with increased risk of AD (McCormick 1985; Read et al. 1994). Ambiguously, many studies do not differentiate between allergic and nonallergic asthma; the elevated risk of asthma after *in utero* growth restriction (IUGR) or low BW may at least partially reflect the effects of impaired lung development or bronchial hyperresponsiveness (Inskip et al. 2006; Paul et al. 2010; Tedner et al. 2012). Data from the Dutch Famine also suggest a link between early- and mid-gestation exposure to famine, resulting in lower birth weight and excess mortality up to the age of 18 years (Painter et al. 2005). In Guinea-Bissau, small thymic size at birth has recently been shown to predict increased infection-related mortality risk in infancy (Aaby et al. 2002). In Gambian infants' study, the maternal nutrition during the hungry period resulted in the birth of babies with smaller sized thymus and was also found to be more likely to develop infections and have higher mortality (Collinson et al. 2007). In addition, animal studies of *in utero* programming of allergy are needed to remove confounding between the frequent comorbidity of IUGR and prematurity (Collinson et al. 2007; Raqib et al. 2007) and more closely examine the underlying mechanisms of fetal programming of immune function.

In animal models, LBW was correlated with increased adult immunoglobulin E (IgE) levels and thyroid autoantibodies may indicate immune dysregulation due to a nutritional insult to the fetal thymus (Pate et al. 2010). While a prospective study carried out in Danish infants did not find any associations between thymic size and head circumference at birth or childhood allergic disease (Benn et al. 2001). Restriction of thymic activity during its establishment of the T-cell repertoire may alternatively lead to defective immunological memory or premature immunosenescence (Kurd and Robey 2016).

Studies have shown pregnant rats exposed to protein-energy malnutrition display a significantly decreased thymus and spleen proliferation in the offspring compared to rats with adequate protein diets (Calder and Yaqoob 2000). A similar study in sheep showed that the ability of sheep to ward off nematode infections reduces drastically on protein malnutrition (Kahn et al. 2003). In humans, protein malnutrition among children in developing countries is linked to diseases such as Kwashiorkor and Marasmus (Cunningham-Rundles et al. 2005). Further, human patients with protein-energy malnutrition were found to be more susceptible to parasitic infection in the stomach. Hence, it can be concluded that protein nourishment from the mother is important to program thymus development and form a vigorous immune system.

The intake of certain food during pregnancy such as margarine, vegetable oils, celery, sweet peppers, and citrus fruits has also been implicated in increasing the risk of allergies such as eczema among infants (Group 2007).

Increasing incidences of allergic diseases in today's industrialized society have been attributed to recent changes in western diets. Earlier, diets in the western world consisted of more or less balanced ratios of omega-3 PUFAs and omega-6 PUFAs (Patterson et al. 2012). However, recent trends point toward imbalanced diets that are now predominantly rich in only omega-6 PUFAs. A propensity toward developing allergies is postulated to result from an abnormal balance between T helper cell type 1 and 2 (Th1 and Th2) pathways during fetal life (Schaub et al. 2008). Consumption of high levels of dietary omega-6 PUFAs advances Th2 differentiation of the immune system during ontogeny and development (Blümer and Renz 2007). Conversely, omega-3 PUFAs alter the T helper cell balance by inhibiting interleukin-13 (IL-13) production. This inhibition is significant as IL-13 is directly related to allergic diseases through its role in inducing IgE synthesis in B cells and Th2-type differentiation in T cells (Bannister and Kouzarides 2011). Therefore, diets high in omega-3 PUFAs not only regulate immune responses but also modulate the development of IgE-mediated allergic disease (Palmer et al. 2012). Of further interest is the fact that PUFAs have been recorded to alter gene expression by either affecting signaling pathways or via direct interaction with nuclear receptors (Nakamura et al. 2004). Omega-3 PUFAs are natural ligands of peroxisome proliferator-activated nuclear receptors such as PPAR-alpha and PPAR-gamma. PPARs are ligand-activated transcription factors present in several cell types, which include the inflammatory cells (Sampath and Ntambi 2005). The binding of omega-3 PUFAs to PPAR-gamma regulates immune and inflammatory responses (Grimm et al. 2002). The omega-3 PUFAs as well directly alter gene expression by altering transcription factor activity such as nuclear factor-kappa B (NF-kB) via inhibition of the inhibitory subunit of NF-kB (Gottrand 2008). In the event of an inflammatory stimulus, the NF-kB modulates the activity of the inflammatory genes – COX-2, ICAM-1, VCAM-1, E-selectin, tumor necrosis factor-alpha, IL-1-beta, inducible nitric oxide synthase (iNOS), and acute-phase protein (Gottrand 2008). Also of import is the ability of omega-3 PUFAs to influence the expression of molecules involved in cell adhesion such as intercellular adhesion molecule-1 (ICAM-1), vascular cell adhesion molecule-1 (VCAM-1), and E-selectin which play a key role in directing leukocyte-endothelium interactions, transendothelial migration of leukocytes, and the trafficking of leukocytes (Grimm et al. 2002).

Vitamin D is also believed to play a role in immune function as its receptor is present in cells of the immune system, including T cells, activated B cells, and dendritic cells (Provvedini et al. 1983). Initially, evidence relating vitamin D to allergic diseases came from investigations showing a correlation between vitamin D receptor (VDR) gene polymorphism and asthma in both adults and children (Poon et al. 2004; Raby et al. 2004). Furthermore, two independent studies showed that wheezing in early childhood was related to insufficient maternal vitamin D intake during pregnancy (Camargo et al. 2007; Devereux et al. 2007). Parallelly, findings have also been recorded implicating vitamin D deficiency in asthma as well. Observations from 44 825 mother–child pairs analyzed in Denmark showed that children of women with a high vitamin D intake during midpregnancy gave birth to children who were 25% less likely to have asthma at seven years when compared to their contemporaries who had less vitamin D prenatal intake (Maslova et al. 2013).

Observational studies suggest that higher dietary intakes of foods rich in antioxidants (such as fresh fruits and vegetables) or higher antioxidant levels (such as selenium; zinc; and vitamins A, C, and E) measured in pregnancy (Bannister and Kouzarides 2011; MolinaSerrano et al. 2019) and early childhood (Pietrocola et al. 2015; Shi and Tu 2015) may decrease the risk of wheezing, asthma, and/or eczema (Tsafriri and Reich 1999; Vega et al. 2000; Seino 2002; Pasqualotto et al. 2004). As of recently, there have been no large-scale efforts to study whether intervention during the early stages of life can directly and conclusively prevent allergies in adulthood. Possible reasons for this redundancy to conduct real-time studies include the presence of two equally weighted but contrasting hypotheses about dietary antioxidant intake and immune outcomes. While one hypothesis posits that antioxidants protect against allergic disease, the other suggests theoretic concern about antioxidant supplementation and an increase in the probability of Th2 differentiation via inhibiting oxidative stress, which, in turn, may lead to the development of asthma and allergic disease (Van Voorhis 1994). The dose, timing, and duration of antioxidant exposure are likely to be critical for the uptake and activity of other nutrients as well.

In both animal and human studies, a maternal diet with high contents of a saturated fat diet has been shown to induce inflammation pathways in the offspring (Perkin and Strachan 2006; Schaub et al. 2009). A recently conducted meta-analysis of 14 high-quality studies observed that children are 30–50% more likely to develop conditions like asthma or wheezing when mothers are obese at conception (Forno et al. 2014). Despite studies linking maternal obesity BMI to asthma or wheezing in children, it must be noted that this relation still lacks complete statistical significance. To explain this tenuous connection, researchers have theorized that the presence of inflammatory cytokines in the blood of obese pregnant women can lead to increased placental phosphorylation of p38-MAPK, STAT3, and IL-β expression. The effect of this placental phosphorylation on the developing fetal immune system is yet to be properly outlined with further statistical validity and analyses (Aye et al. 2014).

15.3.1.3.4.2 Role of Epigenetics Strong evidence is present to suggest the role of epigenetic mechanisms in the regulation of gene expression during the development of the immune system, its cells, and their functions. The epigenetic mechanisms, in turn, are highly likely to be influenced by early-life nutrition; emphasizing this fact are the correlations of folate, vitamins B1, B2, and B12 to DNA methylation. Published evidence implies that epigenetic mechanisms regulate the expression of several transcription factors that control Th1, Th2, and Treg cell lineages. The hypothesis that hypomethylation could prevent allergic airway disease is corroborated by the observation that hypomethylation of naïve CD4+ cells enhances the expression of Forkhead box P3 (Foxp3) and activator (STAT)-4, which expands Treg and Th1 cells (Lee et al. 2006; Wu et al. 2006; Koch et al. 2009; Rowell and Sekimata 2009). This is further evidenced by the hypermethylation of Runx3, a gene involved in the differentiation of CD8+ cells in offspring exposed to methyl donors *in utero*. Runx3 has been shown to be involved in the development and severity of allergic airway diseases (Hollingsworth et al. 2008).

Several studies also suggest that ω-6 and ω-3 PUFAs can affect the synthesis of IgE through the production of prostaglandin E2 (PGE2). PGE2 can increase DNA methyltransferase expression and gene-specific DNA methylation, which consequently regulates the immune system and allergies (Zittermann et al. 2009; Lack 2012; Miles and Calder 2015). Through several genome-wide association studies, demethylation of the promoter region of the thymic stromal lymphopoietin (TSLP) gene is associated with vitamin D-related programming for allergy (Junge et al. 2016).

Findings from animal studies also indicate that total consumption of methyl donors as supplements throughout pregnancy is associated with the increased susceptibility to allergic airway disease. Particularly, mice born to mothers supplemented with folic acid, vitamin B12, methionine, zinc, betaine, and choline experienced significantly higher allergic airway inflammation rates. The mechanisms by which these supplements affect the developing immune system are poorly understood, although animal studies provide some evidence that maternal methyl donor regulates T cell phenotype by hypermethylation and decreased transcriptional activity of the T-cell developmental gene runt-related transcription factor 3 (*RUNX3*) (Hollingsworth et al. 2008). Regardless, a recent meta-analysis found no evidence of an association between maternal folic acid supplementation during the periconceptional period and asthma during childhood (zero to eight years) in the offspring. Thus, it seems that the timing of exposure to folate supplementation *in utero* may be critical with regard to childhood allergic disease outcomes. Others suggest a significant association between perinatal folic acid supplementation and increased risk of wheezing at 18 months of age (Hollingsworth et al. 2008). Hence, the time period in which folate supplements are prescribed is also critical.

In addition, overnutrition can also contribute to the development of chronic inflammation by actively modulating several miRNAs involved in immune function (Cui et al. 2017). Moreover, Vitamin E deficiency in rats reported a reduction in miR-122a and miR-125b which are involved in the regulation of lipid metabolism and inflammation (Gaedicke et al. 2008). A diet based on corn oil-cellulose led to an increased expression of several miRNAs, including miR-21, which is reported to affect the inflammatory pathway NF-kB (Yang and Wang 2016). A recent publication shows that unsaturated fatty acids inhibit the expression of tumor suppressor phosphatase and tensin homolog (*PTEN*) via upregulation of the miR-21. Importantly, AD in both animal models and humans can occur due to miR-21 which promotes Th2 responses by inhibiting *IL-12* in myeloid cells (Lu et al. 2009). Mechanisms for butyrate anti-inflammatory function are also mediated by inhibition of the histone deacetylase (HDAC). Butyrate-induced HDAC inhibition has been shown to regulate macrophage function and promote Treg cell development (Nijhuis et al. 2019). Water-soluble B vitamins, biotin, niacin, and pantothenic acid, also influence histone modification; indeed biotin is a substrate for histone biotinylation and niacin for histone adenosine diphosphate (ADP)-ribosylation (Choi and Friso 2010).

Overall, it is recognized that epigenetic marks provide a mechanistic link between nutrition and the expression of several immune-related genes; these phenomena play a key role in different aspects of health and disease (Figure 15.3).

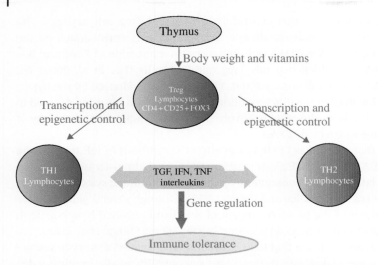

Figure 15.3 An overview of the development of immune tolerance and allergy in the context of developmental programming.

15.3.2 Perinatal Nutrition: Effects on Bone Health and Neurodevelopment

Another critical developmental time window is the perinatal period, the time period immediately before and after birth. It has been shown that maternal diet in late pregnancy and an infant's diet in the beginning weeks can all have significant impacts on gene expression. Therefore, perinatal nutrition is both late-stage *in utero* nutrition and lactation (Gluckman et al. 2008).

15.3.2.1 Epigenetic Contribution to Pre- and Perinatal Nutrition,
Bone Development, and Osteoporosis

Recent interest has focused on the possibility that the perinatal environment also affects skeletal health (Cooper et al. 2006). Osteoporosis is a skeletal metabolic disorder characterized by both low bone mass and loss of the normal bone microarchitecture, which predisposes to fracture (Klibanski et al. 2001). There is growing evidence that osteoporosis occurs when the bone resorption process is faster than bone formation, which is influenced by genes and environments (Rockville 2004). Previous sections in this chapter clearly presented the epidemiological and animal studies that suggested that early life environment determines the development of diseases in adulthood, such as obesity, type 2 diabetes, CVDs, and allergies. In addition, evidence has also accrued that osteoporosis risk might be programmed during intrauterine life (Cooper et al. 2009). Hence, here we focus on evidence for maternal and/or perinatal nutrition and its implications for the developmental origins of osteoporosis in later life.

15.3.2.1.1 Epidemiological Evidences

Several studies support the hypothesis that the perinatal environment, as reflected by birth weight, influences postnatal bone mass, and/or bone size in humans. For example, in young adults, birth weight is positively associated with bone size and bone mineral content (BMC), after controlling for current height, weight, and age (de Bono et al. 2010; Schlüssel et al. 2010). One epidemiological evidence of early-life environment and its implication of osteoporosis indicated that body weight at one year was associated with increased BMC at the femoral neck and lumbar spine at about 20 years old (Cooper et al. 1995). Cooper et al. showed that the growth rate of infancy was associated with skeletal size in adulthood in a cohort aged about 70 years old (Cooper et al. 1997). Dennison et al. also demonstrated that birth weight and body weight at one-year-old determined the bone mass when they were aged around 70 years old (Dennison et al. 2005). A series of clinical studies related to maternal nutrition and the developmental origins of osteoporosis in the United States, Finland (Yarbrough et al. 2000), Sweden (Callréus et al. 2013), Norway (Christoffersen et al. 2017), Australia (Hyde et al. 2017), Netherlands (Leunissen et al. 2008), and India also demonstrated the same phenomenon. However, this association may be confounded by genetics, placental functioning, smoking, and socioeconomic status. Thus, the evidence from genetically identical subjects, in which genetic and environmental factors are likely similar, are considered. For instance, Antoniades et al. showed that birth weight is significantly associated with BMC at weight-bearing sites (spine and hip) in a twin cohort-recruited 4008 females aged about 47.5 years old (Antoniades et al. 2003).

Vitamin D, an important nutrient, can regulate mineral and bone metabolism. A longitudinal, prospective study in Western Australia found that mothers with suboptimal vitamin D status during pregnancy was associated with reduced BMC of total body and BMD in their females' offspring at 9-year-old, 36 and even up to about 20-year-old, 35. Supplementation of pregnant mothers with vitamin D (Brooke et al. 1980), calcium (Raman et al. 1978; Koo et al. 1999), and other micronutrients (Himes et al. 1990) is associated with increased skeletal growth and/or bone mass/density in the offspring.

15.3.2.1.2 Evidences from Animal Models

In addition, numerous studies in animal models involving early-life nutrition provided critical information about the biologic basis for developmental programming of osteoporosis. In the rat maternal protein-deficiency model, Mehta et al. demonstrated that maternal LPD during pregnancy produced offspring with a significantly reduced bone area and BMC, also their growth plate morphology changed in adulthood (Mehta et al. 2002). In the similar rat maternal protein-deficiency model, at four- and eight-week-old, offspring maternal protein restriction downregulated the proliferation and differentiation of bone marrow stromal cells (Oreffo et al. 2003). Further working in the same model, Lanham et al. demonstrated that maternal protein restriction during pregnancy also altered the osteogenic environment of the offspring, with alkaline phosphatase activity peaking earlier, osteocalcin concentration being higher and IGF-1 and 25-OH vitamin D (the active form) levels being significantly lower than in the normal-protein group (Lanham et al. 2008). These changes persisted into adulthood.

In another animal model, feeding a low-vitamin D diet (25 IU vitamin D3/kg diet) during pregnancy and lactation significantly lowered VDR expression, and increased the expression of genes involved in osteoclastogenesis (TNF-a and IL-1b) in the colon of the offspring. Interestingly, maternal consumption of vitamin D during pregnancy and lactation also improved both femur and lumbar vertebra trabecular bone structure in offspring (Villa et al. 2016). Another interesting study showed that presuckling calcium supplements with a normal chow diet in lactating rats during pregnancy produced offspring with greater bone elongation, and increased trabecular BMD even at the age of 27 weeks old (Suntornsaratoon et al. 2015). While Chen et al. demonstrated that maternal HF diet inhibited embryonic bone development at 18.5 days' embryos and the differentiation into mature osteoblasts in offspring rats (Chen et al. 2012).

15.3.2.1.3 Potential Mechanisms Underlying Maternal Nutrition and Osteoporosis in Later Life

The potential events that could underlie the effects of perinatal diet on skeletal acquisition include programming of the growth hormone–IGF-1, hypothalamic pituitary adrenal and PTH–vitamin D axes (Gluckman and Pinal 2003; Tobias and Cooper 2003; Tobias et al. 2005; Kapoor et al. 2006).

The dynamic process of bone remodeling involves the complex and coordinated interaction of osteoblast lineage cells which form bone, and osteoclast lineage cells, which resorb bone. This process occurs at all stages of growth and development throughout the lifespan, and myriad systemic and local factors participate in the regulation of osteoblast and osteoclast functioning. Of particular note, the growth hormone/insulin-like growth factor (GH/IGF) axis plays an important role in the regulation of bone remodeling. The levels of placental GH found in maternal circulation are positively correlated with fetal birth weight; in times of maternal nutrient deprivation, the placental GH secretion is reduced, resulting in LBW offspring (Timasheva et al. 2013). As noted above, there are generalized consequences of birth weight on bone characteristics but LBW due to nutritional deprivation also programs bone through the GH-IGF axis. In rats, post-weaning dietary protein restriction modifies the GH secretory profile, dampening the peak GH rhythms that alter growth and metabolic responses. It is identified that neonatal nutrition programs adult bone mass and bone density is positively associated with peak GH and IGF-1 concentrations. But elevated median GH concentrations, as demonstrated with DR, are negatively associated with bone density (Harel and Tannenbaum 1995; Fall et al. 1998; Cooper et al. 2000). Probably, the effects on bone are owing to the role that GH plays in opening the chromatin surrounding the IGF-1 gene. Furthermore, maternal malnutrition modifies methylation of the GH-responsive promoter 2 of the IGF-1 gene (reviewed in (Oberbauer 2013)) and intrauterine growth restriction is associated with sustained hypermethylation of the IGF-1 promoter in rats, thus augmenting the signaling impairment of GH in the neonate (Fu et al. 2009).

Secondly, bone remodeling is also influenced by the parathyroid hormone (PTH)-Vitamin D axis (Toromanoff et al. 1997). Findings from the mother–offspring cohort study in Pune, India further reinforced the role of maternal calcium homeostasis in the trajectory of intrauterine and early postnatal skeletal development. In this study, offspring of women who consumed calcium-rich food during pregnancy at a higher frequency has higher total and lumbar spine BMC and BMD, independent of parental size, and bone composition. In this cohort, the circulating maternal 25 (OH)-vitamin D concentrations were relatively high and were not associated with childhood skeletal measures. Thus, the calcium-vitamin D axis becomes a more critical determinant of fetal and childhood bone mineral accrual (Ganpule et al. 2006). The calcium needs of the fetus for bone development are mostly acquired by maternofetal calcium transport across the placenta during the third trimester (Kumar and Kaur 2017). Various observational studies have suggested that maternal vitamin D insufficiency during pregnancy might mediate its effects on bone mineral accrual through impairment of placental calcium transport and thus the offspring. Evidence from animal and human studies indicates that placental calcium transport capacity is both regulated by genes and hormones, such as 1,25(OH)2 vitamin D3, PTH, PTH-related protein (PTHrP), and calcitonin (Calvi and Schipani 2000; Karras et al. 2016). The mechanism underlying the association between maternal vitamin D, umbilical cord calcium concentration and offspring bone mass is unclear. However, certain studies suggested that 1,25(OH)-vitamin D (the active form) mediates its effects by first binding to the VDR, then by binding to the retinoic acid receptor (RAR) forming a heterodimer, which subsequently acts upon vitamin D response elements in target genes, initiating gene transcription by either upregulating or downregulating gene products. Vitamin D response elements are DNA sequences found in the promoter region of vitamin D-regulated genes (Pike and Meyer 2010; Harvey et al. 2014). Calcium transporters containing vitamin D response elements are, therefore, of particular interest. Evidence from animal models supports that fetal calcium deficiency may result in stimulation of PTH/PTHrP activity, which, in turn, could decrease mineralization of cortical and trabecular bone differentially. If this change was then tracked into childhood and later life, it might alter the trajectory of skeletal growth (Slatopolsky 1983; Kovacs 2014).

One study has shown that the expression of an active placental calcium transporter (*PMCA3*) gene predicts neonatal whole-body BMC. Earl et al. showed the effects of maternal nutrition-regulated DNA methylation of the promoter region of specific genes, such as PMCA3 and VDRs can regulate bone mass in offspring (Martin et al. 2007).

In addition, various studies also suggested that the epigenetic modulation of the HPA axis by poor maternal nutrition influences bone density and rates of bone loss in adult life (Seckl and Meaney 2004). As previously discussed in this review, animal studies have confirmed that protein restriction during mid- and late pregnancy is associated with reduced methylation of key CpG-rich islands in the promoter region of the gene for the GR, and this results in elevated GR expression and features of hypercortisolism. Recently, the Southampton Women's Survey reported that higher perinatal cyclin-dependent kinase inhibitor 2A (*CDKN2A*) methylation was associated with the lower bone area, BMC, and areal BMD of the whole body minus the head. They further found that each 10% increase in CDKN2A DNA methylation was related to BMC decrease (about 4–9 g) at age four years in offspring (Curtis et al. 2017). However, Fernandez-Rebollo et al. indicate that primary osteoporosis was not associated with DNA methylation or epigenetic modifications in blood obtained from 32 patients (Fernandez-Rebollo et al. 2018). That may be due to the small sample size, stratification of patients by BMD, and variable clinical characteristics. In summary, the aforementioned evidence demonstrates that epigenetic regulation plays a significant role in the *in utero* programming of osteoporosis.

15.3.2.2 Epigenetic Link Between Pre- and Perinatal Nutrition and Neurodevelopmental Disorders

A majority of brain development occurs during the perinatal period. In humans, the brain begins to form ~2-week post-conception and reaches 80% of its adult size by age two years (Tau and Peterson 2010). Early gestation is marked by neuronal proliferation, differentiation, and migration. Synaptogenesis then continues throughout gestation, peaks between gestational week 34 and post-natal year 1, and tapers off just before adolescence. Apoptosis and pruning concurrently counter-act proliferation and synaptogenesis by eliminating redundant and inappropriate connections to fine-tune the neuronal circuitry. These complex and synchronized events are regulated by distinct gene expression patterns followed by various molecular signaling pathways (Stiles and Jernigan 2010). Perturbation of any of these events in this early period can alter neuronal structure and function and may predispose the fetus to NDDs in later life (Linnet et al. 2003; Lyall et al. 2014). It has been well established that apart from genetic makeup, the *in utero* environment significantly influences brain developmental processes. The overall nutritional supply during the preconception and prenatal periods not only provides the basic building blocks for the brain, but may also "program" the brain through epigenetic mechanisms to confer risk or resilience to neurological conditions later in life (Bale et al. 2010; Prado and Dewey 2014).

Several lines of evidence suggest that human IUGR elevates the risk for the development of various NDDs in offspring including intellectual disabilities, communication disorder, Autism Spectrum Disorder (ASD), Attention Deficit Hyperactivity Disorder (ADHD), specific learning disorder, motor disorder, and Schizophrenia (SCZ). The Dutch "Hunger Winter" famine of 1944 ± 1945 provided a stark example of this association in humans, with the surviving children of nutritionally compromised women around the peak of famine close to the periconceptional period and early pregnancy confers an increased risk of neural tube defects such as spina bifida and anencephaly and also with NDDs including different degrees of intellectual disability, ADHD (52) and ASD (53), as well as SCZ in later life (Roseboom et al. 2006; Brown and Susser 2008). Later, two studies in the Chinese Great Leap Forward famine of 1959–1961 noted a long-lasting impact on both physical health and cognitive abilities, including the risks of SCZ, physical disabilities in speech, walking and vision, and measures of mental acuity even half a century after the tragic event (Li and Lumey 2017). However, Chinese studies cannot precisely define the time of exposure. With regard to a direct effect of prenatal famine, it is difficult to attribute outcomes to any single dietary constituent because the diet was deficient in many micro- and macronutrients and both types of deficiency are important causes of neurodevelopmental disorder (Brown et al. 1996).

15.3.2.2.1 Folate

Nevertheless, the Dutch famine cohort based on the co-occurrence of NDDs' risk and schizoid personality disorder with congenital neural defects provides a potentially valuable clue that the folate pathway might be important in the origins of NDDs. In the literature, consistent findings showed an association of lowered ingestion of folic acid during the first trimester of pregnancy with an increased risk for neural tube defects (spina bifida, hydrocephalus, and anencephaly) (Roseboom et al. 2006). A further reason for considering folate as a candidate for an association of neural tube defects and NDDs is the involvement of mutations of the gene coding for 5,10- MTHFR · in increasing liability for neural defects and in patients with NDDs (Yaliwal and Desai 2012). Animal studies have shown that folate deficiency during neurodevelopment results in a decrease in cell proliferation, altered neuron migration, and synaptogenesis by increasing apoptosis in the cerebellum and the hippocampus and by reducing the number of neural progenitor cells in the cortex (Craciunescu et al. 2004; Kruman et al. 2005; Blaise et al. 2007).

With regard to potential mechanisms, there are several scenarios involving factors that intervene between prenatal folate deficiency and the risk of offspring NDDs. First, folate deficiency can hamper the synthesis and repair of DNA and consequently increase the risk of de novo mutations (J.M. McClellan, MD, E. Susser, MD, DrPh, M.C. King, PhD, unpublished data, 2007). Second, folate deficiency can restrain the production of methyl donors and the methylation of DNA and might subsequently downregulate crucial genes such as brain-derived neurotrophic factor (*BDNF*), cAMP response element-binding protein (*CREB*), nerve growth factor (*NGF*) and tyrosine receptor kinase B (*TrkB*), essential for normal brain development and functioning in the offspring (Waterland and Jirtle 2004).

Notably, periconceptional exposure to famine was linked with extensive DNA methylation changes in the blood, whilst the individuals prenatally exposed to famine were compared to their unexposed, same-gender siblings at approximately 60 years of age. The affected genes comprised an imprinted gene *IGF2* as well as other genes implicated in brain growth and differentiation (Heijmans et al. 2008; Tobi et al. 2009). In consistency with this, a recent postmortem study reported a positive correlation between DNA methylation of the *IGF2* locus and brain weight (Pidsley et al. 2012). Further findings show that *IGF2* signaling supports the survival of newborn hippocampal neurons, signifying a vital role for *IGF2* in memory and learning (Chen et al. 2011). Collectively, *IGF2* methylation offers evidence that prenatal nutrition can affect neurodevelopment through epigenetic mechanisms.

Moreover, while SCZ seems to be associated with reduced levels of *IGF2* methylation, *RELN* was reported to be locally hypermethylated and downregulated in the brains of schizophrenic patients (Abdolmaleky et al. 2005; Grayson et al. 2005; Toyokawa et al. 2012). *RELN* facilitates dendrite and dendritic spine development and supports the appropriate neural positioning during brain development by regulating the migration of neural precursor cells (Tissir and Goffinet 2003). In the adult brain, *RELN* is involved in neurogenesis and synaptic plasticity (Pujadas et al. 2010). Remarkably, postmortem brain studies of SCZ patients linked hypermethylation of *RELN* to a local increase in *DNMT1* expression (Veldic et al. 2004; Ruzicka et al. 2007), which may suggest an adaptive response to deficiency of one-carbon nutrients during prenatal development (Kovacheva et al. 2007). These differing methylation patterns at the *IGF2* and *RELN* loci suggest a complex relationship between prenatal nutrition and epigenetic modifications of the genome, including distinct molecular pathways that can impact the epigenetic machinery in an opposing manner (Toyokawa et al. 2012).

Third, folate deficiency can hamper the conversion of hcy to methionine and might thereby lead to accumulation of hcy with negative effects on fetal brain development (Waterland and Jirtle 2004). A decrease in methionine levels and in the ratio of plasma SAM to SAH was found in autistic children whereas an increased level of homocysteine was reported for children affected by intellectual disability and ADHD (Yıldırım et al. 2015; Zhang et al. 2016; Saha et al. 2017).

Nevertheless, the effect of maternal nutritional deficiency also significantly altered the expression of several miRNAs such as miR-22, miR-24, miR-29b, miR-34a, miR-125, miR-344-5p/484, and miR-488 were found to be strongly associated with the genes involved in the metabolic regulation of folate-mediated one-carbon pathway in the offspring (Stone et al. 2011; Koturbash et al. 2013; Franchina et al. 2014). In autistic patients, Sarachana et al. showed a significant upregulation miR-29b in lymphocyte samples is associated with the reduction of its target DNA binding 3 (*ID3*) and Polo-like kinase 2 (*PLK2*). *ID3* and *PLK2* have been associated with circadian rhythm signaling and modulation of synapses, respectively (Seeburg and Sheng 2008; Wieczorek and Balwierz 2015) and both biological mechanisms have been implicated in ASD (Lisé and El-Husseini 2006; Arking et al. 2008; Won et al. 2013). Further analysis corroborated a link between miR-34a and its potential target, metabotropic glutamate receptor 7 (*GRM7*). This has particular relevance to SCZ with *GRM7* as a potential candidate gene and miR-34a displaying increased expression in the peripheral blood mononuclear cell (PBMCs) of SCZ subjects (Beveridge and Cairns 2012). The predicted genes to the miR-22 were enriched in mitogen-activated protein (MAP) kinase signaling pathways in the mediation of intraneuronal signaling, which is implicated in the pathophysiology of SCZ. Furthermore, it was shown that the expression of the N-methyl-d-aspartate receptors (*NMDARs*) subunits genes is regulated partially through mir-125b and multiple alterations. *NMDARs* have pathological consequences and actually lead to intellectual disability and ASDs (Edbauer et al. 2010; Liu et al. 2020). Case-control studies analyzing SNPs in 325 human miRNA regions in a cohort of SCZ patients identified polymorphisms in the miR-22 and this miR-22 was found to regulate several candidate genes such as *BDNF*, Gamma-aminobutyric acid receptor subunit alpha-6 (GABRA6), Cholecystokinin B receptor (*CCKBR*), *POMC*, 5-Hydroxytryptamine receptor 2C *(HTR2C)*, Monoamine oxidase A (*MAOA*) and Regulator of G-protein signaling 2 (*RGS2*), which are associated with anxiety disorders. An RNA sequencing study showed downregulation of miR125b-2-3p in the saliva of ASD patients. An altered mi484 expression appeared in the postmortem brain of SCZ patients (Muiños-Gimeno et al. 2011).

Together, these studies show that perinatal folate deficiency can contribute to the development of various NDDs by inducing long-lasting changes in the offspring's epigenome.

15.3.2.2.2 *Vitamin D*

Vitamin D is also crucial for brain function, via its role in calcium signalling, neurotrophic and neuroprotective actions, as well as its role in neuronal differentiation, maturation, and growth (Groves et al. 2014). There are various other studies suggesting plausible links between maternal vitamin D deficiency (McGrath 1999; McGrath et al. 2003), and adverse neurological outcomes such as ASD, SCZ, depression, multiple sclerosis, and dementia (Eyles et al. 2006; Yates et al. 2018). Recently, a study in Denmark found newborns with vitamin D deficiency had a 44% increased risk of being diagnosed with SCZ as adults compared to those with normal vitamin D levels (Eyles et al. 2018). A rodent model of late gestational developmental vitamin D (DVD) deficiency showed an altered brain development and produced behavioral phenotypes in the offspring of relevance to the positive symptoms of SCZ. This particular critical window of exposure may correspond to the third trimester of human pregnancy (Overeem et al. 2019).

Also, birth cohort studies have provided an association between gestational vitamin D deficiency (based on prenatal maternal sera) with impairment on a range of cognitive outcomes related to language, motor development, and general intelligence (Morales et al. 2012; Whitehouse et al. 2012; Hanieh et al. 2014; Keim et al. 2014). A Netherlands cohort of mother–child dyads ($n = 4229$) reported an association between gestational vitamin D deficiency (defined as 25OHD concentrations less than $25\,\text{nmol}\,\text{l}^{-1}$) and autism-related traits in six-year-old offspring (Vinkhuyzen et al. 2018). A prospective study analyzing data from 1650 mother–child pairs from five birth cohorts embedded in the INMA Project (Spain, 1997–2008) demonstrated that higher maternal circulating levels of Vitamin D (25-hydroxyvitamin D3 [25(OH)D3] in pregnancy are associated with lower risk of developing ADHD-like symptoms in childhood (Morales et al. 2015). Findings from the Stockholm Youth Cohort Study indicate that maternal 25OHD insufficiency ($25 - <50\,\text{nmol/l}$) at ~11 weeks' gestation was associated with 1.58 times higher odds of ASD (95% CI: 1.00, 2.49) as compared with 25OHD sufficiency ($\geq 50\,\text{nmol/l}$). In the same study, neonatal $25\text{OHD} < 25\,\text{nmol/l}$ was associated with 1.33 times higher odds of ASD (95% CI: 1.02, 1.75) as compared with $25\text{OHD} \geq 50\,\text{nmol/l}$. Sibling-matched control analyses indicated these associations were not likely due to familial confounding (Lee et al. 2019).

Further, the developmental vitamin D (DVD) deficiency model as described by Eyles et al. was used to establish the biological plausibility of the associations between maternal vitamin D (VD) deficiency and offspring brain health. In this model, Sprague-Dawley female rats were fed a VD-deficient diet from ~6 weeks before conception until birth. Consequently, the developing fetus was exposed to hypovitaminosis D during gestation. The offspring of DVD-deficient rats exhibited subtle alterations in brain morphology (e.g. significantly enlarged lateral ventricles), increased cell proliferation, reduced expression of *NGF*, glial-derived neurotrophic factor (*GDNF*), and the low-affinity neurotrophin receptor p75NTR (Eyles et al. 2003). Furthermore, as adults, rats exposed to DVD deficiency have shown persisting brain changes, including larger lateral ventricles, reduced NGF protein content, and abnormal expression of genes involved in cytoskeleton maintenance (*MAP2, NF-L*) and neurotransmission (*GABA-Aα4*) (Féron et al. 2005). Additionally, prenatal VD-deficient BALB/c mice reported a reduction in lateral ventricle volume and altered expression of genes involved in neuronal survival, specifically *BDNF* and transforming growth factor-β1 (*Tgf-β1*), and speech and language development, specifically forkhead box protein P2 (*Foxp2*). In DVD-deficient female fetuses, dopamine synthesis was also affected, when both brain tyrosine hydroxylase (*Th*) gene expression and *Th* protein localization were reduced (Hawes et al. 2015). With the use of computational analyses, these impairments were subsequently associated with the pathogenesis of several NDDs like SCZ, ADHD, and autism (Almeras et al. 2007; Eyles et al. 2007).

However, other studies on DVD deficiency point toward hyperlocomotion, impulsivity, lack of control of inhibitory behavior, learning and memory impairments in adult rats, even when pups were fed a VD-replete diet from birth or weaning onward (Burne et al. 2004; Burne et al. 2006; Eyles et al. 2006; Kesby et al. 2006). DVD deficiency from mating to offspring weaning has also been associated with a more anxious and less social phenotype in juvenile Sprague-Dawley rats. Whereas effects related to social behaviors were still present in adulthood, differences pertaining to anxiety-like behaviors did not persist into adulthood. These changes were later related to reduced hippocampal volume in neonatal mice and lower lateral ventricle volumes in adults by MRI assessments (Pan et al. 2014). In fact, some postmortem studies of NDDs have also demonstrated ectopic neurons in the hippocampus and neuroimaging studies of patients with NDDs have shown ventriculomegaly and cortical sulcal prominence, which may be of neurodevelopmental origin (Kroon et al. 2013; Parenti et al. 2020). These data suggest a critical window for prenatal VD effects on offspring brain development and vulnerability to NDDs in later life.

Literature suggests various reasons linking developmental vitamin D deficiency and altered brain development, first by the expression of VDR particularly in dopaminergic-rich brain regions involved in the pathology of NDDs (Cui et al. 2013). Second, in an extensive epidemiological study, Childhood Autism Risks from Genetics and the Environment (CHARGE) showed several functional polymorphisms in genes within the vitamin D pathway, including *Bsm1, Taq1, Cdx2, and FokI* in the VDR gene. Thirdly, nuclear VDR activated by a metabolite of vitamin D, the 1,25-dihydroxyvitamin D(3), cooperates with some chromatin modification enzymes (i.e. HATs and HDACs), taking a role in complex epigenetic events (Sundar and Rahman 2011). Recently, an association between maternal VDD and offspring epigenetic status at imprinted genes was also assessed in humans. Imprinted genes (*H19, IGF2, MEG3, MEG3- IG, MEST, NNAT, PEG3, PLAGL1,* and *SGCE/PEG10*) play vital roles in pre- and postnatal development and health, including brain development. However, the association between maternal 25(OH)D concentrations and cord blood DNA methylation levels at imprinted genes was reported to be nonsignificant (Benjamin Neelon et al. 2018).

15.3.2.2.3 Long-Chain Polyunsaturated Fatty Acids (LCPUFAs)

The LCPUFAs in the n-6 and n-3 series have distinct properties and functions and relatively can be synthesized from shorter PUFAs in the diet. For example, delta 6 desaturase is a key regulatory enzyme required for the conversion of the n-6 PUFA linoleic acid (LA) to arachidonic acid (AA), and employed for the conversion of the n-3 PUFA α-linolenic acid (ALA) to docosahexaenoic acid (DHA) (Sprecher et al. 1995; Sprecher 2002). LCPUFA are principally crucial during the brain growth spurt which occurs during the last trimester of pregnancy with fast growth up to 2 years of age (Dobbing and Sands 1973; Clandinin et al. 1980; Martinez 1992). Throughout pregnancy, AA and DHA are moved across the placenta into fetal venous blood (Campbell et al. 1997; Dutta-Roy 2000). After birth, breast milk is the main source of AA and DHA to the neonate. For the growing infant, there is a high requisite for LCPUFA to build vital cell membrane structures in the central nervous system. DHA is reported to influence cell membrane physical properties (Innis 2008), enzyme activity (Vaidyanathan et al. 1994), ion channels (Poling et al. 1995), and neuroreceptors and their signaling (Delion et al. 1996; Litman and Mitchell 1996; Chalon et al. 1998). On the contrary, variation in brain FA composition, decreased DHA in specific, affects neurodevelopment, alters visual, attention, and cognitive functions, and exhibited symptoms of anxiety, aggression, and depression (Sathyanarayana Rao et al. 2008).

Two studies examined maternal PUFA intake or status in relevance to offspring ASD risk or traits. In the Nurses' Health Study II (NHSII) in the US, total and n-6 PUFA intake before pregnancy was significantly and inversely associated with children's risk of ASD diagnosis as conveyed by mothers, while n-3 PUFA was not suggestively associated with ASD risk (Lyall et al. 2013). In contrast, in the generation R study in The Netherlands, plasma n-6 PUFA levels in midpregnancy were notably and positively associated with children's ASD traits, the ratio of n-3 to n-6 PUFA was inversely associated with the outcome. Alike to NHSII study, plasma n-3 PUFA levels were not related to the outcome. Both studies controlled for a complete set of possible confounders including other features of diet and dietary supplements (Lyall et al. 2013; Steenweg-De Graaff et al. 2016). Both n-3 and n-6 PUFA are essential for prenatal brain development (Yehuda et al. 1999); but, a raised n-6 to n-3 PUFA ratio – typical of modern western diet – could increase inflammatory processes (Schmitz and Ecker 2008; Patterson et al. 2012). Inconsistent results from the two studies possibly may be due to the use of absolute versus relative concentrations of n-3 and n-6 PUFA levels, or differences in the timing of the exposure (before pregnancy vs. mid-pregnancy) and outcome measures (clinical diagnosis vs. trait).

Fish is the main dietary source of DHA – the n-3 PUFA is most relevant for brain development (Martinez 1992). Based on the secondary analysis of the above-mentioned studies on PUFA intake/status, maternal fish intake was not associated with ASD diagnosis/traits (Lyall et al. 2013; Graaff et al. 2015). By contrast, two other studies proposed a potential inverse association between maternal fish intake and offspring ASD risk (Surén et al. 2013; Julvez et al. 2016). Among 1589 children in the Spanish INMA study, maternal total seafood intake in the first trimester was associated with lower autistic traits measured by Childhood Asperger Syndrome Test; similar associations were observed for large fatty fish and lean fish (Julvez et al. 2016). Another study in China of 108 ASD cases and 108 typically developing controls (GAO et al. 2016) found maternal eating of grass carp (>3 times/week) reported four to 17 years after delivery to be associated with a lower risk of ASD. Finally, in the Norwegian Mother and Child Cohort Study, among 85 176 children in (MoBa) (Surén et al. 2013), fish oil supplementation before and in early pregnancy was not associated with ASD risk.

In summary, findings of the associations between maternal PUFA or fish intake and ASD risk are indecisive. Diversity in the PUFA measurement or assessment (i.e. absolute vs. relative concentrations, intake vs. status) and ASD (i.e. clinical diagnosis vs. traits, intake vs. status) made it tough to associate findings across studies. Furthermore, recall bias and potential residual confounding are also of concern.

Neurogenesis is established during gestation in the most brain region and is completed before birth except in the dentate gyrus (DG) of the hippocampal (Huang et al. 2015). The normal development of DG is very vital to learning and memory (Coremans et al. 2010). N-3 PUFAs was demonstrated to have neurogenesis-promoting properties (Lei et al. 2013). On the other hand, maternal dietary n-3 fatty acid deficiency can impair normal neurogenesis in the hippocampus DG in neonatal rats, consequently leading to the impaired learning and memory and a decline in cognitive abilities (Bertrand et al. 2006).

Conceptually, alterations of neurotransmission in the key brain areas play a pivotal role in the development of several NDDs and the useful effects of n-3 PUFAs in these brain-related disorders were, at least moderately, via its modulating effect on neurotransmission (Patrick and Ames 2015). GABA is the major inhibitory neurotransmitter in the central nervous system. GABAergic neurons have been shown to regulate cognitive processing in prefrontal and hippocampal networks (Huang et al. 2014). Recent evidence reported that decreased brain DHA may perhaps reduce presynaptic GLU release and uptake, further lead to degradation of glutamatergic transmission in the hippocampus of aging rats, rather than young rats (Latour et al. 2013). GABA is synthesized in the CNS via decarboxylation of GLU, in a reaction catalyzed by glutamic acid decarboxylase (GAD). The majority of GLU within CNS is produced from glutamine (GLN) via the enzyme glutaminase. Maternal n-3 PUFAs' deficiency prominently reduced the brain concentration of GLN and increased the content of GABA in offspring rats, without altering the level of GLU and the mRNA expression of GAD. Maternal n-3 PUFAs' deficiency gave rise to the failure of the GGC cycle (inhibition of GLN synthesis) in neonatal female rats. This data speculated that the reduced GLN in the deficient group might reflect the degradation of glutamatergic transmission and GABAergic transmission, and the increase in GABA content may be the compensatory mechanism in the organism (Tang et al. 2016).

In another study, exposure to the n-3 fatty acid-deficient diet during the perinatal period (gestation and lactation) resulted in a significant decrease in hypothalamic DHA levels and a reduced male offspring body weight (Khoury et al. 2020). DHA deficiency during the perinatal period significantly increased and prolonged restraint stress-induced changes in colonic temperature and serum corticosterone levels caused a significant increase in γ-aminobutyric acid (GABA$_A$) antagonist-induced heart rate changes and enhanced depressive-like behavior in the forced swimming test and anxiety-like behavior in the plus-maze test in later life. These effects were not seen in male rats fed the n-3 fatty acid-deficient diet during the postweaning period (Chen and Su 2013). These reports suggest that brain development is the critical period in which DHA deficiency leads to might modulate stress-induced *GAD67* expression and alter GABAergic regulation of the HPA axis activity, leading to anxiety- and depression-like behaviors later in life (Mody and Maguire 2012).

It is worth noting that inadequate maternal n-3 PUFAs' diet significantly reduced the brain DA level and significantly altered dopamine receptors and the DOPAC content in neonatal female rats. Since DA plays a key role in governing motivation and reward processing, and alterations to dopamine levels have been linked to the onset of various NDDs including SCZ, ADHD, and depression.

N-3 PUFAs' deficiency during peri-adolescent (P21-90) was reported to display significantly greater 5-hydroxytryptamine (5-HT) content and a significantly reduced **5-Hydroxyindoleacetic acid (5-HIAA)** to 5-HT ratio in the prefrontal cortex and hypothalamus of female adult rats (McNamara et al. 2009; McNamara et al. 2013). Changes in the **5-HIAA** to 5-HT ratio been associated with behavioral disorders (Belay et al. 2011; Kim et al. 2011; Pieper et al. 2011).

Studies indicate that omega-3 fatty acids may affect gene expression changes in the brain through the modulation of transcription factors (Kitajka et al. 2004; Deckelbaum et al. 2006). Animals fed with a diet rich in omega-3 fatty acids have demonstrated lower methylation at *BDNF* exon IV in the brain as compared to the animals fed with a low omega-3 fatty acid diet (Tyagi et al. 2015). Maternal ALA supplementation decreased the methylation of MeCP2 and altered the expression of genes mainly involved in memory and neurogenesis (He et al. 2014). A study has demonstrated an association between major depressive disorder and suicide risk with DNA methylation changes in the genes involved in omega-3 fatty acid biosynthesis (Haghighi et al. 2015). The relation between omega-3 fatty acids and DNA methylation of *BDNF* gene of memory has been established (Niculescu et al. 2013; Hoile et al. 2014). However, limited studies have examined the role of omega-3 fatty acids in influencing epigenetic changes in the brain.

Together, these data suggest that the altered micronutrient intake/disturbed LCPUFA metabolism may cause altered DNA methylation in the brain which may increase the risk for neurological disorders.

15.3.2.2.4 Trace Elements

Trace elements include iron, iodine, zinc, copper, and choline. These elements may be responsible for mediating epigenetic processes in response to the maternal diet because of their role as cofactors and methyl donors. Iron is required for critical neuronal processes such as neurotransmitter production, myelination, and energy metabolism (Beard and Connor 2003). It has a role in learning and memory as it is known to affect the development of the hippocampus. A report indicates that perinatal iron deficiency permanently alters the structure and functioning of the brain consequently may cause anxiety-like behavior in the rat offspring (Li et al. 2011). Additionally, another study demonstrated that fetal iron deficiency was also shown to increase HDAC activity, alter histone methylation, and decrease DNA methylation at exon IV of *Bdnf*, resulting in lower transcription of hippocampal *Bdnf* (Tran et al. 2015). These effects were measured well into adulthood. Similarly, perinatal zinc deficiency is suggested to adversely affect spatial memory in rat offspring by a marked reduction in brain neurotrophins (Grabrucker 2013). Since zinc is required for the catalytic functioning of the majority of HDACs and DNMT1, zinc deficiency may cause decreased histone modification and DNA methylation of brain neurotrophins increasing the risk for NDDs.

Choline is required for the biosynthesis of cell membranes and cholinergic neurotransmission and maternal choline deficiency leads to neural tube defects in infants (Shaw et al. 2004; Zeisel and Da Costa 2009). Choline-deficient diet during gestation is also reported to reduce the proliferation of neural progenitor cells and result in increased hippocampal apoptosis in the fetus (Craciunescu et al. 2003). In addition, choline is involved in the formation of SAM and can modify the gene expression of vital genes in the brain (Bekdash 2016). Nevertheless, gestational choline deficiency affected global and Igf2 gene DNA hypermethylation by upregulation of Dnmt1 and Dnmt 3 expression, suggesting the possible changes in neuronal proliferation and survival, as well as synaptic development (Konishi et al. 1994; Napoli et al. 2008).

15.3.2.2.5 Protein Restriction

A long-term longitudinal Guatemalan investigation of nutrition and mental development which began in 1968 and was recently completed by the Institute of Nutrition of Central America and Panama (INCAP) demonstrated that mothers with severe protein-calorie malnutrition during pregnancy and lactation were associated with reduced intellectual functioning in their offspring at later life (Martorell 2017). In the animal model feeding Wistar rats with a protein-restricted diet (6%) during pregnancy and lactation significantly lowered cortical and hippocampal mass, decreased hippocampal BDNF concentrations, and impaired water maze performance in the young rats. Literature survey shows that maternal LPD during pregnancy and lactation may affect cognitive functioning via epigenetic mechanisms (Wang and Xu 2007).

The renin-angiotensin system (RAS), a peptide hormone, has a marked role in controlling behavioral and cognitive responses. Also, it has been hypothesized that RAS has a pivotal role in some NDDs (Gard 2004; Mertens et al. 2010; Firouzabadi et al. 2016). The implication of RAS in NDDs is supported by the fact that Angiotensin II (Ang II), the ultimate product of RAS, is also assumed to interact with neurotransmitters such as dopamine and serotonin in CNS, which regulate behavioral and cognitive processes (Bohus and de Wied 1999; Gard 2002). Also, brain Ang II has been proposed to induce dopaminergic cell death which has been associated with autism as well as other neurodevelopmental conditions. In addition, two main receptors of angiotensin II type 1 and type 2 receptor have been found to be widely distributed in different areas of the brain associated with cognitive functions including areas affected in autism (Ghanizadeh et al. 2012; Rossignol and Frye 2012). Interestingly, Goyal investigated the epigenetic alterations in gene expression of the brain renin-angiotensin system of the mouse fetus with a perinatal LPD and showed that the CpG islands in the promoter regions of angiotensin-converting enzyme-1 (ACE-1) were hypomethylated. They also found upregulation of the miRNAs, mmu-mir-27a and 27b, which regulate ACE-1 mRNA translation (Goyal et al. 2010). These results suggest that the effect of these epigenetic changes in the developing brain in response to maternal nutrition may play an important role in the brain developmental malformation and other disorders later in life (Figure 15.4).

15.3.3 The Link Between Early Life Nutrition and Breast Cancer Risk

Evidences regarding the effect of early life nutrition on an adult are rather less known than that on the early life origins of metabolic and CVDs. However, the association between proxy markers of the intrauterine environment and risk of specific cancers including breast cancer, and leukaemia and some other nonreproductive cancers is well established. The following discussion will focus on the relationship between birth weight (BW) and later breast cancer risk.

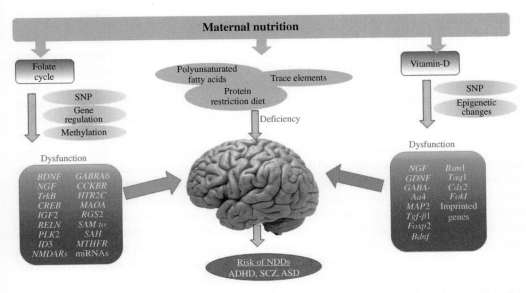

Figure 15.4 Epigenetic linkage of NDDs and maternal nutrition of an offspring as a risk of SCZ, ADHD, and ASD.

Various epidemiological studies have suggested that pre- and perinatal factors may influence the risk for breast cancer later in life. There followed a plethora of studies that reported associations between BW and later breast cancer risk. However, making conclusions regarding the extent of association between BW and later breast cancer risk is challenging, as these studies have differed greatly in their design (Teegarden et al. 2012; Troisi et al. 2013). For instance, whether pre- and postmenopausal women were analyzed together or separately and the extent to which other variables were included in the analysis.

A recent meta-analysis-interpreted data from 26 published studies showed that higher BW was associated with the greatest elevation in risk of breast cancer, predominantly in premenopausal women (Surakasula et al. 2014). The relative risk for breast cancer in premenopausal women compared with high BW to women with low BW was 1.20 (CI 0.91–1.19) for cohort studies and 1.36 (CI 0.66–1.64) for case-control studies. Remarkably, some studies have reported a J- or U-shaped association between BW and disease risk, babies born with BW below 2.5 kg or above 4.5 kg being associated with an increased risk of breast cancer in later life compared to babies born within the normal range (Xiao et al. 2019; López et al. 2020).

The Dutch "Hunger Winter" famine of 1944 ± 1945 provided the best example of this association in humans, with the surviving children of nutritionally compromised women around the peak of famine close to the periconceptional period and early pregnancy confers an increased risk of breast cancer in later life (Stein et al. 1975; Heijmans et al. 2008). Whilst an increase in breast cancer risk was also observed for women who had been exposed to famine during childhood. On the contrary, a decrease in calorie intake during the Second World War in Norway was associated with a decrease in breast cancer risk in women who were born during this period of famine or who were peripubertal at that time (Vin-Raviv et al. 2012; Mahabir 2013). This variation observed between the studies in Norway and the Netherlands may be associated with the severity of the famine in the Netherlands and/or the fact that the famine abruptly in the Netherlands resulting in a period of rapid catch-up growth with normalization of growth factors and hormones which may increase the risk of cancer later in life (Elias et al. 2007). In addition, studies have also pointed that breast-feeding reduces an infant's risk of developing breast cancer before menopause (Anstey et al. 2017). Interestingly, animal models have also shown that diets high in n-3 fatty acids lowered the tumor incidence, thus, suggesting that DHA, present in breast milk, may also influence the development of the mammary gland and, subsequently, cancer risk (Abdelmagid et al. 2016).

Further, animal experiments also supported this hypothesis: feeding an LPD, during pregnancy and lactation, produces LBW offspring, had developed twice the number of early mammary tumors compared to offspring from control-fed dams (Fernandez-Twinn et al. 2007). LP offspring displayed reduced postnatal mammary ductal branching and epithelial invasion at three weeks. This followed rapid development of epithelial density one and two weeks after weaning on to adequate nutrition. This compensatory mammary growth leads to a substantial increase in the risk of early-onset mammary tumors. Conceptually, compensatory mammary epithelial "catch-up" growth may further enhance the rate of transformation and mutagenesis in mammary cells including stem cells or "progenitor" cells. In culture, the rapid growth of mammary epithelial cells may aberrantly hypermethylate the promoter region of a key cell cycle checkpoint regulator, p16INK4a, thereby altering its expression to a detrimental effect. Compensatory mammary growth observed in PR offspring and increased susceptibility to tumor induction is also associated with increased levels of insulin, IGF-1 and estrogen (Fernandez-Twinn et al. 2007). The cross-talk between upregulated estrogen and IGF-1 signaling may further direct transformation (Skandalis et al. 2014).

There are also certain evidences relating overnutrition in early life with an increased risk of mammary tumorigenesis in later life. De AS et al. demonstrated that a HF diet during pregnancy produced offspring, with a higher BW, which increases mammary tumorigenesis in rats. This increase in cancer incidence was accompanied by an increase in the number of terminal end buds (TEBs) and proliferating cells within the mammary glands of the offspring (De Assis et al. 2012). Zheng et al. reported that HF feeding during pregnancy has persistently decreased the expression of the cell cycle inhibitors p16 in the mammary gland of the offspring compared to controls. The decrease in expression was accompanied by a decrease in histone H4 acetylation, decreased HDAC3 binding, but no difference again in DNA methylation levels (Zheng et al. 2012).

Hilakivi-Clarke and her colleagues have demonstrated that maternal intake of diet high in n-6 PUFA increases the risk of chemically induced breast cancer in offspring, possibly by increasing maternal estradiol levels during pregnancy (Hilakivi-Clarke et al. 1997). Feeding a diet high in n-6 PUFA during the peripubertal period in rats also led to an increase in mammary tumor incidence, compared to rats fed a high n-6 PUFA diet post-puberty (MacLennan and Ma 2010), suggesting that the peripubertal along with the prenatal period may be a period of increased susceptibility where nutritional intake may impact cancer risk later in life (Price et al. 2015). In contrast, feeding an n-3 PUFA diet during the peripubertal period resulted in a protective effect against mammary tumorigenesis in rats (Liu and Ma 2014). This decrease in cancer incidence was also accompanied by a reduction in mammary cell proliferation and an increase in apoptosis.

A substantial body of human epidemiological and animal studies has shown that nutrients involved in one-carbon metabolism such as folate, vitamin B6, vitamin B2, vitamin B12, and choline are protective against a number of cancers, although the relationship between folate intake in adulthood and breast cancer risk is complex (Cho et al. 2007). Ly et al. have reported that both maternal and postweaning folic acid supplementation significantly increased the risk of mammary adenocarcinomas in the offspring after DMBA treatment (Ly et al. 2011). In their more recent work, Ly et al. have reported that maternal folic acid supplementation significantly reduced global DNA methylation, whereas postweaning folic acid supplementation significantly decreased DNA methyltransferase activity in non-neoplastic mammary glands of the offspring (Ly et al. 2011; Kim 2016), suggesting that epigenetic processes may be important in determining later cancer risk (Figure 15.5).

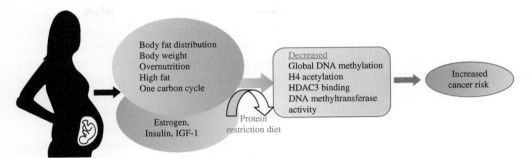

Figure 15.5 The influences of early nutrition and its epigenetic regulation via interaction between estrogen IGF and insulin as a risk factor for cancer.

15.4   Transgenerational Inheritance

As discussed above, both human and animal studies demonstrate that maternal exposures in pregnancy can increase NCDs' predisposition in offspring. This increase in disease risk observed in offspring (F1) is probably due to fetal programming of the vital organs as numerous studies show morphological and molecular alterations in that organ induced by a number of prenatal exposures (Hilakivi-Clarke and de Assis 2006). Nevertheless, it has been reported that *in utero* exposures can also affect developing germ cells in the F1 generation (Gapp et al. 2014), which can cause intergenerational effects and impact the F2 generation's health phenotypes. Those effects can often pass on to the F3 generation and beyond. Effects observed in the F3 generation are the first evidence of environmentally induced transgenerational epigenetic inheritance as they are transmitted through the F2 germline, which was not directly exposed to initial environmental insult in the F0 generation; (Jirtle and Skinner 2007; Horsthemke 2018). The term "transgenerational" epigenetic inheritance is often used rather broadly to describe the transmission of epigenetic markers through the germline between generations in the absence of any environmental exposure. Recently, transgenerational epigenetics have researched due to its ability to prewrite individual epigenetic profiles that lead to implications on the adult phenotype formation and disease onset, which is called the developmental origin of diseases.

Several studies in animal models provide examples that nutritional status in early life can lead to transgenerational inheritance of phenotypes, where transmission of disease risk is passed between generations (Mørkve Knudsen et al. 2018). Transgenerational epigenetic programming has been reported to be involved in a variety of phenotypes, including diabetes, hypertension, cancer, brain development, depression, and, more recently, metabolic syndrome (Zhu et al. 2019).

There is evidence from historical records that female grandchildren (F2) from the paternal grandmother (F0), who experienced dramatic changes in food availability during her own growth, were at higher risk of cardiovascular mortality (Bygren et al. 2014). Similarly, the Dutch famine study found that adult grand-offspring (F2) whose fathers were exposed to famine in utero had higher neonatal adiposity and adverse health outcomes in adulthood. However, the transmission to the third and subsequent generation remains unclear. In the Guatemalan cohort, generations have been studied up to F2 with positive associations seen between improved maternal and F1 nutrition and improved F2 offspring developmental outcomes (Veenendaal et al. 2013). In the China famine, F2 offspring of famine exposed mothers had higher birth weights than did F2 offspring of unexposed mothers. Data from three famines suggest that transgenerational effects of nutrition on offspring phenotype occur via the maternal lineage. However, a historical study of three generations in Overkalix, Sweden revealed that fathers' diets may also play a crucial role. Overnutrition of the fathers during the pre-adolescence period predisposed the sons and grandsons to the risk of diabetics (Pembrey et al. 2014). Evidences have shown that diet-induced paternal obesity can modulate sperm microRNA content and germ methylation status which are potential signals that program offspring health and initiate the transmission of obesity to future generations (Dupont et al. 2019).

Since the data available from retrospective human studies is limited, further understandings into transgenerational programming of NCDs, particularly around alterations in maternal nutrition, have been derived from experimental animal models. It was revealed that transgenerational epigenetic programming can mediate the fetal programming of insulin resistance, which was induced by an HF diet, obesity, or other interventions in F0 offspring (Masuyama et al. 2015; Hanafi et al. 2016; Huypens et al. 2016). Transgenerational epigenetic programming was reported in adipose tissue development. Likewise, transgenerational inheritance of obesity consistent with a leptin-resistant was shown to be induced by transgenerational epigenetic programming of DNA methylome in adipose tissue (Gonzalez-Bulnes et al. 2014; Lecoutre et al. 2018). Significant differential methylation changes in the promoter region of H19 were reported in a multigenerational model of intrauterine growth restriction (IUGR) (Gonzalez-Rodriguez et al. 2016). Thus, nutritional factors with properties that influence epigenetic processes are believed to have effects on multigenerational/transgenerational inheritance of adult-onset disease phenotypes.

15.5 Conclusion

The burden of chronic diseases including obesity and NCDs is rapidly increasing worldwide. Human and experimental animal studies have highlighted that the nutritional environment during developmental periods can influence the risk of the propensity for adult obesity and NCDs. Moreover, evidence exists, at least from animal models, that the late onset of such diseases following earlier transient experiences indicates that developmental programming may have an epigenetic component. As a key and central component of an epigenetic network, DNA methylation or histone tail modifications is labile in response to nutritional influences and could provide a persistent memory of earlier nutritional states. Alterations in DNA methylation profiles can lead to changes in gene expression, resulting in diverse phenotypes with the potential for decreased growth and health. Nevertheless, animal evidence suggests that a history of nutritional insults in the parental generation could lead to multigenerational and transgenerational predispositions for obesity and NCDs. Further studies, however, are needed to fully characterize and confirm this hypothesis in order to apply preventive actions to successfully approach this global health problem.

References

Aaby, P., Marx, C., Trautner, S. et al. (2002). Thymus size at birth is associated with infant mortality: a community study from Guinea-Bissau. *Acta Paediatrica, International Journal of Paediatrics* 91 (6): 698–703.

Abdelmagid, S.A., MacKinnon, J.L., Janssen, S.M., and Ma, D.W.L. (2016). Role of n-3 polyunsaturated fatty acids and exercise in breast cancer prevention: identifying common targets. *Nutrition and Metabolic Insights* 9: 71–84.

Abdolmaleky, H.M., Cheng, K.H., Russo, A. et al. (2005). Hypermethylation of the reelin (RELN) promoter in the brain of schizophrenic patients: a preliminary report. *American Journal of Medical Genetics – Neuropsychiatric Genetics* 134 (1): 60–66.

Alejandro, E.U., Gregg, B., Wallen, T. et al. (2014). Maternal diet-induced microRNAs and mTOR underlie β cell dysfunction in offspring. *Journal of Clinical Investigation* 124 (10): 4395–4410.

Almeras, L., Eyles, D., Benech, P. et al. (2007). Developmental vitamin D deficiency alters brain protein expression in the adult rat: implications for neuropsychiatric disorders. *Proteomics* 7 (5): 769–780.

Altmann, S., Murani, E., Schwerin, M. et al. (2013). Dietary protein restriction and excess of pregnant German Landrace sows induce changes in hepatic gene expression and promoter methylation of key metabolic genes in the offspring. *Journal of Nutritional Biochemistry* 24 (2): 484–495.

Anderson, O.S., Sant, K.E., and Dolinoy, D.C. (2012). Nutrition and epigenetics: an interplay of dietary methyl donors, one-carbon metabolism and DNA methylation. *Journal of Nutritional Biochemistry* 23 (8): 853–859.

Anstey, E.H., Shoemaker, M.L., Barrera, C.M. et al. (2017). Breastfeeding and breast cancer risk reduction: implications for black mothers. *American Journal of Preventive Medicine* 53 (3): S40–S46.

Antoniades, L., MacGregor, A., Andrew, T., and Spector, T.D. (2003). Association of birth weight with osteoporosis and osteoarthritis in adult twins. *Rheumatology* 42 (6): 791–796.

Arking, D.E., Cutler, D.J., Brune, C.W. et al. (2008). A common genetic variant in the neurexin superfamily member CNTNAP2 increases familial risk of Autism. *American Journal of Human Genetics* 82 (1): 160–164.

Armitage, J.A., Lakasing, L., Taylor, P.D. et al. (2005). Developmental programming of aortic and renal structure in offspring of rats fed fat-rich diets in pregnancy. *Journal of Physiology* 565 (1): 171–184.

Aye, I.L.M.H., Lager, S., Ramirez, V.I. et al. (2014). Increasing maternal body mass index is associated with systemic inflammation in the mother and the activation of distinct placental inflammatory pathways. *Biology of Reproduction* 90 (6).

Bale, T.L., Baram, T.Z., Brown, A.S. et al. (2010). Early life programming and neurodevelopmental disorders. *Biological Psychiatry* 68 (4): 314–319.

Bannister, A.J. and Kouzarides, T. (2011). Regulation of chromatin by histone modifications. *Cell Research* 21 (3): 381–395.

Barros, M.A.V., De Brito Alves, J.L., Nogueira, V.O. et al. (2015). Maternal low-protein diet induces changes in the cardiovascular autonomic modulation in male rat offspring. *Nutrition, Metabolism, and Cardiovascular Diseases* 25 (1): 123–130.

Beard, J.L. and Connor, J.R. (2003). Iron status and neural functioning. *Annual Review of Nutrition* 23: 41–58.

Bekdash, R.A. (2016). Choline and the brain: an epigenetic perspective. *Advances in Neurobiology* 12: 381–399.

Belay, H., Burton, C.L., Lovic, V. et al. (2011). Early adversity and serotonin transporter genotype interact with hippocampal glucocorticoid receptor mRNA expression, corticosterone, and behavior in adult male rats. *Behavioral Neuroscience* 125 (2): 150–160.

Benjamin Neelon, S.E., White, A.J., Vidal, A.C. et al. (2018). Maternal Vitamin D, DNA methylation at imprint regulatory regions and offspring weight at birth, 1 year and 3 years. *International Journal of Obesity* 42 (4): 587–593.

Benn, C.S., Jeppesen, D.L., Hasselbalch, H. et al. (2001). Thymus size and head circumference at birth and the development of allergic diseases. *Clinical & Experimental Allergy* 31 (12): 1862–1866.

Bertrand, P.C., O'Kusky, J.R., and Innis, S.M. (2006). Maternal dietary (n-3) fatty acid deficiency alters neurogenesis in the embryonic rat brain. *The Journal of Nutrition* 136 (6): 1570–1575.

Beveridge, N.J. and Cairns, M.J. (2012). MicroRNA dysregulation in schizophrenia. *Neurobiology of Disease* 46 (2): 263–271.

Billet, S., Aguilar, F., Baudry, C., and Clauser, E. (2008). Role of angiotensin II AT1 receptor activation in cardiovascular diseases. *Kidney International* 74 (11): 1379–1384.

Blaise, S.A., Nédélec, E., Schroeder, H. et al. (2007). Gestational vitamin B deficiency leads to homocysteine-associated brain apoptosis and alters neurobehavioral development in rats. *American Journal of Pathology* 170 (2): 667–679.

Blondeau, B., Garofano, A., Czernichow, P., and Breant, B. (1999). Age-dependent inability of the endocrine pancreas to adapt to pregnancy: a long-term consequence of perinatal malnutrition in the rat. *Endocrinology* 140 (09): 4208–4213.

Blondeau, B., Lesage, J., Czernichow, P. et al. (2001). Glucocorticoids impair fetal β-cell development in rats. *American Journal of Physiology. Endocrinology and Metabolism* 281: 44.

Blümer, N. and Renz, H. (2007). Consumption of ω3-fatty acids during perinatal life: role in immuno-modulation and allergy prevention. *Journal of Perinatal Medicine* 35 (SUPPL. 1): S12.

Bohus, B.G.J. and de Wied, D. (1999). The vasopressin deficient Brattleboro rats: a natural knockout model used in the search for CNS effects of vasopressin. *InProgress in brain research* 119: 555–573.

de Bono, S., Schoenmakers, I., Ceesay, M. et al. (2010). Birth weight predicts bone size in young adulthood at cortical sites in men and trabecular sites in women from The Gambia. *Bone* 46 (5): 1316–1321.

Brabin, B.J., Hakimi, M., and Pelletier, D. (2001). Effect of zinc deficiency on methionine metabolism, methylation reactions and protein synthesis in isolated perfused rat liver. *The Journal of Nutrition* 131 (2): 604S–615S.

Brabin, B.J., Hakimi, M., and Pelletier, D. (2001). Assessing the effects of high methionine intake on DNA methylation. *The Journal of Nutrition* 131 (2): 604S–615S.

Brabin, B.J., Hakimi, M., and Pelletier, D. (2001). Methylenetetrahydrofolate reductase C677T polymorphism, folic acid and riboflavin are important determinants of genome stability in cultured human lymphocytes. *The Journal of Nutrition* 131 (2): 604S–615S.

Brakowski, J., Spinelli, S., Dörig, N. et al. (2017). Resting state brain network function in major depression – Depression symptomatology, antidepressant treatment effects, future research. *Journal of Psychiatric Research* 92: 147–159.

Breckler, L.A., Hale, J., Taylor, A. et al. (2008). Pregnancy IFN-γ responses to foetal alloantigens are altered by maternal allergy and gravidity status. *Allergy: European Journal of Allergy and Clinical Immunology* 63 (11): 1473–1480.

Breckler, L.A., Hale, J., Jung, W. et al. (2010). Modulation of in vivo and in vitro cytokine production over the course of pregnancy in allergic and non-allergic mothers. *Pediatric Allergy and Immunology* 21 (PART I): 14–21.

Brenmoehl, J. and Hoeflich, A. (2013). Dual control of mitochondrial biogenesis by sirtuin 1 and sirtuin 3. *Mitochondrion* 13 (6): 755–761.

de Brito Alves, J.L., Nogueira, V.O., Neto, M.P.C. et al. (2015). Maternal protein restriction increases respiratory and sympathetic activities and sensitizes peripheral chemoreflex in male rat offspring. *Journal of Nutrition* 145 (5): 907–914.

Brooke, O.G., Carter, N.D., Brown, I.R.F. et al. (1980). Vitamin D supplements in pregnant Asian women: effects on calcium status and fetal growth. *British Medical Journal* 280 (6216): 751.

Brown, A.S. and Susser, E.S. (2008). Prenatal nutritional deficiency and risk of adult Schizophrenia. *Schizophrenia Bulletin* 34 (6): 1054–1063.

Brown, A.S., Susser, E.S., Butler, P.D. et al. (1996). Neurobiological plausibility of prenatal nutritional deprivation as a risk factor for schizophrenia. *Journal of Nervous and Mental Disease* 184 (2): 71–85.

Burne, T.H.J., Becker, A., Brown, J. et al. (2004). Transient prenatal Vitamin D deficiency is associated with hyperlocomotion in adult rats. *Behavioural Brain Research* 154 (2): 549–555.

Burne, T.H.J., O'Loan, J., McGrath, J.J., and Eyles, D.W. (2006). Hyperlocomotion associated with transient prenatal vitamin D deficiency is ameliorated by acute restraint. *Behavioural Brain Research* 174 (1): 119–124.

Butler, A.A., Kesteson, R.A., Khong, K. et al. (2000). A unique metalolic sysdrone causes obesity in the Melanocortin-3 receptor-deficient mouse. *Endocrinology* 141 (9): 3518–3521.

Bygren, L.O., Tinghög, P., Carstensen, J. et al. (2014). Change in paternal grandmother'searly food supply influenced cardiovascular mortality of the female grandchildren. *BMC Genetics* 15: 12.

Calder, P.C. and Yaqoob, P. (2000). The level of protein and type of fat in the diet of pregnant rats both affect lymphocyte function in the offspring. *Nutrition Research* 20 (7): 995–1005.

Calkins, K. and Devaskar, S.U. (2011). Fetal origins of adult disease. *Current Problems in Pediatric and Adolescent Health Care* 41 (6): 158–176.

Callréus, M., McGuigan, F., and Åkesson, K. (2013). Birth weight is more important for peak bone mineral content than for bone density: the PEAK-25 study of 1,061 young adult women. *Osteoporosis International* 24 (4): 1347–1355.

Calvi, L.M. and Schipani, E. (2000). The PTH/PTHrP receptor in Jansen's metaphyseal chondrodysplasia. *Journal of Endocrinological Investigation* 23 (8): 545–554.

Camargo, C.A. Jr., Rifas-Shiman, S.L., Litonjua, A.A. et al. (2007). Maternal intake of vitamin D during pregnancy and risk of recurrent wheeze in children at 3 year of age. *The American Journal of Clinical Nutrition* 85 (3): 788–795.

Campbell, F.M., Clohessy, A.M., Gordon, M.J. et al. (1997). Uptake of long chain fatty acids by human placental choriocarcinoma (BeWo) cells: role of plasma membrane fatty acid-binding protein. *Journal of Lipid Research* 38 (12): 2558–2568.

Camporeale, G., Giordano, E., Rendina, R. et al. (2006). Drosophila melanogaster holocarboxylase synthetase is a chromosomal protein required for normal histone biotinylation, gene transcription patterns, lifespan. *The Journal of Nutrition* 136 (11): 2735–2742.

Cantó, C., Menzies, K.J., and Auwerx, J. (2015). NAD+ metabolism and the control of energy homeostasis: a balancing act between mitochondria and the nucleus. *Cell Metabolism* 22 (1): 31–53.

Carver, W., Terracio, L., and Borg, T.K. (1993). Expression and accumulation of interstitial collagen in the neonatal rat heart. *The Anatomical Record* 236 (3): 511–520.

Castillo, H., Santos, I.S., and Matijasevich, A. (2015). Relationship between maternal pre-pregnancy body mass index, gestational weight gain and childhood fatness at 6-7 years by air displacement plethysmography. *Maternal & Child Nutrition* 11 (4): 606–617.

Chalon, S., Delion-Vancassel, S., Belzung, C. et al. (1998). Dietary fish oil affects monoaminergic neurotransmission and behavior in rats. *The Journal of Nutrition* 128 (12): 2512–25129.

Chen, H.F. and Su, H.M. (2013). Exposure to a maternal n-3 fatty acid-deficient diet during brain development provokes excessive hypothalamic-pituitary-adrenal axis responses to stress and behavioral indices of depression and anxiety in male rat offspring later in life. *Journal of Nutritional Biochemistry* 24 (1): 70–80.

Chen, D.Y., Stern, S.A., Garcia-Osta, A. et al. (2011). A critical role for IGF-II in memory consolidation and enhancement. *Nature* 469 (7331): 491–499.

Chen, J., Zhang, J., Lazarenko, O.P. et al. (2012). Inhibition of fetal bone development through epigenetic down-regulation of HoxA10 in obese rats fed high-fat diet. *The FASEB Journal* 26 (3): 1131–1141.

Chen, T., Liu, H.-X., Yan, H.-Y. et al. (2016). Developmental origins of inflammatory and immune diseases. *Molecular Human Reproduction* 22 (8): 858–865.

Chen, F., Cao, K., Zhang, H. et al. (2020). Maternal high-fat diet increases vascular contractility in adult offspring in a sex-dependent manner. *Hypertension Research*: 1–11.

Cho, E., Holmes, M., Hankinson, S.E., and Willett, W.C. (2007). Nutrients involved in one-carbon metabolism and risk of breast cancer among premenopausal women. *Cancer Epidemiology, Biomarkers and Prevention* 16 (12): 2787–2790.

Choi, S.W. and Friso, S. (2010). Epigenetics: a new bridge between nutrition and health. *Advances in Nutrition* 1 (1): 8–16.

Christoffersen, T., Ahmed, L.A., Daltveit, A.K. et al. (2017). The influence of birth weight and length on bone mineral density and content in adolescence: the Tromsø study, fit futures. *Archives of Osteoporosis* 12 (1): 1–9.

Clandinin, M.T., Chappell, J.E., Leong, S. et al. (1980). Intrauterine fatty acid accretion rates in human brain: implications for fatty acid requirements. *Early Human Development* 4 (2): 121–129.

Cloos, P.A.C., Christensen, J., Agger, K., and Helin, K. (2008). Erasing the methyl mark: histone demethylases at the center of cellular differentiation and disease. *Genes and Development* 22 (9): 1115–1140.

Coleman, D.N., Vailati-Riboni, M., Elolimy, A.A. et al. (2019). Hepatic betaine-homocysteine methyltransferase and methionine synthase activity and intermediates of the methionine cycle are altered by choline supply during negative energy balance in Holstein cows. *Journal of Dairy Science* 102 (9): 8305–8318.

Collinson, A., Moore, S., Cole, T., and Prentice, A. (2007). Birth season and environmental influences on patterns of thymic growth in rural Gambian infants. *Acta Paediatrica* 92 (9): 1014–1020.

Cooper, C., Cawley, M., Bhalla, A. et al. (1995). Childhood growth, physical activity, and peak bone mass in women. *Journal of Bone and Mineral Research* 10 (6): 940–947.

Cooper, C., Fall, C., Egger, P. et al. (1997). Growth in infancy and bone mass in later life. *Annals of the Rheumatic Diseases* 56 (1): 17–21.

Cooper, C., Walker-Bone, K., Arden, N., and Dennison, E. (2000). Novel insights into the pathogenesis of osteoporosis: the role of intrauterine programming. *Rheumatology* 39 (12): 1312–1315.

Cooper, C., Westlake, S., Harvey, N. et al. (2006). Review: developmental origins of osteoporotic fracture. *Osteoporosis International* 17 (3): 337–347.

Cooper, C., Harvey, N., Cole, Z. et al. (2009). Developmental origins of osteoporosis: the role of maternal nutrition. *Advances in Experimental Medicine and Biology* 646: 31–39.

Coremans, V., Ahmed, T., Balschun, D. et al. (2010). Impaired neurogenesis, learning and memory and low seizure threshold associated with loss of neural precursor cell survivin. *BMC Neuroscience* 11: 1–19.

Costa-Silva, J.H., Silva, P.A., Pedi, N. et al. (2009). Chronic undernutrition alters renal active Na+ transport in young rats: potential hidden basis for pathophysiological alterations in adulthood? *European Journal of Nutrition* 48 (7): 437–445.

Cottrell, E.C., Seckl, J.R., Holmes, M.C., and Wyrwoll, C.S. (2014). Foetal and placental 11β-HSD2: a hub for developmental programming. *Acta Physiologica* 210 (2): 288–295.

Craciunescu, C.N., Albright, C.D., Mar, M.H. et al. (2003). Choline availability during embryonic development alters progenitor cell mitosis in developing mouse hippocampus. *The Journal of Nutrition* 133 (11): 3614–3618.

Craciunescu, C.N., Brown, E.C., Mar, M.H. et al. (2004). Folic acid deficiency during late gestation decreases progenitor cell proliferation and increases apoptosis in fetal mouse brain. *The Journal of Nutrition* 134 (1): 162–166.

Crescenzo, R., Samec, S., Antic, V. et al. (2003). A role for suppressed thermogenesis favoring catch-up fat in the pathophysiology of catch-up growth. *Diabetes* 52 (5): 1090–1097.

Cui, X., Pelekanos, M., Liu, P.Y. et al. (2013). The vitamin D receptor in dopamine neurons; its presence in human substantia nigra and its ontogenesis in rat midbrain. *Neuroscience* 236: 77–87.

Cui, J., Zhou, B., Ross, S.A., and Zempleni, J. (2017). Nutrition, microRNAs, and human health. *Advances in Nutrition* 8 (1): 105–112.

Cunningham-Rundles, S., McNeeley, D.F., and Moon, A. (2005). Mechanisms of nutrient modulation of the immune response. *Journal of Allergy and Clinical Immunology* 115 (6): 1119–1128.

Curtis, E.M., Murray, R., Titcombe, P. et al. (2017). Perinatal DNA methylation at CDKN2A is associated with offspring bone mass: findings from the southampton women's survey. *Journal of Bone and Mineral Research* 32 (10): 2030–2040.

De Assis, S., Warri, A., Cruz, M.I. et al. (2012). High-fat or ethinyl-oestradiol intake during pregnancy increases mammary cancer risk in several generations of offspring. *Nature Communications* 3: 1053.

De Brito Alves, J.L., Nogueira, V.O., De Oliveira, G.B. et al. (2014). Short-and long-term effects of a maternal low-protein diet on ventilation, O2/CO2 chemoreception and arterial blood pressure in male rat offspring. *British Journal of Nutrition* 111 (4): 606–615.

De Mello, W.C. and Frohlich, E.D. (2014). Clinical perspectives and fundamental aspects of local cardiovascular and renal renin-angiotensin systems. *Frontiers in Endocrinology* 5: 6.

Dean, S.V., Lassi, Z.S., Imam, A.M., and Bhutta, Z.A. (2014). Preconception care: nutritional risks and interventions. *Reproductive Health* 11 (3): 1–15.

Deckelbaum, R.J., Worgall, T.S., and Seo, T. (2006). n– 3 fatty acids and gene expression. *The American Journal of Clinical Nutrition* 83 (6): 1520S–1525S.

Delion, S., Chalon, S., Guilloteau, D. et al. (1996). α-Linolenic acid dietary deficiency alters age-related changes of dopaminergic and serotoninergic neurotransmission in the rat frontal cortex. *Journal of Neurochemistry* 66 (4): 1582–1591.

Dennison, E.M., Syddall, H.E., Sayer, A.A. et al. (2005). Birth weight and weight at 1 year are independent determinants of bone mass in the seventh decade: the hertfordshire cohort study. *Pediatric Research* 57 (4): 582–586.

Devereux, G., Litonjua, A.A., Turner, S.W. et al. (2007). Maternal vitamin D intake during pregnancy and early childhood wheezing. *The American Journal of Clinical Nutrition* 85 (3): 853–859.

Devlin, A.M., Arning, E., Bottiglieri, T. et al. (2004). Effect of Mthfr genotype on diet-induced hyperhomocysteinemia and vascular function in mice. *Blood* 103 (7): 2624–2629.

Ding, G.L., Wang, F.F., Shu, J. et al. (2012). Transgenerational glucose intolerance with Igf2/H19 epigenetic alterations in mouse islet induced by intrauterine hyperglycemia. *Diabetes* 61 (5): 1133–1142.

Dobbing, J. and Sands, J. (1973). Quantitative growth and development of human brain. *Archives of Disease in Childhood* 48 (10): 757–767.

Dolinoy, D.C. (2008). The agouti mouse model: an epigenetic biosensor for nutritional and environmental alterations on the fetal epigenome. *Nutrition Reviews* 66 (SUPPL.1): S7.

Dolinoy, D.C. and Jirtle, R.L. (2008). Environmental epigenomics in human health and disease. *Environmental and Molecular Mutagenesis* 49 (1): 4–8.

Dong, E., Agis-Balboa, R.C., Simonini, M.V. et al. (2005). Reelin and glutamic acid decarboxylase67 promoter remodeling in an epeginetic methionine-induced mouse model of schizophrenia. *Proceedings of the National Academy of Sciences of the United States of America* 102 (35): 12578–12583.

Dong, F., Ford, S.P., Fang, C.X. et al. (2005). Maternal nutrient restriction during early to mid gestation up-regulates cardiac insulin-like growth factor (IGF) receptors associated with enlarged ventricular size in fetal sheep. *Growth Hormone & IGF Research* 15 (4): 291–299.

Donohoe, D.R. and Bultman, S.J. (2012). Metaboloepigenetics: interrelationships between energy metabolism and epigenetic control of gene expression. *Journal of Cellular Physiology* 227 (9): 3169–3177.

Ducker, G.S. and Rabinowitz, J.D. (2017). One-carbon metabolism in health and disease. *Cell Metabolism* 25 (1): 27–42.

Dumortier, O., Blondeau, B., Duvillié, B. et al. (2007). Different mechanisms operating during different critical time-windows reduce rat fetal beta cell mass due to a maternal low-protein or low-energy diet. *Diabetologia* 50 (12): 2495–2503.

Dupont, C., Kappeler, L., Saget, S. et al. (2019). Role of miRNA in the transmission of metabolic diseases associated with paternal diet-induced obesity. *Frontiers in Genetics* 10: 336.

Dutta-Roy, A.K. (2000). Transport mechanisms for long-chain polyunsaturated fatty acids in the human placenta. *American Journal of Clinical Nutrition* 71 (1): 315s–322s.

Edbauer, D., Neilson, J.R., Foster, K.A. et al. (2010). Regulation of synaptic structure and function by FMRP-associated MicroRNAs miR-125b and miR-132. *Neuron* 65 (3): 373–384.

Edlow, A.G., Guedj, F., Sverdlov, D. et al. (2019). Significant effects of maternal diet during pregnancy on the murine fetal brain transcriptome and offspring behavior. *Frontiers in Neuroscience* 13: 1335.

Ehlers, M.R. and Todd, R.M. (2017). Genesis and maintenance of attentional biases: the role of the locus coeruleus-noradrenaline system. *Neural Plasticity* 1 (1): 2–3.

Elias, S.G., Peeters, P.H.M., Grobbee, D.E., and Van Noord, P.A.H. (2007). Transient caloric restriction and cancer risk (The Netherlands). *Cancer Causes and Control* 18 (1): 1–5.

Elmquist, J.K., Ahima, R.S., Elias, C.F. et al. (1998). Leptin activates distinct projections from the dorsomedial and ventromedial hypothalamic nuclei. *Proceedings of the National Academy of Sciences of the United States of America* 95 (2): 741–746.

England, L.J., Catalano, P.M., Levine, R.J. et al. (2004). Glucose tolerance and risk of gestational diabetes mellitus in nulliparous women who smoke during pregnancy. *American Journal of Epidemiology* 160 (12): 1205–1213.

Eyles, D., Brown, J., Mackay-Sim, A. et al. (2003). Vitamin D3 and brain development. *Neuroscience* 118 (3): 641–653.

Eyles, D.W., Rogers, F., Buller, K. et al. (2006). Developmental vitamin D (DVD) deficiency in the rat alters adult behaviour independently of HPA function. *Psychoneuroendocrinology* 31 (8): 958–964.

Eyles, D., Almeras, L., Benech, P. et al. (2007). Developmental vitamin D deficiency alters the expression of genes encoding mitochondrial, cytoskeletal and synaptic proteins in the adult rat brain. *Journal of Steroid Biochemistry and Molecular Biology* 103 (3–5): 538–545.

Eyles, D.W., Trzaskowski, M., Vinkhuyzen, A.A.E. et al. (2018). The association between neonatal vitamin D status and risk of schizophrenia. *Scientific Reports* 8 (1): 1–8.

Fall, C., Hindmarsh, P., Dennison, E. et al. (1998). Programming of growth hormone secretion and bone mineral density in elderly men: a Hypothesis 1. *The Journal of Clinical Endocrinology & Metabolism* 83 (1): 135–139.

Fang, M.Z., Wang, Y., Ai, N. et al. (2003). Tea Polyphenol ()-Epigallocatechin-3-Gallate Inhibits DNA Methyltransferase and reactivates methylation-silenced genes in cancer cell lines. *Cancer Research* 63: 7563.

Fang, M., Chen, D., and Yang, C.S. (2007). Dietary polyphenols may affect DNA methylation. *The Journal of Nutrition* 131: 1223S–1228S.

Felekkis, K., Touvana, E., Stefanou, C., and Deltas, C. (2010). MicroRNAs: a newly described class of encoded molecules that play a role in health and disease. *Hippokratia* 14 (4): 236–240.

Férézou-Viala, J., Roy, A.F., Sérougne, C. et al. (2007). Long-term consequences of maternal high-fat feeding on hypothalamic leptin sensitivity and diet-induced obesity in the offspring. *American Journal of Physiology. Regulatory, Integrative and Comparative Physiology* 293 (3): 1056–1062.

Fernandez-Rebollo, E., Eipel, M., Seefried, L. et al. (2018). Primary osteoporosis is not reflected by disease-specific DNA methylation or accelerated epigenetic age in blood. *Journal of Bone and Mineral Research* 33 (2): 356–361.

Fernandez-Twinn, D.S., Ekizoglou, S., Gusterson, B.A. et al. (2007). Compensatory mammary growth following protein restriction during pregnancy and lactation increases early-onset mammary tumor incidence in rats. *Carcinogenesis* 28 (3): 545–552.

Féron, F., Burne, T.H.J., Brown, J. et al. (2005). Developmental Vitamin D3 deficiency alters the adult rat brain. *Brain Research Bulletin* 65 (2): 141–148.

Finer, S., Iqbal, M.S., Lowe, R. et al. (2016). Is famine exposure during developmental life in rural Bangladesh associated with a metabolic and epigenetic signature in young adulthood? A historical cohort study. *BMJ Open* 6 (11): e011768.

Firouzabadi, N., Ghazanfari, N., Alavi Shoushtari, A. et al. (2016). Genetic variants of angiotensin-converting enzyme are linked to autism: a case-control study. *PLoS One* 11 (4): e0153667.

Fleming, T.P., Watkins, A.J., Velazquez, M.A. et al. (2018). Origins of lifetime health around the time of conception: causes and consequences. *The Lancet* 391 (10132): 1842–1852.

Forno, E., Young, O.M., Kumar, R. et al. (2014). Maternal obesity in pregnancy, gestational weight gain, and risk of childhood asthma. *Pediatrics* 134 (2): e535.

Franchina, T., Amodeo, V., Bronte, G. et al. (2014). Circulating miR-22, miR-24 and miR-34a as novel predictive biomarkers to pemetrexed-based chemotherapy in advanced non-small cell lung cancer. *Journal of Cellular Physiology* 229 (1): 97–99.

Friso, S., Carvajal, C.A., Fardella, C.E., and Olivieri, O. (2015). Epigenetics and arterial hypertension: the challenge of emerging evidence. *Translational Research* 165 (1): 154–165.

Friso, S., Udali, S., De Santis, D., and Choi, S.W. (2017). One-carbon metabolism and epigenetics. *Molecular Aspects of Medicine* 54: 28–36.

Froese, D.S., Fowler, B., and Baumgartner, M.R. (2019). Vitamin B_{12}, folate, and the methionine remethylation cycle-biochemistry, pathways, and regulation. *Journal of Inherited Metabolic Disease* 42 (4): 673–685.

Fu, Q., Yu, X., Callaway, C.W. et al. (2009). Epigenetics: intrauterine growth retardation (IUGR) modifies the histone code along the rat hepatic IGF-1 gene. *The FASEB Journal* 23 (8): 2438–2449.

Gaedicke, S., Zhang, X., Schmelzer, C. et al. (2008). Vitamin E dependent microRNA regulation in rat liver. *FEBS Letters* 582 (23–24): 3542–3546.

Gaillard, R., Welten, M., Oddy, W. et al. (2016). Associations of maternal prepregnancy body mass index and gestational weight gain with cardio-metabolic risk factors in adolescent offspring: a prospective cohort study. *BJOG: An International Journal of Obstetrics & Gynaecology* 123 (2): 207–216.

Gali Ramamoorthy, T., Allen, T.J., Davies, A. et al. (2018). Maternal overnutrition programs epigenetic changes in the regulatory regions of hypothalamic Pomc in the offspring of rats. *International Journal of Obesity* 42 (8): 1431–1444.

Ganpule, A., Yajnik, C.S., Fall, C.H.D. et al. (2006). Bone mass in Indian children – relationships to maternal nutritional status and diet during pregnancy: the Pune maternal nutrition study. *Journal of Clinical Endocrinology and Metabolism* 91 (8): 2994–3001.

GAO, L., CUI, S.S., HAN, Y. et al. (2016). Does periconceptional fish consumption by parents affect the incidence of autism spectrum disorder and intelligence deficiency? A case-control study in Tianjin, China. *Biomedical and Environmental Sciences* 29 (12): 885–892.

Gapp, K., Jawaid, A., Sarkies, P. et al. (2014). Implication of sperm RNAs in transgenerational inheritance of the effects of early trauma in mice. *Nature Neuroscience* 17 (5): 667–669.

Gard, P.R. (2002). The role of angiotensin II in cognition and behaviour. *European Journal of Pharmacology* 438 (1–2): 1–14.

Gard, P.R. (2004). Angiotensin as a target for the treatment of Alzheimer's disease, anxiety and depression. *Expert Opinion on Therapeutic Targets* 8 (1): 7–14.

Garofano, A., Czernichow, P., and Bréant, B. (1997). In utero undernutrition impairs rat beta-cell development. *Diabetologia* 40 (10): 1231–1234.

Garofano, A., Czernichow, P., and Bréant, B. (1998). Beta-cell mass and proliferation following late fetal and early postnatal malnutrition in the rat. *Diabetologia* 41 (9): 1114–1120.

Garofano, A., Czernichow, P., and Bréant, B. (1999). Effect of ageing on beta-cell mass and function in rats malnourished during the perinatal period. *Diabetologia* 42 (6): 711–718.

Ghanizadeh, A., Akhondzadeh, S., Hormozi, M. et al. (2012). Glutathione-related factors and oxidative stress in autism, a review. *Current Medicinal Chemistry* 19 (23): 4000–4005.

Ghosh, P., Bitsanis, D., Ghebremeskel, K. et al. (2001). Abnormal aortic fatty acid composition and small artery function in offspring of rats fed a high fat diet in pregnancy. *Journal of Physiology* 533 (3): 815–822.

Gilbert, J.S. and Nijland, M.J. (2008). Sex differences in the developmental origins of hypertension and cardiorenal disease. *American Journal of Physiology. Regulatory, Integrative and Comparative Physiology* 295 (6): 1941–1952.

Gilles, S., Akdis, C., Lauener, R. et al. (2018). The role of environmental factors in allergy: a critical reappraisal. *Experimental Dermatology* 27 (11): 1193–1200.

Gluckman, P.D. and Pinal, C.S. (2003). Regulation of fetal growth by the somatotrophic axis. *The Journal of Nutrition* 133 (5): 1741S–1746S.

Gluckman, P.D., Hanson, M.A., Cooper, C., and Thornburg, K.L. (2008). Effect of in utero and early-life conditions on adult health and disease. *New England Journal of Medicine* 359 (1): 61.

Gluckman, P.D., Hanson, M.A., and Buklijas, T. (2010). A conceptual framework for the developmental origins of health and disease. *Journal of Developmental Origins of Health and Disease* 1 (1): 6–18.

Godfrey, K.M., Sheppard, A., Gluckman, P.D. et al. (2011). Epigenetic gene promoter methylation at birth is associated with child's later adiposity. *Diabetes* 60 (5): 1528–1534.

Gong, L., Pan, Y.X., and Chen, H. (2010). Gestational low protein diet in the rat mediates Igf2 gene expression in male offspring via altered hepatic DNA methylation. *Epigenetics* 5 (7): 619–626.

Gonzalez-Bulnes, A., Astiz, S., Ovilo, C. et al. (2014). Early-postnatal changes in adiposity and lipids profile by transgenerational developmental programming in swine with obesity/leptin resistance. *Journal of Endocrinology* 223 (1): M17–M29.

Gonzalez-Rodriguez, P., Cantu, J., O'Neil, D. et al. (2016). Alterations in expression of imprinted genes from the H19/IGF2 loci in a multigenerational model of intrauterine growth restriction (IUGR). *American Journal of Obstetrics and Gynecology* 214 (5): 625.e1–625.e11.

Gottrand, F. (2008). Long-chain polyunsaturated fatty acids influence the immune system of infants. *The Journal of Nutrition* 138 (9): 1807S–1812S.

Goyal, R., Goyal, D., Leitzke, A. et al. (2010). Brain renin-angiotensin system: fetal epigenetic programming by maternal protein restriction during pregnancy. *Reproductive Sciences* 17 (3): 227–238.

Graaff, J.S.-d., Tiemeier, H., Ghassabian, A. et al. (2015). Maternal fatty acid status during pregnancy and child autistic traits: the generation R study. *Prenatal nutrition and early childhood behaviour* 183 (9): 111.

Grabrucker, A.M. (2013). Environmental factors in autism. *Frontiers in Psychiatry* 3: 118.

Grayson, D.R., Jia, X., Chen, Y. et al. (2005). Reelin promoter hypermethylation in schizophrenia. *Proceedings of the National Academy of Sciences of the United States of America* 102 (26): 9341–9346.

Gregoretti, I.V., Lee, Y.M., and Goodson, H.V. (2004). Molecular evolution of the histone deacetylase family: functional implications of phylogenetic analysis. *Journal of Molecular Biology* 338 (1): 17–31.

Grimm, H., Mayer, K., Mayser, P., and Eigenbrodt, E. (2002). Regulatory potential of n -3 fatty acids in immunological and inflammatory processes. *British Journal of Nutrition* 87 (S1): S59–S67.

Group, L.S. (2007). Maternal diet during pregnancy in relation to eczema and allergic sensitization in the offspring at 2 year of age. *The American Journal of Clinical Nutrition* 85 (2): 530–537.

Groves, N.J., McGrath, J.J., and Burne, T.H.J. (2014). Vitamin D as a neurosteroid affecting the developing and adult brain. *Annual Review of Nutrition* 34: 117–141.

Guay, C. and Regazzi, R. (2015). Role of islet microRNAs in diabetes: which model for which question? *Diabetologia* 58 (3): 456–463.

Guay, C., Jacovetti, C., Nesca, V. et al. (2012). Emerging roles of non-coding RNAs in pancreatic β-cell function and dysfunction. *Diabetes, Obesity and Metabolism* 14 (SUPPL.3): 12–21.

Guéant, J.L., Elakoum, R., Ziegler, O. et al. (2014). Nutritional models of foetal programming and nutrigenomic and epigenomic dysregulations of fatty acid metabolism in the liver and heart. *Pflügers Archiv/European Journal of Physiology* 466 (5): 833–850.

Gujar, H., Weisenberger, D.J., and Liang, G. (2019). The roles of human DNA methyltransferases and their isoforms in shaping the epigenome. *Genes* 10 (2).

Gupta, A., Srinivasan, M., Thamadilok, S., and Patel, M.S. (2009). Hypothalamic alterations in fetuses of high fat diet-fed obese female rats. *Journal of Endocrinology* 200 (3): 293–300.

Gustafsson, C., Mjösberg, J., Matussek, A. et al. (2008). Gene expression profiling of human decidual macrophages: evidence for immunosuppressive phenotype. *PLoS One* 3 (4): e2078.

Habib, S.H. and Saha, S. (2010). Burden of non-communicable disease: global overview. *Diabetes and Metabolic Syndrome: Clinical Research and Reviews* 4 (1): 41–47.

Haghighi, F., Galfalvy, H., Chen, S. et al. (2015). DNA methylation perturbations in genes involved in polyunsaturated fatty acid biosynthesis associated with depression and suicide risk. *Frontiers in Neurology* 6: 92.

Hanafi, M.Y., Saleh, M.M., Saad, M.I. et al. (2016). Transgenerational effects of obesity and malnourishment on diabetes risk in F2 generation. *Molecular and Cellular Biochemistry* 412 (1–2): 269–280.

Hanieh, S., Ha, T.T., Simpson, J.A. et al. (2014). Maternal vitamin D status and infant outcomes in rural vietnam: a prospective cohort study. *PLoS One* 9 (6): e99005.

Harel, Z. and Tannenbaum, G.S. (1995). Long-term alterations in growth hormone and insulin secretion after temporary dietary protein restriction in early life in the rat. *Pediatric Research* 38 (5): 747–753.

Harvey, N.C., Sheppard, A., Godfrey, K.M. et al. (2014). Childhood bone mineral content is associated with methylation status of the RXRA promoter at birth. *Journal of Bone and Mineral Research* 29 (3): 600–607.

Hassa, P.O., Haenni, S.S., Elser, M., and Hottiger, M.O. (2006). Nuclear ADP-ribosylation reactions in mammalian cells: where are we today and where are we going? *Microbiology and Molecular Biology Reviews* 70 (3): 789–829.

Hassan, F.U., Rehman, M.S.U., Khan, M.S. et al. (2019). Curcumin as an alternative epigenetic modulator: mechanism of action and potential effects. *Frontiers in Genetics* 10: 514.

Hawes, J.E., Tesic, D., Whitehouse, A.J. et al. (2015). Maternal vitamin D deficiency alters fetal brain development in the BALB/c mouse. *Behavioural Brain Research* 286: 192–200.

He, F., Lupu, D.S., and Niculescu, M.D. (2014). Perinatal α-linolenic acid availability alters the expression of genes related to memory and to epigenetic machinery, and the Mecp2 DNA methylation in the whole brain of mouse offspring. *International Journal of Developmental Neuroscience* 36: 38–44.

Healy, S., Perez-Cadahia, B., Jia, D. et al. (2009). Biotin is not a natural histone modification. *Biochimica et Biophysica Acta, Gene Regulatory Mechanisms* 1789 (11–12): 719–733.

Heijmans, B.T., Tobi, E.W., Stein, A.D. et al. (2008). Persistent epigenetic differences associated with prenatal exposure to famine in humans. *Proceedings of the National Academy of Sciences of the United States of America* 105 (44): 17046–17049.

Heijmans, B.T., Tobi, E.W., Lumey, L.H., and Slagboom, P.E. (2009). The epigenome: archive of the prenatal environment. *Human Molecular Genetics* 18 (21): 4046–4053.

Hilakivi-Clarke, L. and de Assis, S. (2006). Fetal origins of breast cancer. *Trends in Endocrinology and Metabolism* 17 (9): 340–348.

Hilakivi-Clarke, L., Clarke, R., Onojafe, I. et al. (1997). A maternal diet high in n - 6 polyunsaturated fats alters mammary gland development, puberty onset, and breast cancer risk among female rat offspring. *Proceedings of the National Academy of Sciences of the United States of America* 94 (17): 9372–9377.

Himes, J.H., Caulfield, L.E., Martorell, R., and Delgado, H. (1990). Maternal supplementation and bone growth in infancy. *Paediatric and Perinatal Epidemiology* 4 (4): 436–447.

Ho, S.-M., Johnson, A., Tarapore, P. et al. (2012). Environmental Epigenetics and Its Implication on Disease Risk and Health Outcomes. *ILAR Journal* 53 (3–4): 289–305.

Hoile, S.P., Clarke-Harris, R., Huang, R.C. et al. (2014). Supplementation with n-3 long-chain polyunsaturated fatty acids or olive oil in men and women with renal disease induces differential changes in the DNA methylation of FADS2 and ELOVL5 in peripheral blood mononuclear cells. *PLoS One* 9 (10): e109896.

Hollingsworth, J.W., Maruoka, S., Boon, K. et al. (2008). In utero supplementation with methyl donors enhances allergic airway disease in mice. *The Journal of Clinical Investigation* 118 (10): 3462–3469.

Horsthemke, B. (2018). A critical view on transgenerational epigenetic inheritance in humans. *Nature Communications* 9 (1).

Hou, H. and Yu, H. (2010). Structural insights into histone lysine demethylation. *Current Opinion in Structural Biology* 20 (6): 739–748.

Howie, G.J., Sloboda, D.M., Kamal, T., and Vickers, M.H. (2009). Maternal nutritional history predicts obesity in adult offspring independent of postnatal diet. *Journal of Physiology* 587 (4): 905–915.

Huang, C., Li, Z., Wang, M., and Martorell, R. (2010). Early life exposure to the 1959–1961 chinese famine has long-term health consequences. *The Journal of Nutrition* 140 (10): 1874–1878.

Huang, S., Dai, Y., Zhang, Z. et al. (2014). Docosahexaenoic acid intake ameliorates ketamine-induced impairment of spatial cognition and learning ability in ICR mice. *Neuroscience Letters* 580: 125–129.

Huang, H., Liu, L., Li, B. et al. (2015). Ketamine Interferes with the proliferation and differentiation of neural stem cells in the subventricular zone of neonatal Rats. *Cellular Physiology and Biochemistry* 35 (1): 315–325.

Huang, T., Zheng, Y., Hruby, A. et al. (2017). Dietary protein modifies the effect of the MC4R genotype on 2-year changes in appetite and food craving: the POUNDS lost trial. *The Journal of Nutrition* 147 (3): jn242958.

Hult, M., Tornhammar, P., Ueda, P. et al. (2010). Hypertension, diabetes and overweight: looming legacies of the biafran famine. *PLoS One* 5 (10): e13582.

Huypens, P., Sass, S., Wu, M. et al. (2016). Epigenetic germline inheritance of diet-induced obesity and insulin resistance. *Nature Genetics* 48 (5): 497–499.

Hyde, N.K., Brennan-Olsen, S.L., Wark, J.D. et al. (2017). Maternal dietary nutrient intake during pregnancy and offspring linear growth and bone: the Vitamin D in pregnancy cohort study. *Calcified Tissue International* 100 (1): 47–54.

Ibáñez, L., Ong, K., Dunger, D.B., and de Zegher, F. (2006). Early development of adiposity and insulin resistance after catch-up weight gain in small-for-gestational-age children. *The Journal of Clinical Endocrinology & Metabolism* 91 (6): 2153–2158.

Ingrosso, D., Cimmino, A., Perna, A.F. et al. (2003). Folate treatment and unbalanced methylation and changes of allelic expression induced by hyperhomocysteinaemia in patients with uraemia. *Lancet* 361 (9370): 1693–1699.

Innis, S.M. (2008). Dietary omega 3 fatty acids and the developing brain. *Brain Research* 1237: 35–43.

Inskip, H.M., Godfrey, K.M., Robinson, S.M. et al. (2006). Cohort profile: the Southampton women's survey. *International Journal of Epidemiology* 35 (1): 42–48.

Islam, S.M.S., Purnat, T.D., Phuong, N.T.A. et al. (2014). Non communicable diseases (NCDs) in developing countries: a symposium report. *Globalization and Health* 10 (1): 81.

Janke, R., Dodson, A.E., and Rine, J. (2015). Metabolism and epigenetics. *Annual Review of Cell and Developmental Biology* 31 (1): 473–496.

Jaquet, D., Gaboriau, A., Czernichow, P., and Levy-Marchal, C. (2000). Insulin resistance early in adulthood in subjects born with intrauterine growth Retardation1. *The Journal of Clinical Endocrinology & Metabolism* 85 (4): 1401–1406.

Jiang, Y. and Huang, C. (2015). Polymorphism and cognition: the example of Folate and MTHFR C677T. In: *Diet and Nutrition in Dementia and Cognitive Decline* (eds. C.R. Martin and V.R. Preedy), 357–367. Elsevier Inc.

Jin, B., Li, Y., and Robertson, K.D. (2011). DNA methylation: superior or subordinate in the epigenetic hierarchy? *Genes & Cancer* 2 (6): 607–617.

Jirtle, R.L. and Skinner, M.K. (2007). Environmental epigenomics and disease susceptibility. *Nature Reviews Genetics* 8 (4): 253–262.

Julvez, J., Mendéz, M., Fernandez-Barres, S. et al. (2016). Maternal consumption of seafood in pregnancy and child neuropsychological development: a longitudinal study based on a population with high consumption levels. *American Journal of Epidemiology* 183 (3): 169–182.

Junge, K.M., Bauer, T., Geissler, S. et al. (2016). Increased Vitamin D levels at birth and in early infancy increase offspring allergy risk – evidence for involvement of epigenetic mechanisms. *Journal of Allergy and Clinical Immunology* 137 (2): 610–613.

Kadayifci, F.Z., Zheng, S., and Pan, Y.X. (2018). Molecular mechanisms underlying the link between diet and DNA methylation. *International Journal of Molecular Sciences* 19 (12).

Kahn, L.P., Knox, M.R., Gray, G.D. et al. (2003). Enhancing immunity to nematode parasites in single-bearing Merino ewes through nutrition and genetic selection. *Veterinary Parasitology* 112 (3): 211–225.

Kaiko, G.E., Horvat, J.C., Beagley, K.W., and Hansbro, P.M. (2008). Immunological decision-making: how does the immune system decide to mount a helper T-cell response? *Immunology* 123 (3): 326–338.

Kandi, V. and Vadakedath, S. (2015). Effect of DNA Methylation in various diseases and the probable protective role of nutrition: a mini-review. *Cureus* 7 (8): e309.

Kapoor, A., Dunn, E., Kostaki, A. et al. (2006). Fetal programming of hypothalamo-pituitary-adrenal function: prenatal stress and glucocorticoids. *The Journal of Physiology* 572 (1): 31–44.

Karras, S.N., Fakhoury, H., Muscogiuri, G. et al. (2016). Maternal vitamin D levels during pregnancy and neonatal health: evidence to date and clinical implications. *Therapeutic Advances in Musculoskeletal Disease* 8 (4): 124–135.

Kawamura, M., Itoh, H., Yura, S. et al. (2009). Isocaloric high-protein diet ameliorates systolic blood pressure increase and cardiac remodeling caused by maternal caloric restriction in adult mouse offspring. *Endocrine Journal* 56 (5): 679–689.

Keim, S.A., Bodnar, L.M., and Klebanoff, M.A. (2014). Maternal and cord blood 25(OH)-Vitamin D concentrations in relation to child development and behaviour. *Paediatric and Perinatal Epidemiology* 28 (5): 434–444.

Kesby, J.P., Burne, T.H.J., McGrath, J.J., and Eyles, D.W. (2006). Developmental Vitamin D deficiency alters MK 801-induced hyperlocomotion in the adult rat: an animal model of Schizophrenia. *Biological Psychiatry* 60 (6): 591–596.

Khan, I.Y., Taylor, P.D., Dekou, V. et al. (2003). Gender-linked hypertension in offspring of lard-fed pregnant rats. *Hypertension* 41 (1): 168–175.

Khoury, S., Soubeyre, V., Cabaret, S. et al. (2020). Perinatal exposure to diets with different n-6:n-3 fatty acid ratios affects olfactory tissue fatty acid composition. *Scientific Reports* 10 (1): 1–15.

Kim, Y.I. (2016). Current status of folic acid supplementation on colorectal cancer prevention. *Current Pharmacology Reports* 2 (1): 21–33.

Kim, Y.I., Miller, J.W., da Costa, K.A. et al. (1994). Severe folate deficiency causes secondary depletion of choline and phosphocholine in rat liver. *The Journal of Nutrition* 124 (11): 2197–2203.

Kim, S.J., Kang, J.I., Namkoong, K., and Song, D.H. (2011). The effects of serotonin transporter promoter and monoamine oxidase a gene polymorphisms on trait emotional intelligence. *Neuropsychobiology* 64 (4): 224–230.

Kirk, S.L., Samuelsson, A.M., Argenton, M. et al. (2009). Maternal obesity induced by diet in rats permanently influences central processes regulating food intake in offspring. *PLoS One* 4 (6): e5870.

Kirkland, J.B. (2009). Niacin status impacts chromatin structure. *The Journal of Nutrition* 139 (12): 2397–2401.

Kitajka, K., Sinclair, A.J., Weisinger, R.S. et al. (2004). Effects of dietary omega-3 polyunsaturated fatty acids on brain gene expression. *Proceedings of the National Academy of Sciences of the United States of America* 101 (30): 10931–10936.

Klibanski, A., Adams-Campbell, L., Bassford, T. et al. (2001). Osteoporosis prevention, diagnosis, and therapy. *Journal of the American Medical Association* 285 (6): 785–795.

Koch, M.A., Perdue, N.R., Killebrew, J.R. et al. (2009). The transcription factor T-bet controls regulatory T cell homeostasis and function during type 1 inflammation. *Nature Immunology* 10 (6): 595.

Konishi, Y., Takahashi, K., Chui, D.H. et al. (1994). Insulin-like growth factor II promotes in vitro cholinergic development of mouse septal neurons: comparison with the effects of insulin-like growth factor I. *Brain Research* 649 (1–2): 53–61.

Koo, W.W.K., Walters, J.C., Esterlitz, J. et al. (1999). Maternal calcium supplementation and fetal bone mineralization. *Obstetrics and Gynecology* 94 (4): 577–582.

Koturbash, I., Melnyk, S., James, S.J. et al. (2013). Role of epigenetic and miR-22 and miR-29b alterations in the downregulation of Mat1a and Mthfr genes in early preneoplastic livers in rats induced by 2-acetylaminofluorene. *Molecular Carcinogenesis* 52 (4): 318–327.

Koupil, I., Shestov, D.B., Sparén, P. et al. (2007). Blood pressure, hypertension and mortality from circulatory disease in men and women who survived the siege of Leningrad. *European Journal of Epidemiology* 22 (4): 223–234.

Kovacheva, V.P., Mellott, T.J., Davison, J.M. et al. (2007). Gestational choline deficiency causes global and Igf2 gene DNA hypermethylation by up-regulation of Dnmt1 expression. *Journal of Biological Chemistry* 282 (43): 31777–31788.

Kovacs, C.S. (2014). Bone development and mineral homeostasis in the fetus and neonate: roles of the calciotropic and phosphotropic hormones. *Physiological Reviews* 94 (4): 1143–1218.

Kroon, T., Sierksma, M.C., and Meredith, R.M. (2013). Investigating mechanisms underlying neurodevelopmental phenotypes of autistic and intellectual disability disorders: a perspective. *Frontiers in Systems Neuroscience* 7: 75.

Kruman, I.I., Mouton, P.R., Emokpae, R. et al. (2005). Folate deficiency inhibits proliferation of adult hippocampal progenitors. *NeuroReport* 16 (10): 1055–1059.

Kulkarni, A., Dangat, K., Kale, A. et al. (2011). Effects of altered maternal folic acid, vitamin B_{12} and docosahexaenoic acid on placental global DNA methylation patterns in wistar rats. *PLoS One* 6 (3).

Kumar, A. and Kaur, S. (2017). Calcium: a nutrient in pregnancy. *Journal of Obstetrics and Gynecology of India* 67 (5): 313–318.

Kumar, R., Singh, V.P., and Baker, K.M. (2007). The intracellular renin-angiotensin system: a new paradigm. *Trends in Endocrinology and Metabolism* 18 (5): 208–214.

Kurd, N. and Robey, E.A. (2016). T-cell selection in the thymus: a spatial and temporal perspective. *Immunological Reviews* 271 (1): 114–126.

Lack, G. (2012). Update on risk factors for food allergy. *Journal of Allergy and Clinical Immunology* 129 (5): 1187–1197.

Lafontan, M., Moro, C., Sengenes, C. et al. (2005). An unsuspected metabolic role for atrial natriuretic peptides: the control of lipolysis, lipid mobilization, and systemic nonesterified fatty acids levels in humans. *Arteriosclerosis, Thrombosis, and Vascular Biology* 25 (10): 2032–2042.

Laker, R.C., Wlodek, M.E., Connelly, J.J., and Yan, Z. (2013). Epigenetic origins of metabolic disease: the impact of the maternal condition to the offspring epigenome and later health consequences. *Food Science and Human Wellness* 2 (1): 1–11.

Langley-Evans, S.C. (2015). Nutrition in early life and the programming of adult disease: a review. *Journal of Human Nutrition and Dietetics* 28 (s1): 1–14.

Lanham, S.A., Roberts, C., Cooper, C., and Oreffo, R.O.C. (2008). Intrauterine programming of bone. Part 1: alteration of the osteogenic environment. *Osteoporosis International* 19 (2): 147–156.

Latour, A., Grintal, B., Champeil-Potokar, G. et al. (2013). Omega-3 fatty acids deficiency aggravates glutamatergic synapse and astroglial aging in the rat hippocampal CA1. *Aging Cell* 12 (1): 76–84.

Lecoutre, S., Petrus, P., Rydén, M., and Breton, C. (2018). Transgenerational epigenetic mechanisms in adipose tissue development. *Trends in Endocrinology and Metabolism* 29 (10): 675–685.

Lee, G.R., Kim, S.T., Spilianakis, C.G. et al. (2006). T helper cell differentiation: regulation by cis elements and epigenetics. *Immunity* 24 (4): 369–379.

Lee, B.K., Eyles, D.W., Magnusson, C. et al. (2019). Developmental vitamin D and autism spectrum disorders: findings from the Stockholm Youth Cohort. *Molecular Psychiatry*: 1–11.

Lei, X., Zhang, W., Liu, T. et al. (2013). Perinatal supplementation with Omega-3 polyunsaturated fatty acids improves sevoflurane-induced neurodegeneration and memory impairment in neonatal rats. *PLoS One* 8 (8): e70645.

Leunissen, R.W.J., Stijnen, T., Boot, A.M., and Hokken-Koelega, A.C.S. (2008). Influence of birth size and body composition on bone mineral density in early adulthood: the PROGRAM study. *Clinical Endocrinology* 69 (3): 386–392.

Li, C. and Lumey, L.H. (2017). Exposure to the Chinese famine of 1959–61 in early life and long-term health conditions: a systematic review and meta-analysis. *International Journal of Epidemiology* 46 (4): 1157–1170.

Li, Y., Kim, J., Buckett, P.D. et al. (2011). Severe postnatal iron deficiency alters emotional behavior and dopamine levels in the prefrontal cortex of young male rats. *Journal of Nutrition* 141 (12): 2133–2138.

Lillycrop, K.A., Phillips, E.S., Torrens, C. et al. (2008). Feeding pregnant rats a protein-restricted diet persistently alters the methylation of specific cytosines in the hepatic PPARα promoter of the offspring. *British Journal of Nutrition* 100 (2): 278–282.

Linnet, K.M., Dalsgaard, S., Obel, C. et al. (2003). Maternal lifestyle factors in pregnancy risk of attention deficit hyperactivity disorder and associated behaviors: review of the current evidence. *American Journal of Psychiatry* 160 (6): 1028–1040.

Lisé, M.F. and El-Husseini, A. (2006). The neuroligin and neurexin families: from structure to function at the synapse. *Cellular and Molecular Life Sciences* 63 (16): 1833–1849.

Litman, B.J. and Mitchell, D.C. (1996). A role for phospholipid polyunsaturation in modulating membrane protein function. *Lipids* 31 (3 SUPPL): S193–S197.

Liu, J. and Ma, D.W.L. (2014). The role of n-3 polyunsaturated fatty acids in the prevention and treatment of breast cancer. *Nutrients* 6 (11): 5184–5223.

Liu, Z., Xie, Z., Jones, W. et al. (2009). Curcumin is a potent DNA hypomethylation agent. *Bioorganic and Medicinal Chemistry Letters* 19 (3): 706–709.

Liu, Y., Ji, Y., Li, M. et al. (2018). Integrated analysis of long noncoding RNA and mRNA expression profile in children with obesity by microarray analysis. *Scientific Reports* 8 (1): 1–13.

Liu, Z.-G., Li, Y., Jiao, J.-H. et al. (2020). MicroRNA regulatory pattern in spinal cord ischemia-reperfusion injury. *Neural Regeneration Research* 15 (11): 2123.

López, A., Garmendia, M.L., Shepherd, J. et al. (2020). Effect of excessive gestational weight on daughters' breast density at the end of puberty onset. *Scientific Reports* 10 (1): 1–8.

Lu, T.X., Munitz, A., and Rothenberg, M.E. (2009). MicroRNA-21 Is up-regulated in allergic airway inflammation and regulates IL-12p35 expression. *The Journal of Immunology* 182 (8): 4994–5002.

Lumey, L.H., Stein, A.D., Kahn, H.S. et al. (2007). Cohort profile: the Dutch Hunger Winter families study. *International Journal of Epidemiology* 36 (6): 1196–1204.

Lumey, L.H., Stein, A.D., Kahn, H.S., and Romijn, J.A. (2009). Lipid profiles in middle-aged men and women after famine exposure during gestation: the Dutch Hunger Winter families study. *American Journal of Clinical Nutrition* 89 (6): 1737–1743.

Lumey, L.H., Stein, A.D., and Susser, E. (2011). Prenatal famine and adult health. *Annual Review of Public Health* 32 (1): 237–262.

Ly, A., Lee, H., Chen, J. et al. (2011). Effect of maternal and postweaning folic acid supplementation on mammary tumor risk in the offspring. *Cancer Research* 71 (3): 988–997.

Lyall, K., Munger, K.L., O'Reilly, É.J. et al. (2013). Maternal dietary fat intake in association with autism spectrum disorders. *American Journal of Epidemiology* 178 (2): 209–220.

Lyall, K., Schmidt, R.J., and Hertz-Picciotto, I. (2014). Maternal lifestyle and environmental risk factors for autism spectrum disorders. *International Journal of Epidemiology* 43 (2): 443–464.

MacLennan, M. and Ma, D.W.L. (2010). Role of dietary fatty acids in mammary gland development and breast cancer. *Breast Cancer Research* 12 (5): 211.

Mahabir, S. (2013). Association between diet during preadolescence and adolescence and risk for breast cancer during adulthood. *Journal of Adolescent Health* 52: S30eS35.

Maric-Bilkan, C., Symonds, M., Ozanne, S., and Alexander, B. (2011). Impact of maternal obesity and diabetes on long-term health of the offspring. *Journal of Diabetes Research*: 1–2.

Martin, R., Harvey, N.C., Crozier, S.R. et al. (2007). Placental calcium transporter (PMCA3) gene expression predicts intrauterine bone mineral accrual. *Bone* 40 (5): 1203–1208.

Martinez, M. (1992). Tissue levels of polyunsaturated fatty acids during early human development. *The Journal of Pediatrics* 120 (4): S129–S138.

Martino, D.J. and Prescott, S.L. (2011). Maternal Fibre and prebiotic intake during pregnancy and early lactation in allergy prevention View project Methylation-sensitive genes in food allergy View project. Elsevier.

Martín-Orozco, E., Norte-Muñoz, M., and Martínez-García, J. (2017). Regulatory T cells in allergy and asthma. *Frontiers in Pediatrics* 5: 1.

Martins, R., Lithgow, G.J., and Link, W. (2016). Long live FOXO: unraveling the role of FOXO proteins in aging and longevity. *Aging Cell* 15 (2): 196–207.

Martorell, R. (2017). Improved nutrition in the first 1000 days and adult human capital and health. *American Journal of Human Biology* 29 (2): e22952.

Maslova, E., Hansen, S., Jensen, C.B. et al. (2013). Vitamin D intake in mid-pregnancy and child allergic disease – a prospective study in 44,825 Danish mother-child pairs. *BMC Pregnancy and Childbirth* 13 (1): 199.

Masuyama, H., Mitsui, T., Nobumoto, E., and Hiramatsu, Y. (2015). The effects of high-fat diet exposure in utero on the obesogenic and diabetogenic traits through epigenetic changes in Adiponectin and Leptin gene expression for multiple generations in female mice. *Endocrinology* 156 (7): 2482–2491.

McCormick, M.C. (1985). The contribution of low birth weight to infant mortality and childhood morbidity. *New England Journal of Medicine* 312 (2): 82–90.

McCurdy, C.E., Bishop, J.M., Williams, S.M. et al. (2009). Maternal high-fat diet triggers lipotoxicity in the fetal livers of nonhuman primates. *Journal of Clinical Investigation* 119 (2): 323–335.

McGrath, J. (1999). Hypothesis: is low prenatal vitamin D a risk-modifying factor for schizophrenia? *Schizophrenia Research* 40 (3): 173–177.

McGrath, J., Eyles, D., Mowry, B. et al. (2003). Low maternal vitamin D as a risk factor for schizophrenia: a pilot study using banked sera. *Schizophrenia Research* 63 (1–2): 73–78.

McMillen, I.C. and Robinson, J.S. (2005). Developmental origins of the metabolic syndrome: prediction, plasticity, and programming. *Physiological Reviews* 85 (2): 571–633.

McNamara, R.K., Able, J., Liu, Y. et al. (2009). Omega-3 fatty acid deficiency during perinatal development increases serotonin turnover in the prefrontal cortex and decreases midbrain tryptophan hydroxylase-2 expression in adult female rats: dissociation from estrogenic effects. *Journal of Psychiatric Research* 43 (6): 656–663.

McNamara, R.K., Able, J.A., Liu, Y. et al. (2013). Omega-3 fatty acid deficiency does not alter the effects of chronic fluoxetine treatment on central serotonin turnover or behavior in the forced swim test in female rats. *Pharmacology Biochemistry and Behavior* 114–115: 1–8.

Meems, L.M.G., Mahmud, H., Buikema, H. et al. (2016). Parental vitamin d deficiency during pregnancy is associated with increased blood pressure in offspring via panx1 hypermethylation. *American Journal of Physiology - Heart and Circulatory Physiology* 311 (6): H1459–H1469.

Mehta, G., Roach, H.I., Langley-Evans, S. et al. (2002). Intrauterine exposure to a maternal low protein diet reduces adult bone mass and alters growth plate morphology in rats. *Calcified Tissue International* 71 (6): 493–498.

Mentch, S.J. and Locasale, J.W. (2016). One-carbon metabolism and epigenetics: understanding the specificity. *Annals of the New York Academy of Sciences* 1363 (1): 91–98.

Mertens, B., Vanderheyden, P., Michotte, Y., and Sarre, S. (2010). The role of the central renin-angiotensin system in Parkinson's disease. *Journal of the Renin-Angiotensin-Aldosterone System* 11 (1): 49–56.

Miles, E.A. and Calder, P.C. (2015). Maternal diet and its influence on the development of allergic disease. *Clinical and Experimental Allergy* 45 (1): 63–74.

Mody, I. and Maguire, J. (2012). The reciprocal regulation of stress hormones and GABA A receptors. *Frontiers in Cellular Neuroscience* 6: 4.

MolinaSerrano, D., Kyriakou, D., and Kirmizis, A. (2019). Histone modifications as an intersection between diet and longevity. *Frontiers in Genetics* 10: 192.

Moosavi, A. and Ardekani, A.M. (2016). Role of epigenetics in biology and human diseases. *Iranian Biomedical Journal* 20 (5): 246–258.

Morales, E., Guxens, M., Llop, S. et al. (2012). Circulating 25-hydroxyvitamin D3 in pregnancy and infant neuropsychological development. *Pediatrics* 130 (4): e913–e920.

Morales, E., Julvez, J., Torrent, M. et al. (2015). Vitamin D in pregnancy and attention deficit hyperactivity disorder-like symptoms in childhood. *Epidemiology* 26 (4): 458–465.

Morales, S., Monzo, M., and Navarro, A. (2017). Epigenetic regulation mechanisms of microRNA expression. *Biomolecular Concepts* 8 (5–6): 203–212.

Mørkve Knudsen, T., Rezwan, F.I., Jiang, Y. et al. (2018). Transgenerational and intergenerational epigenetic inheritance in allergic diseases. *Journal of Allergy and Clinical Immunology* 142 (3): 765–772.

Motta, M.C., Divecha, N., Lemieux, M. et al. (2004). Mammalian SIRT1 Represses Forkhead Transcription Factors. *Cell* 116 (4): 551–563.

Muhlhausler, B.S., Adam, C.L., Findlay, P.A. et al. (2006). Increased maternal nutrition alters development of the appetite-regulating network in the brain. *The FASEB Journal* 20 (8): E556–E565.

Muhlhausler, B.S., Duffield, J.A., and McMillen, I.C. (2007). Increased maternal nutrition stimulates peroxisome proliferator activated receptor-γ, adiponectin, and leptin messenger ribonucleic acid expression in adipose tissue before birth. *Endocrinology* 148 (2): 878–885.

Muiños-Gimeno, M., Espinosa-Parrilla, Y., Guidi, M. et al. (2011). Human microRNAs miR-22, miR-138-2, miR-148a, and miR-488 are associated with panic disorder and regulate several anxiety candidate genes and related pathways. *Biological Psychiatry* 69 (6): 526–533.

Muñoz-Durango, N., Fuentes, C.A., Castillo, A.E. et al. (2016). Role of the renin-angiotensin-aldosterone system beyond blood pressure regulation: molecular and cellular mechanisms involved in end-organ damage during arterial hypertension. *International Journal of Molecular Sciences* 17 (7): 797.

Münzberg, H., Huo, L., Nillni, E.A. et al. (2003). Role of signal transducer and activator of transcription 3 in regulation of hypothalamic Proopiomelanocortin gene expression by leptin. *Endocrinology* 144 (5): 2121–2131.

Nakahata, Y., Kaluzova, M., Grimaldi, B. et al. (2008). The NAD +-dependent deacetylase SIRT1 modulates CLOCK-mediated chromatin remodeling and circadian control. *Cell* 134 (2): 329–340.

Nakamura, M.T., Cheon, Y., Li, Y., and Nara, T.Y. (2004). Mechanisms of regulation of gene expression by fatty acids. *Lipids* 39 (11): 1077–1083.

Napoli, I., Blusztajn, J.K., and Mellott, T.J. (2008). Prenatal choline supplementation in rats increases the expression of IGF2 and its receptor IGF2R and enhances IGF2-induced acetylcholine release in hippocampus and frontal cortex. *Brain Research* 1237: 124–135.

Nathanielsz, P.W., Ford, S.P., Long, N.M. et al. (2013). Interventions to prevent adverse fetal programming due to maternal obesity during pregnancy. *Nutrition Reviews* 71 (SUPPL1): S78.

Nesca, V., Guay, C., Jacovetti, C. et al. (2013). Identification of particular groups of microRNAs that positively or negatively impact on beta cell function in obese models of type 2 diabetes. *Diabetologia* 56 (10): 2203–2212.

Newman, J.C. and Verdin, E. (2014). Ketone bodies as signaling metabolites. *Trends in Endocrinology and Metabolism* 25 (1): 42–52.

Nian, H., Delage, B., Ho, E., and Dashwood, R.H. (2009). Modulation of histone deacetylase activity by dietary isothiocyanates and allyl sulfides: studies with sulforaphane and garlic organosulfur compounds. *Environmental and Molecular Mutagenesis* 50 (3): 213–221.

Nicolas, E., Roumillac, C., and Trouche, D. (2003). Balance between Acetylation and Methylation of Histone H3 Lysine 9 on the E2F-Responsive Dihydrofolate Reductase Promoter. *Molecular and Cellular Biology* 23 (5): 1614–1622.

Niculescu, M.D., Lupu, D.S., and Craciunescu, C.N. (2013). Perinatal manipulation of α-linolenic acid intake induces epigenetic changes in maternal and offspring livers. *The FASEB Journal* 27 (1): 350–358.

Nijhuis, L., Peeters, J.G.C., Vastert, S.J., and Van Loosdregt, J. (2019). Restoring T cell tolerance, exploring the potential of histone deacetylase inhibitors for the treatment of juvenile idiopathic arthritis. *Frontiers in Immunology* 10: 151.

O'Garra, A. and Vieira, P. (2004). Regulatory T cells and mechanisms of immune system control. *Nature Medicine* 10 (8): 801–805.

Oberbauer, A.M. (2013). The regulation of IGF-1 gene transcription and splicing during development and aging. *Frontiers in Endocrinology* 4 (MAR): 39.

Oreffo, R.O.C., Lashbrooke, B., Roach, H.I. et al. (2003). Maternal protein deficiency affects mesenchymal stem cell activity in the developing offspring. *Bone* 33 (1): 100–107.

Overeem, K., Alexander, S., Burne, T.H.J. et al. (2019). Developmental Vitamin D deficiency in the rat impairs recognition memory, but has no effect on social approach or Hedonia. *Nutrients* 11 (11): 2713.

Ozaki, T., Nishina, H., Hanson, M.A., and Poston, L. (2001). Dietary restriction in pregnant rats causes gender-related hypertension and vascular dysfunction in offspring. *Journal of Physiology* 530 (1): 141–152.

Pacurari, M. and Tchounwou, P.B. (2015). Role of microRNAs in renin-angiotensin-aldosterone system-mediated cardiovascular inflammation and remodeling. *International Journal of Inflammation* 2015: 101527.

Padoan, A., Rigano, S., Ferrazzi, E. et al. (2004). Differences in fat and lean mass proportions in normal and growth-restricted fetuses. *American Journal of Obstetrics and Gynecology* 191 (4): 1459–1464.

Painter, R.C., Roseboom, T.J., and Bleker, O.P. (2005). Prenatal exposure to the Dutch famine and disease in later life: an overview. *Reproductive Toxicology* 20 (3): 345–352.

Pallos, J., Bodai, L., Lukacsovich, T. et al. (2008). Inhibition of specific HDACs and sirtuins suppresses pathogenesis in a Drosophila model of Huntington's disease. *Human Molecular Genetics* 17 (23): 3767–3675.

Palmer, D.J., Sullivan, T., Gold, M.S. et al. (2012). Effect of n-3 long chain polyunsaturated fatty acid supplementation in pregnancy on infants' allergies in first year of life: randomised controlled trial. *BMJ (Online)* 344 (7845): 14.

Pan, P., Jin, D.H.S., Chatterjee-Chakraborty, M. et al. (2014). The effects of vitamin D3 during pregnancy and lactation on offspring physiology and behavior in Sprague-Dawley rats. *Developmental Psychobiology* 56 (1): 12–22.

Paparo, L., Di Costanzo, M., Di Scala, C. et al. (2014). The influence of early life nutrition on epigenetic regulatory mechanisms of the immune system. *Nutrients* 6 (11): 4706–4719.

Parenti, I., Rabaneda, L.G., Schoen, H., and Novarino, G. (2020). Neurodevelopmental disorders: from genetics to functional pathways. *Trends in Neurosciences* 43 (8): 608–621.

Parlee, S.D. and MacDougald, O.A. (2014). Maternal nutrition and risk of obesity in offspring: the Trojan horse of developmental plasticity. *Biochimica et Biophysica Acta – Molecular Basis of Disease* 1842 (3): 495–506.

Pasqualotto, E.B., Agarwal, A., Sharma, R.K. et al. (2004). Effect of oxidative stress in follicular fluid on the outcome of assisted reproductive procedures. *Fertility and Sterility* 81 (4): 973–976.

Pasyukova, E.G. and Vaiserman, A.M. (2017). *HDAC Inhibitors: A New Promising Drug Class in Anti-Aging Research*. Elsevier.

Pate, M.B., Smith, J.K., Chi, D.S., and Krishnaswamy, G. (2010). Regulation and dysregulation of immunoglobulin E: a molecular and clinical perspective. *Clinical and Molecular Allergy* 8: 3.

Patel, A.R., Patra, F., Shah, N.P., and Shukla, D. (2017). Biological control of mycotoxins by probiotic lactic acid bacteria. *Dynamism in dairy industry and consumer demands* 2015 (February): 2–4.

Patrick, R.P. and Ames, B.N. (2015). Vitamin D and the omega-3 fatty acids control serotonin synthesis and action, part 2: relevance for ADHD, bipolar disorder, schizophrenia, and impulsive behavior. *FASEB Journal* 29 (6): 2207–2222.

Patterson, E., Wall, R., Fitzgerald, G.F. et al. (2012). Health implications of high dietary omega-6 polyunsaturated fatty acids. *Journal of nutrition and metabolism* 2012: 539426.

Paul, I.M., Camera, L., Zeiger, R.S. et al. (2010). Relationship between infant weight gain and later asthma. *Pediatric Allergy and Immunology* 21 (PART I): 82–89.

Pembrey, M., Saffery, R., and Bygren, L.O. (2014). Human transgenerational responses to early-life experience: potential impact on development, health and biomedical research. *Journal of Medical Genetics* 51 (9): 563–572.

Perkin, M.R. and Strachan, D.P. (2006). Which aspects of the farming lifestyle explain the inverse association with childhood allergy? *Journal of Allergy and Clinical Immunology* 117 (6): 1374–1381.

Pidsley, R., Fernandes, C., Viana, J. et al. (2012). DNA methylation at the Igf2/H19 imprinting control region is associated with cerebellum mass in outbred mice. *Molecular Brain* 5 (1): 42.

Pieper, S., Out, D., Bakermans-Kranenburg, M.J., and van Ijzendoorn, M.H. (2011). Behavioral and molecular genetics of dissociation: the role of the serotonin transporter gene promoter polymorphism (5-HTTLPR). *Journal of Traumatic Stress* 24 (4): 373–380.

Pietrocola, F., Galluzzi, L., Bravo-San Pedro, J.M. et al. (2015). Acetyl coenzyme A: a central metabolite and second messenger. *Cell Metabolism* 21 (6): 805–821.

Pike, J.W. and Meyer, M.B. (2010). The vitamin D receptor: new paradigms for the regulation of gene expression by 1,25-dihydroxyvitamin D3. *Endocrinology and Metabolism Clinics of North America* 39 (2): 255–269.

Pinney, S.E., Jaeckle Santos, L.J., Han, Y. et al. (2011). Exendin-4 increases histone acetylase activity and reverses epigenetic modifications that silence Pdx1 in the intrauterine growth retarded rat. *Diabetologia* 54 (10): 2606–2614.

Piper, M.D. and Bartke, A. (2008). Diet and aging. *Cell Metabolism* 8 (2): 99–104.

Pogribny, I.P., Ross, S.A., Wise, C. et al. (2006). Irreversible global DNA hypomethylation as a key step in hepatocarcinogenesis induced by dietary methyl deficiency. *Mutation Research, Fundamental and Molecular Mechanisms of Mutagenesis* 593 (1–2): 80–87.

Poling, J., Karanian, J., Salem, N., and Vicini, S. (1995). Time-and voltage-dependent block of delayed rectifier potassium channels by docosahexaenoic acid. *Molecular Pharmacology* 47 (2): 381–390.

Poojary, K.V., Kong, Y.C.M., and Farrar, M.A. (2010). Control of Th2-mediated inflammation by regulatory T cells. *American Journal of Pathology* 177 (2): 525–531.

Poon, A.H., Laprise, C., Lemire, M. et al. (2004). Association of vitamin D receptor genetic variants with susceptibility to asthma and atopy. *American Journal of Respiratory and Critical Care Medicine* 170 (9): 967–973.

Poston, L., Harthoorn, L.F., and Van Der Beek, E.M. (2011). Obesity in pregnancy: implications for the mother and lifelong health of the child. A consensus statement. *Pediatric Research* 69 (2): 175–180.

Prado, E.L. and Dewey, K.G. (2014). Nutrition and brain development in early life. *Nutrition Reviews* 72 (4): 267–284.

Prescott, S.L. (2016). Early nutrition as a major determinant of "immune health": implications for allergy, obesity and other noncommunicable diseases. *Nestle Nutrition Institute Workshop Series* 85: 1–17.

Prescott, S.L. and Clifton, V. (2009). Asthma and pregnancy: emerging evidence of epigenetic interactions in utero. *Current Opinion in Allergy and Clinical Immunology* 9 (5): 417–426.

Prescott, S. and Saffery, R. (2011). The role of epigenetic dysregulation in the epidemic of allergic disease. *Clinical Epigenetics* 2 (2): 223–232.

Price, K.C. and Coe, C.L. (2000). Maternal constraint on fetal growth patterns in the rhesus monkey (Macaca mulatta): the intergenerational link between mothers and daughters. *Human Reproduction* 15 (2): 452–457.

Price, K.C., Hyde, J.S., and Coe, C.L. (1999). Matrilineal transmission of birth weight in the rhesus monkey (Macaca mulatta) across several generations. *Obstetrics and Gynecology* 94 (1): 128–134.

Price, R.J., Burdge, G.C., and Lillycrop, K.A. (2015). The link between early life nutrition and cancer risk. *Current Nutrition Reports* 4 (1): 6–12.

Provvedini, D.M., Tsoukas, C.D., Deftos, L.J., and Manolagas, S.C. (1983). 1,25-Dihydroxyvitamin D3 receptors in human leukocytes. *Science* 221 (4616): 1181–1183.

Pujadas, L., Gruart, A., Bosch, C. et al. (2010). Reelin regulates postnatal neurogenesis and enhances spine hypertrophy and long-term potentiation. *Journal of Neuroscience* 30 (13): 4636–4649.

Qiu, H. and Schlegel, V. (2015). Chronic nutrition overtake can lead to the onset of multiple diseases. *Nutrition Reviews* 73 (2): 97–109.

Quintanilha, B.J., Reis, B.Z., Silva Duarte, G.B. et al. (2017). Nutrimiromics: role of micrornas and nutrition in modulating inflammation and chronic diseases. *Nutrients* 9 (11): 1168.

Raby, B.A., Lazarus, R., Silverman, E.K. et al. (2004). Association of vitamin D receptor gene polymorphisms with childhood and adult asthma. *American Journal of Respiratory and Critical Care Medicine* 170 (10): 1057–1065.

Raghupathy, R., Makhseed, M., Azizieh, F. et al. (1999). Maternal Th1- and Th2-type reactivity to placental antigens in normal human pregnancy and unexplained recurrent spontaneous abortions. *Cellular Immunology* 196 (2): 122–130.

Raman, L., Rajalakshmi, K., Krishnamachari, K.A., and Sastry, J.G. (1978). Effect of calcium supplementation to undernourished mothers during pregnancy on the bone density of the neonates. *The American Journal of Clinical Nutrition* 31 (3): 466–469.

Rangel, M., Dos Santos, J.C., Ortiz, P.H.L. et al. (2014). Modification of epigenetic patterns in low birth weight children: importance of hypomethylation of the ACE gene promoter. *PLoS One* 9 (8): 106138.

Raqib, R., Alam, D.S., Sarker, P. et al. (2007). Low birth weight is associated with altered immune function in rural Bangladeshi children: a birth cohort study. *The American Journal of Clinical Nutrition* 85 (3): 845–852.

Raychaudhuri, N., Raychaudhuri, S., Thamotharan, M., and Devaskar, S.U. (2008). Histone code modifications repress glucose transporter 4 expression in the intrauterine growth-restricted offspring. *Journal of Biological Chemistry* 283 (20): 13611–13626.

Read, J.S., Clemens, J.D., and Klebanoff, M.A. (1994). Moderate low birth weight and infectious disease mortality during infancy and childhood. *American Journal of Epidemiology* 140 (8): 721–733.

Remely, M., Ferk, F., Sterneder, S. et al. (2017). EGCG prevents high fat diet-induced changes in gut microbiota, decreases of DNA strand breaks, and changes in expression and DNA methylation of Dnmt1. *Oxidative Medicine and Cellular Longevity* 2017: 1–17.

Rhizobium, G.E. (2013). Complete genome sequence of the sesbania symbiont and rice. *Nucleic Acids Research* 1 (1256879): 13–14.

Rivière, G., Lienhard, D., Andrieu, T. et al. (2011). Epigenetic regulation of somatic angiotensin-converting enzyme by DNA methylation and histone acetylation. *Epigenetics* 6 (4): 478–489.

Robertson, S.A., Guerin, L.R., Bromfield, J.J. et al. (2009). Seminal fluid drives expansion of the CD4+CD25+ T regulatory cell pool and induces tolerance to paternal alloantigens in Mice1. *Biology of Reproduction* 80 (5): 1036–1045.

Rockville, M. (2004). *The Basics of Bone in Health and Disease*. US Department of Health and Human Services.

Rodgers, J.T. and Puigserver, P. (2007). Fasting-dependent glucose and lipid metabolic response through hepatic sirtuin 1. *Proceedings of the National Academy of Sciences of the United States of America* 104 (31): 12861–12866.

Rodriguez, A. (2010). Maternal pre-pregnancy obesity and risk for inattention and negative emotionality in children. *Journal of Child Psychology and Psychiatry, and Allied Disciplines* 51 (2): 134–143.

Rogers, I. (2003). The influence of birthweight and intrauterine environment on adiposity and fat distribution in later life. *International Journal of Obesity* 27 (7): 755–777.

Roseboom, T., de Rooij, S., and Painter, R. (2006). The Dutch famine and its long-term consequences for adult health. *Early Human Development* 82 (8): 485–491.

Ross, M.G. and Desai, M. (2005). Gestational programming: population survival effects of drought and famine during pregnancy. *American Journal of Physiology. Regulatory, Integrative and Comparative Physiology* 288: 25–33.

Rossignol, D.A. and Frye, R.E. (2012). A review of research trends in physiological abnormalities in autism spectrum disorders: immune dysregulation, inflammation, oxidative stress, mitochondrial dysfunction and environmental toxicant exposures. *Molecular Psychiatry* 17 (4): 389–401.

Rothstein, M.A., Cai, Y., and Marchant, G.E. (2009). The ghost in our genes: legal and ethical implications of epigenetics. *Health matrix (Cleveland, Ohio: 1991)* 19 (1): 1–62.

Rowell, E. and Sekimata, M. (2009). Epigenetic control of T-helper-cell differentiation. *Nature Reviews Immunology* 9 (2): 91–105.

Ruzicka, W.B., Zhubi, A., Veldic, M. et al. (2007). Selective epigenetic alteration of layer I GABAergic neurons isolated from prefrontal cortex of schizophrenia patients using laser-assisted microdissection. *Molecular Psychiatry* 12 (4): 385–397.

Saha, T., Chatterjee, M., Sinha, S. et al. (2017). Components of the folate metabolic pathway and ADHD core traits: an exploration in eastern Indian probands. *Journal of Human Genetics* 62 (7): 687–695.

Sampath, H. and Ntambi, J.M. (2005). Polyunsaturated fatty acid regulation of genes of lipid metabolism. *Annual Review of Nutrition* 25: 317–340.

Samuelsson, A.M., Matthews, P.A., Argenton, M. et al. (2008). Diet-induced obesity in female mice leads to offspring hyperphagia, adiposity, hypertension, and insulin resistance: a novel murine model of developmental programming. *Hypertension* 51 (2): 383–392.

Samuelsson, A.M., Matthews, P.A., Jansen, E. et al. (2013). Sucrose feeding in mouse pregnancy leads to hypertension, and sex-linked obesity and insulin resistance in female offspring. *Frontiers in Physiology* 4: 14.

Sandovici, I., Smith, N.H., Nitert, M.D. et al. (2011). Maternal diet and aging alter the epigenetic control of a promoter-enhancer interaction at the Hnf4a gene in rat pancreatic islets. *Proceedings of the National Academy of Sciences of the United States of America* 108 (13): 5449–5454.

Sathyanarayana Rao, T., Asha, M., Ramesh, B., and Jagannatha Rao, K. (2008). Understanding nutrition, depression and mental illnesses. *Indian Journal of Psychiatry* 50 (2): 77.

Schaub, B., Liu, J., Höppler, S. et al. (2008). Impairment of T-regulatory cells in cord blood of atopic mothers. *Journal of Allergy and Clinical Immunology* 121 (6): 1491.

Schaub, B., Liu, J., Höppler, S. et al. (2009). Maternal farm exposure modulates neonatal immune mechanisms through regulatory T cells. *Journal of Allergy and Clinical Immunology* 123 (4): 774.

Schlüssel, M.M., de Castro, J.A.S., Kac, G. et al. (2010). Birth weight and bone mass in young adults from Brazil. *Bone* 46 (4): 957–963.

Schmitz, G. and Ecker, J. (2008). The opposing effects of n-3 and n-6 fatty acids. *Progress in Lipid Research* 47 (2): 147–155.

Seeburg, D.P. and Sheng, M. (2008). Activity-induced polo-like kinase 2 is required for homeostatic plasticity of hippocampal neurons during epileptiform activity. *Journal of Neuroscience* 28 (26): 6583–6591.

Seckl, J.R. (2004). Prenatal glucocorticoids and long-term programming. *European Journal of Endocrinology, Supplement* 151 (3): U49.

Seckl, J.R. and Meaney, M.J. (2004). Glucocorticoid programming. *Annals of the New York Academy of Sciences* 1032 (1): 63–84.

Seino, T. (2002). Eight-hydroxy-2′-deoxyguanosine in granulosa cells is correlated with the quality of oocytes and embryos in an in vitro fertilization-embryo transfer program. *Fertility and Sterility* 77 (6): 1184–1190.

Sferruzzi-Perri, A.N. and Camm, E.J. (2016). The programming power of the placenta. *Frontiers in Physiology* 7 (MAR): 33.

Shaw, G.M., Carmichael, S.L., Yang, W. et al. (2004). Periconceptional dietary intake of choline and betaine and neural tube defects in offspring. *American Journal of Epidemiology* 160 (2): 02–109.

Shivapurkar, N. and Poirier, L.A. (1983). Tissue levels of S-adenosylmethionine and S-adenosylhomocysteine in rats fed methyl-deficient, amino acid-defined diets for one to five weeks. *Carcinogenesis* 4 (8): 1051–1057.

Shi, L. and Tu, B.P. (2015). Acetyl-CoA and the regulation of metabolism: mechanisms and consequences. *Current Opinion in Cell Biology* 33: 125–131.

Sivanand, S., Viney, I., and Wellen, K.E. (2018). Spatiotemporal control of Acetyl-CoA metabolism in chromatin regulation. *Trends in Biochemical Sciences* 43 (1): 61–74.

Skandalis, S.S., Afratis, N., Smirlaki, G. et al. (2014). Cross-talk between estradiol receptor and EGFR/IGF-IR signaling pathways in estrogen-responsive breast cancers: focus on the role and impact of proteoglycans. *Matrix Biology* 35: 182–193.

Slatopolsky, E. (1983). Pathophysiology of calcium, magnesium, and phosphorus metabolism. In: *The Kidney and Body Fluids in Health and Disease* (ed. S. Klahr), 269–330. Springer.

Sprecher, H. (2002). The roles of anabolic and catabolic reactions in the synthesis and recycling of polyunsaturated fatty acids. *Prostaglandins, Leukotrienes, and Essential Fatty Acids* 67 (2–3): 79–83.

Sprecher, H., Luthria, D.L., Mohammed, B.S., and Baykousheva, S.P. (1995). Reevaluation of the pathways for the biosynthesis of polyunsaturated fatty acids. *Journal of Lipid Research* 36 (12): 2471–2477.

Stacchiotti, A., Favero, G., and Rezzani, R. (2019). Resveratrol and SIRT1 activators for the treatment of aging and age-related diseases. In: *Resveratrol – Adding Life to Years, Not Adding Years to Life* (ed. F.A. Badria), 117–136. IntechOpen.

Steenweg-De Graaff, J., Tiemeier, H., Ghassabian, A. et al. (2016). Maternal fatty acid status during pregnancy and child autistic traits: the generation R study. *American Journal of Epidemiology* 183 (9): 792–799.

Stein, A.D., Kahn, H.S., Rundle, A. et al. (2007). Anthropometric measures in middle age after exposure to famine during gestation: evidence from the Dutch famine. *The American Journal of Clinical Nutrition* 85 (3): 869–876.

Stein, Z., Susser, M., Saenger, G., and Marolla, F. (1972). Nutrition and mental performance. *Science* 178 (4062): 708–713.

Stein, Z., Susser, M., Saenger, G., and Marolla, F. (1975). Famine and human development: the Dutch hunger winter of 1944-1945. *Annals of Internal Medicine* 83 (2): 290.

Stewart, R.J.C., Preece, R.F., and Sheppard, H.G. (1975). Twelve generations of marginal protein deficiency. *British Journal of Nutrition* 33 (2): 233–253.

Stewart, R.J.C., Sheppard, H., Preece, R., and Waterlow, J.C. (1980). The effect of rehabilitation at different stages of development of rats marginally malnourished for ten to twelve generations. *British Journal of Nutrition* 43 (3): 403–412.

Stiles, J. and Jernigan, T.L. (2010). The basics of brain development. *Neuropsychology Review* 20 (4): 327–348.

Stone, N., Pangilinan, F., Molloy, A.M. et al. (2011). Bioinformatic and genetic association analysis of microrna target sites in One-Carbon metabolism genes. *PLoS One* 6 (7): 21851.

Strakovsky, R.S., Lezmi, S., Flaws, J.A. et al. (2014). Genistein exposure during the early postnatal period favors the development of obesity in female, but not male rats. *Toxicological Sciences* 138 (1): 161–174.

Suntornsaratoon, P., Krishnamra, N., and Charoenphandhu, N. (2015). Positive long-term outcomes from presuckling calcium supplementation in lactating rats and the offspring. *American Journal of Physiology – Endocrinology and Metabolism* 308 (11): E1010–E1022.

Sundar, I.K. and Rahman, I. (2011). Vitamin D and susceptibility of chronic lung diseases: role of epigenetics. *Frontiers in Pharmacology* 2: 50.

Surakasula, A., Nagarjunapu, G., and Raghavaiah, K. (2014). A comparative study of pre- and post-menopausal breast cancer: risk factors, presentation, characteristics and management. *Journal of Research in Pharmacy Practice* 3 (1): 12.

Surén, P., Roth, C., Bresnahan, M. et al. (2013). Association between maternal use of folic acid supplements and risk of autism spectrum disorders in children. *JAMA: The Journal of the American Medical Association* 309 (6): 570–577.

Suter, M.A., Chen, A., Burdine, M.S. et al. (2012). A maternal high-fat diet modulates fetal SIRT1 histone and protein deacetylase activity in nonhuman primates. *FASEB Journal* 26 (12): 5106–5114.

Symonds, M.E., Sebert, S.P., Hyatt, M.A., and Budge, H. (2009). Nutritional programming of the metabolic syndrome. *Nature Reviews Endocrinology* 5 (11): 604–610.

Tang, M., Zhang, M., Cai, H. et al. (2016). Maternal diet of polyunsaturated fatty acid altered the cell proliferation in the dentate gyrus of hippocampus and influenced glutamatergic and serotoninergic systems of neonatal female rats. *Lipids in Health and Disease* 15 (1): 71.

Tappia, P.S., Nijjar, M.S., Mahay, A. et al. (2005). Phospholipid profile of developing heart of rats exposed to low-protein diet in pregnancy. *American Journal of Physiology. Regulatory, Integrative and Comparative Physiology* 289 (5): R1400–R1406.

Tau, G.Z. and Peterson, B.S. (2010). Normal development of brain circuits. *Neuropsychopharmacology* 35 (1): 147–168.

Teegarden, D., Romieu, I., and Lelièvre, S.A. (2012). Redefining the impact of nutrition on breast cancer incidence: is epigenetics involved? *Nutrition Research Reviews* 25 (1): 68–95.

Tedner, S.G., Örtqvist, A.K., and Almqvist, C. (2012). Fetal growth and risk of childhood asthma and allergic disease. *Clinical & Experimental Allergy* 42 (10): 1430–1447.

Tehlivets, O., Malanovic, N., Visram, M. et al. (2013). S-adenosyl-L-homocysteine hydrolase and methylation disorders: yeast as a model system. *Biochimica et Biophysica Acta – Molecular Basis of Disease* 1832 (1): 204–215.

Teng, Y.W., Mehedint, M.G., Garrow, T.A., and Zeisel, S.H. (2011). Deletion of betaine-homocysteine S-methyltransferase in mice perturbs choline and 1-carbon metabolism, resulting in fatty liver and hepatocellular carcinomas. *Journal of Biological Chemistry* 286 (42): 36258–36267.

Tiffon, C. (2018). The impact of nutrition and environmental epigenetics on human health and disease. *International Journal of Molecular Sciences* 19 (11).

Timasheva, Y., Putku, M., Kivi, R. et al. (2013). Developmental programming of growth: genetic variant in GH2 gene encoding placental growth hormone contributes to adult height determination. *Placenta* 34 (11): 995–1001.

Timpka, S., Macdonald-Wallis, C., Hughes, A.D. et al. (2016). Hypertensive disorders of pregnancy and offspring cardiac structure and function in adolescence. *Journal of the American Heart Association* 5 (11).

Tissir, F. and Goffinet, A.M. (2003). Reelin and brain development. *Nature Reviews Neuroscience* 4 (6): 496–505.

Tobi, E.W., Lumey, L.H., Talens, R.P. et al. (2009). DNA methylation differences after exposure to prenatal famine are common and timing-and sex-specific. *Human Molecular Genetics* 18 (21): 4046–4053.

Tobi, E.W., Slieker, R.C., Stein, A.D. et al. (2015). Early gestation as the critical time-window for changes in the prenatal environment to affect the adult human blood methylome. *International Journal of Epidemiology* 44 (4): 1211–1223.

Tobias, J.H. and Cooper, C. (2003). Perspective: PTH/PTHrP activity and the programming of skeletal development in utero. *Journal of Bone and Mineral Research* 19 (2): 177–182.

Tobias, J.H., Steer, C.D., Emmett, P.M. et al. (2005). Bone mass in childhood is related to maternal diet in pregnancy. *Osteoporosis International* 16 (12): 1731–1741.

Toromanoff, A., Ammann, P., Mosekilde, L. et al. (1997). Parathyroid hormone increases bone formation and improves mineral balance in Vitamin D-deficient female rats. *Endocrinology* 138 (6): 2449–2457.

Tosh, D.N., Fu, Q., Callaway, C.W. et al. (2010). Epigenetics of programmed obesity: alteration in IUGR rat hepatic IGF1 mRNA expression and histone structure in rapid vs. delayed postnatal catch-up growth. *American Journal of Physiology – Gastrointestinal and Liver Physiology* 299 (5): G1023–G1029.

Tran, P.V., Kennedy, B.C., Lien, Y.C. et al. (2015). Fetal iron deficiency induces chromatin remodeling at the Bdnf locus in adult rat hippocampus. *American Journal of Physiology. Regulatory, Integrative and Comparative Physiology* 308 (4): R276–R282.

Troisi, R., Grotmol, T., Jacobsen, J. et al. (2013). Perinatal characteristics and breast cancer risk in daughters: a Scandinavian population-based study. *Journal of Developmental Origins of Health and Disease* 4 (1): 35–41.

Toyokawa, S., Uddin, M., Koenen, K.C., and Galea, S. (2012). How does the social environment "get into the mind"? Epigenetics at the intersection of social and psychiatric epidemiology. *Social Science and Medicine* 74 (1): 67–74.

Tsafriri, A. and Reich, R. (1999). Molecular aspects of mammalian ovulation. *Experimental and Clinical Endocrinology and Diabetes* 107 (1): 1–11.

Tyagi, E., Zhuang, Y., Agrawal, R. et al. (2015). Interactive actions of Bdnf methylation and cell metabolism for building neural resilience under the influence of diet. *Neurobiology of Disease* 73: 307–318.

Vaidyanathan, V.V., Rao, K.V.R., and Sastry, P.S. (1994). Regulation of diacylglycerol kinase in rat brain membranes by docosahexaenoic acid. *Neuroscience Letters* 179 (1–2): 171–174.

Van Straten, E.M.E., Bloks, V.W., Huijkman, N.C.A. et al. (2010). The liver X-receptor gene promoter is hypermethylated in a mouse model of prenatal protein restriction. *American Journal of Physiology. Regulatory, Integrative and Comparative Physiology* 298 (2): R275.

Van Voorhis, B.J. (1994). Nitric oxide: an autocrine regulator of human granulosa-luteal cell steroidogenesis. *Endocrinology* 135 (5): 1799–1806.

Veenendaal, M.V.E., Painter, R.C., De Rooij, S.R. et al. (2013). Transgenerational effects of prenatal exposure to the 1944-45 Dutch famine. *BJOG: An International Journal of Obstetrics and Gynaecology* 120 (5): 548–554.

Vega, M., Urrutia, L., Iniguez, G. et al. (2000). Nitric oxide induces apoptosis in the human corpus luteum in vitro. *Molecular Human Reproduction* 6 (8): 681–687.

Veldic, M., Caruncho, H.J., Liu, W.S. et al. (2004). DNA-methyltransferase 1 mRNA is selectively overexpressed in telencephalic GABAergic interneurons of schizophrenia brains. *Proceedings of the National Academy of Sciences of the United States of America* 101 (1): 348–353.

Vickers, M.H. (2014). Early life nutrition, epigenetics and programming of later life disease. *Nutrients* 6 (6): 2165–2178.

Villa, C.R., Chen, J., Wen, B. et al. (2016). Maternal Vitamin D beneficially programs metabolic, gut and bone health of mouse male offspring in an obesogenic environment. *International Journal of Obesity* 40 (12): 1875–1883.

Vin-Raviv, N., Barchana, M., Linn, S., and Keinan-Boker, L. (2012). Severe caloric restriction in young women during World War II and subsequent breast cancer risk. *International Journal of Clinical Practice* 66 (10): 948–958.

Vinkhuyzen, A.A.E., Eyles, D.W., Burne, T.H.J. et al. (2018). Gestational Vitamin D deficiency and autism-related traits: the generation R study. *Molecular Psychiatry* 23 (2): 240–246.

Wan, L., Li, Y., Zhang, Z. et al. (2018). Methylenetetrahydrofolate reductase and psychiatric diseases. *Translational Psychiatry* 8 (1): 242.

Wang, Z., Song, J., Li, C. et al. (2020). DNA methylation of the INSR gene as a mediator of the association between prenatal exposure to famine and adulthood waist circumference. *Scientific Reports* 10 (1): 1–8.

Wang, L. and Xu, R.-J. (2007). The effects of perinatal protein malnutrition on spatial learning and memory behaviour and brain-derived neurotrophic factor concentration in the brain tissue in young rats. *Asia Pacific Journal of Clinical Nutrition* 16 (1): 467–472.

Wang, P.X., Wang, J.J., Lei, Y.X. et al. (2012). Impact of fetal and infant exposure to the chinese great famine on the risk of hypertension in adulthood. *PLoS One* 7 (11): e49720.

Wadley, G.D., McConell, G.K., Goodman, C.A. et al. (2013). Growth restriction in the rat alters expression of metabolic genes during postnatal cardiac development in a sex-specific manner. *Physiological Genomics* 45 (3): 99–105.

Waterland, R.A. and Jirtle, R.L. (2004). Early nutrition, epigenetic changes at transposons and imprinted genes, and enhanced susceptibility to adult chronic diseases. *Nutrition* 20 (1): 63–68.

Whitehouse, A.J.O., Holt, B.J., Serralha, M. et al. (2012). Maternal serum vitamin D levels during pregnancy and offspring neurocognitive development. *Pediatrics* 129 (3): 485–493.

Wieczorek, A. and Balwierz, W. (2015). The role of Id2 protein in Neuroblatoma in children. *Pathology and Oncology Research* 21 (4): 999–1004.

Wilson, M.J., Shivapurkar, N., and Poirier, L.A. (1984). Hypomethylation of hepatic nuclear DNA in rats fed with a carcinogenic methyl-deficient diet. *Biochemical Journal* 218 (3): 987–990.

Woods, L.L., Ingelfinger, J.R., and Rasch, R. (2005). Modest maternal protein restriction fails to program adult hypertension in female rats. *American Journal of Physiology. Regulatory, Integrative and Comparative Physiology* 289: 58.

Woods, L.L., Ingelfinger, J.R., Nyengaard, J.R., and Rasch, R. (2001). Maternal protein restriction suppresses the newborn renin-angiotensin system and programs adult hypertension in rats. *Pediatric Research* 49 (4): 460–467.

Woods, L.L. and Rasch, R. (1998). Perinatal ANG II programs adult blood pressure, glomerular number, and renal function in rats. *American Journal of Physiology. Regulatory, Integrative and Comparative Physiology* 275: 544–545.

Woods, L.L., Weeks, D.A., and Rasch, R. (2004). Programming of adult blood pressure by maternal protein restriction: role of nephrogenesis. *Kidney International* 65 (4): 1339–1348.

Won, J.L., Shim, J.Y., and Zhu, B.T. (2005). Mechanisms for the inhibition of DNA methyltransferases by tea catechins and bioflavonoids. *Molecular Pharmacology* 68 (4): 1018–1030.

Won, H., Mah, W., and Kim, E. (2013). Autism spectrum disorder causes, mechanisms, and treatments: focus on neuronal synapses. *Frontiers in Molecular Neuroscience* 6: 1–24, Article 19.

Wu, S., Zhang, J., Li, F. et al. (2019). One-carbon metabolism links nutrition intake to embryonic development via epigenetic mechanisms. *Stem Cells International* 2019: 3894101.

Wu, Y., Borde, M., Heissmeyer, V. et al. (2006). FOXP3 controls regulatory T cell function through cooperation with NFAT. *Cell* 126 (2): 375–381.

Xiao, Y., Xia, J., Li, L. et al. (2019). Associations between dietary patterns and the risk of breast cancer: a systematic review and meta-analysis of observational studies. *Breast Cancer Research* 21 (1): 16.

Yan, X., Huang, Y., Zhao, J.-X. et al. (2011). Maternal obesity-impaired insulin signaling in sheep and induced lipid accumulation and fibrosis in skeletal muscle of Offspring1. *Biology of Reproduction* 85 (1): 172–178.

Yang, Y. and Wang, J.K. (2016). The functional analysis of MicroRNAs involved in NF-kB signaling. *European Review for Medical and Pharmacological Sciences* 20: 1764–1774.

Yaliwal, L.V. and Desai, R.M. (2012). Methylenetetrahydrofolate reductase mutations, a genetic cause for familial recurrent neural tube defects. *Indian Journal of Human Genetics* 18 (1): 122–124.

Yarbrough, D.E., Barrett-Connor, E., and Morton, D.J. (2000). Birth weight as a predictor of adult bone mass in postmenopausal women: the Rancho Bernardo study. *Osteoporosis International* 11 (7): 626–630.

Yates, N.J., Tesic, D., Feindel, K.W. et al. (2018). Vitamin D is crucial for maternal care and offspring social behaviour in rats. *Journal of Endocrinology* 237 (2): 73–85.

Yehuda, S., Rabinovitz, S., and Mostofsky, D.I. (1999). Essential fatty acids are mediators of brain biochemistry and cognitive functions. *Journal of Neuroscience Research* 56 (6): 565–570.

Yıldırım, A., Keleş, F., Özdemir, G. et al. (2015). Homocysteine levels in normotensive children of hypertensive parents. *Anatolian Journal of Cardiology* 15 (12): 1008–1013.

Zambrano, E. and Nathanielsz, P.W. (2013). Mechanisms by which maternal obesity programs offspring for obesity: evidence from animal studies. *Nutrition Reviews* 71 (SUPPL1): S42.

Zampieri, M., Ciccarone, F., Calabrese, R. et al. (2015). Reconfiguration of DNA methylation in aging. *Mechanisms of Ageing and Development* 151: 60–70.

Zeisel, S.H., Zola, T., daCosta, K.A., and Pomfret, E.A. (1989). Effect of choline deficiency on S-adenosylmethionine and methionine concentrations in rat liver. *The Biochemical Journal* 259: 725–729.

Zeisel, S.H. and Da Costa, K.A. (2009). Choline: an essential nutrient for public health. *Nutrition Reviews* 67 (11): 615–623.

Zempleni, J., Liu, D., and Xue, J. (2013). Nutrition, histone epigenetic marks, and disease. *Human Health*: 197–217.

Zempleni, J., Li, Y., Xue, J., and Cordonier, E.L. (2011). The role of holocarboxylase synthetase in genome stability is mediated partly by epigenomic synergies between methylation and biotinylation events. *Epigenetics* 6 (7): 892–894.

Zhang, N. (2015). Epigenetic modulation of DNA methylation by nutrition and its mechanisms in animals. *Animal Nutrition* 1 (3): 144–151.

Zhang, N. (2018). Role of methionine on epigenetic modification of DNA methylation and gene expression in animals. *Animal Nutrition* 4 (1): 11–16.

Zhang, L., Chen, W., Dai, Y. et al. (2016). Detection of expressional changes induced by intrauterine growth restriction in the developing rat pancreas. *Experimental Biology and Medicine* 241 (13): 1446–1456.

Zhang, B.K., Lai, Y.Q., Niu, P.P. et al. (2013). Epigallocatechin-3-gallate inhibits homocysteine-induced apoptosis of endothelial cells by demethylation of the DDAH2 gene. *Planta Medica* 79 (18): 1715–1719.

Zhang, H., Liu, Z., Ma, S. et al. (2016). Ratio of S-adenosylmethionine to S-adenosylhomocysteine as a sensitive indicator of atherosclerosis. *Molecular Medicine Reports* 14 (1): 289–300.

Zhang, S., Rattanatray, L., Morrison, J.L. et al. (2011). Maternal obesity and the early origins of childhood obesity: weighing up the benefits and costs of maternal weight loss in the periconceptional period for the. *Experimental Diabetes Research* 2011: 1–10.

Zhang, J., Zhang, F., Didelot, X. et al. (2009). Maternal high fat diet during pregnancy and lactation alters hepatic expression of insulin like growth factor-2 and key microRNAs in the adult offspring. *BMC Genomics* 10: 478.

Zheng, S., Li, Q., Zhang, Y. et al. (2012). Histone deacetylase 3 (HDAC3) participates in the transcriptional repression of the p16INK4a gene in mammary gland of the female rat offspring exposed to an early-life high-fat diet. *Epigenetics* 7 (2): 183–190.

Zhou, D. and Pan, Y.X. (2011). Gestational low protein diet selectively induces the amino acid response pathway target genes in the liver of offspring rats through transcription factor binding and histone modifications. *Biochimica et Biophysica Acta, Gene Regulatory Mechanisms* 1809 (10): 549–556.

Zhubi, A., Chen, Y., Dong, E. et al. (2014). Increased binding of MeCP2 to the GAD1 and RELN promoters may be mediated by an enrichment of 5-hmC in autism spectrum disorder (ASD) cerebellum. *Translational Psychiatry* 4 (1): e349.

Zhu, Z., Cao, F., and Li, X. (2019). Epigenetic programming and fetal metabolic programming. *Frontiers in Endocrinology* 10: 764.

Zittermann, A., Tenderich, G., and Koerfer, R. (2009). Vitamin D and the adaptive immune system with special emphasis to allergic reactions and allograft rejection. *Inflammation & Allergy Drug Targets* 8 (2): 161–168.

16

Surfactant and Polymer-Based Self-Assemblies for Encapsulation, Protection, and Release of Nutraceuticals

Saima Afzal[1], Mohd Sajid Lone[1], Pawandeep Kaur[1], Firdous Ahmad Ahanger[1], Nighat Nazir[2], and Aijaz Ahmad Dar[1]

[1] *Soft Matter Research Group, Department of Chemistry, University of Kashmir, Srinagar, Jammu and Kashmir, India*
[2] *Department of Chemistry, Islamia College of Science and Commerce, Hawal, Jammu and Kashmir, India*

16.1   Introduction

Customer satisfaction regarding the effect of the general well-being of food products on human health has been gaining increasing importance due to the advent of more food processing techniques. In contemporary times, it is possible to fabricate palatable foods by employing different bioengineering methods through various encapsulation methods and carriers, which has opened up a huge food service industry across the globe. Owing to the rapid advancements in the nanoscopic imaging and other related physicochemical characterization techniques, the revelations about the very captivating microstructure of the food has been on the rise (Livney 2015). This has greatly enhanced our abilities to understand and manipulate the food microstructure for obtaining better food properties and functionalities. The elaborate relation between food and health has been the driving force behind the rapid and inclusive increase in scientific literature to alleviate the occurrence of diseases like obesity, cancer, and diabetes. The term "nutraceutical" is a link between food and medicine derived from the combination of terms "nutrition" and "pharmaceutics." The famous quote by Hippocrates (400 BC), "Let food be thy medicine and medicine be thy food" sums up the entire significance of nutraceuticals and underscores their importance and familiarity among the masses since time immemorial (Helal et al. 2019). Pertinently, in the recent past the nutraceutical industry has picked up pace so fast that its estimated market is expected to reach about 49 billion USD in 2023 (Chen and Hu 2020). Nutraceuticals are not essential for life, but they have a significant effect on the human health depending on their amount and type present within a living body. A significant body of literature points toward the fact that nutraceuticals enhance the human resistance to the diseases and hence promote good health (Asghar et al. 2018). Owing to their beneficial effects, they have been used as treatments against different health ailments, like cancer, inflammation, atherosclerosis, obesity, and diabetes in addition to having antiaging and antioxidant properties (Table 16.1). (Bourbon et al. 2018; Zhang et al. 2019)

The nutraceuticals are quite often the bioactive molecules or molecules derived from plant sources. Such molecules suffer from lots of challenges that have been on the forefront confronting scientists for harvesting their health benefits like the low aqueous solubility, chemical instabilities

Handbook of Nutraceuticals and Natural Products: Biological, Medicinal, and Nutritional Properties and Applications,
Volume 1, First Edition. Edited by Sreerag Gopi and Preetha Balakrishnan.

Table 16.1 Some common nutraceuticals with benefits and common problems associated with them.

Nutraceutical	Reported health benefits	Limitations in applications	References
Curcumin	Major antioxidant, anti-inflammatory effects, Alzheimer's disease	Very low solubility in water and low bioavailability, degradation in alkaline pH conditions, unstable in light	Hewlings and Kalman (2017)
Lycopene	Anticarcinogenic, antioxidant	Extremely low soluble in water, isomerization under light	Shi et al. (2008)
Soy protein	Bone protective, lowering of blood pressure, obesity and diabetic prevention	Solubility and viscosity of dispersions is affected by pH, ionic strength	Arrese et al. (1991)
Linoleic acid, Palmitic acid	Involved in the synthesis of hormones, cardiovascular effects, AIDS prevention	Solubility is very low water, poor absorption in gut	Lee et al. (2009)
Quercetin	Antioxidant, anti-inflammation, antitumor	Extreme low solubility in water, unstable under light, low permeability	Anand David et al. (2016)
Resveratrol	Cardioprotective activities, anti-inflammation, chemoprevention	Susceptible to oxidation, short shelf-life	Lu et al. (2016)
Caffeine	Orthostatic hypotension, migraine headache treatment	Mildly soluble in room temperature water	Velikov and Pelan (2008)
Saponins	Antimutagenic and antitumor activities	Low bioavailability due to its extensive H-bonding capability	Lipinski et al. (2012)
Ascorbic Acid	Antioxidant, ROS scavenger, anticancerous	Undergoes oxidation to diketogulonic acid, xylonic acid	de Carvalho Melo-Cavalcante et al. (2019)
Lutein	Prevents cataract, prevents other eye-related diseases	Extremely insoluble in water	Buscemi et al. (2018)
Silymarin	Cures liver diseases of various types	Low bioavailability due to low solubility	Dixit et al. (2007)
Rutaecarpine	Cures diarrhea, headaches, hemorrhages, as well as GI disorders	Susceptible to radical generation and degradation, low solubility	Lee et al. (2008)

(due to the changes in pH, ionic strength, etc. along the gut), and their targeted delivery (Chen and Hu 2020). The developments in the food nanotechnology hold a promising future in order to provide with the new and effective strategies in combating such challenges related to the bioavailability and stability of the nutraceuticals.

16.1.1 Solubility Characteristics

Most of the nutraceuticals are hydrophobic in nature, i.e. water hating, as a result of which they tend to have low water solubility and are not easily dissolved in water at the required concentration to be effective in a particular dose. As a result, their bioavailability is significantly reduced (McClements 2015). Conversely, these nutraceuticals have high oil solubility, i.e. they can be solubilized and transported from one place to another within the living systems encapsulated in an oil phase. This can be advantageous for the development of nutraceutical carriers in living systems and to form selective barriers for the mass transport of such nutraceuticals across a living membrane or from one region to another.

16.1.2 Stability Characteristics

It has been found that most of the nutraceuticals are chemically and physically vulnerable to the external conditions like pH, ionic strength, temperature, light, and oxygen as mentioned in Table 16.1 (Abbas et al. 2012). Due to the presence of multiple number of constituents in foods or beverages, the interactions between such constituents have been found to promote precipitation of some proteins and gelation of some polysaccharides (Pitkowski et al. 2009) The utility of nano assemblies of soft matter in a bid to prevent chemical and physical complications is one of the better ways to isolate the food components from one another and from the external potentially deleterious environment (Burey et al. 2008). In recent times, the development and formulation of the multi-compartment encapsulating systems like multiple emulsions and composite nanoparticles have increased the stability and functionality of the foods and beverages manifold.

16.1.3 Targeted Delivery

After the encapsulation of nutraceutical within the nano colloidal systems, their apt delivery at the appropriate site within the living body is as essential as their protection from the external conditions. For example, some nutraceutical if released in the buccal cavity give very distasteful flavors upon interaction with the enzymes and mucin of the buccal cavity. For some nutraceuticals, the acidic environment of the stomach and small intestines leads to the denaturation or hydrolysis of the enzymes. Therefore, it is imperative to design the encapsulating cum delivery systems, which can achieve the targeted delivery of the nutraceuticals at specific sites within the gut. For example, the nutraceutical could be well trapped within the internal environment of the encapsulating system when it is in the mouth cavity and could be released, once the nanocarrier, with loaded nutraceuticals, reaches stomach or colon.

The problems as discussed above, related to the bioaccessbility of the nutraceuticals, arise because of the fact that such nutraceuticals are often administered orally into the human body as this mode of administration is both economical and convenient to the humans. However, once taken orally, the human body poses some challenges along the gastrointestinal (GI) tract owing primarily to the diverse chemical and physical conditions along the GI tract, which has the potential to alter the chemical structure of the nutraceuticals and turn it into a less benign chemical or even into a malignant species (Acosta 2009). In lieu of the above mentioned factors, McClements ascribed the total bioavailability to different factors such as (i) the nature of hydrophobic portion of the nutraceutical, (ii) the penetrating power of the nutraceutical through small intestines, and (iii) the resistance of the nutraceuticals toward the possible disintegration while passing through the circulatory system (McClements et al. 2015a). The net bioavailability of a nutraceutical is judged and calculated based on the above three factors after which the data obtained is used to formulate the encapsulating, protecting, and delivery systems within the human body.

For the alleviation of the above discussed problems related to the moderated bioavailability and hence nutritional values of the nutraceuticals, various nanoscale systems have been employed ranging from nanoemulsions to solid lipid particles (Wang et al. 2008b; Sachdeva et al. 2015). These nanoformulations, by virtue of their nanosize, are widely acclaimed for circumventing the obstacles of poor pharmacokinetics. Among them, the self-assembled soft systems based on surfactants, polymers including emulsions, and hydrogels have gained utmost importance primarily owing to their biocompatibility, easy mode of preparation, cost-effectiveness, and broad range of applicability in various food and beverage formulations. The very nature of surfactants and polymers in possessing the intrinsic duality of hydrophobicity and hydrophilicity leads to the formation of wide variety of self-assembled nano and microstructures (Lone et al. 2017) with disparate shapes and structures like spherical micelles, rod micelles, vesicles, hydrogel matrices, etc. (Figure 16.1).

It is pertinent to mention here that the system required for preparing the encapsulating, protecting, and release vehicles should fulfill some of desirable characteristics for carrying out the required processes:

a) *Food grade*: It is highly desirable that the system is of food grade quality as approved by the relevant authorities of the concerned country.

b) *Cost effective*: The systems should be economically viable preferably manufactured from the cheap ingredients.

c) *Highly biocompatible:* The delivery systems apart from increasing the bioavailability of the foods should also be biocompatible itself in nature. Furthermore, the system should be compatible with the surrounding food matrix, i.e. it should not change the appearance, texture, and flavor of the food in question.

d) *Resistant against the food matrix environment*: Besides protecting the encapsulated nutraceutical, the system itself should be resistant against all the changing environments of the GI tract.

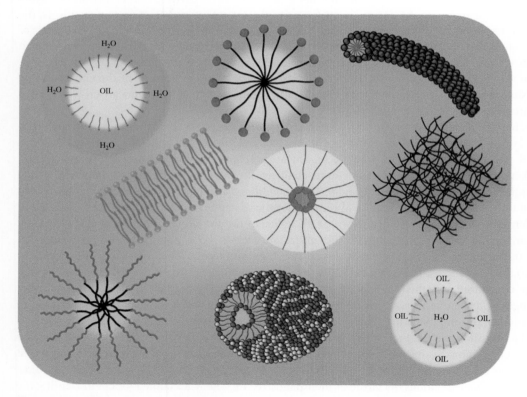

Figure 16.1 Different nano and microstructures formed due to self-assembly of surfactants and polymers.

Owing to their significant flexibility both prior to and after their incorporation in the food systems, the self-assembled soft systems based on surfactants and polymers have proved to possess the potential to fulfill all the above mentioned requirements in order to make a successful and efficient encapsulating, protecting, and releasing vehicle for neutraceuticals. Here in this chapter, we take a look at some of the most commonly employed soft materials in the food industry, which have been employed to encapsulate, protect, and release the important nutraceuticals.

16.2 Micelles, Liposomes, and Emulsions as Encapsulating, Protecting, and Releasing Agents for the Nutraceuticals

16.2.1 Micelles

Surfactants are the amphiphilic low-molecular-weight molecules that are associated with the food and welfare industry for a very long time (Dar et al. 2007). These molecules can self-assemble into different association colloids, for example micelles, worm like micelles, vesicles, reverse micelles, and bilayers. The main driving force for the formation of such microstructures is the hydrophobic effect, which prompts the monomer surfactant molecules to self-assemble into different structures as shown in Figure 16.1. Based on the nature of the head group charge, the surfactants are classified into anionic, nonionic, cationic, and zwitterionic (dipolar) surfactants. The self-assembling tendency of the surfactants is only realized above a certain concentration known as the critical micelle concentration (cmc), below which they get adsorbed on to the interface and decrease the free energy by decreasing the interfacial tension. The micelles thus formed possess the capability to encapsulate the hydrophobic nutraceuticals inside their hydrophobic regions (Lone et al. 2019), which is primarily because of the tendency to form a thermodynamically stable and uniform solution and sometimes assisted by the favorable interactions between the micelles itself and the encapsulated nutraceutical. The nature and efficiency of solubilization has been shown to be a function of different factors, like the head group charge, the tail length of the surfactant, pH, temperature, and ionic strength of the solution (Torchilin 2001). Furthermore, the site of solubilization of the nutraceuticals has been evaluated to be a crucial factor in determining its solubilization within the micellar systems. The different solubilization sites offered by the micellar systems are core, the palisade layer and the interfacial region, which can be occupied by the nutraceuticals of varying polarities (Maswal and Dar 2013). For example, the nonpolar substances like alkanes prefer to occupy the core region of the micelles, the comparatively less polar substances like alcohols prefer to be located within the palisade layer, while as the significantly polar species are most likely to be found in the interfacial regions of the micelles (Figure 16.2).

Surfactants have been used in the encapsulation, protection, and release of lipophilic nutraceuticals to affect their bioavailability in the GIT via numerous methods either by affecting the membrane permeability or by shaping the digesting ability of certain enzymes like amylase, lipase, or protease (McClements et al. 2015b). In one of such studies, Vinarov et al. have demonstrated the effect of various low-molecular-weight surfactants on the lipolysis of triglycerides by pancreatic lipase. The maximum activity was found to be when the surfactant micelles were mixed with the bile salt micelles with the efficiency decreasing in the order anionic > cationic > nonionic surfactants (Vinarov et al. 2012). Bachar et al. have developed a micellar system based on bovine β-casein, which is an amphiphilic molecule having a strong tendency to self-assemble into micelles and used it as a carrier for the delivery of hydrophobic nutraceutical moiety. Dai et al (Dai et al. 2018) have successfully increased the bioavailability of curcumin when it was encapsulated

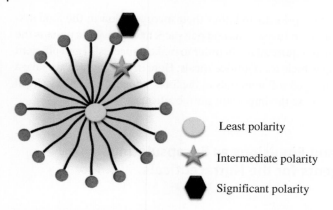

Least polarity

Intermediate polarity

Significant polarity

Figure 16.2 Schematic depiction of the site of solubilization for the nutraceuticals of varying polarity.

in a protein/polysaccharide complex aided by the surfactants like rhamnolipid and lecithin. Owing to the combined interactions like electrostatic, hydrogen bonding, and hydrophobic between the curcumin (Cur) and zein (Z)/propylene glycol alginate (P)/rhamnolipid (R), lecithin (L), the encapsulation efficiency increased in the following order for different combinations: Z-Cur (21%); Z-P-Cur (67%); Z-P-R-Cur (92%); and Z-P-L-Cur (94%). Further, it was observed that the surfactants improved the photostability and bioaccessbility of curcumin significantly. Another natural surfactant-like substance, casein, has been used by many authors to encapsulate, protect, and release some important nutraceuticals like quercetin, curcumin, and β-carotene. Semo et al. (2007) demonstrated for the first time the encapsulating and protecting nature of the casein micelles by taking the example of a model hydrophobic nutraceutical vitamin D2. As such, they established a protocol for the encapsulation process into the casein micelles and found in this study that the casein micelles increased the concentration of vitamin D2 to about 5.5 times within themselves compared with the outside of the micelles, i.e. the serum with a simultaneous protection against the UV-light-induced degradation for vitamin D2. Moreover, Ghayour et al. (2019) nanoencapsulated both quercetin and curcumin in the casein reassembled micelles and reported the enhanced chemical stability and encapsulation, which hit over 90% for both the nutraceuticals. On similar lines, Sáiz-Abajo et al. Sáiz-Abajo et al. (2013) have employed the casein micelles to encapsulate and protect the β-carotene, which is liable to degradation during different food processing techniques like heat stabilization, high pressure processing, etc.

Reverse micelles has equally been found to have promising applications in encapsulating, protection, and delivery of the nutraceuticals. Wang et al. (2009) have shown, by simulation studies, that the reverse micelles formed from CTAB do retain their characteristics when they are transferred to vacuum. This preservation of the micellar structure has been shown to retain the protecting abilities of the encapsulated nutraceuticals within such micelles. Following this study, Fang et al. (2010) have seen formation of reverse micelles in a gas phase from NaAOT surfactants and their utility in the encapsulation and protection of glycine. They verified that the aggregation number of the reverse micelles was somehow directly proportional to the number of glycine molecules being encapsulated within them, which subsequently was affecting the overall stability and encapsulation of the glycine molecules.

Encapsulation of the polyphenols (antioxidants) by the micellar aggregates has also been dealt, which has been monitored through the reduction potential of these polyphenols toward 2,2-diphenyl-1-picrylhydrazyl (DPPH) radical (Laguerre et al. 2014). Chat et al. (2011) have studied the effect of various surfactant systems, which included cationic (CTAB, TTAB, DTAB), nonionic (Brij78, Brij58, Brij35), and anionic surfactant systems (SDS) on the radical scavenging activity of rutin by using DPPH radical. The encapsulation of the micellar systems toward both the molecules followed the order: cationic > nonionic > anionic. In general, they found that the radical scavenging activity of rutin was higher within the ionic micelles than in nonionic micelles; however, the antioxidant activity of rutin was found to be higher in the mixed cationic–nonionic micelles compared to any other single micellar system. Similar observations were also found in another study related to the effect of the surfactant systems on the radical scavenging activity of antioxidant "quercetin" toward hydroxyl radical by Jabeen et al. (2013). In this report they found that the radical scavenging activity of quercetin was higher in ionic micelles than in nonionic micelles with the mixed systems of DTPB-Brij30 exhibiting even higher activity compared to the single surfactant micellar systems.

Micelles have also been used as the stabilizers to enhance the shelf-life toward some of the flavoring agents like citral and limonene, which have the liability to get degraded by the external conditions in order to increase their shelf-life. In this direction, various studies have been carried out, for example Maswal et al. have demonstrated the protecting capabilities of polyoxyethylene alkylether-based nonionic surfactants toward citral (Maswal and Dar 2013). It was concluded from the studies that the nonionic surfactants, which have less number of oxyethylene units, are better candidates in protecting citral from the external acidic conditions that was attributed to the differential hydration of the palisade layers, which resulted in the segregation of encapsulated nutraceutical (citral) from the external acidic aqueous conditions (Figure 16.3).

In another parallel study by Choi et al. (2010), it was shown that the rate of citral degradation decreased with the increase in the concentration of Tween 80 from 1 to 5% in both aqueous solutions and in emulsions suggesting that the nano-encapsulation of citral was the main factor determining the chemical stability of citral. Furthermore, Ribeiro et al.(Ribeiro et al. 2009) have shown that the solubilization of quercetin and rutin was significantly increased in a mixture of a block copolymer of ethylene oxide styrene oxide.

Curcumin is another nutraceutical, which has attracted significant attention in terms of its encapsulation and protection from the alkaline medium by the colloidal science fraternity. It is a phytochemical isolated from the rhizome of *Curcuma longa L.* with important pharmacological properties but suffers from the lack of solubility in aqueous medium and liability toward degradation in alkaline medium as mentioned in Table 16.1. Micellar systems have been the preferable

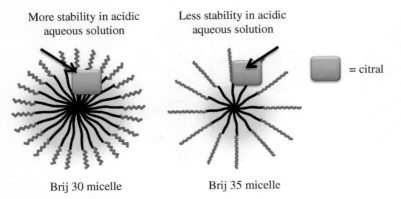

Figure 16.3 Schematic representation of the two nonionic micellar systems in stabilizing citral molecules in acidic aqueous environment.

candidates to solve these problems in order to increase the bioavailability of curcumin (Leung et al. 2008). The nature of the encapsulation of curcumin in micellar systems is significantly dependent on the head group charge of the surfactant monomers. For example, Leung et al. (2008) have shown that the cationic micellar systems, CTAB and DTAB, were very effective in inhibiting the degradation close to 90% compared to the anionic SDS micellar system, wherein no such inhibition was observed. The results were correlated with the electrostatic interactions between the curcumin and ionic head groups of the micelles (Figure 16.4). Pertinently, Iwunze (2004) demonstrated the inhibition of degradation of curcumin in CTAB micelles owing to the spontaneous transfer of it from aqueous phase to the hydrophobic micellar phase with a free energy change of −21.79 KJ/mol. This type of behavior was further confirmed by Wang and Gao (2018), wherein they demonstrated that more hydrophobic environment for curcumin in tween 60 compared to the tween 80 micellar systems protects it significantly.

This was attributed to the presence of unsaturation in the alkyl units of the tween 80 surfactant monomers compared to the tween 60 monomers, which provide a glimpse of hydrophilicity to the curcumin molecules in the former micellar system. The very nature of the micellar systems allows for their fine tuning vis-à-vis the encapsulation of curcumin and hence its degradation inhibition in such systems. This was demonstrated by the Patra and Barakat (2011) wherein they tuned the micellar-forming tendency of cationic, anionic, and nonionic micellar systems and their interactions with curcumin, in presence of hydrophilic ionic liquid, 1-butyl-3-methylimidazolium tetrafluoroburate, to alter their encapsulation and protecting abilities for curcumin. The stabilization of curcumin was highest in nonionic micellar systems due to the predominance of hydrophobic interactions between the [bmim][BF4] and the head group of the surfactants. It is a well-known fact that the mixed micelles possess superior physico-chemical properties compared to the single micellar systems, and this fact was utilized by Patil et al. (2015), wherein they achieved a 3-fold improvement in its cytotoxic activity and 55-fold increase in bioavailability by employing the mixed micellar systems based on Pluronic F-127 (PF127) and Gelucire 44/14 (GL44). The results were attributed again to the enhanced solubilization of curcumin inside the micellar cores.

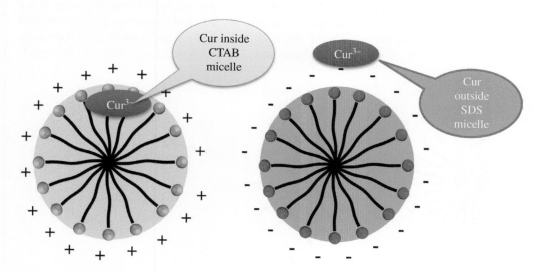

Figure 16.4 Schematic depiction for the stabilization of curcumin in CTAB micelles compared to the SDS micelles.

16.2.2 Liposomes

Liposomes are a class of self-assembled microstructures, which enclose a water pool inside a bilayer of surfactant molecules. Liposomal encapsulating systems have exhibited promising approach toward the bioavailability of nutraceuticals mainly due to the enhanced membrane permeability and cellular absorption (Zhang et al. 2013). Mohanraj et al. (2010) developed a liposomal system based on 1,2-dipalmitoyl-sn-glycero-3-phosphocholine and cholesterol. The as-formulated system was decorated with the silica nanoparticles on its surface and used for encapsulation, protection, and release of insulin. The authors demonstrated that the protection and release behavior of the liposomes was enhanced significantly when they were decorated with the silica nanoparticles compared to the uncoated liposomes. The study demonstrated that the encapsulating and protecting ability of the liposomes can be enhanced drastically by the careful engineering of the interfacial region of such microstructures in order to make up the smart and efficient excipients. In yet another related study, the liposomes were coated with the thiolated chitosan particles in order to alter its physico-chemical properties for better penetration through the intestinal mucus layer. The release behavior of the modified liposomes toward encapsulated salmon calcitonin was monitored through the fluorescence of fluoresceinisothiocyanate-labeled salmon calcitonin (Gradauer et al. 2013). Thirawong et al. (2008) studied the bioavailability of calcitonin by following its encapsulation and release from the cationic liposomes, which were modified with the pectin polymer. The enhanced absorption of the calcitonin was attributed to the significant change in the size of the liposomal particles and a significant shift in the zeta potential from positive to negative upon the incorporation of pectin into the cationic liposomes. Kumar et al. (2016) have demonstrated the enhanced antioxidant activity and biocompatibility of curcumin in the mixed surfactant vesicles. The authors employed fluorescence spectroscopy to determine the position of curcumin inside the vesicular structures and was found to be in the palisade layers of such assemblies. The formulation was successful in inhibiting the curcumin degradation to above 70% in about 10 hours at pH 13.

The anticancer activity of various nutraceuticals like curcumin, resveratrol, fisetin, etc. (Dutta et al. 2018) has been found to be significantly dependent on the nature of encapsulating liposome. The nutraceutical encapsulated liposome has been used to target various forms of cancer like cervical (Saengkrit et al. 2014), prostrate (Thangapazham et al. 2008), colorectal (Pandelidou et al. 2011), pancreatic (Li et al. 2005), ovarian (Phan et al. 2013), and breast (Halwani et al. 2015), and the results have been encouraging as far as the improvement in the anticancer activity of the encapsulated nutraceuticals is concerned. Liposomes were formulated by employing a large number of amphiphilic molecules like didodecyl dimethyl ammonium bromide (DDAB), cholesterol, phosphatidyl choline, dioleyl phosphatidylethanolamine, etc. (Dutta et al. 2018).

16.2.3 Emulsions

Emulsions are defined as the dispersions, which are made by mixing of two immiscible liquid phases, i.e. oil phase and aqueous phase using mechanical shear and a surfactant. Surfactants are basically the amphiphilic surface-active molecules that are used as surface tension reducing agents. Thus emulsions are composed of aqueous phase, oil phase, surfactant, and a co-surfactant if needed. Surfactant facilitates the process of dispersion during preparation of microemulsion by lowering the interfacial tension to negligible value (Saini et al. 2014). In food industries, these emulsion systems are used for the solubilization of oil soluble or hydrophobic nutraceuticals or drugs, for their enhancement in absorption within the body, in masking their disagreeable odor and/or taste, enhancing palatability of nutrient oils, etc. (Yaqoob Khan et al. 2006). Thus, emulsions can be used to encapsulate, protect, and deliver the nutraceuticals at the target site of gastrointestinal tract (GIT). However, due to less stability, short shelf-life, cracking, creaming, flocculation, phase inversion, and some other problems (Kale and Deore 2017), in recent years, use of new concept formulations emerged in emulsions, which include microemulsion, nanoemulsion, double emulsion, and Pickering emulsion. They are good in terms of not only stability but also effectively encapsulate, protect, and release the nutraceuticals. A brief discussion of these is given below:

16.2.3.1 Microemulsions

The concept of microemulsion was first introduced by Hoar and Schulman in 1943 (Hoar and Schulman 1943). Microemulsions are defined as a colloidal, optically isotropic, transparent, or slightly opalescent formulations, consisting of surfactant, co-surfactant, oil, and water (Chen et al. 2006a). Surfactants get adsorbed at the oil–water interface, where they achieve dual affinity with hydrophilic and hydrophobic groups located in aqueous and oil phases of the emulsion, respectively. They also reduce mismatching with solvent by micellization process (Paul and Moulik 1997). Most of the times, oil–water interfacial tension is not sufficiently reduced by single chain surfactants invoking the need of a co-surfactant (most preferably short to medium chain length alcohols), which accumulates substantially at interfacial layer, penetrates the surfactant layer, and therefore increases the fluidity of interfacial film (Graf et al. 2008). The main points of difference between emulsion and microemulsion lies in the size and shape of the droplets that are dispersed in the continuous phase. Droplet size is smaller in the case of microemulsions (10–200 nm) than those of conventional emulsions (1–20 µm). Other important differences include emulsions being cloudy, require a large input of energy, consist of roughly spherical droplets of one phase dispersed into the other, whereas microemulsions are clear or translucent, do not require large energy inputs, and constantly evolve between various structures ranging from droplet-like swollen micelles to bi-continuous structures (Kreilgaard 2002). These are basically classified into three types, viz., oil-in-water microemulsions (o/w) wherein oil droplets are dispersed in the continuous aqueous phase; water-in-oil microemulsions (w/o) wherein water droplets are dispersed in the continuous oil phase; and bi-continuous microemulsions wherein the microdomains of both oil and water are interdispersed within the system (Helal et al. 2019). As far as their method of preparation are concerned, there are two such methods – phase titration method and phase inversion method. The former method involves spontaneous emulsification, whereas the latter involves addition of excess of dispersed phase, leading to phase inversion and hence ultimately radical physical change in droplet size that alters the release of a nutraceutical (Henri et al. 1988). In food industry, oil-in-water microemulsions are particularly suitable for the encapsulation of hydrophobic nutraceuticals because they can be easily manufactured using food-grade ingredients and readily manufactured by widely used and sophisticated production techniques (McClements 2012b). Many food products already exist in the form of oil-in-water emulsions (such as beverages, sauces, soups, desserts, dressings, and yogurts), and so it is relatively easy to incorporate nutraceutical-loaded emulsions into them. Moreover, by using freeze- or spray-drying emulsions, these can easily be converted into a powdered form, which means that encapsulated nutraceuticals can also be incorporated into solid foods such as baked foods, cereals, and confectionaries (Kharat et al. 2017). The nutraceuticals encapsulated within nanosized capsules are reported to favor the stability, duration, and interactions with different matrices, thereby facilitating their promising protection and controlled release. Since the utilization of curcumin as a nutraceutical in food and supplement products is often limited because of its low aqueous solubility, low oral bioavailability, and poor chemical stability, there has been lots of efforts to use microemulsions as the encapsulating vehicles. Kharat et al. (2017) in 2016 examined the impact of pH, storage temperature, and molecular environment on the physical and chemical stability of pure curcumin in aqueous solutions and in oil-in-water emulsions. The results suggested that emulsion-based delivery systems may be suitable for improving the water dispersibility and chemical stability of curcumin, which would facilitate its application in foods and supplements. Choi et al. (2009a) examined the impact of organic phase composition-triacetin and medium chain triacylglycerols on the oil–water partitioning and chemical degradation of citral in oil-in-water emulsions. Triacetin was present as microemulsion droplets ($d \approx 10$ nm) that may have been able to protect the citral by incorporating it within their hydrophobic internal regions, whereas medium chain triacylglycerol was present as emulsion droplets ($d \approx 900$ nm) that acted as sinks for the citral, thereby protecting it from chemical degradation in the acidic aqueous phase.

16.2.3.2 Nanoemulsion

There exists both similarity and dissimilarity between a nano- and a microemulsion (Table 16.2). Both are dispersions of nanoscale particles, but the former is obtained by mechanical force, whereas the latter is formed spontaneously (Talegaonkar et al. 2008). The main difference between a micro- and nanoemulsion is that the former is thermodynamically stable, whereas latter is only kinetically stable. There are primarily two broad categories of techniques for the preparation of nanoemulsions, viz., low-energy methods and high-energy methods (Fryd and Mason 2012). In low-energy methods, when the system undergoes a phase inversion in response to changes in composition or temperature, the smaller droplets are formed and pass through a state of low interfacial tension. The two most widely used low-energy methods are emulsion inversion point (EIP) or phase inversion composition (PIC) and phase inversion temperature (PIT) (Izquierdo et al. 2002). The high energy methods involve high-pressure homogenization (HPH) and ultrasonication (Wooster et al. 2008). Figure 16.5 summarizes the preparation methods for o/w nanoemulsion via the HPH, ultrasonication, EIP, and PIT routes. Other preparation methods include bubble bursting at an oil/water interface, evaporative ripening, and microfluidization (Fryd and Mason 2010). Various advantages of nanoemulsions are to improve water solubility and ultimately bioavailability of lipophilic molecules. They have gained popularity over the past decade because of their exceptional properties such as large surface area, robust stability, transparent appearance, and tunable rheology. Stability issues like creaming, flocculation, coalescence, and sedimentation are rarely observed (Wu et al. 2013). The very small particle size of nanoemulsion delivery systems is a promising advantage over conventional emulsions. These systems, therefore, have optically transparent appearances and show greater stability against droplet flocculation and coalescence (Qian and McClements 2011). Encapsulation of nutraceuticals in nanoemulsion systems also increase the physio-chemical stability of encapsulated compounds. The physio-chemical properties of nanoemulsion systems improve bioactivity of encapsulated components and have wide application for delivery of antibiotics, disinfectants, antiseptics, and anticancer agents (Karthik et al. 2017). O/W vitamin and other neutraceutical nanoemulsions facilitate solubilization of these hydrophobic bioactive food components in GIT, therefore increasing bioavailability (Komaiko and McClements 2016). Being almost transparent systems, they barely scatter the light, which makes them suitable to be incorporated in clear drinks and foods (McClements 2002). Due to their reduced droplet size, they are considered to be more stable in terms of coalescence, gravitational separation, or particle aggregation (Mason et al. 2006). It has been recently pointed out that nanoemulsions may also enhance the transport of active ingredients through biological membranes, thus intensifying the bioavailability of bioactive compounds (Acosta 2009) or the bactericidal

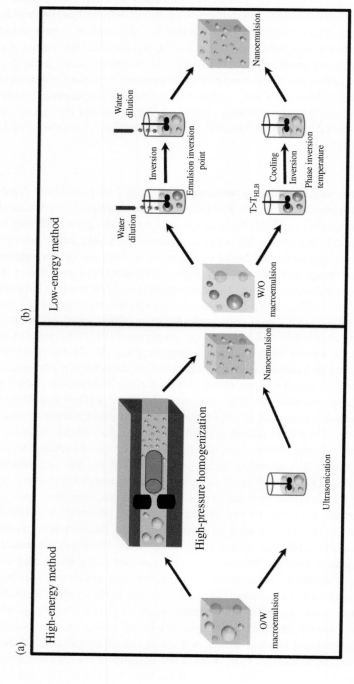

Figure 16.5 Schematic diagram showing high-energy and low-energy methods for preparing O/W nanoemulsions. (a) High energy such as HPH and ultrasonication break macroemulsion drops into smaller droplets. (b) Low-energy methods commence with w/o macroemulsions and break emulsions into small droplets as they pass through a state of low interfacial tension during phase inversion. *Source:* Adopted from Gupta et al. (2016) after permission from Royal Society of Chemistry.

Table 16.2 Comparison of macroemulsions, nanoemulsions (also referred to as miniemulsions), and microemulsions with respect to size, shape, stability, method of preparation, and polydispersity.

Emulsion type	Macroemulsions	Nanoemulsions	Microemulsions
Size	1–100 μm	20–500 nm	10–100 nm
Shape	Spherical	Spherical	Spherical, lamellar
Stability	Thermodynamically unstable, weak kinetic stability	Thermodynamically unstable, kinetically stable	Thermodynamically stable
Method of preparation	High- and low-energy methods	High- and low-energy methods	Low energy Method
Polydispersity	Often high (>40%)	Typically low (<10–20%)	Typically low (<10%)

activity of antimicrobials (Donsì et al. 2011). Thus, nanoemulsion delivery systems are promising methods for better formulation of food ingredients and their targeted delivery.

16.2.3.3 Pickering Emulsions

Pickering emulsions are among the most well-studied alternative strategies used for successful encapsulation and release of nutraceuticals. These were first proposed by S.U. Pickering. They employed solid particles alone as stabilizers, which accumulate at the interface of two immiscible liquid phases, i.e. oil and water phase, and stabilize droplets against coalescence (Pickering 1907). Pickering emulsions improve the protection of the food-grade neutraceutical from degradation due to the presence of barrier created by solid particles around the droplets (Wang et al. 2015a). They not only have outstanding stability but also satisfy the demand for intelligent stimuli-responsive emulsions because of functional nanoparticles anchored at the water/oil interface such as spherical nanoparticles, nanocrystals, and nanotubes (Cho et al. 2018). All emulsification processes used to prepare emulsions stabilized by surfactants can be applied to prepare Pickering emulsions. However, rotor-stator homogenization, HPH, and sonication are most commonly used for their formulation (Canselier et al. 2002). Various unique advantages include (i) solid particles bring about higher stability to emulsions by reducing the possibility of coalescence, (ii) many solid particles can endow useful characteristics such as porosity, conductivity, responsiveness, and so on; (iii) food-grade solid particles have lower or no toxicity at all (Yang et al. 2017). Since curcumin has numerous biological and pharmacological activities like antioxidant, anti-inflammatory, anti-bacterial, antiviral, anticancerous and so on, it is prone to degradation at high temperature, light, and neutral to alkaline media. The starch-based Pickering emulsion efficiently retained and protected curcumin from degradation during storage and simulated in vitro oral, gastric, and intestinal digestions (Marefati et al. 2017). Shah et al. encapsulated curcumin in the oil droplets of emulsions stabilized by chitosan nanoparticles by using tripolyphosphate as the cross-linker. Better protection of curcumin against degradation during storage and slower release rate were obtained with such Pickering emulsions than with classical emulsions (Shah et al. 2016). Few years back, some newly structure-modified celluloses such as NFC (nanofibrilated mangosteen cellulose) and ANC (aminated nanocellulose) have been explored for the stabilization of green Pickering emulsions as novel oral delivery systems for both curcumin and vitamins (Winuprasith et al. 2018). Liu and Tang (2016), Shao and Tang (2016) and Tan et al. (2017) encapsulated β-carotene in the oil droplets of Pickering emulsions respectively stabilized by three different types of protein particles – soy protein particles, pea protein particles, and gelatin particles. In all the three cases, the emulsion droplets had approximately the same size (ranging from a few to tens of micrometers). Their study regarding the release of β-carotene during in vitro digestion found an additional stability and sustained release.

16.2.3.4 Multiple or Double Emulsions

Multiple emulsions are complex heterogeneous systems in which simple emulsions (O/W or W/O) are further dispersed in oil or water to form water-oil-water (W/O/W) or oil-water-oil (O/W/O) emulsions, respectively, in the presence of two stabilizing surfactants, one hydrophilic and the other lipophilic (Vasudevan and Naser 2002). The surfactants rearrange at the interface of the dispersed droplets to expose their hydrophilic moieties to the aqueous phase and their hydrophobic moieties to the nonaqueous or oil phase (Kronberg and Lindman 2003). In the food industry, double emulsions have a number of potential applications that make them commercially attractive, including (i) encapsulation of vitamins, aromas, nutraceuticals, flavors, or enzymes to enhance their water-solubility, increase their activity, mask off-flavors, improve their stability, and control their release (Serdaroğlu et al. 2016); and (ii) a reduction of the amount of fat in W/O/W emulsions compared to conventional O/W emulsions makes it feasible to produce low-fat foods (Choi et al. 2009b). For the encapsulation of many molecules of interest that need to be protected from external stresses before being released, double emulsions are very beneficial. In the food processing industry, the high potential of multiple emulsions to encapsulate and protect relatively unstable, sensitive, and reactive compounds such as flavors, vitamins, or minerals has been demonstrated (O'Regan and Mulvihill 2010). In most cases, the preparation of double emulsions requires a combination of hydrophilic and hydrophobic surfactants to stabilize the W/O, as well as the O/W interface, and also a two-step emulsification process that introduces many destabilization pathways and lead to emulsions with short-term stability (Garti 1997). To overcome unstability problems, many formulation approaches need to be deployed. Most common approaches involve selection of sophisticated combinations of emulsifiers, optimization of the proportions of the two types of emulsifiers, addition of appropriate co-surfactants, and so on (Garti and Benichou 2004). However, there still appears a limitation to its large-scale application, which arises due to the lack of control of emulsions morphology and encapsulation rate, the complexity of their multistep formulation route, and the necessity of using appropriate amounts of surfactants to obtain stable multiple emulsions (Dickinson 2011). In recent years, double emulsions have been used to encapsulate, stabilize, and deliver both hydrophilic and hydrophobic food components, including minerals, vitamins, polyphenols, flavors, peptides, probiotics, and sweeteners. Even two different nutraceuticals like hydrophilic one and hydrophobic one can be simultaneously encapsulated within the same double emulsion. For example, both hydrophilic (catechin) and hydrophobic (curcumin) active agents were simultaneously encapsulated into a single emulsion, which proved to be of great advantage for certain applications (Aditya et al. 2015; Xiao et al. 2017).

16.3   Self-assemblies of Polymers Including Hydrogels as Encapsulating, Protecting, and Delivery Systems for Nutraceuticals

16.3.1   Polymers

In the encapsulation, stability, and controlled release of lipophilic food components such as ω-3 rich oils, conjugated linoleic acid (CLA), oil-soluble vitamins, flavors, colors, and nutraceuticals, natural polymers find great application as these are generally biodegradable and are generally recognized as safe (GRAS). The biopolymers such as proteins and polysaccharides have been used unceasingly since long for the micro and nanoencapsulation of these functional food materials so as to ensure their stability (against harsh conditions of gastrointestinal tract such as pH, temperature, ionic strength) and controlled release at the site of action. Researchers have fabricated different colloid-based delivery systems for the encapsulation, protection, and controlled release of these lipophilic components, which has emerged as a promising technique in food industry (Aguilera 2000; Augustin et al. 2001; McClements et al. 2007). Such colloid-based delivery systems need to be prepared from food-grade ingredients using economical and reliable approach. The use of biopolymers like proteins and polysaccharides are the building blocks for the production of such systems and has been one among the most promising methods (Matalanis et al. 2011). The micro or nanoencapsulation of nutraceuticals by biopolymers is achieved by employing different procedures which include spray-drying, emulsion techniques, ionotropic gelation etc. The biopolymer based micro and nanoencapsulation processes have a great importance in food industry due their ability to incorporate different bioactive materials such as lipids, enzymes, phytochemicals, vitamins, flavors and probiotics in food products thereby adding many advantages in their preservation and contribution in developing functional foods (Kwak 2014; Quirós-Sauceda et al. 2014; Gutiérrez and Álvarez 2017). The priority of micro- and nanoencapsulation technologies by biopolymers lies in improving the physicochemical and biological properties of the functional ingredients entrapped, in a variety of ways which involves (i) masking the organoleptic properties such as taste, color, and odor of the functional components, (ii) guarding the encapsulated substance from external conditions during processing and stowage inside food system, (3) ensuring the sustained, targeted, and controlled release of the bioactive component, and (4) providing better uptake, absorption, and bioavailability of specific nutrients in the body (Ray et al. 2016).

16.3.1.1 Rules Governing the Selection of Biopolymer-Derived Micro or Nanoparticle-Based Encapsulant or Delivery Systems

Advances have been fast in the development of biopolymer derived micro as well as nanoparticle based delivery system to encapsulate, protect, and release nutraceutical type of bioactives or functional foods over the past few years. In polysaccharides, these include the micro and nanoencapsulants formed from chitosan, pectin, alginates, gum Arabic, agar, and many others. In proteins, micro and nanoencapsulants are developed from caseins, whey proteins, gelatin, zein, albumin, etc. From lipids, beeswax, candelilla waxes, carnauba waxes, phospholipids, and glycolipids are some examples of micro and nanoencapsulants. In addition to these many hybrid micro and nanoencapsulants formed by polysaccharide–protein, protrein–protein, or protein–lipid mixtures have also been developed for improved protection and delivery in comparison to single biopolymer. However, in choosing a particular material for encapsulation, one has to ensure that the material finds a widespread use in food industry as micro or nanoparticle-based delivery system and in order to be so the encapsulating material or the encapsulant or the delivery system must fulfil the following requirements (McClements 2012a).

- The encapsulant must be formulated from legally acceptable ingredients and processing methods. The processes involved should be economic as well.
- There should be compatibility between the encapsulant and the food matrix, i.e. the properties of the product such as appearance, texture, flavor, rheology, or shelf life should not get affected undesirably.
- The encapsulant formulated must be able to render the hydrophobic bioactives, e.g. lipids aqueous soluble in aqueous-based food products such as beverages, desserts, dressing, sauce and so on. At the same time, the encapsulated compound being prone to chemical degradation should be stabilized against factors like oxygen, pH, high ionic strength, temperature, etc.

- The encapsulant should have the ability to enclose a sufficiently large amount of functional components per unit mass of delivery system and should retain them until the functional compound is delivered.
- The encapsulant should be designed such that it releases the food component at a controlled rate in response to a specific environmental stimulus such as pH, ionic strength, enzyme activity, or temperature.
- The encapsulant should improve (or at least not adversely affect) the bioavailability/bioactivity of the functional food. Also the delivery system must survive the human digestive system to significant extent to protect the functional food and maintaining its bioavailability until it reaches the target site(s).
- The encapsulant should have the quality of being manufactured from economically inexpensive ingredients. In this sense, the benefits gained from encapsulating a food ingredient within a micro or nanosystem such as shelf life improvement, marketability enhancement, novel functionality, and better bioavailability should outweigh the additional costs associated with encapsulation.

16.3.1.2 Encapsulation Process

The encapsulation of functional materials like nutraceuticals is carried out by fabrication of capsules in which the nutraceutical is incorporated as a core material inside a wall material manufactured from biopolymer-based colloidal particles. The morphology of the capsule is a function of nature of inner core material and the position of wall material. Based on this, different types of capsules are fabricated, which include (i) single-core capsule (a core that is surrounded by a wall of the polymer material), (ii) dispersed core in polymer network (a core that is entrapped within a continuous polymer network). Some other variations in these morphologies include multilayered capsules and dual-core or dual-layer capsules (Figure 16.6) (Augustin and Hemar 2009). The capsules are also classified based on their size, in macrocapsules (>5000 μm), microcapsules (0.2–5000 μm), and nanocapsules (< 0.2 μm), and hence the encapsulations are categorized accordingly as macroencapsulation, microencapsulation, and nanoencapsulation, respectively (Silva et al. 2014).

The nature of core material actually governs the type of wall material and the suitable method for encapsulation (Dias et al. 2017). Therefore, the core material attributes such as thermal stability, viscosity in case of a liquid, particle size, and shape in case of a solid, density, reactivity, and solubility determine the effective design and development of the preferred micro- and

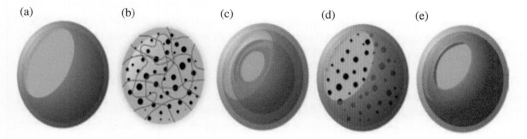

Figure 16.6 Morphologies of capsules: (a) single-core capsule; (b) dispersed core in polymer network; (c) multilayered capsule; (d) dual-core capsule; (e) dual-layer capsule. *Source:* Adapted from Augustin and Hemar (2009) after permission from Royal Society of Chemistry.

nanocapsule (Mishra 2016). The wall material, on the other hand, should possess the capability of forming a cohesive film with the core material so that it determines the inner core's degree of protection, have a positive influence on stability of capsules that can be micro or nanocapsule and enhances the efficiency of the encapsulation process (Bakry et al. 2016). A wall material is considered excellent if it (i) remains unreactive toward the core for very long durations, (ii) seals and sustains the core efficiently inside the micro or nanocapsule, (iii) have a pleasing taste when taken as food, (iv) provides best protection to the core from external unfavorable environmental factors, and (v) is economic (Kwak 2014). Keeping in view these requirements of wall material, palatable polymers such as polysaccharides, proteins, and lipids come out to be the best candidates for encapsulation processes of nutraceutical type of functional components. However, the type of polymer chosen for encapsulation process is determined on the basis of physical and chemical properties of the type of nutraceutical to be encapsulated (Shit and Shah 2014).

16.3.1.3 Different Types of Biopolymers Used for Micro and Nanoencapsulation of Nutraceuticals

As discussed earlier, the incorporation of functional foods through micro- or nanoencapsulation methods are a function of specific molecular properties of the functional foods such as conformation, weight, and polarity. Therefore, selection of an adequate encapsulating material improves the efficacy of these bioactive compounds significantly (Suganya and Anuradha 2017). Materials fulfilling these properties are edible polymers, i.e. carbohydrates, proteins, and lipids as already discussed. The commonly used carbohydrates, proteins, and lipids for micro and nanoencapsulation processes of bioactive foods are presented in Figure 16.7.

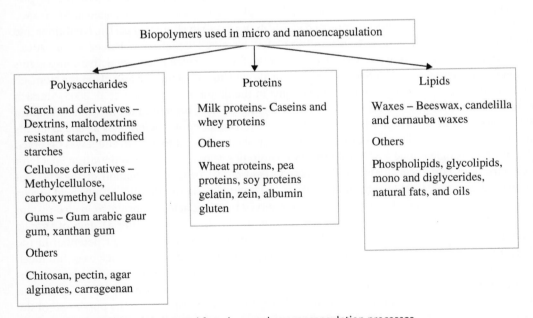

Figure 16.7 Some biopolymers used for micro- and nanoencapsulation processes.

Carbohydrates Carbohydrate polymers consist of sugar residues and/or their derivatives bonded by specific linkages called O-glycosidic linkages. This linkage can occur between any of the hydroxyl groups of sugar monomers resulting in linear and branched chain polysaccharides. The nature of a polymer's structure governs its functional properties, such as solubility, gel forming, and surface properties. Commercially, for their use in the food industry, the polysaccharide polymers are accessible as thickening and gelling agents, stabilizers, crystallization inhibitors, and as the wall material or carrier in encapsulations (de Vos et al. 2014). Polysaccharides are classified in different categories based on their biological origin. For example, starch, cellulose, pectin, gum arabic, inulin, and guar gum have a plant origin, while as agar, alginate, and carrageenan have algal origin, and chitosan and xanthan are from animal and microbial origin, respectively (Figure 16.7) (Liu et al. 2015). The polymers based on polysaccharides have emerged as potential candidates for micro- and nanoencapsulation due to several attributes associated with them such as (i) forming an integral part of many food systems, (ii) cost-effective, (iii) variable available polymer sizes, and (iv) having desirable physicochemical properties such as solubility, melting and phase change, low viscosity, wall-forming ability, and efficient drying properties (Fathi et al. 2014). Alginates, chitosan, pectins, dextran, starch, and inulin are some most commonly used polysaccharides in micro- and nanoencapsulation (Ishak et al. 2017). During micro- and nanoencapsulation processes, they retain a functional component by a unique mechanism involving physicochemical interactions depending on molecular association by hydrogen bonding (Cook et al. 2012).

Numerous reports have been made till date where different types of polysaccharides or their derivatives have been used for micro- and nanoencapsulation of bioactive compounds for their protection and controlled delivery. Enhanced protection of probiotic lactobacilli (Lactobacillus plantarum LAB12) against low pH and high temperature have been achieved by immobilizing the probiotic within polymeric matrix containing alginate (Alg) along with supplementation of cellulose derivatives (methylcellulose (MC), sodium carboxymethyl cellulose (NaCMC), or hydroxypropyl methylcellulose (HPMC)). It was observed that L. plantarum LAB12 encapsulated in Alg-HPMC (1.0) and Alg-MC (1.0) produced improved survivability (91%) in simulated gastric conditions and facilitated maximal release (~100%) in simulated intestinal conditions (Fareez et al. 2018). Chitosan, a very interesting polysaccharide, is known for its targeted release of active components to living cells. Usually, it is blended together with alginate to withstand the low pH in the stomach and to facilitate the release of active components in the ileum or colon (Iyer et al. 2005; Marsich et al. 2008) for example, blends from alginate and chitosan have been used to encapsulate vitamin B2 (Azevedo et al. 2014). In other work, chitosan-alginate based nanolaminates as encapsulants were successfully used for photoprotection and controlled release of folic acid, and it was observed that the encapsulated folic acid within the nanolaminates were more stable under ultraviolet light exposure than non-encapsulated ones (Acevedo-Fani et al. 2018). Investigation of the effect of alginate-pectin-poly (ethylene oxide) (PEO) electrospun fibers on the stability of folic acid in gastrointestinal tract has also been carried. It was observed that folic acid encapsulated in electrospun fibers achieved close to 100% retention when stored in the dark at pH 3 after 41 days of storage (Alborzi et al. 2013). The plant-derived polymers, starch, and inulin find their potential in the delivery of active food/drug components owing to their inherent advantages, such as economical, relative ease of handling, and can be applied in combination with almost all encapsulation techniques. Due to their stability toward hydrolysis, they have been used as materials for encapsulation of micro- or nanoparticles for their targeted delivery to colon and survival in the upper part of the gastrointestinal tract (Macfarlane and Englyst 1986; Gibson et al. 2004). For example, in the spray-drying encapsulation process of essential oils from oregano and rosemary using inulin as encapsulating material, the results showed that inulin-based microcapsules formed were regular, smooth, uninjured, and spherical, with size in the range of 3–4.5 μm and provided significant protection to these oils in upper gastrointestinal tract (da Costa et al. 2012; Beirão-da-Costa et al. 2013). Moreover, in studying the impact of the partial or total replacement of gum arabic by modified starch, maltodextrin, or inulin on properties of microcapsules with rosemary essential oil, it was noticed that the particles containing inulin were characterized by smoother surface. One more class of polysaccharide biopolymers are the gums, which are being used in microencapsulation because of their film forming and emulsion stabilization properties. Among all gums, acacia gum (gum arabic), due to its excellent emulsification properties, stands mostly used. It is a polymer consisting of D-glucuronic acid, L-rhamnose, D-galactose, and L-arabinose, with approximately 2% protein. It is the occurrence of this 2% protein which gives it excellent emulsification properties (Dickinson 2003). For the encapsulation of cardamom oleoresin, gum arabic was found to be a better wall material than maltodextrins and modified starch, and the obtained microcapsules exhibited a free-flowing character (Krishnan et al. 2005). It was also recently reported that gum arabic is good wall material for encapsulation of cumin oleoresin by spray-drying (Kanakdande et al. 2007). It has been observed that gum arabic produces stable emulsions with most oils over a wide pH range due to its film-forming properties, and consequently it has been in frequent use to encapsulate lipids (Kenyon 1995).

Proteins Proteins are the natural macromolecules of linear chains of amino acids that have a number of applications including micro- and nanoencapsulation processes (Lam and Nickerson 2013). The protein polymers have the compositions resulting from various combinations of 20 amino acids giving them enormous variety of sequences. Even though proteins are of natural origin, certain properties associated with them like fibers and hydrogels are comparable to those of synthetic materials. The properties associated with proteins such as biocompatibility, biodegradability, good water solubility, film-forming and barrier properties, ability for adhesion, and acting as organic solvents make them much suitable materials for encapsulation of lipophilic functional foods such as nutraceuticals (Riaz and Masud 2013). Like carbohydrates, proteins too have different types based on their origin. Some of the most commonly employed proteins in the micro- and nanoencapsulation processes are caseins, whey proteins, and gelatin having animal origin; and pea, soy proteins, zein, and wheat proteins having vegetable origin.

For the sake of protection and controlled release of nutraceutical, use of protein-based biopolymers have been reported enormously. In one study regarding the encapsulation by proteins, α-tocopherol was encapsulated using β-lactoglobulin as shell material (Liang et al. 2011), while in another study curcumin was encapsulated by incorporating it into gelatin, which served as a wall material (Gómez-Estaca et al. 2015). The casein proteins have been potentially used as natural nanovehicles in the form of casein micelles for hydrophobic nutraceuticals (Semo et al. 2007). For example, a study Haham et al. (2012) reported the use of casein micelles to encapsulate vitamin D so as to evaluate the protection conferred by them against thermal and oxidative degradation of vitamin D. Some vegetable origin proteins such as soy protein and pea protein have been used to encapsulate α-tocopherol and flaxseed oil (Nesterenko et al. 2014; Bajaj et al. 2017). Zein a cereal protein is an attractive novel material that is used in a wide range of protecting applications of bioactive components such as polyphenols, vitamins, and omega-3 fatty polymeric amphiphile, which enables the encapsulation and dispersion of oil-based microspheres (Wang et al. 2008a). Because of its extremely high surface area and trapping efficiency, zein creates a protective layer around hydrophobic bioactives when they are coprecipitated with it (Luo and Wang 2014). Being resistant to digestive enzymes, zein made capsules result in a slower digestibility in the gastrointestinal tract; hence, a controlled release of functional components loaded in zein colloidal particles can be achieved (Patel and Velikov 2014). A watersoluble chitosan derivative, carboxymethyl chitosan (CM-chitosan), is used to form coatings on the zein surface. This CM-chitosan coating confers pH and thermal stability to zein nanoparticles, as a result these complex nanoparticles provide excellent protection of labile nutraceuticals against thermal degradation and oligomerization (Luo and Wang 2014). The zein–chitosan complex acids function as nanoparticle is tailored in two ways for different applications. One is based on the hydrophobicity of zein shell, which prevents dissolution of chitosan in the low pH conditions of stomach; as a result, the zein–chitosan complex nanoparticles bring improvement in the encapsulation efficiency and slower release of hydrophilic nutrients in the gastrointestinal tract. In the second way, the zein nanoparticles are poured into chitosan solution in such a way that the zein–chitosan complex delivery system so formed gets tuned to encapsulate and deliver the hydrophobic drugs and nutrients (Luo and Wang 2014). There are various other reports where polysaccharides and proteins have been used in combination in order to fabricate micro- and nanoparticle delivery systems. For example, the combination of polysaccharides such as carboxymethyl cellulose and pectin with whey proteins has been significantly helpful during microencapsulation of antioxidants from Roselle extract, in improving emulsifying and film-forming properties (Serrano-Cruz et al. 2013). Similarly, the combination of pea protein isolate with sodium alginate, carrageenan, and gellan gum has been used in the encapsulation of many bioactives (Varankovich et al. 2015). Certain other types of nontoxic, non-immunogenic, biocompatible, and biodegradable proteins called globular proteins have shown interesting properties in developing polyunsaturated fatty acid (PUFA)-based delivery systems. One of the most studied globular protein is β-lactoglobulin, the binding properties of which have received considerable attention due to its potential uses in PUFA-delivery strategies (Livney 2010).

Lipids Lipids are the fats and oils, consisting of monoglycerides, phospholipids, triacylglycerol, cholesterol, and other groups of compounds (Shishir et al. 2018). Due to their less toxicity, good surface activity, and biocompatibility, lipid-based micro and nano-delivery systems have excellent functionality in emulsification, film formation, and encapsulation of bioactive compounds (Fathi et al. 2012). Phospholipids, glycolipids, natural fats and oils, mono and di-glycerides, beeswax, candelilla, and carnauba waxes are some commonly employed lipids as wall materials (Figure 16.2) in micro- and nanoencapsulation of lipophilic bioactives such as nutraceuticals to protect them from extreme conditions of temperature or moisture (Fathi et al. 2012). In contrast to micro, the lipid-based nano-delivery systems are extensively employed in food and pharmaceutical industry due to their excellent abilities to encapsulate, stabilize, and improvement in controlled and sustained release. Solid lipid nanoparticles (SLNs), nanostructure lipid carriers (NLCs), nanoemulsions, and nanoliposomes are some of the lipid-based nano-delivery systems among which the SLNs and NLCs have gained extraordinary attention (Fathi et al. 2012).

In recent times, there has been enormous increase in the reports where lipid-based micro- and nano-delivery systems have been employed for protection and controlled release of food components. For example, hydrophobic micronutrients such as resveratrol and quercetin have been encapsulated within the lipid droplets in nanoemulsions to increase their bioavailability (Pool et al. 2013; Sessa et al. 2014). In another study, double emulsions with different lipid sources, i.e. chia oil, sunflower oil, olive oil, or rendered pork back fat, were used to encapsulate riboflavin where chia oil proved to be the most efficient encapsulant (Bou et al. 2014). Solid lipid nanoparticles (SLNs) provide higher encapsulation efficiency and greater protection to both lipophilic and hydrophilic compounds from unfavorable conditions. For example, SLNs obtained from hydrogenated canola oil have shown high retention of vitamin B2, a hydrophilic bioactive compound (Couto et al. 2017). Likewise, there have been other reports recently regarding the usage of SLNs in encapsulation, e.g. encapsulation of β-carotene, vitamin A (acetate), and ω-3 fish oil (Salminen et al. 2016), encapsulation of curcumin (Ayan et al. 2017), and encapsulation of astaxanthin (Bakry et al. 2016). To overcome certain limitations associated with SLNs, i.e. low loading capacity, to overcome the burst release of active compounds, and to enhance the sustained release profile, SLNs are modified to nanostructured lipid carriers (NLCs), by replacing 5–40% of solid lipid phase of SLNs by liquid lipid phase (Wang et al. 2017). In a study, three lipid-based delivery systems, i.e. solid lipid nanoparticles (SLNs), nanostructured lipid carriers (NLCs), and lipid nanoemulsions (LNEs) in order to evaluate their bioavailability by using incorporation of quercetin (Aditya et al. 2014). The results showed that quercetin-loaded NLCs had the smallest particle size, maximum bioaccessibility, and transparency with high encapsulation efficiency (>90%). Many lipid-based vesicular carriers have been developed, which include liposomes, niosomes, bilosomes, transferosomes, ethosomes, and phytosomes, among which liposomes are the most used lipid vesicular carriers in food and pharmaceutical industries (Aditya et al. 2017). Liposomes show excellent ability to encapsulate hydrophobic, hydrophilic, and amphiphilic bioactive compounds simultaneously. This property of liposomes arises from their structure and composition. These are phospholipid vesicles, having a lipid bilayer formed by hydrophilic-hydrophobic interactions that segregate the inner aqueous phase from the external continuous water phase. Liposomes have successfully been studied as good bioactive carrier for anthocyanin, lutein, quercetin, and vitamins (Zhao et al. 2017).

16.3.2 Hydrogels

Hydrogels are the three-dimensional polymeric networks in which the polymeric chains are either physically or chemically crosslinked to give the network a rigid structure. Hydrogels owing to their porous structure have the capability to absorb and lock plenty of the water molecules inside the structure and interestingly become insoluble in the aqueous media. Hydrogels possess the excellent biocompatibility and display versatility in their structure and properties. Hence, it is appealing to use hydrogels as the most feasible and intelligent class of materials for protection and sustained carrier of proteins, lipids, polysaccharides, and other nutraceuticals in order to make them biologically efficacious (Lima et al. 2012). The hydrogels are tunable to different modifications in the chemical structure and the surface properties in order to serve the specific functions. However, the applications of hydrogels in the food industry require preparation of safe hydrogels suitable for the consumption. This signals the use of natural macromolecules, which include proteins like gelatin, zein, gliadin, and carbohydrates such as starch, chitosan, and gum (Klein and Poverenov 2020) to develop hydrogels to be used in the food industry for the preservation and bioaccessibility of the nutraceuticals. Such biological macromolecules offer many advantages such as enhanced solubility and stability of nutraceuticals, bioaccessibility, compatibility with the food systems, and controlled release at targeted site in human body (Asghar et al. 2018).

16.3.2.1 Characteristics of Hydrogel for Encapsulation, Protection, and Release of the Nutraceuticals

Since there are the three main stages in the process of enhancing bioaccessibility of the nutraceuticals, viz., encapsulation, protection, and release of the cargo, the hydrogels possess the unique properties, which augment all the three stages and hence have been rendered as versatile and desirable platform for their use as delivery systems, which are summed up as below.

Porosity   The porous structure of the hydrogels plays an important role in the encapsulation of the nutraceuticals and is highly desirable for the use in the sustained delivery. Encapsulation is an effective approach to entrap the nutraceuticals within the delivery systems, which can protect and improve the solubility of these active molecules from the harsh intra and extracellular environmental conditions via partitioning of the molecules from the bulk phase to the colloidal phase. Hydrogels offer an excellent and versatile route for encapsulation of the food ingredients, which have resulted in remarkable solubility and protection of the encapsulated molecules. The porous network allows the active molecules to diffuse into the gel matrix and their subsequent release at a controlled rate upon the triggering conditions. The permeability of a food ingredient into the hydrogel can be easily tuned as it highly depends on the pore size, which in turn can be tuned by controlling the composition and the degree of cross-linking in the gel matrix (LaNasa et al. 2011). It has been seen that effective retention and sustained release occur when the pore size is greater than the size of the encapsulated molecule. Hence, the encapsulation, retention, and release from the hydrogels can be tailored by tuning the nature of the biopolymer and crosslinking density. In a study carried out by Zeeb et al. (2015), the rate of release of curcumin-loaded lipid droplets encapsulated in the calcium alginate hydrogel beads showed high dependence on the pore size of the hydrogel, which was regulated by changing alginate and calcium concentrations.

Degradability   Two of the most important aspects of the nutraceutical bioavailability are the retention and release of the encapsulated nutraceutical. Generally, a nutraceutical must be retained in its active form within the hydrogel matrix until it comes in contact with certain environmental conditions causing the disintegration/hydrolysis of the hydrogel resulting in the release of the nutraceutical. For the commercial food applications, the biodegradability of the hydrogels is emphasized so as to control their release properties. Therefore, the polymeric components chosen for the synthesis of hydrogels should be biodegradable either by enzymatic actions, chemisorption or hydrolysis in the physiological processes. The polymers like chitosan, sodium alginate, dextran, gum arabic, cellulose, etc. are considered to be superior and preferable candidates for the formulation of hydrogels due to their biocompatibility and biodegradability attributed to their amide or glycosidic linkages, which make them susceptible to hydrolysis (Abedini et al. 2018). Therefore, controlling the biodegradability of the hydrogels, the release rate, and the fate of the encapsulated nutraceutical in the GIT can be tuned. My-Le et al. (2020) have investigated the effect of incorporating alginate into N,O-carboxymethyl chitosan (NOCC)-aldehyde hyaluronic acid (AHA) network on the degradation and biocompatibility of the hybrid hydrogel. The incorporation of alginate proved to significantly enhance the system stability and prolong degradation time.

Mechanical Strength   Poor mechanical strength of the delivery systems lays huge obstruction in their utilization in the food fortification applications. Hydrogels offer excellent mechanical properties to withstand the environmental stress and tear. In this context, a vast research has been carried out to tune the mechanical properties of the hydrogels to be used as delivery systems. Many strategies have been followed by the researchers to improve the mechanical properties of hydrogels such as to introduce the cross linkers in the polymeric network (Okumura and Ito 2001) and develop composite hydrogels with nanoparticles and graphene oxide (Amalraj et al. 2018). For example, a composite hydrogel developed by combining two prolamin proteins, hordein, and zein exhibited outstanding mechanical strength (Wang et al. 2019).

Water Content and Swelling Character   The high water content in the hydrogels induces the likeness of being similar to the soft biological tissues and overcome the brittle nature of hydrogels, which limits their use in food companies. The water content of hydrogels can be easily accommodated by tuning the non-covalent crosslink density (Wojtecki et al. 2011). The water content influences the permeation of nutrients (Hoffman 2012) and the mechanical strength of the hydrogels (Pasqui et al. 2012). Nowadays, the formulation of ultrahigh water content hydrogels has attracted the attention of researchers. In one report, Maciel et al. (2019) reacted aldehyde group modified cashew gum with gelatin through a Schiff base reaction to produce a hydrogel with high capacity for water absorption.

Bioadhesion The adherence of hydrogels to biological tissues is an important characteristic of the delivery systems. Hydrogels with porous structure have the excellent absorbing tendency and can thus absorb the extracellular proteins efficiently which provides the base for cell adhesion. Moreover, a gel-like layer of mucin, a negatively charged glycoprotein, covers the intestinal lining and acts as a barrier for the nutraceutical absorption (Bansil and Turner 2006). Thus, it is necessary to induce the adhesion between the encapsulant and mucin called as mucoadhesion to improve the efficacy of nutraceuticals (Thongborisute and Takeuchi 2008). This mucoadhesive property of polymers is very beneficial for developing the delivery systems for oral or intestinal mucosa by which they increase the contact time of nutraceutical at the absorption site with the mucosa and surmount the shortcomings of low biological half-life and high dosing frequency. Cationic polymers such as chitosan exhibits strong mucoadhesive capacity due to its electrostatic attraction with mucin (Claesson and Ninham 1992).

The natural macromolecules are highly recommended to be used in the formulation of food-grade hydrogels due to their biocompatibility and biodegradability and as such proteins and polysaccharides having high nutritional value and generally recognized as safe (GRAS) status have been often used in the formulation of the delivery systems for encapsulation of bioactive molecules by the food companies (Miao et al. 2018). The hydrogels as delivery systems for the food ingredients can be broadly divided into two categories.

16.3.2.2 Protein-Based Hydrogels

Proteins are the main nutritional components acting as the source of amino acids and bioactive peptides. At the same time, proteins possess multiple functional groups that can undergo different interactions such as hydrogen bonding, π–π, electrostatic, or hydrophobic interactions within themselves leading to the formation of hydrogels or with the other molecules and result in their encapsulation and stabilization (Chen et al. 2006b). They possess excellent emulsifying and gelling properties favorable for the formation of hydrogels or hydrogel emulsions with controllable droplet size (Chen and Subirade 2009). Therefore, the protein hydrogels have been also referred to as smart hydrogels as they are highly sensitive to the environmental conditions such as pH, temperature, light, or solvent and inducing different responses in the hydrogel network. Hence, protein-based hydrogels have emerged as an interesting strategy to encapsulate the nutraceuticals in order to enhance the solubility, preserve the biological activity, and control their release. There are a number of proteins such as gelatin, zein, soy, whey, casein, gliadin, and so on, which can be used for the hydrogel formulation with different morphology, texture, pore size, and different chemical structure having diverse functionalities, pH, and temperature specificity, which can be modulated to achieve desirable encapsulation, protection, stabilization, and release of the nutraceuticals beneficial for the fortification of foods. For instance, Maltais et al. (2009) have developed the particulate and filamentous type of hydrogels from soy protein and investigated the encapsulation and release of riboflavin under gastric (pH 1.2) and intestinal (pH 7.5) conditions. This study revealed that under the SGF conditions, the release of riboflavin is initially faster for one hour in the particulate gel than that in the filamentous gel due to the presence of larger pore in the former as shown in Figure 16.8a. While as under the SIF conditions, riboflavin release from both the gels is very high reaching up to 80–100% in 6 hours (Figure 16.8b). It was also observed that both the hydrogels protected riboflavin in the presence of pepsin at pH 1.2 for 6 hours, while as the digestion was observed in presence of pancreatin at pH 7.5. Thus, such type of hydrogel can be used to transport the nutraceuticals through GIT and deliver them in small intestines.

In another study by Chen and Subirade (2009), hydrogel microspheres were synthesized using soy protein isolate (SPI), viz., zein and SPI/zein blend for the encapsulation and release of riboflavin in simulated gastric and intestinal fluids at pH 1.2 and 7.4. An encapsulation efficiency of 79–88% was obtained for all microspheres with loading efficiency ranging from 9.0 to 9.8%. The riboflavin release showed burst release for the first 15 minutes from both pure SPI and zein microspheres (Figure 16.9) at both the pHs followed by steady release from 15 minutes to 4 hours. It was also observed that at pH 1.2, faster release of riboflavin occurs from the SPI microspheres than at pH 7.4, while a slow release was observed from the zein microspheres at both the pHs. On blending the two proteins together, the release rate can be controlled by adjusting the SPI/zein ratio as shown in Figure 16.10a,b and the rate of release of riboflavin decreased progressively on increasing

(a)

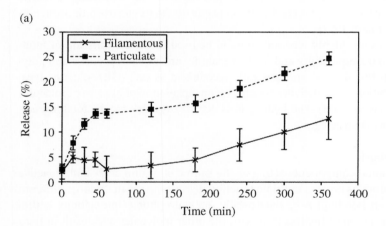

(b)

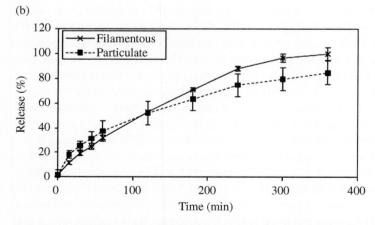

Figure 16.8 Riboflavin release from the filamentous and particulate gels in (a) SGF (pH 1.2) in presence of pepsin and (b) in SIF (pH 7.5) in presence of pancreatin during a 6-hour dissolution test. *Source*: Adapted from Maltais et al. (2009) after permission from Elsevier.

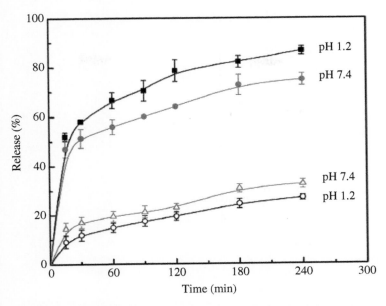

Figure 16.9 Release of riboflavin from pure SPI (solid symbol) and pure zein (hollow symbol) microspheres in simulated gastric (pH 1.2) and intestinal (pH 7.4) fluids. *Source*: Adapted from Chen and Subirade (2009) after permission from American Chemical Society.

the zein content. Thus, the blending of two polymers aid in controlling the nutrient release from the hydrogel microspheres in GIT conditions.

16.3.2.3 Polysaccharide-Based Hydrogels

Polysaccharides are nontoxic, safe, hypoallergenic, highly available, biocompatible, and biodegradable polymers containing numerous hydroxyl and other functional groups that undergo chemical and/or physical interactions (Zhang et al. 2010). Pectin, gum arabic, starch, chitosan, alginate, carrageenan, agar, starch, dextran, hyaluronic acid, and cellulose derivatives are examples of polysaccharides utilized for the preparation of biocompatible hydrogels (Klein and Poverenov 2020). The encapsulation, stabilization, and release properties of the hydrogels can be modulated by varying the composition of the hydrogel, which can be also achieved by blending two or more polysaccharides together. Hydrogels based on chitosan/alginate polyelectrolyte complexes have been widely employed for the encapsulation of nutraceuticals with promising results. In one study chitosan/alginate hydrogel prepared at different pHs and compositions has been utilized for the encapsulation of citral, which is a natural flavoring compound widely used as a food additive (Afzal et al. 2018). Its encapsulation by the synthesized hydrogels revealed that the hydrogels prepared at different pHs with different weight percentage of alginate and chitosan exhibit different citral encapsulation and loading capabilities which was found to be maximum at pH 7 and increased with the increase in the chitosan weight percent (EE ≈ 71%). Therefore, these hydrogels are envisioned to be applicable for the solubilization of nutraceuticals. Polyunsaturated fatty acids (PUFAs) are also highly liable to chemical degradation due to lipid oxidation giving rise to undesirable rancidity and toxic reaction products (McClements and Decker 2000). Studies have shown that hydrogel beads are proficient systems to protect the PUFA-rich lipid droplets from oxidation (Chen et al. 2017a, b; Huang et al. 2020). Other studies have also illustrated that calcium alginate hydrogel beads (Zhang et al. 2016a) and the beads of starch crosslinked by sodium trimetaphosphate (Wang et al. 2015b) enhance the chemical stability of the carotenoid-enriched lipid

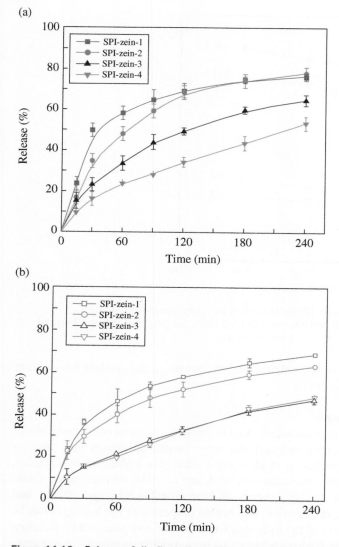

(a)

(b)

Figure 16.10 Release of riboflavin from SPI/zein (Red: 8:2; Green: 6:4; Blue: 5:5; Cyan: 3:7) microspheres in (a) simulated gastric fluid and (b) simulated intestinal fluid. *Source*: Adapted from Chen and Subirade (2009) after permission from American Chemical Society.

droplets via encapsulation, which were found to be retained by the beads in the mouth and released in the small intestines (Zhang et al. 2016b). Carotenoids are also highly susceptible to degradation by temperature, light, or pH. Therefore, many of the polysaccharide-based hydrogels have been studied for their efficiency to protect the carotenoids. In one study (Zhang et al. 2016a), β-carotene was entrapped into three different delivery systems: free lipid droplets; filled hydrogel beads formed using 0.5 and 1% alginate, and it was found that β-carotene encapsulated in free lipid droplets was highly unstable to chemical degradation when stored at 55 °C temperature, while β-carotene loaded in hydrogel beads had improved chemical stability (Figure 16.11). The figure indicated that the relative amount of β-carotene dropped immediately from an initial value of 100% to about 0.2, 0.2, 38%, and 55% for the nanoemulsions, 1% beads and 0.5% beads, respectively, after storage for 12 days. Moreover, the release of free fatty acid from the β-carotene-loaded delivery systems studied and was found to be rapid (over 76% in 5 minutes) in the nanoemulsions, while as the release rate in the filled hydrogels was much slower depending upon the alginate concentration (Figure 16.12). The chemical stability of β-carotene is shown in Figure 16.13 from which it is obvious that the hydrogel beads proved effective in improving the chemical stability within the GIT, which also enhances with increase in the alginate content.

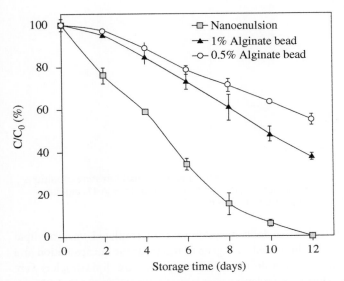

Figure 16.11 Degradation rates of β-carotene loaded in different delivery systems (nanoemulsions and hydrogel beads) during storage at 55 °C. *Source*: Adapted from Zhang et al. (2016a) after permission from Elsevier.

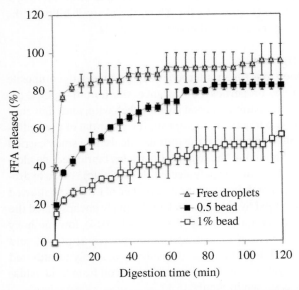

Figure 16.12 Release of fatty acids from β-carotene delivery systems: (a) nanoemulsions, (b) nanoemulsions in 0.5% alginate beads, and (c) nanoemulsions in 1% alginate beads. *Source*: Adapted from Zhang et al. (2016a) after permission from Elsevier.

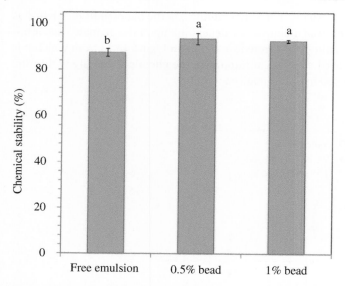

Figure 16.13 Chemical stability (%) of β-carotene after exposure to simulated small intestine conditions in (a) nanoemulsions, (b) nanoemulsions in 0.5% alginate beads, and (c) nanoemulsions in 1% alginate beads. *Source*: Adapted from Zhang et al. (2016a) after permission from Elsevier.

In another instance (Zhang et al. 2016b), three delivery systems were formulated, viz., free lipid droplets, lipid-loaded alginate beads, and lipid-loaded carrageenan beads for the encapsulation and release of curcumin. The study revealed that under simulated GIT conditions, free lipid droplets were quickly disintegrated than the hydrogel beads and released over 60% of fatty acid in the first 10 minutes. Moreover, carrageenan beads partly disintegrated and released fatty acid (46%) faster than that of the robust alginate beads, which released only 33% of fatty acid after 2 hours as shown in Figure 16.14a. Moreover, the curcumin bioaccessibility followed the order: free lipid droplets (73%) > carrageenan beads (33%) > alginate beads (16%) (Figure 16.14b). Thus, the bioavailability of the nutraceuticals can be modulated by also altering the composition of the hydrogels.

16.3.2.4 Mixed Protein and Polysaccharide Hydrogels

Proteins and polysaccharides can be combined to form an interpenetrating network or composite hydrogels to obtain the hydrogels with modified properties. For instance, silk fibroin–agarose gel formulated by Singh et al. exhibited immune compatibility, good swelling behavior, and high elasticity (Singh et al. 2016). Hence, blending the two together can improve the potential of the hydrogel not only in transport but also in enhancing the stability of the nutraceuticals. In a study carried out by Zhang et al. (2015), corn oil was incorporated in the hydrogel particles fabricated via electrostatic complexation of a protein (casein) and an anionic polysaccharide (alginate). These hydrogel particles underwent aggregation at lower pH and disintegration at higher pH while as showed stability in the pH range of four to five. The blended hydrogel particles effectively encapsulated the lipid and were feasible for its oral delivery. In an another study (Zhang et al. 2014), low-methoxy pectin and caseinate were utilized for the formation of hydrogel microspheres at pH 4.5 and applied to study the encapsulation, chemical stability, and lipase digestibility of a polyunsaturated lipid, fish oil. It should be noted that the hydrogel effectively protected the fish oil from lipid oxidation over the studied duration of seven days as shown in Figure 16.15.

Somchue et al. (2009) also reported the encapsulation of α-tocopherol in the salt induced gels of β-lactoglobulin (BLG) and hen egg white (HEW). The encapsulation efficiency of α-tocopherol was

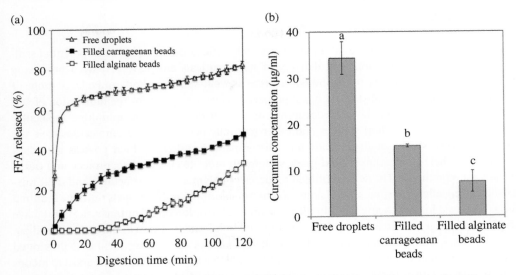

Figure 16.14 (a) Release of free fatty acid from free lipid droplets, filled alginate beads, and filled carrageenan beads, and (b) amount of curcumin present in the mixed micelle phase for free lipid droplets, filled alginate beads, and filled carrageenan beads after in vitro digestion. *Source*: Adapted from Zhang et al. (2016b) after permission from Elsevier.

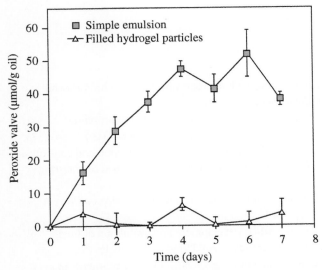

Figure 16.15 Concentration of hydroperoxides formed from fish oil during the seven-day storage in simple oil-in-water emulsions and in filled hydrogel particles. *Source*: Adapted from Zhang et al. (2014) after permission from Elsevier.

about 20 and 32% in BLG and HEW gels, respectively. Moreover, it was found that 86 and 93% of the encapsulated α-tocopherol was released after 2 hours in simulated gastric conditions from BLG and HEW gels, respectively. However, when the gels were coated with sodium alginate, the release rate got reduced in simulated gastric fluid and enhanced in the intestinal environment with the increase in alginate concentration.

16.4 Conclusion

In conclusion, the soft systems based on polymers and surfactants have proven as potential scaffolds for entrapment, protection, and delivery of nutraceuticals and have displayed promising results and excellent reliability in the industrial areas as well. Many methods and a large range of constituents having diverse physicochemical properties have been used for the fabrication of soft systems in order to realize the bioaccessibility of the nutraceuticals. Amphiphilic molecules derived from animal and plant sources and other naturally occurring macromolecules have the capability to form stable, biodegradable, and biocompatible systems, which possess abundant advantages for their application in food-grade systems in order to encapsulate, protect, and transport the food ingredients. The self-assembled matrices of polymers and surfactants and their mixtures such as micelles, liposomes, emulsions, polymeric solutions, and hydrogels fulfil the required criteria to be used for enhancing the solubilization and stabilization of the nutraceuticals and have been primarily targeted toward the enhancement in the retainment of nutritional value, stabilization against oxidation, bioavailability, and controlled release of the nutraceuticals. As illustrated above, these designed systems have the tunable physicochemical properties, which assist to modulate the biological fate of the encapsulated nutraceuticals in the GIT and thereby lead to reduction in their toxicity and upgradation of their bio-efficacy. The composite systems involving the complexation between two or more constituents have the synced properties, which have led to improve both the nutraceutical dosage and the dose interval by achieving a controllable release properties of the system.

References

Abbas, S., Da Wei, C., Hayat, K. et al. (2012). Ascorbic acid: microencapsulation techniques and trends — a review. *Food Reviews International 28* (4): 343–374.

Abedini, F., Ebrahimi, M., Roozbehani, A.H. et al. (2018). Overview on natural hydrophilic polysaccharide polymers in drug delivery. *Polymers for Advanced Technologies 29* (10): 2564–2573.

Acevedo-Fani, A., Soliva-Fortuny, R., and Martín-Belloso, O. (2018). Photo-protection and controlled release of folic acid using edible alginate/chitosan nanolaminates. *Journal of Food Engineering 229*: 72–82.

Acosta, E. (2009). Bioavailability of nanoparticles in nutrient and nutraceutical delivery. *Current Opinion in Colloid & Interface Science 14* (1): 3–15.

Aditya, N.P., Macedo, A.S., Doktorovova, S. et al. (2014). Development and evaluation of lipid nanocarriers for quercetin delivery: a comparative study of solid lipid nanoparticles (SLN), nanostructured lipid carriers (NLC), and lipid nanoemulsions (LNE). *LWT-Food Science and Technology 59* (1): 115–121.

Aditya, N.P., Aditya, S., Yang, H. et al. (2015). Co-delivery of hydrophobic curcumin and hydrophilic catechin by a water-in-oil-in-water double emulsion. *Food Chemistry 173*: 7–13.

Aditya, N.P., Espinosa, Y.G., and Norton, I.T. (2017). Encapsulation systems for the delivery of hydrophilic nutraceuticals: Food application. *Biotechnology Advances 35* (4): 450–457.

Afzal, S., Maswal, M., and Dar, A.A. (2018). Rheological behavior of pH responsive composite hydrogels of chitosan and alginate: characterization and its use in encapsulation of citral. *Colloids and Surfaces B: Biointerfaces 169*: 99–106.

Aguilera, J.M. (2000). Microstructure and food product engineering. *Food Technology 54*: 56-X.

Alborzi, S., Lim, L.-T., and Kakuda, Y. (2013). Encapsulation of folic acid and its stability in sodium alginate-pectin-poly (ethylene oxide) electrospun fibres. *Journal of Microencapsulation 30* (1): 64–71.

Amalraj, A., Gopi, S., Thomas, S. et al. (2018). *Cellulose Nanomaterials in Biomedical, Food, and Nutraceutical Applications: A Review*, 1e, vol. 380, 1800115. Wiley Online Library.

Anand David, A.V., Arulmoli, R., and Parasuraman, S. (2016). Overviews of biological importance of quercetin: a bioactive flavonoid. *Pharmacognosy Reviews 10* (20): 84–89.

Arrese, E.L., Sorgentini, D.A., Wagner, J.R. et al. (1991). Electrophoretic, solubility and functional properties of commercial soy protein isolates. *Journal of Agricultural and Food Chemistry 39* (6): 1029–1032.

Asghar, A., Randhawa, M.A., Masood, M.M. et al. (2018). Chapter 10 – nutraceutical formulation strategies to enhance the bioavailability and efficiency: an overview. In: *Role of Materials Science in Food Bioengineering* (eds. A.M. Grumezescu and A.M. Holban), 329–352. Academic Press.

Augustin, M.A. and Hemar, Y. (2009). Nano- and micro-structured assemblies for encapsulation of food ingredients. *Chemical Society Reviews 38* (4): 902–912.

Augustin, M.A., Sanguansri, L., Margetts, C. et al. (2001). Encapsulation of food ingredients. *Food Australia 53*: 220–223.

Ayan, A.K., Yenilmez, A., and Eroglu, H. (2017). Evaluation of radiolabeled curcumin-loaded solid lipid nanoparticles usage as an imaging agent in liver-spleen scintigraphy. *Materials Science and Engineering: C 75*: 663–670.

Azevedo, M.A., Bourbon, A.I., Vicente, A.A. et al. (2014). Alginate/chitosan nanoparticles for encapsulation and controlled release of vitamin B2. *International Journal of Biological Macromolecules 71*: 141–146.

Bajaj, P.R., Bhunia, K., Kleiner, L. et al. (2017). Improving functional properties of pea protein isolate for microencapsulation of flaxseed oil. *Journal of Microencapsulation 34* (2): 218–230.

Bakry, A.M., Abbas, S., Ali, B. et al. (2016). Microencapsulation of oils: a comprehensive review of benefits, techniques, and applications. *Comprehensive Reviews in Food Science and Food Safety 15* (1): 143–182.

Bansil, R. and Turner, B.S. (2006). Mucin structure, aggregation, physiological functions and biomedical applications. *Current Opinion in Colloid & Interface Science 11* (2–3): 164–170.

Beirão-da-Costa, S., Duarte, C., Bourbon, A.I. et al. (2013). Inulin potential for encapsulation and controlled delivery of Oregano essential oil. *Food Hydrocolloids 33* (2): 199–206.

Bou, R., Cofrades, S., and Jiménez-Colmenero, F. (2014). Physicochemical properties and riboflavin encapsulation in double emulsions with different lipid sources. *LWT-Food Science and Technology 59* (2): 621–628.

Bourbon, A.I., Pinheiro, A.C., Cerqueira, M.A. et al. (2018). in vitro digestion of lactoferrin-glycomacropeptide nanohydrogels incorporating bioactive compounds: Effect of a chitosan coating. *Food Hydrocolloids 84*: 267–275.

Burey, P., Bhandari, B.R., Howes, T. et al. (2008). Hydrocolloid gel particles: formation, characterization, and application. *Critical Reviews in Food Science and Nutrition 48* (5): 361–377.

Buscemi, S., Corleo, D., Di Pace, F. et al. (2018). The effect of lutein on eye and extra-eye health. *Nutrients 10* (9): 1321.

Canselier, J.P., Delmas, H., Wilhelm, A.M. et al. (2002). Ultrasound emulsification – an overview. *Journal of Dispersion Science and Technology 23* (1-3): 333–349.

de Carvalho Melo-Cavalcante, A.A., da Rocha Sousa, L., Alencar, M.V.O.B. et al. (2019). Retinol palmitate and ascorbic acid: role in oncological prevention and therapy. *Biomedicine & Pharmacotherapy 109*: 1394–1405.

Chat, O.A., Najar, M.H., Mir, M.A. et al. (2011). Effects of surfactant micelles on solubilization and DPPH radical scavenging activity of Rutin. *Journal of Colloid and Interface Science 355* (1): 140–149.

Chen, J. and Hu, L. (2020). Nanoscale delivery system for nutraceuticals: preparation, application, characterization, safety, and future trends. *Food Engineering Reviews 12* (1): 14–31.

Chen, L. and Subirade, M. (2009). Elaboration and characterization of soy/zein protein microspheres for controlled nutraceutical delivery. *Biomacromolecules 10* (12): 3327–3334.

Chen, H., Chang, X., Du, D. et al. (2006a). Microemulsion-based hydrogel formulation of ibuprofen for topical delivery. *International Journal of Pharmaceutics 315* (1): 52–58.

Chen, L., Remondetto, G.E., and Subirade, M. (2006b). Food protein-based materials as nutraceutical delivery systems. *Trends in Food Science & Technology 17* (5): 272–283.

Chen, F., Fan, G.-Q., Zhang, Z. et al. (2017a). Encapsulation of omega-3 fatty acids in nanoemulsions and microgels: impact of delivery system type and protein addition on gastrointestinal fate. *Food Research International 100*: 387–395.

Chen, F., Liang, L., Zhang, Z. et al. (2017b). Inhibition of lipid oxidation in nanoemulsions and filled microgels fortified with omega-3 fatty acids using casein as a natural antioxidant. *Food Hydrocolloids 63*: 240–248.

Cho, Y.-J., Kim, D.-M., Song, I.-H. et al. (2018). An oligoimide particle as a pickering emulsion stabilizer. *Polymers 10* (10): 1071.

Choi, S.J., Decker, E.A., Henson, L. et al. (2009a). Stability of citral in oil-in-water emulsions prepared with medium-chain triacylglycerols and triacetin. *Journal of Agricultural and Food Chemistry 57* (23): 11349–11353.

Choi, S.J., Decker, E.A., and McClements, D.J. (2009b). Impact of iron encapsulation within the interior aqueous phase of water-in-oil-in-water emulsions on lipid oxidation. *Food Chemistry 116* (1): 271–276.

Choi, S.J., Decker, E.A., Henson, L. et al. (2010). Inhibition of citral degradation in model beverage emulsions using micelles and reverse micelles. *Food Chemistry 122* (1): 111–116.

Claesson, P.M. and Ninham, B.W. (1992). pH-dependent interactions between adsorbed chitosan layers. *Langmuir 8* (5): 1406–1412.

Cook, M.T., Tzortzis, G., Charalampopoulos, D. et al. (2012). Microencapsulation of probiotics for gastrointestinal delivery. *Journal of Controlled Release 162* (1): 56–67.

da Costa, S.B., Duarte, C., Bourbon, A.I. et al. (2012). Effect of the matrix system in the delivery and in vitro bioactivity of microencapsulated Oregano essential oil. *Journal of Food Engineering 110* (2): 190–199.

Couto, R., Alvarez, V., and Temelli, F. (2017). Encapsulation of Vitamin B2 in solid lipid nanoparticles using supercritical CO2. *The Journal of Supercritical Fluids 120*: 432–442.

Dai, L., Wei, Y., Sun, C. et al. (2018). Development of protein-polysaccharide-surfactant ternary complex particles as delivery vehicles for curcumin. *Food Hydrocolloids 85*: 75–85.

Dar, A.A., Rather, G.M., and Das, A.R. (2007). Mixed micelle formation and solubilization behavior toward polycyclic aromatic hydrocarbons of binary and ternary cationic–nonionic surfactant mixtures. *The Journal of Physical Chemistry B 111* (12): 3122–3132.

Dias, D.R., Botrel, D.A., Fernandes, R.V.D.B. et al. (2017). Encapsulation as a tool for bioprocessing of functional foods. *Current Opinion in Food Science 13*: 31–37.

Dickinson, E. (2003). Hydrocolloids at interfaces and the influence on the properties of dispersed systems. *Food Hydrocolloids 17* (1): 25–39.

Dickinson, E. (2011). Double emulsions stabilized by food biopolymers. *Food Biophysics 6* (1): 1–11.

Dixit, N., Baboota, S., Kohli, K. et al. (2007). Silymarin: a review of pharmacological aspects and bioavailability enhancement approaches. *Indian Journal of Pharmacology 39* (4): 172–179.

Donsì, F., Annunziata, M., Sessa, M. et al. (2011). Nanoencapsulation of essential oils to enhance their antimicrobial activity in foods. *LWT-Food Science and Technology 44* (9): 1908–1914.

Dutta, S., Moses, J.A., and Anandharamakrishnan, C. (2018). Encapsulation of nutraceutical ingredients in liposomes and their potential for cancer treatment. *Nutrition and Cancer 70* (8): 1184–1198.

Fang, Y., Bennett, A., and Liu, J. (2010). Multiply charged gas-phase NaAOT reverse micelles: Formation, encapsulation of glycine, and collision-induced dissociation. *International Journal of Mass Spectrometry 293* (1): 12–22.

Fareez, I.M., Lim, S.M., Zulkefli, N.A.A. et al. (2018). Cellulose derivatives enhanced stability of alginate-based beads loaded with Lactobacillus plantarum lab12 against low pH, high temperature and prolonged storage. *Probiotics Antimicrobial Proteins 10* (3): 543–557.

Fathi, M., Mozafari, M.R., and Mohebbi, M. (2012). Nanoencapsulation of food ingredients using lipid based delivery systems. *Trends in Food Science Technology 23* (1): 13–27.

Fathi, M., Martin, A., and McClements, D.J. (2014). Nanoencapsulation of food ingredients using carbohydrate based delivery systems. *Trends in Food Science & Technology 39* (1): 18–39.

Fryd, M.M. and Mason, T.G. (2010). Time-dependent nanoemulsion droplet size reduction by evaporative ripening. *The Journal of Physical Chemistry Letters 1* (23): 3349–3353.

Fryd, M.M. and Mason, T.G. (2012). Advanced nanoemulsions. *Annual Review of Physical Chemistry 63* (1): 493–518.

Garti, N. (1997). Double emulsions — scope, limitations and new achievements. *Colloids and Surfaces A: Physicochemical and Engineering Aspects 123–124*: 233–246.

Garti, N. and Benichou, A. (2004). Recent developments in double emulsions for food applications. *Food Emulsions 35*.

Ghayour, N., Hosseini, S.M.H., Eskandari, M.H. et al. (2019). Nanoencapsulation of quercetin and curcumin in casein-based delivery systems. *Food Hydrocolloids 87*: 394–403.

Gibson, G.R., Probert, H.M., Loo, J.V. et al. (2004). Dietary modulation of the human colonic microbiota: updating the concept of prebiotics. *Nutrition Research Reviews 17* (2): 259–275.

Gómez-Estaca, J., Gavara, R., and Hernández-Muñoz, P. (2015). Encapsulation of curcumin in electrosprayed gelatin microspheres enhances its bioaccessibility and widens its uses in food applications. *Innovative Food Science Emerging Technologies 29*: 302–307.

Gradauer, K., Barthelmes, J., Vonach, C. et al. (2013). Liposomes coated with thiolated chitosan enhance oral peptide delivery to rats. *Journal of Controlled Release 172* (3): 872–878.

Graf, A., Ablinger, E., Peters, S. et al. (2008). Microemulsions containing lecithin and sugar-based surfactants: nanoparticle templates for delivery of proteins and peptides. *International Journal of Pharmaceutics 350* (1–2): 351–360.

Gupta, A., Eral, H.B., Hatton, T.A. et al. (2016). Nanoemulsions: formation, properties and applications. *Soft Matter 12* (11): 2826–2841.

Gutiérrez, T.J. and Álvarez, K. (2017). Biopolymers as microencapsulation materials in the food industry. *Advances in Physicochemical Properties of Biopolymers: Part 2*: 296–322.

Haham, M., Ish-Shalom, S., Nodelman, M. et al. (2012). Stability and bioavailability of vitamin D nanoencapsulated in casein micelles. *Food function 3* (7): 737–744.

Halwani, M., Hossain, Z., Khiyami, M.A. et al. (2015). Liposomal β-glucan: preparation, characterization and anticancer activities. *Journal of Nanomedicine & Nanotechnology 6* (5): 1–7.

Helal, N.A., Eassa, H.A., Amer, A.M. et al. (2019). Nutraceuticals' novel formulations: the good, the bad, the unknown and patents involved. *Recent Patents on Drug Delivery & Formulation 13* (2): 105–156.

Hewlings, S.J. and Kalman, D.S. (2017). Curcumin: A Review of Its' Effects on Human Health. *Foods 6* (10): 1–11.

Hoar, T.P. and Schulman, J.H. (1943). Transparent water-in-oil dispersions: the oleopathic hydro-micelle. *Nature 152* (3847): 102–103.

Hoffman, A.S. (2012). Hydrogels for biomedical applications. *Advanced Drug Delivery Reviews 64*: 18–23.

Huang, J., Wang, Q., Chu, L. et al. (2020). Liposome-chitosan hydrogel bead delivery system for the encapsulation of linseed oil and quercetin: preparation and in vitro characterization studies. *LWT 117*: 108615.

Ishak, K., Annuar, M.M., and Ahmad, N. (2017). Nano-delivery systems for nutraceutical application. In: *Nanotechnology Applications in Food* (eds. A.E. Oprea and A.M. Grumezescu), 179–202. Elsevier.

Iwunze, M.O. (2004). Binding and distribution characteristics of curcumin solubilized in CTAB micelle. *Journal of Molecular Liquids 111* (1): 161–165.

Iyer, C., Phillips, M., and Kailasapathy, K. (2005). Release studies of Lactobacillus casei strain Shirota from chitosan-coated alginate-starch microcapsules in ex vivo porcine gastrointestinal contents. *Letters in Applied Microbiology 41* (6): 493–497.

Izquierdo, P., Esquena, J., Tadros, T.F. et al. (2002). Formation and stability of nano-emulsions prepared using the phase inversion temperature method. *Langmuir 18* (1): 26–30.

Jabeen, S., Chat, O.A., Rather, G.M. et al. (2013). Investigation of antioxidant activity of Quercetin (2-(3, 4-dihydroxyphenyl)-3,5,7-trihydroxy-4H-chromen-4-one) in aqueous micellar media. *Food Research International 51* (1): 294–302.

Kale, S.N. and Deore, S.L. (2017). Emulsion micro emulsion and nano emulsion: a review. *Systematic Reviews in Pharmacy 8* (1): 39.

Kanakdande, D., Bhosale, R., and Singhal, R.S. (2007). Stability of cumin oleoresin microencapsulated in different combination of gum arabic, maltodextrin and modified starch. *Carbohydrate Polymers 67* (4): 536–541.

Karthik, P., Ezhilarasi, P.N., and Anandharamakrishnan, C. (2017). Challenges associated in stability of food grade nanoemulsions. *Critical Reviews in Food Science and Nutrition 57* (7): 1435–1450.

Kenyon, M.M. (1995). *Modified Starch, Maltodextrin, and Corn Syrup Solids as Wall Materials for Food Encapsulation*. ACS Publications.

Kharat, M., Du, Z., Zhang, G. et al. (2017). Physical and chemical stability of curcumin in aqueous solutions and emulsions: impact of pH, temperature, and molecular environment. *Journal of Agricultural and Food Chemistry 65* (8): 1525–1532.

Klein, M. and Poverenov, E. (2020). Natural biopolymer-based hydrogels for use in food and agriculture. *Journal of the Science of Food and Agriculture 100* (6): 2337–2347.

Komaiko, J.S. and McClements, D.J. (2016). Formation of food-grade nanoemulsions using low-energy preparation methods: a review of available methods. *Comprehensive Reviews in Food Science and Food Safety 15* (2): 331–352.

Kreilgaard, M. (2002). Influence of microemulsions on cutaneous drug delivery. *Advanced Drug Delivery Reviews 54*: S77–S98.

Krishnan, S., Bhosale, R., and Singhal, R.S. (2005). Microencapsulation of cardamom oleoresin: Evaluation of blends of gum arabic, maltodextrin and a modified starch as wall materials. *Carbohydrate Polymers 61* (1): 95–102.

Kronberg, B. and Lindman, B. (2003). *Surfactants and Polymers in Aqueous Solution*. Chichester: John Wiley & Sons Ltd.

Kumar, A., Kaur, G., Kansal, S.K. et al. (2016). Enhanced solubilization of curcumin in mixed surfactant vesicles. *Food Chemistry 199*: 660–666.

Kwak, H.-S. (2014). Overview of nano- and microencapsulation for foods. In: *Nano- and Microencapsulation for Foods* (ed. H.-S. Kwak), 1–14. Chichester: Wiley Blackwell.

Laguerre, M., Hugouvieux, V., Cavusoglu, N. et al. (2014). Probing the micellar solubilisation and inter-micellar exchange of polyphenols using the DPPH free radical. *Food Chemistry 149*: 114–120.

Lam, R.S. and Nickerson, M.T. (2013). Food proteins: a review on their emulsifying properties using a structure–function approach. *Food Chemistry 141* (2): 975–984.

LaNasa, S.M., Hoffecker, I.T., and Bryant, S.J. (2011). Presence of pores and hydrogel composition influence tensile properties of scaffolds fabricated from well-defined sphere templates. *Journal of Biomedical Materials Research Part B: Applied Biomaterials 96* (2): 294–302.

Le, A.N.-M., Nguyen, T.T., Ly, K.L. et al. (2020). Modulating biodegradation and biocompatibility of in situ crosslinked hydrogel by the integration of alginate into N, O-carboxylmethyl chitosan–aldehyde hyaluronic acid network. *Polymer Degradation and Stability*: 109270.

Lee, S.H., Son, J.-K., Jeong, B.S. et al. (2008). Progress in the studies on rutaecarpine. *Molecules (Basel, Switzerland) 13* (2): 272–300.

Lee, D.Y., Lin, X., Paskaleva, E.E. et al. (2009). Palmitic acid is a novel CD4 fusion inhibitor that blocks HIV entry and infection. *AIDS Research and Human Retroviruses 25* (12): 1231–1241.

Leung, M.H.M., Colangelo, H., and Kee, T.W. (2008). Encapsulation of curcumin in cationic micelles suppresses alkaline hydrolysis. *Langmuir 24* (11): 5672–5675.

Li, L., Braiteh, F.S., and Kurzrock, R. (2005). Liposome-encapsulated curcumin: in vitro and in vivo effects on proliferation, apoptosis, signaling, and angiogenesis. *Cancer 104* (6): 1322–1331.

Liang, L., Tremblay-Hébert, V., and Subirade, M. (2011). Characterisation of the β-lactoglobulin/α-tocopherol complex and its impact on α-tocopherol stability. *Food Chemistry 126* (3): 821–826.

Lima, A.C., Sher, P., and Mano, J.F. (2012). Production methodologies of polymeric and hydrogel particles for drug delivery applications. *Expert Opinion on Drug Delivery 9* (2): 231–248.

Lipinski, C.A., Lombardo, F., Dominy, B.W. et al. (2012). Experimental and computational approaches to estimate solubility and permeability in drug discovery and development settings. *Advanced Drug Delivery Reviews 64*: 4–17.

Liu, F. and Tang, C.-H. (2016). Soy glycinin as food-grade Pickering stabilizers: Part. III. Fabrication of gel-like emulsions and their potential as sustained-release delivery systems for β-carotene. *Food Hydrocolloids 56*: 434–444.

Liu, J., Willför, S., Xu, C. et al. (2015). A review of bioactive plant polysaccharides: biological activities, functionalization, and biomedical applications. *Bioactive Carbohydrates 5* (1): 31–61.

Livney, Y.D. (2010). Milk proteins as vehicles for bioactives. *Current Opinion in Colloid Interface Science 15* (1–2): 73–83.

Livney, Y.D. (2015). Nanostructured delivery systems in food: latest developments and potential future directions. *Current Opinion in Food Science 3*: 125–135.

Lone, M.S., Bhat, P.A., Shah, R.A. et al. (2017). A green pH-switchable amino acid based smart wormlike micellar system for efficient and controlled drug delivery. *ChemistrySelect 2* (3): 1144–1148.

Lone, M.S., Chat, O.A., Vashishtha, M. et al. (2019). Transition from competitive to non-competitive solubilization with the decrease in number of oxyethylene (OE) units of non-ionic surfactants towards polycyclic aromatic hydrocarbons. *Bulletin of the Chemical Society of Japan 92* (1): 115–123.

Lu, W., Kelly, A.L., and Miao, S. (2016). Emulsion-based encapsulation and delivery systems for polyphenols. *Trends in Food Science & Technology 47*: 1–9.

Luo, Y. and Wang, Q. (2014). Zein-based micro-and nano-particles for drug and nutrient delivery: a review. *Journal of Applied Polymer Science 131* (16).

Macfarlane, G. and Englyst, H. (1986). Starch utilization by the human large intestinal microflora. *Journal of Applied Bacteriology 60* (3): 195–201.

Maciel, J.S., Azevedo, S., Correia, C.R. et al. (2019). Oxidized cashew gum scaffolds for tissue engineering. *Macromolecular Materials and Engineering 304* (3): 1800574.

Maltais, A., Remondetto, G.E., and Subirade, M. (2009). Soy protein cold-set hydrogels as controlled delivery devices for nutraceutical compounds. *Food Hydrocolloids 23* (7): 1647–1653.

Marefati, A., Bertrand, M., Sjöö, M. et al. (2017). Storage and digestion stability of encapsulated curcumin in emulsions based on starch granule Pickering stabilization. *Food Hydrocolloids 63*: 309–320.

Marsich, E., Borgogna, M., Donati, I. et al. (2008). Alginate/lactose-modified chitosan hydrogels: A bioactive biomaterial for chondrocyte encapsulation. *Journal of Biomedical Materials Research Part A 84* (2): 364–376.

Mason, T.G., Wilking, J.N., Meleson, K. et al. (2006). Nanoemulsions: formation, structure, and physical properties. *Journal of Physics: Condensed Matter 18* (41): R635.

Maswal, M. and Dar, A.A. (2013). Inhibition of citral degradation in an acidic aqueous environment by polyoxyethylene alkylether surfactants. *Food Chemistry 138* (4): 2356–2364.

Matalanis, A., Jones, O.G., and McClements, D.J. (2011). Structured biopolymer-based delivery systems for encapsulation, protection, and release of lipophilic compounds. *Food Hydrocolloids 25* (8): 1865–1880.

McClements, D.J. (2002). Colloidal basis of emulsion color. *Current Opinion in Colloid & Interface Science 7* (5): 451–455.

McClements, D.J. (2012a). 1 - Requirements for food ingredient and nutraceutical delivery systems. In: *Encapsulation Technologies and Delivery Systems for Food Ingredients and Nutraceuticals* (eds. N. Garti and D.J. McClements), 3–18. Woodhead Publishing.

McClements, D.J. (2012b). Advances in fabrication of emulsions with enhanced functionality using structural design principles. *Current Opinion in Colloid & Interface Science 17* (5): 235–245.

McClements, D.J. (2015). Encapsulation, protection, and release of hydrophilic active components: potential and limitations of colloidal delivery systems. *Advances in Colloid and Interface Science 219*: 27–53.

McClements, D.J. and Decker, E.A. (2000). Lipid oxidation in oil-in-water emulsions: impact of molecular environment on chemical reactions in heterogeneous food systems. *Journal of Food Science 65* (8): 1270–1282.

McClements, D.J., Decker, E.A., and Weiss, J. (2007). Emulsion-based delivery systems for lipophilic bioactive components. *Journal of Food Science 72* (8): R109–R124.

McClements, D.J., Li, F., and Xiao, H. (2015a). The nutraceutical bioavailability classification scheme: classifying nutraceuticals according to factors limiting their oral bioavailability. *Annual Review of Food Science and Technology 6*: 299–327.

McClements, D.J., Zou, L., Zhang, R. et al. (2015b). Enhancing nutraceutical performance using excipient foods: designing food structures and compositions to increase bioavailability. *Comprehensive Reviews in Food Science and Food Safety 14* (6): 824–847.

Miao, T., Wang, J., Zeng, Y. et al. (2018). Polysaccharide-based controlled release systems for therapeutics delivery and tissue engineering: from bench to bedside. *Advanced Science 5* (4): 1700513.

Mishra, M. (2016). *Degradation of Polymers. Handbook of Encapsulation and Controlled Release.* Taylor & Francis Group.

Mohanraj, V.J., Barnes, T.J., and Prestidge, C.A. (2010). Silica nanoparticle coated liposomes: a new type of hybrid nanocapsule for proteins. *International Journal of Pharmaceutics 392* (1): 285–293.

Nesterenko, A., Alric, I., Silvestre, F. et al. (2014). Comparative study of encapsulation of vitamins with native and modified soy protein. *Food Hydrocolloids 38*: 172–179.

O'Regan, J. and Mulvihill, D.M. (2010). Sodium caseinate–maltodextrin conjugate stabilized double emulsions: encapsulation and stability. *Food Research International 43* (1): 224–231.

Okumura, Y. and Ito, K. (2001). The polyrotaxane gel: a topological gel by figure-of-eight cross-links. *Advanced Materials 13* (7): 485–487.

Pandelidou, M., Dimas, K., Georgopoulos, A. et al. (2011). Preparation and characterization of lyophilised egg PC liposomes incorporating curcumin and evaluation of its activity against colorectal cancer cell lines. *Journal of Nanoscience and Nanotechnology 11* (2): 1259–1266.

Pasqui, D., De Cagna, M., and Barbucci, R. (2012). Polysaccharide-based hydrogels: the key role of water in affecting mechanical properties. *Polymers 4* (3): 1517–1534.

Patel, A.R. and Velikov, K. (2014). Zein as a source of functional colloidal nano-and microstructures. *Current Opinion in Colloid Interface Science 19* (5): 450–458.

Patil, S., Choudhary, B., Rathore, A. et al. (2015). Enhanced oral bioavailability and anticancer activity of novel curcumin loaded mixed micelles in human lung cancer cells. *Phytomedicine 22* (12): 1103–1111.

Patra, D. and Barakat, C. (2011). Unique role of ionic liquid [bmin][BF4] during curcumin–surfactant association and micellization of cationic, anionic and non-ionic surfactant solutions. *Spectrochimica Acta Part A: Molecular and Biomolecular Spectroscopy 79* (5): 1823–1828.

Paul, B.K. and Moulik, S.P. (1997). Microemulsions: an overview. *Journal of Dispersion Science and Technology 18* (4): 301–367.

Phan, V., Walters, J., Brownlow, B. et al. (2013). Enhanced cytotoxicity of optimized liposomal genistein via specific induction of apoptosis in breast, ovarian and prostate carcinomas. *Journal of Drug Targeting 21* (10): 1001–1011.

Pickering, S.U. (1907). CXCVI.— emulsions. *Journal of the Chemical Society, Transactions 91* (0): 2001–2021.

Pitkowski, A., Nicolai, T., and Durand, D. (2009). Stability of caseinate solutions in the presence of calcium. *Food Hydrocolloids 23* (4): 1164–1168.

Pool, H., Mendoza, S., Xiao, H. et al. (2013). Encapsulation and release of hydrophobic bioactive components in nanoemulsion-based delivery systems: impact of physical form on quercetin bioaccessibility. *Food & Function 4* (1): 162–174.

Qian, C. and McClements, D.J. (2011). Formation of nanoemulsions stabilized by model food-grade emulsifiers using high-pressure homogenization: Factors affecting particle size. *Food Hydrocolloids 25* (5): 1000–1008.

Quirós-Sauceda, A.E., Ayala-Zavala, J.F., Olivas, G.I. et al. (2014). Edible coatings as encapsulating matrices for bioactive compounds: a review. *Journal of Food Science and Technology 51* (9): 1674–1685.

Ray, S., Raychaudhuri, U., and Chakraborty, R. (2016). An overview of encapsulation of active compounds used in food products by drying technology. *Food Bioscience 13*: 76–83.

Riaz, Q.U.A. and Masud, T. (2013). Recent trends and applications of encapsulating materials for probiotic stability. *Critical Reviews in Food Science Nutrition 53* (3): 231–244.

Ribeiro, M.E.N.P., Vieira, Í.G.P., Cavalcante, I.M. et al. (2009). Solubilisation of griseofulvin, quercetin and rutin in micellar formulations of triblock copolymers E62P39E62 and E137S18E137. *International Journal of Pharmaceutics 378* (1): 211–214.

Henri, L.R., Cavallo, J.L., Chang, D.L. et al. (1988). Microemulsions: a commentary on their preparation. *Journal of the Society of Cosmetic Chemists 39*: 201–209.

Sachdeva, A.K., Misra, S., Pal Kaur, I. et al. (2015). Neuroprotective potential of sesamol and its loaded solid lipid nanoparticles in ICV-STZ-induced cognitive deficits: Behavioral and biochemical evidence. *European Journal of Pharmacology 747*: 132–140.

Saengkrit, N., Saesoo, S., Srinuanchai, W. et al. (2014). Influence of curcumin-loaded cationic liposome on anticancer activity for cervical cancer therapy. *Colloids and Surfaces B: Biointerfaces 114*: 349–356.

Saini, J.K., Nautiyal, U., Kumar, M. et al. (2014). Microemulsions: a potential novel drug delivery system. *International Journal of Pharmaceutical and Medicinal Research 2* (1): 15–20.

Sáiz-Abajo, M.-J., González-Ferrero, C., Moreno-Ruiz, A. et al. (2013). Thermal protection of β-carotene in re-assembled casein micelles during different processing technologies applied in food industry. *Food Chemistry 138* (2): 1581–1587.

Salminen, H., Gömmel, C., Leuenberger, B.H. et al. (2016). Influence of encapsulated functional lipids on crystal structure and chemical stability in solid lipid nanoparticles: Towards bioactive-based design of delivery systems. *Food Chemistry 190*: 928–937.

Semo, E., Kesselman, E., Danino, D. et al. (2007). Casein micelle as a natural nano-capsular vehicle for nutraceuticals. *Food Hydrocolloids 21* (5): 936–942.

Serdaroğlu, M., Öztürk, B., and Urgu, M. (2016). Emulsion characteristics, chemical and textural properties of meat systems produced with double emulsions as beef fat replacers. *Meat Science 117*: 187–195.

Serrano-Cruz, M.R., Villanueva-Carvajal, A., Rosales, E.J.M. et al. (2013). Controlled release and antioxidant activity of Roselle (Hibiscus sabdariffa L.) extract encapsulated in mixtures of carboxymethyl cellulose, whey protein, and pectin. *LWT-Food Science Technology 50* (2): 554–561.

Sessa, M., Balestrieri, M.L., Ferrari, G. et al. (2014). Bioavailability of encapsulated resveratrol into nanoemulsion-based delivery systems. *Food Chemistry 147*: 42–50.

Shah, B.R., Li, Y., Jin, W. et al. (2016). Preparation and optimization of Pickering emulsion stabilized by chitosan-tripolyphosphate nanoparticles for curcumin encapsulation. *Food Hydrocolloids 52*: 369–377.

Shao, Y. and Tang, C.-H. (2016). Gel-like pea protein Pickering emulsions at pH3.0 as a potential intestine-targeted and sustained-release delivery system for β-carotene. *Food Research International 79*: 64–72.

Shi, J., Dai, Y., Kakuda, Y. et al. (2008). Effect of heating and exposure to light on the stability of lycopene in tomato purée. *Food Control 19* (5): 514–520.

Shishir, M.R.I., Xie, L., Sun, C. et al. (2018). Advances in micro and nano-encapsulation of bioactive compounds using biopolymer and lipid-based transporters. *Trends in Food Science Technology 78*: 34–60.

Shit, S.C. and Shah, P.M. (2014). Edible polymers: challenges and opportunities. *Journal of Polymers 2014*.

Silva, P., Fries, L., Menezes, C. et al. (2014). Microencapsulation: concepts, mechanisms, methods and some applications in food technology. *Ciência Rural 44*: 1304–1311.

Singh, Y.P., Bhardwaj, N., and Mandal, B.B. (2016). Potential of agarose/silk fibroin blended hydrogel for in vitro cartilage tissue engineering. *ACS Applied Materials & Interfaces 8* (33): 21236–21249.

Somchue, W., Sermsri, W., Shiowatana, J. et al. (2009). Encapsulation of α-tocopherol in protein-based delivery particles. *Food Research International 42* (8): 909–914.

Suganya, V. and Anuradha, V. (2017). Microencapsulation and nanoencapsulation: a review. *International Journal of Pharmaceutical and Clinical Research 9* (3): 233–239.

Talegaonkar, S., Azeem, A., Ahmad, F.J. et al. (2008). Microemulsions: a novel approach to enhanced drug delivery. *Recent Patents on Drug Delivery & Formulation 2* (3): 238–257.

Tan, H., Zhao, L., Tian, S. et al. (2017). Gelatin particle-stabilized high-internal phase emulsions for use in oral delivery systems: protection effect and in vitro digestion study. *Journal of Agricultural and Food Chemistry 65* (4): 900–907.

Thangapazham, R.L., Puri, A., Tele, S. et al. (2008). Evaluation of a nanotechnology-based carrier for delivery of curcumin in prostate cancer cells. *International Journal of Oncology 32* (5): 1119–1123.

Thirawong, N., Thongborisute, J., Takeuchi, H. et al. (2008). Improved intestinal absorption of calcitonin by mucoadhesive delivery of novel pectin-liposome nanocomplexes. *Journal Control Release 125* (3): 236–245.

Thongborisute, J. and Takeuchi, H. (2008). Evaluation of mucoadhesiveness of polymers by BIACORE method and mucin-particle method. *International Journal of Pharmaceutics 354* (1–2): 204–209.

Torchilin, V.P. (2001). Structure and design of polymeric surfactant-based drug delivery systems. *Journal of Controlled Release 73* (2): 137–172.

Varankovich, N.V., Khan, N.H., Nickerson, M.T. et al. (2015). Evaluation of pea protein–polysaccharide matrices for encapsulation of acid-sensitive bacteria. *Food Research International 70*: 118–124.

Vasudevan, T.V. and Naser, M.S. (2002). Some aspects of stability of multiple emulsions in personal cleansing systems. *Journal of Colloid and Interface Science 256* (1): 208–215.

Velikov, K.P. and Pelan, E. (2008). Colloidal delivery systems for micronutrients and nutraceuticals. *Soft Matter 4* (10): 1964–1980.

Vinarov, Z., Tcholakova, S., Damyanova, B. et al. (2012). Effects of emulsifier charge and concentration on pancreatic lipolysis: 2 interplay of emulsifiers and biles. *Langmuir 28* (33): 12140–12150.

de Vos, P., Lazarjani, H.A., Poncelet, D. et al. (2014). Polymers in cell encapsulation from an enveloped cell perspective. *Advanced Drug Delivery Reviews 67–68*: 15–34.

Wang, X. and Gao, Y. (2018). Effects of length and unsaturation of the alkyl chain on the hydrophobic binding of curcumin with Tween micelles. *Food Chemistry 246*: 242–248.

Wang, Q., Yin, L., and Padua, G.W. (2008a). Effect of hydrophilic and lipophilic compounds on zein microstructures. *Food Biophysics 3* (2): 174–181.

Wang, X., Jiang, Y., Wang, Y.-W. et al. (2008b). Enhancing anti-inflammation activity of curcumin through O/W nanoemulsions. *Food Chemistry 108* (2): 419–424.

Wang, Y., Larsson, D.S.D., and van der Spoel, D. (2009). Encapsulation of myoglobin in a cetyl trimethylammonium bromide micelle in vacuo: a simulation study. *Biochemistry 48* (5): 1006–1015.

Wang, L.-J., Hu, Y.-Q., Yin, S.-W. et al. (2015a). Fabrication and characterization of antioxidant pickering emulsions stabilized by zein/chitosan complex particles (ZCPs). *Journal of Agricultural and Food Chemistry 63* (9): 2514–2524.

Wang, S., Chen, X., Shi, M. et al. (2015b). Absorption of whey protein isolated (WPI)-stabilized β-Carotene emulsions by oppositely charged oxidized starch microgels. *Food Research International 67*: 315–322.

Wang, T., Xue, J., Hu, Q. et al. (2017). Preparation of lipid nanoparticles with high loading capacity and exceptional gastrointestinal stability for potential oral delivery applications. *Journal of Colloid and Interface Science 507*: 119–130.

Wang, J.J., Wang, Y., Wang, Q. et al. (2019). Mechanically strong and highly tough prolamin protein hydrogels designed from double-cross-linked assembled networks. *ACS Applied Polymer Materials 1* (6): 1272–1279.

Winuprasith, T., Khomein, P., Mitbumrung, W. et al. (2018). Encapsulation of vitamin D3 in pickering emulsions stabilized by nanofibrillated mangosteen cellulose: impact on in vitro digestion and bioaccessibility. *Food Hydrocolloids 83*: 153–164.

Wojtecki, R.J., Meador, M.A., and Rowan, S.J. (2011). Using the dynamic bond to access macroscopically responsive structurally dynamic polymers. *Nature Materials 10* (1): 14–27.

Wooster, T.J., Golding, M., and Sanguansri, P. (2008). Impact of oil type on nanoemulsion formation and ostwald ripening stability. *Langmuir 24* (22): 12758–12765.

Wu, Y., Li, Y.-H., Gao, X.-H. et al. (2013). The application of nanoemulsion in dermatology: an overview. *Journal of Drug Targeting 21* (4): 321–327.

Xiao, J., Lu, X., and Huang, Q. (2017). Double emulsion derived from kafirin nanoparticles stabilized Pickering emulsion: fabrication, microstructure, stability and in vitro digestion profile. *Food Hydrocolloids 62*: 230–238.

Yang, Y., Fang, Z., Chen, X. et al. (2017). An overview of Pickering emulsions: solid-particle materials, classification, morphology, and applications. *Frontiers in Pharmacology 8*: 287.

Yaqoob Khan, A., Talegaonkar, S., Iqbal, Z. et al. (2006). Multiple emulsions: an overview. *Current Drug Delivery 3* (4): 429–443.

Zeeb, B., Saberi, A.H., Weiss, J. et al. (2015). Formation and characterization of filled hydrogel beads based on calcium alginate: Factors influencing nanoemulsion retention and release. *Food Hydrocolloids 50*: 27–36.

Zhang, X., Huang, J., Chang, P.R. et al. (2010). Structure and properties of polysaccharide nanocrystal-doped supramolecular hydrogels based on cyclodextrin inclusion. *Polymer 51* (19): 4398–4407.

Zhang, L., Wang, S., Zhang, M. et al. (2013). Nanocarriers for oral drug delivery. *Journal of Drug Targeting 21* (6): 515–527.

Zhang, Z., Decker, E.A., and McClements, D.J. (2014). Encapsulation, protection, and release of polyunsaturated lipids using biopolymer-based hydrogel particles. *Food Research International 64*: 520–526.

Zhang, Z., Zhang, R., Decker, E.A. et al. (2015). Development of food-grade filled hydrogels for oral delivery of lipophilic active ingredients: pH-triggered release. *Food Hydrocolloids 44*: 345–352.

Zhang, Z., Zhang, R., and McClements, D.J. (2016a). Encapsulation of β-carotene in alginate-based hydrogel beads: impact on physicochemical stability and bioaccessibility. *Food Hydrocolloids 61*: 1–10.

Zhang, Z., Zhang, R., Zou, L. et al. (2016b). Encapsulation of curcumin in polysaccharide-based hydrogel beads: Impact of bead type on lipid digestion and curcumin bioaccessibility. *Food Hydrocolloids 58*: 160–170.

Zhang, X., Liu, J., Qian, C. et al. (2019). Effect of grafting method on the physical property and antioxidant potential of chitosan film functionalized with gallic acid. *Food Hydrocolloids 89*: 1–10.

Zhao, L., Temelli, F., and Chen, L. (2017). Encapsulation of anthocyanin in liposomes using supercritical carbon dioxide: Effects of anthocyanin and sterol concentrations. *Journal of Functional Foods 34*: 159–167.

17

Encapsulation and Delivery of Nutraceuticals and Bioactive Compounds by Nanoliposomes and Tocosomes as Promising Nanocarriers

Narges Shahgholian

Food Machinery Division, Department of Biosystems Engineering, Shahid Chamran University of Ahvaz, Ahvaz, Iran

List of Abbreviations

ACN	anthocyanin
BHT	butylated hydroxyl toluene
CD	cyclodextrin
CH	chitosan
DBV	double bilayer membranes
DRV	dehydration–rehydration vesicles
EE	encapsulation efficiency
FATMLV	frozen and thawed multi lamellar vesicle
GUV	giant unilamellar vesicles
HM	heating method
IV	Iodine value
LE	loading efficiency
LUV	large unilamellar vesicles
MCV	microencapsulation vesicle method
MLV	multilamellar vesicles
MVV	multivesicular vesicles
NH	neohesperidin
NL	nanoliposome
OLV	oligo-lamellar vesicle
P	pectin
PC	phosphatidylcholine
PE	phosphatidylethanolamine
PI	phosphatidyl inositol
PL	phospholipid
PS	phosphatidylserine
Quer	quercetin
RPE/REV	reverse phase evaporation
RSM	response surface method
SGF	simulated gasterointestinal fluids

Handbook of Nutraceuticals and Natural Products: Biological, Medicinal, and Nutritional Properties and Applications,
Volume 1, First Edition. Edited by Sreerag Gopi and Preetha Balakrishnan.
© 2022 John Wiley & Sons, Inc. Published 2022 by John Wiley & Sons, Inc.

SPLV   stable pluri lamellar vesicle
SUV   small unilamellar vesicles
TAG   triacyglycerol
TP   tocopheryl phosphate
T$_2$P   di-tocopheryl phosphate
VET   vesicle prepared by extrusion technique

17.1 Introduction

Micronutrients' administration by fortification of staple and complementary foods is a followed strategy to coping with malnutrition and micronutrient deficiencies. There is a great industrial interest in the preparation of formulations for joint administration of vitamins, minerals, low-soluble herbal drugs, natural antioxidants, for providing bone and teeth support, promoting heart health and helping boost immunity (Dalmoro et al. 2019).

In recent years, there has been increased attention to adding micronutrient interventions using new approaches, on top of the other common food-based fortification. Recommended intake dose for several micronutrients according to a certain age and physiologic groups have been formed. The term "lipid-based nutrient supplements" (LNS) refers generically to a range of fortified, lipid-based products, including:

1) "Ready-to-use" therapeutic foods (RUTF): (a large daily ration with relatively low micronutrient concentration) which have been successfully used for management of severe acute malnutrition (SAM) among children or *prevention* of malnutrition in smaller doses.
2) "Point-of-use" fortification contains highly concentrated supplements (1–4 teaspoons/day, providing <100 kcal/day) (Chaparro and Dewey 2010).

It is necessary to design desired nutritional formulation of LNS for different target groups, taking into account the expected bioavailability of relevant nutrients, toxicity concerns, stability and shelf-life considerations, production, packaging, cost, and distribution of LNS in the context of emergencies. They target the population as a whole or supplementary (selective) feeding program (SFP). For nutritionally vulnerable or malnourished individuals, most vulnerable groups (e.g. infants and children between 6 and 24 months of age, and pregnant and lactating women [PLW]) or people in emergency settings are groups of interest. Emergency settings include general food distribution (GFD) rations in logistical and operational challenges (Chaparro and Dewey 2010).

Among advanced types of food fortification, encapsulation of intended bioactive compounds using different kind of polymers is the best approach. These encapsulated compounds can be used alone or in different kinds of food. Encapsulation of bioactive compounds and nutraceuticals in different "lipid-based carriers" such as nanoemulsions, nanoliposomes, nanonoisome, solid lipid nanoparticles (SLNs) and nanostructured lipid carriers (NLCs), surfactant systems, and polymer/lipid encapsulation in hybrid systems have been reported. Lipid-based nanocarriers (LNCs) represent a class of lipid particles, in nanoscale dimension with improved characteristics compared with conventional formulations (Pauli et al. 2019).

Liposomes (derived from the Greek words lypo [fat] and soma [body]) are small spherical vesicles in which one or more aqueous compartments are completely enclosed by a bilayer of amphiphilic molecules, such as phospholipids (PLs) and cholesterol. They have been identified by Alec Bangham and his group at Babraham Institute of Animal Physiology in the 1960s as Multilayer vesicles consisting of lipid compounds in an aqueous environment. Later this building was named Liposome (Bangham et al. 1974).

Liposome is a general terminology covering many classes of vesicles in a broad range of diameter, range from tens of nanometers to several micrometers (Mozafari 2010; Weissig 2010). Liposome as a microscopic vesicle contains a phospholipid layer that surrounds a fluid space. The bilayers are typically from 3 to 6 nm thick and the liposome can range from about 50 nm to 50 microns in diameter (Zasadzinski et al. 2011).

The term "nanoliposome" has been introduced recently to specifically refer to nanoscale bilayer lipid vesicles (Mozafari 2010; Weissig 2010). With the progress in the field of nanoscience and nanotechnology, the term "nanoliposome" has been introduced to exclusively refer to nanoscale lipid vesicles since "liposome" is a general word covering many classes of lipid vesicles with diameters in the size range of tens of nanometers to several micrometers (Mohammadabadi and Mozafari 2018). These nanometric versions of liposomes are similar to a spherical vesicle consisting of one or more phospholipid bilayer membranes surrounding an aqueous core. NLs are one of the most applied encapsulation and drug delivery systems (Shishir et al. 2019).

Liposomes' encapsulation has drawn great attention due to their low intrinsic toxicity and immunogenicity and their capability to prolong shelf life and improve the bioavailability of a wide variety of hydrophilic and hydrophobic molecules. These features led to the introduction of liposomes as a very suitable carrier in modern pharmaceutical systems (Zasadzinski et al. 2011).

These tiny structures look like packages or capsules that can be used to carry bioactive molecules to different parts of the body by encapsulating them. The similarity of their structure to that of cell membranes helps the penetration and overcoming of biological barriers to cellular and tissue uptake of entrapped nutrients.

Liposomes and NLs share the same chemical, structural, and thermodynamic properties. Nevertheless, compared to liposomes, NLs provide more surface area and have the potential to increase solubility and bioavailability, improve the controlled release and enable precision targeting of the encapsulated material to a greater extent. Among the major parameters in the NL formulation, lipid composition and cholesterol content are the most important (Mozafari 2010; Weissig 2010).

Due to the amphipathic properties of its constituent elements, it makes it possible for liposomes to coadminister hydrophilic and hydrophobic molecules. In other words, as nanoliposomal vesicles have both water and lipid phase, they can easily encapsulate hydrophobic, hydrophilic or amphiphilic molecules. The hydrophilic and lipophilic molecules can be encapsulated in the inner aqueous phase and the region between the lipid bilayer of the liposomal carrier, respectively, while amphiphilic molecules can be entrapped in the water/lipid phase (Shishir et al. 2019). The structure of bioactive-loaded NLs based on the positioning of bioactive dispersion are divided into three groups including homo-/heterogeneous core and membrane model, bioactive-enriched membrane model, and bioactive-enriched core model (Balamurugan and Chintamani 2018).

Liposomes are colloidal particles with at least two layers of phospholipid membranes. Due to their amphiphilic nature of PLs, they can have such a two-layer architecture.

It is now possible to engineer a wide range and different self-assembled structures of NLs of different sizes, with diverse phospholipid compositions and surface properties.

17.2 PLs' Characteristics

17.2.1 PLs in Original Food Materials

PLs are commonly found in soy lecithin, egg lecithin, as well as in other sources such as milk fat globule membrane (MFGM) (Toniazzo and Pinho 2016).

In the fish, phosphatidyl ethanol amine (PE) fraction, has high source of eicosatetraenoic acid (ETA) in particularly and is also rich in docosahexaenoic acid (DHA) (Bandarra et al. 2001).

Most PLs obtained during the degumming of edible oils are unsuitable for human use. They are added back to the extracted meal and used as feed. It is reported that only soybean lecithin has a quality sufficient for human food and industrial uses. PLs from animal sources, mainly egg yolk PLs, can be used similarly as soybean lecithin; however, these are very expensive. For this reason, they are used only for pharmaceutical products or for biochemical research (Pokorný and Schmidt 2010).

17.2.2 Structure and Charge of PLs

The basic molecular building block of a cell membrane as well as a typical liposomal membrane is a phospholipid. PLs are built on a glycerol backbone (interface) and phosphorylated molecules are esterified to C_3 of the glycerol, forming a polar group. Fatty acids are esterified to C_1 and C_2 of the glycerol. PLs are known as polar lipids because the phosphorylated portion is water-soluble while fatty acid tails of the molecules are nonpolar or fat-soluble. The chain length can vary from 3 to 24 carbons either saturated or unsaturated fatty acids. The most common natural PLs contain palmitic and oleic acids. However, synthetic ones can be synthesized with any combination of fatty acids. Some PLs carry additional charges in addition to the negative charge at the phosphate residue. In phosphatidylcholine (PC) (lecithin) and phosphatidylethanolamine (PE) (cephalin), the amino alcohol is positively charged. As a whole, these two phosphatides, therefore, appear to be neutral. In contrast, phosphatidylserine (PS), with one additional positive charge and one additional negative charge in the serine residue and phosphatidylinositol (PI) (with no additional charge), have a negative net charge, due to the phosphate residue (Koolman and Röhm 2005; Pokorný and Schmidt 2010).

17.2.3 Biological and Physicochemical Activities of PLs

PLs are ubiquitous in all organisms and there has recently been evidence presented that the nutritional value of PLs is higher than that of triacylglycerols (TAGs). It has been demonstrated that PC can decreased lymphatic cholesterol absorption (Jiang et al. 2001). Vegetable lecithin (PC) can modulate lipoprotein metabolism, decrease hepatic lipogenesis and blood cholesterol, and act as a potential preventive or therapeutic for cardiometabolic diseases (Robert et al. 2020), PE caused a decrease in serum cholesterol (Imaizumi et al. 1983), and PI increased the level of HDL-cholesterol in rabbits and humans (Adamczak and Bednarski 2010; Stamler et al. 2000).

17.2.4 Thermal Characteristics of PLs

The interaction between PLs and water takes place at a temperature above the gel to liquid-crystalline phase transition temperature (T_C), which represents the melting point of the acyl chains. T_c is at temperatures lower than their final melting point (T_m), also known as gel-to-liquid crystalline transition temperature, is a temperature at which the lipidic bilayer loses much of its ordered packing while its fluidity increases. When fully hydrated, most PLs exhibit a phase change from L-β gel crystalline to the L-α crystalline state at T_C. All PLs have a characteristic T_C which depends on the nature of the lipids.

It is necessary to know more about fluidity and phase transition of PLs membrane for rational manufacturing and utilization of liposomes.

The physicochemical properties of NLs depend on several factors including pH, ionic strength, type, and essence of ingredients such as lipids, sterols, PLs, and temperature.

17.3 Mechanism of NLs' Formation

17.3.1 Arrangement of Building Blocks of NLs

PLs are the building blocks of liposomes and NLs. Amphiphilic molecules come together in such a way that their hydrophobic tails/groups oriented toward the inner layers of the sphere escape from the core and their hydrophilic head is directed toward the two outer and inner surfaces of the sphere. In this way, a double-layer spherical membrane is formed. As a result, a completely closed spherical membrane is formed. This orientation provides the possibility of loading hydrophilic molecules in the core while hydrophobic bioactive compounds anchor in the liposome shell or between bilayers (Gregoriadis 1984).

PLs are often depicted/drawn as a ball representing the head group (negative phosphoryl group) with two tails attached to hydrophobic fatty acids. In an aqueous medium/environment, PLs orient themselves into a thermal dynamically stable structure called the bilayer. This flat sheet of lipids then curves into a geometric structure that has no edges, sphere (Figure 17.1).

These carriers are formed through the hydration of surfactants (e.g. PLs) when they are mixed in the water under little shear forces. Phospholipid molecules initially form regular sheets, which, after interconnection of hydrophobic tails, form a bilayer membrane resulting in some water entrapped in the interior of phospholipid vesicles (Katouzian et al. 2017).

There are many different self-assembly structures of PLs due to their amphiphilic character. These structures include lamellar, micellar, cubic, and hexagonal mesophases self-assembly structure of bilayer to the liposome.

17.3.2 Classifications of NLs Based on Morphology and Size

Liposomes are generally classified by categorizing them based upon their size, lamellarity (number of lamellae and number of internalized vesicles), surface charge, and functionality.

Depending on the lipid composition and method of production, liposomes can be classified. These properties can be tuned to substantially changing composition and/or method of preparation. Based on their ingredients and preparation method, different types of liposomes and NLs can be manufactured in the form of unilamellar or multilamellar vesicles.

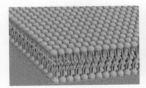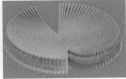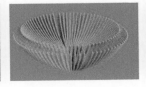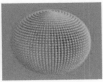

Figure 17.1 Self-assembly structure of bilayer to vesicular liposome (from left to right). *Source:* Copyright permission was obtained from Encapsula Nanosciences (encapsula.com).

Fundamentally, all liposomes are classified based on their size and morphology, as follows:

1) Liposomes with single bilayer membrane class (which itself has three types):
    a) Small unilamellar vesicles (SUV having average diameter d ~ 20–100 nm),
    b) Large unilamellar vesicles (LUV, $d > 100$ nm),
    c) Giant unilamellar vesicles (GUV, $d > 1000$ nm).
2) Liposomes composed of more than one bilayer:
    a) Multilamellar vesicles (MLV),
    b) Multivesicular vesicles (MVV).

MLVs consist of five or more concentric lamellae with an average diameter range from 0.5 to 5 μm. MLVs can be several microns in diameter. MVVs consist of small vesicles trapped within the large vesicles or vesicles enclosing many smaller vesicles (liposomes within liposomes) and whose diameters are usually larger than 1 μm (Lasic 1988; Toniazzo and Pinho 2016; Zhang 2017). The schematic representation of MVV is depicted in Figure 17.2.

In a more detailed classification of liposomes, the other two groups are double bilayer vesicle (DBV, composed of two bilayer membranes, >300 nm) and oligolamellar vesicle (OLV, composed of ~three to five bilayers). With respect to their size range and number of lamellae, DBV and OLV are located between two subclasses of LUV and GUV. So, logically, MLV is composed of more than five concentric bilayer vesicles (Figure 17.3). Due to their size limitations, NLs (submicron lipid vesicles) can only be in the form of SUV, LUV, DBV, or OLV, while liposomes can be in the form of LUV, DBV, OLV, MLV, GUV, or MVV (Mohammadabadi and Mozafari 2018).

17.3.3 Classification of Liposomes and NLs Based on Preparation Method

There are diverse methods of liposome preparation. The choice of the best method depends on the physicochemical characteristics of the components, the concentration of the loaded substance, type of the dispersion medium, desired size and the half-life for the successful application, costs, reproducibility, and applicability regarding large-scale production (Gomez-Hens and Fernandez-Romero 2006; Reza Mozafari et al. 2008; Wagner and Vorauer-Uhl 2011).

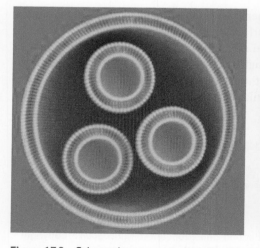
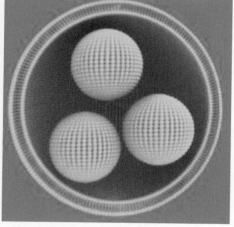

Figure 17.2 Schematic representation of multivesicular vesicles (MVV). *Source:* Copyright permission was obtained from Encapsula Nanosciences (encapsula.com).

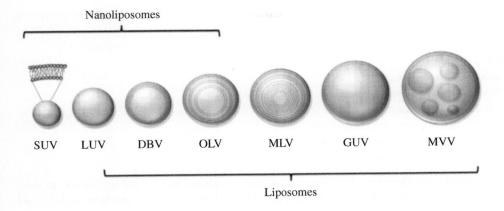

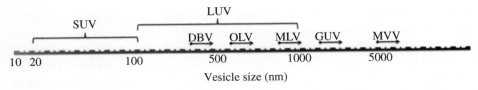

Figure 17.3 Different types of liposomes and nanoliposomes according to their size, number of lamellae, and number of internalized vesicles. An enlarged section of phospholipid bilayer is depicted on top of SUV. *Source:* Copyright permission was obtained from Mohammadabadi and Mozafari (2018).

There is the versatility of the developed preparation protocol to achieve tailored liposomes in terms of size and EE. The process used to generate the liposome will impact its size and lamellarity (Pauli et al. 2019). Likewise, choosing various lipids with different properties in the formulation can affect/change the properties of liposomes (such as size, drug release kinetics, biocompatibility, surface charge, and cell targeting).

The two main categories of liposome preparation are top-bottom and bottom-up. The first includes homogenization, extrusion, high shear mixing, and sonication, and the latter covers the procedures such as solvent injection, supercritical fluids, inkjet, and microfluidics (Perrie et al. 2017).

Barenholz and Lasic (2018) categorized the main methods for preparing different liposomes into five main groups including mechanical methods, replacement of organic solvent by aqueous media, detergent/surfactant displacement, size transformation, and fusion and pH adjustment. It is suggested to refer to the reference for more information (Barenholz and Lasic 2018).

Physical dispersion, solvent dispersion, and detergent solubilization are the three basic categories of liposomes and NL preparations. The subunits of these three categories are listed below:

1) **Physical dispersion**
   a) Lipid film hydration/dehydration–rehydration vesicles (DRV)
      i) Hand-shaking MLVs
      ii) Nonshaking LUVs (Thin film hydration)
      iii) Size transformation ("Freeze-dried MLVs" and "Frozen and thawed multilamellar vesicle" [FATMLV])
      iv) Proliposomes/dried reconstitute vesicles

    b) High pressure and vesicle prepared by extrusion technique (VET)/membrane extrusion techniques

    c) Heating method (HM-liposomes) and Mozafari method (modified heating method)

2) **Solvent dispersion**

    a) Ethanol/ether injection

    b) Water organic phase

      i) Double emulsion method

      ii) Reverse phase evaporation (RPE/REV)

      iii) Stable plurilamellar vesicle (SPLV)

3) **Detergent solubilization**

It is worth mentioning that some techniques have been employed to help reduce the size of vesicles, for instance, sonication and microfluidization. The first two categories are more widely used in the food sector and in the following, some of them are discussed.

17.3.3.1 Physical Dispersion

17.3.3.1.1 Thin Film Hydration (Bangham Method/Non-Shaking LUVs) The simplest method for the preparation of liposomes is the hydration of dry lipids. Lipids are dissolved in organic solvent all along with any soluble compounds to be incorporated into the liposomes. The solvent is commonly removed by rotary evaporation resulting in thin-film hydration of dry lipid. Thin lipid films or lipid cakes are hydrated and stacks of liquid crystalline bilayers become fluid and swell, and the liposomes are formed. The hydrated lipid sheets detach during agitation and self-close to form LMVs, with each lipid bilayer separated by a water layer. The spacing between lipid layers is determined by the composition and highly charged layers are farther apart based on electrostatic repulsion. This method produces large and nonhomogeneous MLVs that require sonication or extrusion processes to be produced in homogeneous SUVs (Bozzuto and Molinari 2015).

Hydration of the dry lipid film is accomplished by adding an aqueous medium (including water-soluble bioactive material) to the container of dry lipid and agitating them while the temperature of the added medium is above the gel-liquid crystal of the lipid with the highest T_c of the used lipids. After the addition of the hydrating medium, the lipid suspension should be maintained at a temperature above the T_c during the hydration period by placing the round bottom flask on a rotary evaporation system spinning the round bottom flask in the warm water bath without a vacuum.

These features guarantee the lipid to hydrate in its fluid phase with adequate agitation. An average hydration time of one hour with vigorous shaking, mixing, or stirring is recommended. It is suggested to stand the vesicle suspension overnight (aging) prior to downsizing makes to improve the homogeneous dispersion, while it is not suggested to use high transition lipids because of the probability of the increase in lipid hydrolysis with elevated temperatures (Dr. Stephen Burgess, Chief Scientific Officer at Avanti® Polar Lipids).

17.3.3.1.2 Proliposomes Proliposomes are particulate systems of dry, free-flowing PLs, which contain the bioactive to be encapsulated in their lipid matrix. Liposome vesicles are obtained after the hydration of the formulated suspension/dispersion under controlled conditions of temperature and agitation. To verify the feasibility of producing proliposomes containing curcumin, coating of micronized sucrose using mixtures of purified and unpurified PLs have been reported (Chaves and Pinho 2018, 2019; Parhizkar et al. 2018; Waghule et al. 2020).

In one research, the ethanolic solution of PLs (P90H : LS40 in different ratios) and curcumin, simultaneously have been sonicated and added dropwise to the micronized sucrose in a rotary evaporator, while maintaining the temperature at 55 °C to evaporate ethanol. Liposomes were then prepared by adding 2 g of proliposomes containing curcumin to 100 ml of deionized water while subjected to ultra-agitation (at 13 000 rpm for five minutes at 65 °C). Subsequently, the dispersions were immediately cooled to 25 °C for the addition of 0.1% carbohydrates under magnetic stirring. Proliposomes had a very irregular shape with many agglomerates. The images revealed that the micronized sucrose was efficiently coated by the PLs. According to the averzage hydrodynamic diameters of hydrated proliposomes (ranged from 207 to 222 nm), they are in the category of LUVs while the vesicles produced using the hydration of the proliposomes method are usually multilamellar (≥500 nm). Research showed tighter packing in the membranes containing PC, decreases the vesicle size. The short storage time observed for the dispersions suggests the need for more study for the optimization of the process parameters (Chaves and Pinho 2019).

17.3.3.1.3 Freeze and Thaw Method To overcome the limitation of low EE and vehiculation of hydrophilic, amphiphilic, or lipophilic compounds, a common procedure is freezing the liposomes/NLs with liquid nitrogen (−196 °C) and thawing at a temperature above the phase transition temperature of the lipids. In the preparation of liposomes, freeze–thaw cycling is used to reduce the lamellarity of liposomes, disrupt the liposomal bilayer to allow molecules to diffuse into the liposome, and increase encapsulation. To eliminate any effects related to polydispersity and/or multiple lipid lamellae, a monodispersed population of unilamellar, preformed empty (PFE) liposomes (diameter of 166.8 ± 39.8 nm) were chosen. Factors chosen for evaluation include thawing and annealing temperatures as well as annealing duration (Costa et al. 2014).

17.3.3.1.4 Heating Method (HM) The majority of NLs' manufacturing techniques involves the utilization of potentially toxic solvents or high-shear force procedures. These hurdles can be overcome by employing alternative methods such as the heating method by which liposomes and NLs can be prepared using a single apparatus in the absence of toxic solvents. The nanoliposomal ingredients may be hydrated together or separately according to their solubility and T_c. The heating method can be easily adapted from small to industrial scales. The heating method has flexibility for the entrapment of various drugs and other bioactive compounds with respect to their temperature sensitivities (Mozafari 2010).

17.3.3.1.5 Mozafari Method (Modified Heating Method) Most recently introduced and one of the simplest methods without the need for the prehydration of ingredients material and without employing toxic solvents or detergents from small scales to large industrial scales is Mozafari method. The Mozafari method has recently been used successfully for the encapsulation of the food-grade antimicrobial nisin (Mozafari 2010).

17.3.3.2 Solvent Dispersion

17.3.3.2.1 Ethanol/Ether Injection (Phase Separation Method) NLs' preparation using the ethanol injection method is easy to scale up. PL and cholesterol amounts indicated a significant influence on liposome size and EE. Comparing bioactive compounds or drugs with different hydrophobicities, the higher EE was for the hydrophobic drug rather than for the hydrophilic ones (case study: EE of hydrophobic [beclomethasone dipropionate; BDP] vs. a hydrophilic [cytarabine; Ara-C] was reported 100 : 16) (Jaafar-Maalej et al. 2010).

Ishii et al. in Japan offered a unique perspective on liposome preparation using the coacervation (phase separation) technique to prepare microcapsules in agrochemicals and other fields. They claimed that this simple and reproducible method is valuable as a drug carrier for encapsulation and sustained release of various drugs within the body. The coacervation method is a unique way of forming NLs in various types and sizes, without the need for special equipment or even without involving sonication steps, which are difficult to scale up. To form the coacervate droplets under agitation at constant temperature (20 °C), water was added dropwise to the PL-alcohol solutions with various concentrations (ranging from 0.1 to 50% W/V). To optimize the coacervation conditions, a triangular phase diagram of the coacervation system was developed. The dialysis tube containing lipid vesicles was then dialyzed three times with distilled water for one hour. In this study, when ethanol was used as a solvent, fluidized precipitation of PL was observed. They found optimum level of ethanol for the preparation of liposome by the coacervation method with PL (Ishii 2018).

17.3.3.2.2 Microencapsulation Vesicle (MCV) Method (Parallel to Double Emulsion Method) The MCV method is considered parallel to several methods using double emulsion techniques. A prominent feature of the MCV method is solvent evaporation from $W_1/O/W_2$ double emulsions.

The MCV method was originally reported by Ishii et al. (1988). In this method, liposomes are formed through a two-step emulsification process. First, PLs are dissolved in an organic solvent that is immiscible in water, then mixed with a solution containing hydrophilic substances to be encapsulated. The W_1/O emulsion prepared by mechanical agitation of the mixture is then added to another water phase to form $W_1/O/W_2$ emulsion. Stirring was continued at a constant temperature under a stream of nitrogen gas until the solvent was evaporated. After solvent evaporation from the surface of the mother liquid, lipid films are formed and liposomal suspension is created. The structure of the liposomes prepared by the MCV method was unilamellar vesicles (Nii and Ishii 2006) (Figure 17.4).

17.3.3.2.3 Reverse Phase Evaporation (RPE) Among the methods for preparing liposomes, RPE is a typical approach. The "reverse-phase evaporation" technique is composed of inverted micelles or W/O emulsions in which the water phase contains the interested bioactive compounds and the organic phase (isopropyl/diethyl ether) consists of the lipids to form a liposomal bilayer. After adding this lipid mixture to a flask and evaporate the solvent, the lipid films are obtained as shown in Figure 17.5. Then the gained lipid film after evaporation is redissolved in an organic phase. The addition of the water phase leads to a two-phase system following the subsequent sonication results in a homogeneous dispersion. The organic solvent was slowly removed by the reduced pressure method, initially leading to the conversion of the dispersion into a viscous gel, which finally formed a liposomal suspension. Compared to the thin-film hydration method, the RPE technique shows an advantage of higher internal aqueous loading. Dialysis and centrifugation can be applied to remove the remaining solvent (Seth and Misra 2002; Szoka et al. 1980; Szoka and Papahadjopoulos 1978).

Removal of organic solvent causes the production of single, oligolamellar, or multilamellar vesicles (LUV, OLV, and MLV). Chlorinated solvents, diethyl ether or methanol, are toxic and prone to a possible risk for human health and influence the stability of the vesicles. An alternative solvent such as ethanol, ethyl acetate, and two mixtures of ethanol/ethyl acetate, for the production of liposomes, have been introduced (Cortesi 1999).

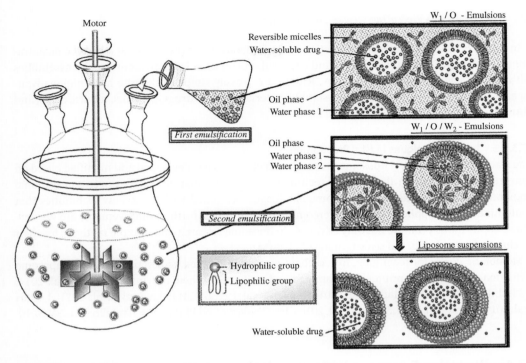

Figure 17.4 Preparation of a lipid vesicle suspension by the MCV method, *Source:* Copyright permission was obtained from Nii and Ishii (2006).

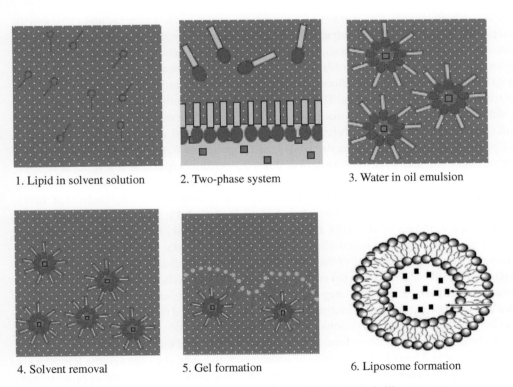

1. Lipid in solvent solution

2. Two-phase system

3. Water in oil emulsion

4. Solvent removal

5. Gel formation

6. Liposome formation

Figure 17.5 Flow chart of nanoliposomes' preparation by RPE technique. Lollipop structures are representative of dissolved lipids and, squares (at the end of the arrows), display compound to be encapsulated. *Source:* Copyright permission was obtained from Piramal Healthcare Group.

In the RPE method, a substantial fraction of the aqueous phase (up to 65% at low salt concentrations) is entrapped within the vesicles and encapsulation of even large macromolecular assemblies with high efficiency is accessible. Thus, RPE as a relatively simple technique has unique advantages for encapsulating valuable water-soluble materials such as drugs, proteins, nucleic acids, and other biochemical reagents (Shi and Qi 2018).

17.3.3.3 Latest Techniques in NLs' Preparation

The state of the art of novel liposome preparation techniques has developed and modified based on conventional methods. Although new techniques have particular advantages over conventional preparation methods, there are still some challenges associated with these new techniques that could hinder their applications. For overcoming those hurdles, further improvements are needed. These applications promote not only advances in liposome research, but also the methods for their production on an industrial scale (Huang et al. 2014).

Membrane contactor technique, freeze–thaw–annealing method, supercritical assisted liposome formation and an inkjet printer are examined and evaluated in new researches (Costa et al. 2014; Hauschild et al. 2005; Huang et al. 2014; Jaafar-Maalej et al. 2011; Laouini et al. 2011; Lestari et al. 2019; Perrie et al. 2017; Sebaaly et al. 2016a, b, c; Toniazzo and Pinho 2016; Trucillo et al. 2019a, b).

17.4 Bioactive Compounds' Encapsulation in Nanoliposomal Carriers

Bioactive compounds including pigments (anthocyanins, carotenoids, lycopene, and chlorophyll), herbal polyphenols and flavonoids extract (ginger, garlic, tea, turmeric,. . .), essential oils and omegas, flavors, enzymes, vitamins and minerals, probiotics and prebiotics, dietary compounds, and bioactive peptides and different natural antioxidants have been used and investigated to increase their efficiency, stability, or bioavailability by liposomal/nanoliposomal encapsulation systems. Some of these interesting cases are mentioned here. These compounds have different or similar properties to prevent, delay, or fight against different diseases in our body, most of them related to inflammation.

Different foods with diverse texture and pH have been fortified or suggested to enrich with nanoliposomal ingredients including dairy products (skimmed milk, fermented milk, cheese, and yogurt powder) (Alkhalaf et al. 1988; Ding et al. 2010; Gulzar and Benjakul 2020a; Jafari et al. 2019; Laridi et al. 2003; Mohammadi et al. 2015; Toniazzo et al. 2014), mayonnaise (Rafiee et al. 2018), beverages (orange juice) (Mohammadi Ghanbarzadeh and Hamishehkar 2014; Poudel et al. 2019), chocolate (Gültekin-Özgüven et al. 2016), bread (Amoah et al. 2019; Narsaiah et al. 2019; Ojagh and Hasani 2018; Pinilla et al. 2019), minced beef (Tometri et al. 2020), cooked beef sausage (Khatib et al. 2020), margarines and oils (Rasti et al. 2017; Yasufuku et al. 1988), gummi candy, free-flowing powdery foods like coffee and confectionary (Amjadi et al. 2018; Gulzar and Benjakul 2020b), flavor sweets and bakeries and as preservatives (Keivani Nahr et al. 2019).

Liposome-encapsulated peptides may offer the possibility of application in areas such as food science and technology in order to increase the nutritional value and shelf life of food products, as well as for the development of functional foods (Corrêa et al. 2019).

Liquid compositions of liposome formulations are not widely used due to the instability of PLs in high temperature and low pH. Formulation of liposomes with a long shelf life at room temperature can be achieved by freeze-drying. This formulation in a powdered form, known as proliposome, stops lipid degradation and destabilization (Bankole et al. 2020; Ren et al. 2017; Wang et al. 2018).

The following is a description of some nanoformula of bioactive compounds in NLs.

17.4.1 Vitamin and Mineral Supplements

Nanoliposomal formulation of ferrous sulfate (Bochicchio et al. 2020), micronutrient (Dalmoro et al. 2019), and vitamins (Matheus Andrade Chaves et al. 2018; Janssens 2017; Maurya et al. 2020; Parhizkar et al. 2018) have been reported which are good alternatives for conventional supplements.

17.4.1.1 Nanoliposomal Vitamin D

Vitamins are classified into two categories – water-soluble and fat-soluble ones. They are essential micronutrients as they cannot be synthesized by a living organism so that it is indispensable that they are assumed with food in adequate quantities to impede the development of a deficiency syndrome (Gueli et al. 2012). In recent years, vitamin D is a controversial vitamin worldwide for its deficiency in diets. The problem of vitamin D results in some critical diseases such as rickets, osteomalacia, and osteoporosis. Vitamin D, as an important liposoluble vitamin, travels in the blood bound to an alpha globulin and is present in two forms: (i) ergocalciferol (vitamin D_2) and (ii) cholecalciferol (vitamin D_3). The principal functions of this vitamin are an augmentation of intestinal absorption of calcium and promotion of normal bone formation and mineralization. The blood level of vitamin D_3 in the plasma, of a healthy human body (in the range of 30–100 ng/ml), is found in elevated quantities in fish liver oil and egg yolk (Gueli et al. 2012). The possible causes of vitamin D deficiency including a reduction in skin synthesis and absorption, hepatic failure, malabsorption, nephrotic syndrome, and chronic renal failure. The biological effects of vitamin D are as follows: prevention of different diseases including autoimmune diseases (immunomodulators), like multiple sclerosis and diabetes type 1, cancers, and metastases, also improvement in depression and schizophrenia, and strengthening of skeleton and muscles (Gueli et al. 2012).

Nutritionists believe that fortification of food products through this micronutrient is the best method to solve this problem. Yogurt powders fortified with nanoliposomal encapsulated vitamin D were evaluated and reported. The average particle size of nanoliposomal vitamin D was about 120 nm. The addition of maltodextrin caused spherical powder particles with an even distribution in the matrix including yogurt and drying aids (Jafari et al. 2019).

17.4.2 Nanoliposomal Flavonoids

Plants are a rich source of phenolic compounds (phenolic acids, flavonoids, and tannins) which are the most important natural antioxidants. Antioxidants in the diet are important in protecting the body against oxidative stress and maintaining good health. The antioxidant activity of these plants is directly related to the amount of phenolic compounds and total flavonoids.

Anthocyanin (ACN), quercetin (Quer), and neohesperidin (NH) belong to a parent class of molecules called flavonoids synthesized via the phenyl propanoid pathway.

When these flavonoids are added directly into the food matrix, they may cause disagreeable taste and color, as well as possible aggregation/precipitation phenomena in protein foods. Such limitations could be overcome using delivery systems for encapsulation, protection, and controlled release of flavonoids, as has been recently reported (Silva-Weiss et al. 2018). The aim of polyphenolic-nutrient nanoencapsulation is to protect and transport these active components and ensure their maximum bioavailability (Milinčić et al. 2019).

17.4.2.1 Quer-in-Cyclodextrin (CD)-in-NLs

The flavonol Quer is the most abundant flavonoid with low aqueous solubility (about 0.01 mg/ml at 25 °C), bitter taste, and reduced chemical stability cause a reduction of its use in the food industry. Azzi et al. used the technique of entrapment of cyclodextrin (CD)/Quer inclusion complexes, into the internal core of liposomes, to combine the advantages of both carriers and to limit their disadvantage (Azzi et al. 2018). CD has a truncated cone shape with a hydrophilic outside and an apolar cavity, able to form reversible inclusion complexes with nonpolar molecules (Szejtli 1997). Liposomes' preparation was carried out using the ethanol injection method. They concluded that egg lecithin (Lipoid E80) has more potent to form smaller liposomes with narrow size distribution in comparison to soya lecithins (either natural or hydrogenated, i.e. Lipoid S100 and Phospholipon 90H, respectively). The mean diameter of the particles increases with the decrement of the zeta potential value. The best LR% value was obtained with Lipoid E80 (15.0 ± 0.3%) which is ~1.8 and 2.4 fold higher than that of Lipoid S100 and Phospholipon 90H, respectively. This may be due to the presence of PE that may form hydrogen bonds with hydroxyl groups of Quer. Besides, PE is preferably localized in the outer monolayer when mixed with PC at low concentrations (below 10% mol), thus favoring the incorporation of Quer. Lipoid E80 (IV = 65–69) liposomes were the most efficient in protecting Quer from UV-light followed by Lipoid S100 (IV = 97–105) and Phospholipon 90H. Among five different types of CD evaluated in this research, highly charged derivatives of CD, i.e. SBE-β-CD (sulfobutylether-β-cyclodextrin) inclusion in liposome containing Lipoid E80, provide the highest binding affinity toward Quer with more photostability and protective against simulated gastrointestinal fluids (SGF). Any type of CD/Quer is reported to have more stability in nanoliposomes compared to conventional liposomes. A higher affinity of a Quer to CD than to lipid membrane may delay the drug release. The percentage distribution and the mean particle size of the nanometric populations in Quer-loaded Lipoid E80:Chol: SBE-β-CD liposomes were 68% and 150 nm, respectively (Azzi et al. 2018).

17.4.2.2 ACNs-in-NLs (Fortification of Milk)

ACNs are in the flavonoid class of water-soluble, vacuolar edible pigments, depending on their pH, may appear red, purple, blue, or black. ACNs are highly susceptible to degradation in high pH, light, heat, and oxygen, enzyme, and metal ions during processing and storage. The high instability and low bioavailability of ACNs limit their application during food processing and storage. For overcoming these shortcomings, different encapsulation methods have been suggested.

Chi et al. (2019) prepared nanoliposomal ACNs by combining ethanol injection method and ultrasonication, using response surface methodology (RSM) to optimize the parameters. Based on the experimental results, the optimal levels of lecithin concentration of 10.75 g/l, lecithin-to-cholesterol ratio of 5.98 and 0.15 g of ACNs were chosen as optimized independent variables (with desired minimum particle size and maximum ACNs' retention rate). The ACNs displayed higher stability when encapsulated in nanoliposomes compared with free ACNs under different storage conditions. The resulting mean particle size of ACNs was 53.80 nm and the ACNs' retention rate was 82.38%. In addition, the optimized nanoliposomes had encapsulation efficiency of 91.13%, polydispersity index of 0.190 and zeta potential of −42.69.

For the first time in this work, the stability and retention rate of liposomal and free ACNs have been evaluated in two phases of simulated gastric (SGF) and intestinal fluids (SIF). The difference between the free and liposomal forms of ACNs was more significant during incubation under the simulated intestinal phase (72.76% for the encapsulated ACNs and 52.01% for the free ACNs).

The stability of ACNs in the liposome and in the free form was compared in different storage conditions (retention rate of ACN in encapsulated versus free form) have been reported as follows:

In the dark at 4 °C after 28 days: 83.34 vs. 76.63%

In the dark at 25 °C after 28 days: 66.80 vs. 48.53%

Test in milk at 4 °C for 5 days: 89.01 vs. 83.06%

Under white fluorescent light at 25 °C, at three pH levels (3.0, 5.0, and 7.0) over five days: 93.79, 89.67, and 60.60% vs. 88.24, 80.34, and 40.81%, respectively (Chi et al. 2019).

17.4.2.3 ACNs-in-Chitosan-Coated NLs (Fortification of Dark Chocolate)

In the practical study, fortification of dark chocolate with chitosan-coated liposomal powder containing ACNs of black mulberry waste extract (BME) have been done. They explored the capability of liposomal delivery systems to retain ACNs' content against increased pH and temperature during the industrial production of dark chocolate. Naked and BME-loaded liposomes were prepared using a microfluidizer (five times' passage at homogenization pressure of 25 000 psi). Spray-dried chitosan-coated liposomal powder containing BME and maltodextrin (with positive zeta potential and mean diameter >400 nm) was added to natural (pH 4.5) and alkalized cocoa liquor samples (pH 6 and 7.5) at temperatures of 40, 60, and 80 °C, respectively. ACN retention of spray-dried liposomal powder was $56.19 \pm 4.8\%$. The results showed that the chitosan layer protected ACNs compared to the BME dried in the presence of only maltodextrin ($p < 0.05$) (Gültekin-Özgüven et al. 2016). To mimic chocolate production, powders were mixed in the last hour of conching to get maximum viscosity reduction which means keeping lecithin on the surface of the particles. Chocolate was fortified with liposomes containing a maximum 76.8% of added ACNs, depending on conching temperature and pH. The percentage of loss of ACNs in chitosan-coated liposomes was in the range of 32.4 and 49.8% with increasing temperature from 40 and 80 °C at pH 4.5. However, increasing pH from 4.5 to 7.5 resulted in higher ACNs' loss in all samples (Gültekin-Özgüven et al. 2016).

This mentioned method of liposomal preparation has the advantage of mucoadhesive properties of chitosan also giving slow release behavior while passing the gastric fluid. The desired nanoliposomes should not only protect ACNs from adverse environmental conditions but also slow down their release in SGF. Stable shell-core nanostructures, with mucoadhesive properties, are capable of controlled release of the active encapsulated compounds.

17.4.2.4 NH in Pectin (P) – and Chitosan (CH) – Conjugated NH in NLs

NH is a flavanone glycoside found in citrus fruits, possessing diverse biological activities such as anti-inflammation, neuroprotection, gastric protection, antidiabetic, antiallergic, and anticancer. Nevertheless, NH is unstable in physiological condition and poorly soluble in water. To overcome these shortcomings and facilitate the delivery of NH in the simulated gastrointestinal (GI) tract, a nanoliposome delivery system was prepared using thin-film hydration method combined with probe sonication. For enhancing cellular uptake, conjugation of CH and P onto the surface of nanoliposomes by the electrostatic layer-by-layer self-assembled approach had been used. Results showed the nanoliposome diameter was in the range of 87–225 nm. Well-encapsulation of NH-P-CH-conjugated-nanoliposomes (P-CH-NL) significantly controlled the NH release followed by anomalous diffusion mechanism and preserved around 72–78% of NH in GI condition. This study investigated the antioxidant activities of NH and NH-loaded carriers both before and after GI digestion. *In vitro* cytotoxicity and cellular uptake studies were carried out using human Caco-2 cells. Their results showed that the biopolymer-conjugated nanoliposomal system can show enhanced cellular uptake with reduced cytotoxicity and greater biological activity. Deposition of P and CH molecules simultaneously onto NLs provided better shelter to the nanoliposomal membrane from the GI degradation in comparison with CH alone, thereby enhancing the controlled release profile of NH (Shishir et al. 2019).

Table 17.1 demonstrates a list of nanoliposomal bioactive compounds, mentioning the method of preparation for their applications in food systems, where most of these systems have been developed and used in laboratory-scale situations.

Table 17.1 List of some nanoliposomal nutraceuticals (*bioactives-loaded NLs*).

Bioactive compound	The results and application (s)	Method of preparation	Size (nm), PDI, zeta potential, EE	References
Orthosiphon stamineus (OS)	• Improving the solubility of the lipophilic flavones • Improvement of the bioavailability and the overall pharmacological activity of OS extracts • Increasing extract's solubility from 956 ± 34 to 3979 ± 139 µg/ml	Conventional film method	152.5 ± 1.1 nm ξ; −49.8 ± 1.0 mv EE: 66.2 ± 0.9%	Aisha et al. (2014)
Rutin flavonoids	• Purification of food-grade crude soybean lecithin was obtained and it is advantageous and economical for large-scale production • Preparation of the spherical and unilamellar NLs • Formation of the hydrogen bonds between hydroxyl groups of rutin with the polar head groups of the PLs in the bilayer of the liposomes • Higher packing density of the bilayer and a lower rutin permeability • The slow-release rate of the rutin from the liposome. • Lyophilized liposomes showed a significant increase in the diameter while helping to maintain the encapsulated rutin for a longer time • Preventing damage to the liposome bilayer and maintaining the spherical structure after 56 days of storage	Heating/homogenization (ultrasound) method	102–184 nm ξ; −40 mv EE: 81.9%	Lopez-Polo et al. (2020)
Clove essential oil (CEO)/ Eugenol	• Obtaining homogeneous, stable, nanometric-sized and multilamellar liposomes with high EE and ability to scale-up, employing *hydrogenated or non-hydrogenated soybean PC* • Similar vesicles mean size, PDI, and zeta potential values were obtained for Eug- and CEO-loaded Phospholipon • Highest EE values of Eug in unsaturated Lipoid S100 liposomes compared with the saturated Phospholipon 90H liposomes	Ethanol injection method: 1) At the intermediate volume (600 ml): a membrane contactor 2) At a pilot scale (3l): a membrane for injection (Tubular SPG membrane, hydrophilic with a mean pore size of 0.9 mm). 36 vs. 360 s	Eug: 194 nm ξ; −6.3 mv EE: 94.4 ± 4.1% *for Lipoid S100 vs. 82.6 ± 4.3% for phospholipon 90H* liposomes.	Sebaaly et al. (2016c)

Compound	Description	Method	Characteristics	Reference
Satureja khuzestanica essential oils (SKEO)	• Formulation of a novel biodegradable meat-coating containing nanoliposomal SKEO with prolonged antimicrobial and antiseptic activity in lamb meat extending the shelf-life of lamb meat with chitosan coating containing encapsulated SKEO • Improved sensory attributes, mitigating the sensory impact of essential oils, decreasing their diffusion rate and modulating the release of SEKO	Thin-film hydration-sonication method	93–96 nm PDI: 0.83–0.88 EE: 46–69%	Pabast et al. (2018)
Phytostrols (from canola oil deodorizer distillate containing brassica-sterol, campesterol and β-sitosterol along with α-, γ-, and δ-tocopherol)	• Lyophilized liposome (with sucrose as cryo-protectant), was used for incorporation in model juice • Optimum liposomes in the model orange juice showed adequate stability after pasteurization (72 °C for 15 s) for a month • The optimum ratio of bioactive/lipid was selected 1 : 5 for formulations prepared by the Mozafari method	1) Thin-film hydration-homogenization, 2) Thin-film hydration-ultrasonication 3) Mozafari method	<200 nm in *Homogenization/ Ultrasonication methods* vs. 260 nm in *Mozafari method* ξ: −9 to −14 mv EE: >89% (by all three methods)	Poudel et al. (2019)
Tea polyphenols (TP) and vitamin E (VE)	• Co-encapsulation of soluble and insoluble ingredients, simultaneously: TP-VE complex liposome • Optimized condition: 4 : 1 mass ratio of SPC to cholesterol and 3 : 1 volume ratio of organic phase to aqueous phase loaded with 10 mg/ml of TP and 15 mg of VE • The entrapment efficient of TP was significantly enhanced by adding a certain amount of phosphate-buffered saline (PBS: 6.7 mmol/l)	Reverse-phase evaporation (RPE) method	197–213 nm PDI: 0.24 ξ: −46 mv *EE of VE:* 50.81 ± 1.91% *EE of TP:* 94.05 ± 3.45%	Ma et al. (2009)
Green tea polyphenols	• Enhancement of bioavailability of tea polyphenols, oxygen and light stability (which is suitable for more widespread application including processing, storage) • Optimum polyphenols/lecithin ratio was 0.125 : 1 and lecithin/cholesterol ratio was 4 : 1 • Optimum pH of 6.62, and ultrasonic time of 3.5 min, introduced as optimal	Thin-film, ultrasonic dispersion method	160.4 nm ξ: −67.2 mv EE: 60.36%	Lu et al. (2011)

(Continued)

Table 17.1 (Continued)

Bioactive compound	The results and application (s)	Method of preparation	Size (nm), PDI, zeta potential, EE	References
Tea polyphenol (EGCG)	• First report of high entrapment of hydrophilic compound in liposomes prepared with HPH • The presence of the EGCG in the liposomes dispersion did not affect size or stability of particles up to 5 mg/ml • At the most concentrated PL in the sample, the molar ratio of PL to EGCG was approximately 10 • The extent of release of tea polyphenols during storage was lower for milk PL nanoliposomes compared with liposomes containing soy PLs (with larger size and lower EE)	High-pressure homogenization (HPH)	Nanoliposomes with milk PL: 140 nm ξ: −20 mv EE: 58%	Gülseren and Corredig (2013)
EGCG	• Optimum conditions for preparation: • PC-to-cholesterol ratio of 4.00 • EGCG concentration of 4.88 mg/ml • Tween 80 concentration of 1.08 mg/ml • Compared with free nanoliposomes, nanoliposomal EGCG enhanced its inhibitory effect on tumor cell viability at higher concentrations • Prepared EGCG nanoliposomes were stable and fit for use in oral administration	RPE method	180 nm ± 4 nm EE: 85.79 ± 1.65%	Luo et al. (2014)
Green tea extract (GTE)	• Antibacterial activity (strongest antibacterial activity was seen against listeria monocytogenes) • Prebiotic activity, enhanced growth rate of Lactobacillus casei and Bifidobacterium lactis to a significant extent 97%	Thin-film sonication method	44.7 ± 1.9 nm PDI: 0.203 ± 0.014	Noudoost et al. (2015)
Ginger extract (GE)	• Used as an antioxidant in sunflower oil • Higher antioxidant activities of ginger extract nanoliposomes (NGE) as compared with GE and BHT in all tests • The NGE at 1000 ppm concentration had the higher antioxidant activity	Heating method	164.5 nm PDI: 0.186 EE: 89.8%	Ganji and Sayyed-Alangi (2017)
Turmeric extract	• Having antioxidant activity in functional drinks significantly lower release of turmeric in a drink model with pH = 6.8 than that with pH = 3.5 and 4.5, and inhibition of bacterial activity at ambient temperature for over 40 days	Thin layer hydration, method coupled with: high shear homogenization and sonication	92 nm PDI: 0.4 EE: 95 ± 2a% LC: 45%	Karimi et al. (2019)

Pistachio Green Hull's extracts (PGHE)	• Natural source of bio-preservatives for mayonnaise without adverse effect on sensory properties, produced by inexpensive soybean lecithin as a natural source of PLs, considered for large-scale production • The samples containing nanoliposomal PGHE were the most preferred sensory acceptance • Gradual release of polyphenols • 1000 mg PGH/kg freshly prepared mayonnaise exhibited higher antioxidant activity than 200 mg/kg of BHT • Microbial population was within permissible level after four months of storage	Extrusion through polycarbonate membrane with a pore size of 100 nm (above the phase transition temperature of vesicles)	90.76–95.35 nm (LUVs) PDI: 0.2 and ζ-potential value ranged from −40.8 to −50.6 mv EE: 37–52.93%	Rafiee et al. (2018)
Proteinase form *B. subtilis* (Neutrase)	• Accelerated model cheese ripening, provided desired texture and flavor in cheese, because of adequate control of pH and calcium loss at draining and satisfactory proteolysis • Liposome retention rate in cheese matrix correlated to liposome size, i.e. the smaller size of REV allows a greater exclusion of these liposomes from the curd matrix • Bitterness development, a critical defect in enzyme added cheese, could be delayed and minimized texture defects • Peptide analysis in the whey indicated that no casein hydrolysis occurred in REV-treated cheeses due to Neutrase activity *during the first hours* of cheese-making. This indicates that liposomes were stable enough to prevent enzyme leakage • REV allowed a higher entrapment rate than MLV, and its proteolysis were more stable at dairy products	Reverse phase evaporation vesicles (REV)	Multilamellar vesicles (MLVs) EE: 30%	Alkhalaf et al. (1988)
Bovine Casein hydrolysate (rich in oligopeptides)	• The encapsulation in liposomes was able to mask the bitterness and was also able to reduce the hydrophobicity keeping the chemical stability during 60 days of storage at 25 °C • The UV spectrometry with second-derivative transformation was efficient in measuring the encapsulation rates of casein hydrolysates	RPE method	500–1000 nm EE: 56–62%	Morais et al. (2005)

(Continued)

Table 17.1 (Continued)

Bioactive compound	The results and application (s)	Method of preparation	Size (nm), PDI, zeta potential, EE	References
Whey peptide fractions	• Soy lecithin-derived nanoliposomes were found to encapsulate peptides with high EE • No apparent difference in EE for different-sized peptides • The net negatively charged peptide fraction had a significantly lower EE than the other fractions • The hydrophilic peptide fraction resulted in unstable liposome suspension, with the lowest ζ-potential • Prevention of maillard reaction in foods and bitter taste • There was no obvious correlation between liposome dimensions and the molecular weight of the peptide fractions used, as the same for surface hydrophobicity and size • Strong correlation between the surface charge and mean particle diameter of the liposomes • Loading smaller peptides into liposomes can improve their stability in aqueous suspensions by increasing the electrostatic repulsion between them • Nanoliposomes prepared appear to be stable without the addition of cholesterol	Film hydration method	Size <200 nm *medium-to-large unilamellar vesicles* (from all whey peptide fractions, regardless of their molecular weight ranges) ξ: −55 to −71 mv EE: >80%.	Mohan et al. (2018)
Bioactive peptides (sheep whey hydrolysates by the bacterial protease P7)	• The antioxidant activity values were the highest in fractions 7 and 8 (48.6 and 38.6% ABST scavenging, respectively), corresponding to a molecular weight around 4500 Da • Both antioxidant and ACE-I-inhibitory activities of hydrolysates were detected in the liposomes • In liposomal form of bioactive peptides: more stability, with consequent lower degradation of peptides, have been observed • The residual antioxidant activity was 87% after 30 days storage, suggesting the bioactive peptides are stable in nanoliposomes	Thin film evaporation	166 nm ξ: −17 mv EE: 48% (1 mg/ml peptide)	Corrêa et al. (2019)

Note:

Encapsulation efficiency (EE) is representative of the amount of a bioactive compound trapped within or on a carrier surface compared to the initial amount of the used bioactive material (encapsulated vs. first feeding). Although EE value depends on the conditions in which encapsulation is carried out and encapsulation technique or production method utilized, but the EE value may be associated with the concentration of bioactive compounds in the formulation.

An important feature in the field of micro-/nanoencapsulation researchers should pay attention to is that loading efficiency (LE) is more important than EE, in reporting nanocarrier capability for loading of intended bioactive compounds. LE is dependent on the "core-to-wall material molar ratio" and varies for the different initial amount of the same compound.

LE is a good and reliable indicator of the capacity of wall material to encapsulate a definite amount of bioactive compound. It is necessary to report LE for comparison between different nanocarriers in order to choose the best wall material or the best encapsulant.

As an example, the extent of encapsulation of tea polyphenols increased with tea polyphenol concentration up to about 4 mg/ml. At polyphenol concentrations ≥6 mg/ml, the liposome dispersions were no longer stable (Gülseren and Corredig 2013). Another study showed that different whey peptide fractions had similar encapsulation efficiencies in soy lecithin liposomes, despite differences in their molecular weights, molecular heterogeneities, and surface hydrophobicity (Mohan et al. 2018).

17.5 Loading of Bioactive Compounds in NLs

17.5.1 Types of Encapsulated Bioactive Compounds in NLs

NLs can encapsulate both water-soluble and fat-soluble drugs, which are slowly released as the liposome is broken down by enzymes and acids found in tissues and cells. Water-soluble molecules enclose/entrap in NLs internal sphere cavity. Many fat-soluble compounds can be incorporated into the PL bilayer. Incorporating the cholesterol into the membrane can increase the chemical stability of unsaturated PLs.

17.5.2 Trend of Loading Bioactive Compounds

To encapsulate bioactive compounds into NLs, two methods have been implemented; passive and active loading. In passive encapsulation, the formation of liposomes and encapsulation of bioactive compounds is performed co-currently during the lipid hydration step, i.e. lipids and bioactive compounds/drugs are mixed with each other in one step. This method is referred to as co-current loading. In this method, the loading capacity and stability are poor, leading to burst drug leakage (Pauli et al. 2019). The disadvantages of passive loading include burst and quick release of bioactive compounds due to weak association of drugs into a liposome, poor drug retention and poor storage stability and, in most cases, the typical drug-to-lipid ratio (D/L) is less than 0.05% (w/w) (Gubernator 2011).

In active encapsulation, loading is done after the liposomes are produced and referred to remote loading. The driving force of loading is basically pH (developed by Deamer and Nicols) (Deamer et al. 1972) or ionic gradients (first using ammonium sulfate gradients) (Haran et al. 1993).

An amphipathic drug dissolved in the exterior aqueous phase, permeates across the phospholipid bilayers, then interactions with a trapping agent in the core lead to lock-in the drug (Pauli et al. 2019). This method is superior for amphipathic compounds having high solubility and membrane permeability. For hydrophobic compounds, use of excipients such as β-cyclodextrin and supersaturated solutions have been used to increase loading efficiency. More discussion of these techniques is beyond the scope of this chapter.

In both cases, the unloaded "free" agent has to be removed and separated from the liposomes using differences in charge, size, or other properties (physical, chemical, or biological properties) (Barenholz and Lasic 2018).

To produce loaded liposomes, three basic steps are used: (i) lipid hydration; (ii) regulation of liposome size; (iii) removal of nonencapsulated drug.

Methods for controlling liposome size generally include fractionation (centrifugation and size exclusion chromatography) and homogenization (capillary pore membrane extrusion and ceramic extrusion).

17.6 NLs' Surface Coating

17.6.1 Modification of Nanoliposomal Surface

Although the advantages of using liposomes rather than other delivery systems are their low intrinsic toxicity and immunogenicity (Bochicchio et al. 2016), stability is a general problem with liposomes. The phenomenon of less stability and leakage of the encapsulated bioactive materials in liposomes is attributed to the easy oxidative damage of phospholipid bilayer during storage and hydrolytic degradation of phospholipid under low pH and enzymatic conditions (Shishir et al. 2019). Liposomes have a short circulation half-life after intravenous administration and prone to adhere to each other and fuse to form larger vesicles in suspension (Mady et al. 2009). Surface modification is needed to modify liposomes' characterization. Liposomes have the flexibility to couple with site-specific ligands in order to achieve active targeting (Bochicchio et al. 2016). Biopolymer conjugation could minimize the permeability of phospholipid bilayers and enhancing the stability of the drug-loaded liposomal system through the formation of electrostatic bridges between phospholipid and biopolymer molecule (Shishir et al. 2019) to wrap nanoliposomes to obtain hybrid nanostructures with a shell–core (polymeric-lipid) architecture (Bochicchio et al. 2018).

The coating of dipalmitoylphosphatidylcholine (DPPC) liposome by CH layer resulted in an increase in liposomal size as well as positive charge almost three times and change in the natural membrane permeation properties. Coating of liposomes with CH would cause an increase in the DPPC liposomes' plastic viscosity (Mady et al. 2009).

Covered NLs were prepared using an innovative continuous method based on microfluidic principles. Liposomes were enwrapped by CH to achieve stable shell–core nanostructures. The proposed simil-microfluidic method led to the production of stable and completely CH-covered liposomes that avoided the disadvantages of the conventional method (Bochicchio et al. 2018).

CH-lipid hybrid delivery system through a novel continuous simil-microfluidic method was used to put a polymeric layer, surrounding nanoliposomal indomethacin. This method provided a thicker and smoother layer than that achievable by the dropwise method and improving their storage stability. The gastroretentive behavior of nanoliposomal delivery system in SGF and SIF shows appropriateness for the oral-controlled release of indomethacin (Dalmoro et al. 2018).

Pectin from apple has the ability to inhibit the adhesion of *Helicobacter pylori* to human stomach cells and can be considered a novel type of multifunctional liposomal carriers for local antibiotic therapy against *H. pylori* (Gottesmann et al. 2020).

β-Carotene molecules-loaded NLs have been confirmed for additional UV photostability with electrospun fiber using electrospinning performance. In this approach, the mixed polymer solutions containing polyvinyl alcohol and polyethylene oxide electrospun has been used to produce hybrid nanoliposome-loaded ultrathin fibers (de Freitas Zômpero et al. 2015).

17.7 Tocosome

17.7.1 Definition

Tocosome is a novel nanocarrier system and defined as a colloidal and vesicular delivery system similar to nanoliposomes, introduced by Mozafari et al. for the first time (Mozafari et al. 2017). Tocosomes consist of two derivatives of vitamin E that differentiate them from liposomes. Two index ingredients in tocosome comprise α-Tocopheryl phosphate (TP) and di-α-Tocopheryl phosphate (*bis*-tocopherol phosphate ester) (T_2P). TP is a phosphoric acid ester of α-tocopherol, esterified at the hydroxyl group of tocopherol while T_2P molecule can be synthesized through the esterification of two tocopherol moieties and one phosphate group (Mozafari et al. 2017). Both TP and T_2P molecules consist of a chroman head (with two rings: one phenolic and one heterocyclic) and a phytyl tail and are able to self-assemble into vesicular structures in aqueous environments (Figure 17.6).

17.7.2 Resources and Health Benefits of TP

The detected α-tocopheryl phosphate in biological tissues includes liver and adipose tissue and in a variety of foods, suggesting a ubiquitous presence in animal and plant tissues (Gianello et al. 2005). It has been reported that TP is present in dairy products, green vegetables, fruits, and cereals as well as in some seeds and nuts (Gianello et al. 2005; Libinaki et al. 2006; Munteanu et al. 2004).

The ingredients of tocosomes possess more health benefits compared to PLs. TP/T_2P, as potent antioxidants in tocosomes, accompanied with another antioxidant encapsulated, will construct a multicomponent, synergistic antioxidant delivery formulation. So, tocosome is a good candidate for applications in different food systems. Being composed of molecules with exquisite strong antioxidant activities, tocosomes have great potential for applications in the formulation of functional

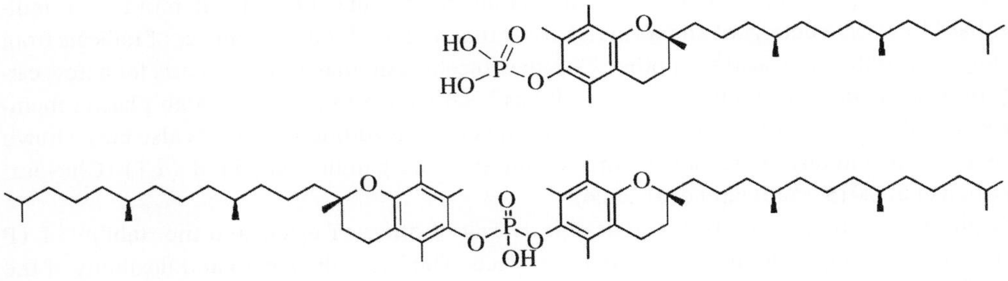

Figure 17.6 Chemical structure of the phosphorylated tocopherols, tocopheryl phosphate (TP), and di-α- tocopheryl phosphate ester (T_2P) that make up tocopheryl phosphate mixture (TPM). *Source*: Copyright permission was obtained from Gavin et al. (2017).

food, dietary foods, beverages, supplements, and nutraceutical products. In some cases, TP and T_2P are erroneously referred to as PLs, while in a phospholipid molecule, the presence of phosphate group, two fatty acid tails, and a glycerol linker is necessary. Tocopherols and their derivatives do not contain the glycerol group as an indispensable chemical part of PLs. The tocopheryl phosphates are composed of a chroman head (with two rings: one phenolic and the other heterocyclic) and a phytyl tail with three isoprene side-chains (Zarrabi et al. 2020).

Clinical investigations have shown that TP and T_2P molecules have different kinds of health benefits because of being strong antioxidant activities. These benefits including anti-inflammatory and antidepressant effects, atherosclerotic-preventing, and cardioprotective properties. Libinaki et al. (2006) conducted a series of toxicological tests (both *in vivo* and *in vitro*) on mixed tocopheryl phosphates (MTP) intended for use as a dietary supplement and for dermal applications in humans and animals to evaluate the safety of formulation. Daily administration of MTP for 28 days by gavage in rats, at doses up to 955 mg/kg bw/day (780 mg tocopherol equivalents/kg bw/day), produced no consistent, dose-dependent adverse effects (Libinaki et al. 2006).

17.7.3 Limitations and Benefits of Using Vitamin E and Its Derivatives

Vitamin E is easily oxidized when subjected to heat, light, and alkaline conditions, but esters including acetate, nicotinate, succinate, and phosphate are less susceptible to oxidation and, therefore, more appropriate for food, cosmetic, and pharmaceutical applications compared to the free form. Vitamin E in dietary supplements and fortified foods is often esterified to prolong its shelf life while protecting its antioxidant properties (Niki and Abe 2019).

Vitamin E isomers, including α-T, are all fat-soluble vitamins, while α-TP is a naturally occurring water-soluble form of vitamin E (Michael Eskin 2013). Water-soluble precursors of vitamin E, such as its esters with phosphate (α-TP), have increased solubility in water and stability against reaction with free radicals, but they are rapidly converted during their uptake into the lipid-soluble vitamin E (Zingg 2018). α-TP molecule is resistant to both acid and alkaline hydrolysis, making it undetectable using standard assays for vitamin E (Gianello et al. 2005).

Water-soluble derivatives of vitamin E including α-TP are increasingly used as components of nanocarriers for enhanced and targeted delivery of drugs and other molecules (vitamins, including αT and αTP, vitamin D_3, carnosine, caffeine, docosahexaenoic acid [DHA], insulin) and cofactors such as coenzyme Q10 (Zingg 2018).

17.7.4 The Role of TP/T_2P in Membrane Bilayers and Their Geometric Shape

All-rac-vitamin E phosphate (TP) decreases membrane fluidity in contrast to vitamin E. This indicates that TP acts as a detergent and forms a barrier that might inhibit the transfer of radicals from one polyunsaturated fatty acid to another. This new mechanism may form the basis for a new category of antioxidants (Rezk et al. 2004). α-TP has been shown to passes through plasma membranes and affect several important intracellular processes. In addition, α-TP has also been shown to possess a potentially more potent antioxidant than its parent compound (α-T) (Ghayour-Mobarhan et al. 2015; Munteanu et al. 2004).

The phosphate group of TP is not as flexible as that of other αT esters and the stability of TP could explain its antiproliferative and apoptotic effects. The lesser the length and flexibility of the terminal carboxyl moiety, the more the apoptotic activity (Rezk et al. 2007).

The geometric shape of TP molecule is cylindrical (similar to the PC molecule), while the geometric shape of T_2P molecule is conical (unlike to the PLs). This cylindrical configuration of TP is

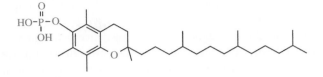

α-Tocopheryl Phosphate (TP)

Molecular formula: $C_{29}H_{51}O_5P$
Average mass: 510.69 Da
Monoisotopic mass: 510.347412 Da

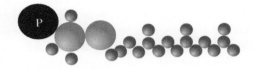

(2R)-2,5,7,8-Tetramethyl-2-[4R, 8R]-4,8,12-trimethyltridecyl]-3,4-dihydro-2H-chromen-6-yl dihydrogen phosphate

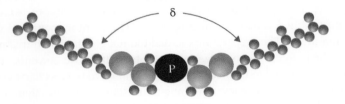

Di-α-Tocopheryl Phosphate (T_2P)

Molecular formula: $C_{58}H_{99}O_6P$ Average mass: 923.54 Da

Figure 17.7 Chemical structure of α-tocopheryl phosphate (TP) and di-α-tocopheryl phosphate (T_2P). The angle of alignment of phytyl tails of T_2P molecule created an inverted truncated cone molecule with a critical packing parameter (CPP) >1. *Source:* Copyright permission was obtained from Zarrabi et al. (2020).

related to the phosphate head group attached to one hydrophobic phytyl tail made of three iso-prene units, while T_2P is composed of two phytyl chains, cannot align in parallel position or even with a small angle due to the presence of bulky isoprene side-chains (Figure 17.7), (Zarrabi et al. 2020).

The most important factor in determining which kind of diverse self-assembled structure is formed through preparation is the shape of the used molecules, which is arising from the critical packing parameter (CPP) (Zarrabi et al. 2020). Double-chain lipids with large head group areas and fluid chains, formed packaging shape of a truncated cone and packing parameter range between ½ to 1, make lamellar flexible vesicle/bilayers (Williams 1972). Amphipathic molecules, i.e. PLs (in the case of nanoliposome) and tocopheryl phosphates (in the case of tocosome), arrange and self-assemble themselves as spherical bilayer structures in aqueous media and under certain conditions of temperature, pH, pressure, and agitation, via hydrophilic/hydrophobic and Van der Waals interactions form tocosomes or nanoliposomes. These self-assembled structures may contain proteins and carbohydrates in their structure to increase their stability or targeting techniques (Mozafari et al. 2017; Zarrabi et al. 2020).

17.7.5 Formulation of Tocosome

Despite the differences in the chemical constituents of tocosomes and nanoliposomes, these nano-carriers are both bilayer colloidal systems composed of amphiphilic molecules, so they can be utilized for the encapsulation of different types of bioactive compounds either with a hydrophobic or hydrophilic entity.

Mozafari et al. (2017) designed a novel drug delivery system named tocosome, using tocopheryl phosphate molecules (TP and T_2P molecules ratio of TP/T_2P was 2 : 1). The potential of this nanocarrier was investigated and some promising results have been obtained so far, which by itself is an ideal antioxidant system (Mozafari et al. 2017). This team has been investigated the use of TP and T_2P in the encapsulation and release of a number of pharmaceutical and nutraceutical compounds via different routes of administration with promising results (Mozafari et al. 2017). Tocosomal drug delivery systems composed of different ingredients including α-tocopheryl phosphate disodium salt (TP), soy phosphatidylcholine (PC), stearyl amine (SA), cholesterol (Chol), and glycerol.

Mozafari et al., as a pioneer, reported and introduced the successful formulation of "tocosome" vesicles. Tocosome containing TP, T_2P, and different lipids/PLs (stearyl amine and phosphatidylcholine: Phospholipon 90H, Phospholipon 100H) with and without cholesterol were prepared using Mozafari method (modified version of heating method) for entrapment and controlled-release of the drug 5-fluorouracil. The preparation method did not require harsh treatments such as sonication and high-shear force homogenization or potentially toxic solvents. Tocosomes, containing 5-fluorouracil (as a model anticancer drug), were shown to possess narrow size distribution, acceptable encapsulation efficiency and long-term stability (more than two years). Formulation of TP and T_2P without other excipients causes thread-like structures. Confocal and fluorescent microscopy observations showed that without other ingredients, TP and T_2P couldn't form stable vesicles and the formulation, collapse, or forms gel within hours after preparation. Among the different number of excipients studied, PLs proved to be the best excipients and stable vesicles were formed both in the presence and absence of the positively charged stearyl amine and cholesterol. It was reported that the configuration of the conical shape of T_2P is not proper for the formation of stable spherical or oval structures. Adding TP to T_2P molecules also did not result in the construction of spherical vesicles. The inclusion of positively charged stearyl amine changes the tocosome sizes to a larger one while adding cholesterol to the formulation had no effect on tocosome sizes and both these excipients cause a decrease in PDI (Mozafari et al. 2017).

17.7.6 Related Research to Tocopheryl Phosphate as a Carrier

Tocopheryl phosphate mixture (TPM) as a combination of α-tocopheryl phosphate (TP) and di-α-tocopheryl phosphate (T_2P) formulations have been used to evaluate its potential to facilitate the transport of a range of actives with different sizes and chemistries, into and across the skin.

Small and larger lipophilic molecules (vitamin D_3 and CoQ_{10}) as well as small hydrophilic drugs (caffeine) and dipeptides (carnosine) were included. The TPM/drug/ethanol solution was added slowly to the warm water whilst being stirred. The formulation was cooled to room temperature while mixing over 20 minutes. Vesicles with a new class of highly deformable and elastic (or ultra-flexible) are formable. The formulation components are important in dictating the particle size and deformability, while the TP/T_2P ratio can alter the internal particle morphology. A noticeable discovered issue in one study was the feasibility of changing the flexibility in size and elasticity of vesicles by altering the ratio of TP : T_2P. It was reported that vesicles high in TP are prone to be more deformable than those rich in T_2P. TPM produced a significant ($p < 0.05$) increase of 2.4–3.4-fold in the absorption of mentioned bioactive materials into or through the skin. As the amount of T_2P was increased in the formulation, the force required to pass the particles through the filter increased significantly. Results show that TPM self-assembles to form vesicular structures in hydro-ethanolic solutions in the approximate range size of 100–250 nm (depending on the amount of TPM and ethanol present in the formulation). The high rate of entrapment was related to the lipophilicity of the molecules and their relatively poor solubility in the dispersive medium. So, caffeine and carnosine as more soluble compounds were, therefore, not driven to be encapsulated within the TPM particles at high efficiency. TPM encapsulates poorly soluble molecules at high efficiency. Authors suggested that this TPM delivery platform has the significant potential to deliver a diverse range of actives with differing size and solubility profile (Gavin et al. 2017).

In another work, it has been shown that incorporation of the tocopherol-based excipient, TPM, into a medium-chain triglyceride (MCT)-based lipid formulation, improve the solubilization of Coenzyme Q_{10} (CoQ_{10}) as a lipophilic molecule during *in vitro* digestion which is strongly correlated with enhanced exposure *in vivo* (Pham et al. 2019). The addition of TPM at 10% (w/w) of the total MCT + TPM provided optimal performance in terms of CoQ_{10} solubilization during digestion. Pham et al. investigated the other derivatives of tocopheryl, D-α-tocopheryl polyethylene glycol 1000 succinate (TPGS), in enhancing the solubilization of CoQ_{10} during digestion. The results further highlight the potential of TPM as an additive in lipid formulations to improve the solubilization and oral bioavailability of poorly water-soluble compounds (Pham et al. 2019).

There are some *in vitro* biological data from tests with TPM that show it has anti-inflammatory properties (Libinaki et al. 2006).

17.8 From the Laboratory to the Manufacturing Plant

The formulation process of NLs often involves the use of organic solvents, high-speed homogenization, sonication, milling, emulsification, evaporation of organic solvents, centrifugation, filtration, and lyophilization. Some obstacles were related to nanoliposomal scale-up issues including lipid peroxidation, endotoxin and free drug removal, size distribution, trace organic solvent, and sterilization.

Depending on conditions, the process may lead to the altered chemical structure of bioactives/lipids and a substantial amount of impurities. Different preparation methods lead to creating liposomes with different lamellarities. There is a risk of being damaged by sterilization techniques (irradiation or autoclaving), especially when biological materials are involved.

The FDA states that "liposome drug products are sensitive to changes in the manufacturing conditions, including changes in scale. This should be considered during the development process and manufacturing parameters (i.e. scale, temperature, shear force,. . .) should be identified and evaluated."

A chain of interrelated issues from a chain of raw material accessibility to process requirements (reproducibility and sterilization), chemical and physical stability in long-term storage, and quality control validation, slowed down the development of large-scale production and stability assessment.

17.8.1 Manufacturing Challenges and Scale-up Issues

The cosmetic industry was the first pioneer to solve the manufacturing process and trade development of liposomes because of its need for large-scale preparations of liposomes, while in the pharmaceutical industry with the concern of higher dosage requirements, it took much longer to resolve these issues at the standards required (Barenholz and Lasic 2018). Despite extensive and noticeable progress in the commercial application of nanotechnology in the field of pharmaceutical and cosmetics industries, there has been less development of NL and tocosome technology in the food and nutraceutical industries. However, it is believed that the agricultural sector has a great potential for the use of NLs and other nanocarriers (Verma 2017).

Today, the production of nanoliposomes on an industrial scale has become a reality and different techniques have been introduced. Heating method, spray-drying, freeze-drying, supercritical fluid processing, and modified ethanol-injection are among important techniques. Process control and reproducibility are among the most important challenges in the industrialization of methods (Laouini et al. 2012).

The heating method and Mozafari method are suggested as good methods for encapsulation of heat-resistant material in NL and coacervation method for labile bioactive material.

On top of that, the microfluidic-based method is an emerging technology for liposome synthesis that allows for strict control of the lipid-hydration process. Microfluidics is a method to manipulate liquid flows in channels with dimensions of tens to hundreds of micrometers. In the matter of equipment, microfluidizer processor can produce nanomaterials with a wide variety of multiphase applications. Through the demonstrated case studies, microfluidizer technology has been proven to be superior to conventional technology, very efficient and reliable, offering precise, repeatable, and scalable results. This technology results in uniform droplet and particle size reduction (often submicron), which allows the production of stable NLs and nanoencapsulated bioactive compounds. Production-scale models use the same microfluidizer proprietary continuous high shear fluid processing technology. Dalmoro et al. reported NL as a carrier for encapsulation of vitamins D_3 and K, both as hydrophobic compounds, with simil-microfuidic technique with the advantages of massive production (Dalmoro et al. 2019).

Another feasible scaleable method for food applications is the hydration of proliposomes. Proliposomes are aqueous-soluble dry PL particles with loading ingredients that, on hydration above transition temperatures and appropriate agitation, result in the formation of liposomes (Toniazzo and Pinho 2016).

The limited application of NLs in the food industry section is not only related to difficulties in finding safe, low-cost ingredients, but also to the economical processing and batch-to-batch consistency methods suitable for producing large volumes of NLs/tocosomes.

Two positive points that should be considered in the issue of large-scale production and using of NL are as follows:

- The recent development in liposome preparation including Mozafari method (Colas et al. 2007; Poudel et al. 2019) and pro-liposome techniques (Patel et al. 2019) offers possible solutions to use in different food processing while overcoming its challenges and problems.
- Application of cost-effective commercial lecithin ingredients may lead to suitably low product costs (Zarrabi et al. 2020). On the subject of supply of raw materials, crude soybean lecithin contains 65–75% PLs, together with triglycerides and small amounts of other ingredients such as carbohydrates, pigments, sterols, and sterol glycosides (Scholfield 1981). The cost of crude soybean PLs is only 5% of the pure one, which makes unpurified soybean PLs a good alternative and attractive choice (Aisha et al. 2014). As NLs were produced by soybean lecithin as an inexpensive, safe and natural source of PLs in nanometric particle size, they can be considered for large-scale use and promotion of biofunctional activities of phenolic compounds in food, pharmaceutical, and cosmetics applications (Rafiee et al. 2018).

References

Adamczak, M. and Bednarski, W. (2010). Lipids with special biological and physicochemical activities. In: *Chemical, Biological, and Functional Aspects of Food Lipids* (ed. Z.Z.E. Sikorski and A. Kolakowska), 423–442. CRC Press.

Aisha, A.F., Majid, A.M.S.A., and Ismail, Z. (2014). Preparation and characterization of nano liposomes of *Orthosiphon stamineus* ethanolic extract in soybean phospholipids. *BMC Biotechnology* 14 (23): 1–11.

Alkhalaf, W., Piard, J.C., El Soda, M. et al. (1988). Liposomes as proteinase carriers for the accelerated ripening of Saint-Paulin type cheese. *Journal of Food Science* 53 (6): 1674–1679.

Amjadi, S., Ghorbani, M., Hamishehkar, H., and Roufegarinejad, L. (2018). Improvement in the stability of betanin by liposomal nanocarriers: its application in gummy candy as a food model. *Food Chemistry* 256: 156–162.

Amoah, I., Cairncross, C., Sturny, A., and Rush, E. (2019). Towards improving the nutrition and health of the aged: the role of sprouted grains and encapsulation of bioactive compounds in functional bread–a review. *International Journal of Food Science & Technology* 54 (5): 1435–1447.

Azzi, J., Jraij, A., Auezova, L. et al. (2018). Novel findings for quercetin encapsulation and preservation with cyclodextrins, liposomes, and drug-in-cyclodextrin-in-liposomes. *Food Hydrocolloids* 81: 328–340.

Balamurugan, K. and Chintamani, P. (2018). Lipid nano particulate drug delivery: an overview of the emerging trend. *The Pharma Innovation Journal* 7: 779–789.

Bandarra, N.M., Batista, I., Nunes, M.L., and Empis, J.M. (2001). Seasonal variation in the chemical composition of horse-mackerel (Trachurus trachurus). *European Food Research and Technology* 212 (5): 535–539.

Bangham, A.D., Hill, M.W., and Miller, N. (1974). Preparation and use of liposomes as models of biological membranes. In: *Methods in Membrane Biology* (ed. E.D. Korn), 1–68. Springer.

Bankole, V.O., Osungunna, M.O., Souza, C.R.F. et al. (2020). Spray-dried proliposomes: an innovative method for encapsulation of *Rosmarinus officinalis* L. polyphenols. *AAPS PharmSciTech* 21 (143): 1–17.

Barenholz, Y. and Lasic, D.D. (ed.) (2018). An overview of liposome scaled-up production and quality control. In: *Handbook of Nonmedical Applications of Liposomes. Volume 3, From Design to Microreactors*, 23–30. CRC Press.

Bochicchio, S., Barba, A.A., Grassi, G., and Lamberti, G. (2016). Vitamin delivery: carriers based on nanoliposomes produced via ultrasonic irradiation. *LWT-Food Science and Technology* 69: 9–16.

Bochicchio, S., Dalmoro, A., Bertoncin, P. et al. (2018). Design and production of hybrid nanoparticles with polymeric-lipid shell–core structures: conventional and next-generation approaches. *RSC Advances* 8 (60): 34614–34624.

Bochicchio, S., Dalmoro, A., Lamberti, G., and Barba, A.A. (2020). Advances in nanoliposomes production for ferrous sulfate delivery. *Pharmaceutics* 12 (5): 445.

Bozzuto, G. and Molinari, A. (2015). Liposomes as nanomedical devices. *International Journal of Nanomedicine* 10: 975.

Williams, D.E. (1972). Molecular packing analysis. *Acta Crystallographica Section A: Crystal Physics, Diffraction, Theoretical and General Crystallography* 28 (6): 629–635.

Chaparro, C.M. and Dewey, K.G. (2010). Use of lipid-based nutrient supplements (LNS) to improve the nutrient adequacy of general food distribution rations for vulnerable sub-groups in emergency settings. *Maternal & Child Nutrition* 6: 1–69.

Chaves, M. and Pinho, S. (2018). Effect of phospholipid composition on the structure and physicochemical stability of proliposomes incorporating curcumin and cholecalciferol. *21st International Drying Symposium,* Valencia, Spain (11–14 September 2018). http://hdl.handle.net/10251/106925.

Chaves, M.A. and Pinho, S.C. (2019). Curcumin-loaded proliposomes produced by the coating of micronized sucrose: influence of the type of phospholipid on the physicochemical characteristics of powders and on the liposomes obtained by hydration. *Food Chemistry* 291: 7–15.

Chaves, M.A., Oseliero Filho, P.L., Jange, C.G. et al. (2018). Structural characterization of multilamellar liposomes coencapsulating curcumin and vitamin D_3. *Colloids and Surfaces A: Physicochemical and Engineering Aspects* 549: 112–121.

Chi, J., Ge, J., Yue, X. et al. (2019). Preparation of nanoliposomal carriers to improve the stability of anthocyanins. *LWT* 109: 101–107.

Colas, J.-C., Shi, W., Rao, V.M. et al. (2007). Microscopical investigations of nisin-loaded nanoliposomes prepared by Mozafari method and their bacterial targeting. *Micron* 38 (8): 841–847.

Corrêa, A.P.F., Bertolini, D., Lopes, N.A. et al. (2019). Characterization of nanoliposomes containing bioactive peptides obtained from sheep whey hydrolysates. *LWT* 101: 107–112.

Cortesi, R. (1999). Preparation of liposomes by reverse-phase evaporation using alternative organic solvents. *Journal of Microencapsulation* 16 (2): 251–256.

Costa, A.P., Xu, X., and Burgess, D.J. (2014). Freeze–anneal–thaw cycling of unilamellar liposomes: effect on encapsulation efficiency. *Pharmaceutical Research* 31 (1): 97–103.

Dalmoro, A., Bochicchio, S., Nasibullin, S.F. et al. (2018). Polymer-lipid hybrid nanoparticles as enhanced indomethacin delivery systems. *European Journal of Pharmaceutical Sciences* 121: 16–28.

Dalmoro, A., Bochicchio, S., Lamberti, G. et al. (2019). Micronutrients encapsulation in enhanced nanoliposomal carriers by a novel preparative technology. *RSC Advances* 9 (34): 19800–19812.

Deamer, D.W., Prince, R.C., and Crofts, A.R. (1972). The response of fluorescent amines to pH gradients across liposome membranes. *Biochimica et Biophysica Acta (BBA)-Biomembranes* 274 (2): 323–335.

Ding, B.-M., Zhang, X.-M., and Xia, S.-Q. (2010). Effect of ferrous glycinate nanoliposomes on chemical oxidation and sensory quality of fortified milk. *Journal of Food Science and Biotechnology* 4: 7.

de Freitas Zômpero, R.H., López-Rubio, A., de Pinho, S.C. et al. (2015). Hybrid encapsulation structures based on β-carotene-loaded nanoliposomes within electrospun fibers. *Colloids and Surfaces B: Biointerfaces* 134: 475–482.

Ganji, S. and Sayyed-Alangi, S.Z. (2017). Encapsulation of ginger ethanolic extract in nanoliposome and evaluation of its antioxidant activity on sunflower oil. *Chemical Papers* 71 (9): 1781–1789.

Gavin, P.D., El-Tamimy, M., Keah, H.H., and Boyd, B.J. (2017). Tocopheryl phosphate mixture (TPM) as a novel lipid-based transdermal drug delivery carrier: formulation and evaluation. *Drug Delivery and Translational Research* 7 (1): 53–65.

Ghayour-Mobarhan, M., Saghiri, Z., Ferns, G., and Sahebkar, A. (2015). α-Tocopheryl phosphate as a bioactive derivative of vitamin E: a review of the literature. *Journal of Dietary Supplements* 12 (4): 359–372.

Gianello, R., Libinaki, R., Azzi, A. et al. (2005). α-Tocopheryl phosphate: a novel, natural form of vitamin E. *Free Radical Biology and Medicine* 39 (7): 970–976.

Gomez-Hens, A. and Fernandez-Romero, J. (2006). Analytical methods for the control of liposomal delivery systems. *TrAC Trends in Analytical Chemistry* 25 (2): 167–178.

Gottesmann, M., Goycoolea, F.M., Steinbacher, T. et al. (2020). Smart drug delivery against *Helicobacter pylori*: pectin-coated, mucoadhesive liposomes with antiadhesive activity and antibiotic cargo. *Applied Microbiology and Biotechnology* 104 (13): 5943–5957. https://doi.org/10.1007/s00253-020-10647-3.

Gregoriadis, G. (1984). *Liposome Technology: Preparation of Liposomes*, vol. 1. CRC.

Gubernator, J. (2011). Active methods of drug loading into liposomes: recent strategies for stable drug entrapment and increased in vivo activity. *Expert Opinion on Drug Delivery* 8 (5): 565–580.

Gueli, N., Verrusio, W., Linguanti, A. et al. (2012). Vitamin D: drug of the future. A new therapeutic approach. *Archives of Gerontology and Geriatrics* 54 (1): 222–227.

Gülseren, I.b. and Corredig, M. (2013). Storage stability and physical characteristics of tea-polyphenol-bearing nanoliposomes prepared with milk fat globule membrane phospholipids. *Journal of Agricultural and Food Chemistry* 61 (13): 3242–3251.

Gültekin-Özgüven, M., Karadağ, A., Duman, Ş. et al. (2016). Fortification of dark chocolate with spray dried black mulberry (*Morus nigra*) waste extract encapsulated in chitosan-coated liposomes and bioaccessability studies. *Food Chemistry* 201: 205–212.

Gulzar, S. and Benjakul, S. (2020a). Fortification of skim milk with nanoliposomes loaded with shrimp oil: properties and storage stability. *Journal of the American Oil Chemists' Society* 97 (8): 929–940.

Gulzar, S. and Benjakul, S. (2020b). Nanoliposome powder containing shrimp oil increases free flowing behavior and storage stability. *European Journal of Lipid Science and Technology* 122 (6): 2000049.

Haran, G., Cohen, R., Bar, L.K., and Barenholz, Y. (1993). Transmembrane ammonium sulfate gradients in liposomes produce efficient and stable entrapment of amphipathic weak bases. *Biochimica et Biophysica Acta (BBA)-Biomembranes* 1151 (2): 201–215.

Hauschild, S., Lipprandt, U., Rumplecker, A. et al. (2005). Direct preparation and loading of lipid and polymer vesicles using inkjets. *Small* 1 (12): 1177–1180.

Huang, Z., Li, X., Zhang, T. et al. (2014). Progress involving new techniques for liposome preparation. *Asian Journal of Pharmaceutical Sciences* 9 (4): 176–182.

Imaizumi, K., Mawatari, K., Murata, M. et al. (1983). The contrasting effect of dietary phosphatidylethanolamine and phosphatidylcholine on serum lipoproteins and liver lipids in rats. *The Journal of Nutrition* 113 (12): 2403–2411.

Ishii, F. (2016). The Preparation of Lipid Vesicles (Liposomes) Using the Coacervation Technique. *In Liposome Technology* (pp. 43–56). CRC Press.

Ishii, F., Takamura, A., and Ogata, H. (1988). Preparation conditions and evaluation of the stability of lipid vesicles (liposomes) using the microencapsulation technique. *Journal of Dispersion Science and Technology* 9 (1): 1–15.

Jaafar-Maalej, C., Diab, R., Andrieu, V. et al. (2010). Ethanol injection method for hydrophilic and lipophilic drug-loaded liposome preparation. *Journal of Liposome Research* 20 (3): 228–243.

Jaafar-Maalej, C., Charcosset, C., and Fessi, H. (2011). A new method for liposome preparation using a membrane contactor. *Journal of Liposome Research* 21 (3): 213–220.

Jafari, S.M., Vakili, S., and Dehnad, D. (2019). Production of a functional yogurt powder fortified with nanoliposomal vitamin D through spray drying. *Food and Bioprocess Technology* 12 (7): 1220–1231.

Janssens, B. (2017). Encapsulation of vitamin D_3 and vitamin K_2 in chitosan coated liposomes. Master dissertation. Ghent University/Università degli Studi di Salerno (UNISA).

Jiang, Y., Noh, S.K., and Koo, S.I. (2001). Egg phosphatidylcholine decreases the lymphatic absorption of cholesterol in rats. *The Journal of Nutrition* 131 (9): 2358–2363.

Karimi, N., Ghanbarzadeh, B., Hajibonabi, F. et al. (2019). Turmeric extract loaded nanoliposome as a potential antioxidant and antimicrobial nanocarrier for food applications. *Food Bioscience* 29: 110–117.

Katouzian, I., Esfanjani, A. F., Jafari, S. M., & Akhavan, S. (2017). Formulation and application of a new generation of lipid nano-carriers for the food bioactive ingredients. *Trends in Food Science & Technology,* 68, 14–25.

Keivani Nahr, F., Ghanbarzadeh, B., Hamishehkar, H. et al. (2019). Investigation of physicochemical properties of essential oil loaded nanoliposome for enrichment purposes. *LWT* 105: 282–289.

Khatib, N., Varidi, M.J., Mohebbi, M. et al. (2020). Replacement of nitrite with lupulon-xanthohumol loaded nanoliposome in cooked beef-sausage: experimental and model based study. *Journal of Food Science and Technology* 57 (7): 2629–2639.

Koolman, J. and Röhm, K.-H. (2005). *Color Atlas of Biochemistry*. Stuttgart: Thieme.

Laouini, A., Jaafar-Maalej, C., Sfar, S. et al. (2011). Liposome preparation using a hollow fiber membrane contactor—application to spironolactone encapsulation. *International Journal of Pharmaceutics* 415 (1–2): 53–61.

Laouini, A., Jaafar-Maalej, C., Limayem-Blouza, I. et al. (2012). Preparation, characterization and applications of liposomes: state of the art. *Journal of Colloid Science and Biotechnology* 1 (2): 147–168.

Laridi, R., Kheadr, E., Benech, R.-O. et al. (2003). Liposome encapsulated nisin Z: optimization, stability and release during milk fermentation. *International Dairy Journal* 13 (4): 325–336.

Lasic, D.D. (1988). The mechanism of vesicle formation. *Biochemical Journal* 256 (1): 1–11.

Lestari, S.D., Machmudah, S., Winardi, S. et al. (2019). Particle micronization of *Curcuma mangga* rhizomes ethanolic extract/biopolymer PVP using supercritical antisolvent process. *The Journal of Supercritical Fluids* 146: 226–239.

Libinaki, R., Ogru, E., Gianello, R. et al. (2006). Evaluation of the safety of mixed tocopheryl phosphates (MTP)—a formulation of α-tocopheryl phosphate plus α-di-tocopheryl phosphate. *Food and Chemical Toxicology* 44 (7): 916–932.

Lopez-Polo, J., Silva-Weiss, A., Giménez, B. et al. (2020). Effect of lyophilization on the physicochemical and rheological properties of food grade liposomes that encapsulate rutin. *Food Research International* 130: 108967.

Lu, Q., Li, D.-C., and Jiang, J.-G. (2011). Preparation of a tea polyphenol nanoliposome system and its physicochemical properties. *Journal of Agricultural and Food Chemistry* 59 (24): 13004–13011.

Luo, X., Guan, R., Chen, X. et al. (2014). Optimization on condition of epigallocatechin-3-gallate (EGCG) nanoliposomes by response surface methodology and cellular uptake studies in Caco-2 cells. *Nanoscale Research Letters* 9 (1): 291.

Ma, Q., Kuang, Y., Hao, X., and Gu, N. (2009). Preparation and characterization of tea polyphenols and vitamin E loaded nanoscale complex liposome. *Journal of Nanoscience and Nanotechnology* 9 (2): 1379–1383.

Mady, M.M., Darwish, M.M., Khalil, S., and Khalil, W.M. (2009). Biophysical studies on chitosan-coated liposomes. *European Biophysics Journal* 38 (8): 1127–1133.

Marsanasco, M., Chiaramoni, N.S., and del Valle Alonso, S. (2017). Liposomes as matrices to hold bioactive compounds for drinkable foods: their ability to improve health and future prospects. In: *Functional Food – Improve Health Through Adequate Food*, 1e (ed. M.C. Hueda), 185–208. London: IntechOpen.

Maurya, V.K., Bashir, K., and Aggarwal, M. (2020). Vitamin D microencapsulation and fortification: trends and technologies. *The Journal of Steroid Biochemistry and Molecular Biology* 196: 105489.

Michael Eskin, N. (2013). Vitamin E and the role of water-soluble α-tocopheryl phosphate. *Vitamins and Minerals* 3 (1): 1000e123.

Milinčić, D.D., Popović, D.A., Lević, S.M. et al. (2019). Application of polyphenol-loaded nanoparticles in food industry. *Nanomaterials* 9 (11): 1629.

Mohammadabadi, M. and Mozafari, M. (2018). Enhanced efficacy and bioavailability of thymoquinone using nanoliposomal dosage form. *Journal of Drug Delivery Science and Technology* 47: 445–453.

Mohammadi, M., Ghanbarzadeh, B., and Hamishehkar, H. (2014). Formulation of nanoliposomal vitamin D_3 for potential application in beverage fortification. *Advanced Pharmaceutical Bulletin* 4 (Suppl 2): 569–575.

Mohammadi, R., Mahmoudzadeh, M., Atefi, M. et al. (2015). Applications of nanoliposomes in cheese technology. *International Journal of Dairy Technology* 68 (1): 11–23.

Mohan, A., Rajendran, S.R., Thibodeau, J. et al. (2018). Liposome encapsulation of anionic and cationic whey peptides: influence of peptide net charge on properties of the nanovesicles. *LWT* 87: 40–46.

Morais, H., De Marco, L., Oliveira, M., and Silvestre, M. (2005). Casein hydrolysates using papain: peptide profile and encapsulation in liposomes. *Acta Alimentaria* 34 (1): 59–69.

Mozafari, M. (2010). Nanoliposomes: preparation and analysis. In: *Liposomes, Methods in Molecular Biology*, vol. 605 (ed. V. Weissig), 29–50. Humana Press https://doi.org/10.1007/978-1-60327-360-2_2.

Mozafari, M., Javanmard, R., and Raji, M. (2017). Tocosome: novel drug delivery system containing phospholipids and tocopheryl phosphates. *International Journal of Pharmaceutics* 528 (1–2): 381–382.

Munteanu, A., Zingg, J.-M., Ogru, E. et al. (2004). Modulation of cell proliferation and gene expression by α-tocopheryl phosphates: relevance to atherosclerosis and inflammation. *Biochemical and Biophysical Research Communications* 318 (1): 311–316.

Narsaiah, K., Sharma, M., Sridhar, K., and Dikkala, P. (2019). Garlic oil nanoemulsions hybridized in calcium alginate microcapsules for functional bread. *Agricultural Research* 8 (3): 356–363.

Nii, T. and Ishii, F. (2006). The novel liposome preparation methods based on in-water drying and phase separation: microencapsulation vesicle method and coacervation method. *Advances in Planar Lipid Bilayers and Liposomes* 5: 41–61.

Niki, E. and Abe, K. (2019). Vitamin E: structure, properties and functions. In: *Vitamin E: Chemistry and Nutritional Benefits* (ed. E. Niki), 1–11. Royal Society of Chemistry https://doi.org/10.1039/9781788016216-00001.

Noudoost, B., Noori, N., Amo Abedini, G. et al. (2015). Encapsulation of green tea extract in nanoliposomes and evaluation of its antibacterial, antioxidant and prebiotic properties. *Journal of Medicinal Plants* 3 (55): 66–78.

Ojagh, S.M. and Hasani, S. (2018). Characteristics and oxidative stability of fish oil nano-liposomes and its application in functional bread. *Journal of Food Measurement and Characterization* 12 (2): 1084–1092.

Pabast, M., Shariatifar, N., Beikzadeh, S., and Jahed, G. (2018). Effects of chitosan coatings incorporating with free or nano-encapsulated Satureja plant essential oil on quality characteristics of lamb meat. *Food Control* 91: 185–192.

Parhizkar, E., Rashedinia, M., Karimi, M., and Alipour, S. (2018). Design and development of vitamin C-encapsulated proliposome with improved in-vitro and ex-vivo antioxidant efficacy. *Journal of Microencapsulation* 35 (3): 301–311.

Patel, S., Patel, R., and Dharamsi, A. (2019). A review: proliposomes as a stable novel drug delivery. *World Journal of Pharmaceutical Research* 8: 638–651.

Pauli, G., Tang, W.-L., and Li, S.-D. (2019). Development and characterization of the solvent-assisted active loading technology (SALT) for liposomal loading of poorly water-soluble compounds. *Pharmaceutics* 11 (9): 465.

Perrie, Y., Kastner, E., Khadke, S. et al. (2017). Manufacturing methods for liposome adjuvants. In: *Vaccine Adjuvants: Methods and Protocols, Methods in Molecular Biology*, vol. 1494 (ed. C.B. Fox), 127–144. New York, NY: Humana Press https://doi.org/10.1007/978-1-4939-6445-1_9.

Pham, A., Gavin, P.D., Libinaki, R. et al. (2019). Differential effects of TPM, a phosphorylated tocopherol mixture, and other tocopherol derivatives as excipients for enhancing the solubilization of co-enzyme Q10 as a lipophilic drug during digestion of lipid-based formulations. *Current Drug Delivery* 16 (7): 628–636.

Pinilla, C.M.B., Thys, R.C.S., and Brandelli, A. (2019). Antifungal properties of phosphatidylcholine-oleic acid liposomes encapsulating garlic against environmental fungal in wheat bread. *International Journal of Food Microbiology* 293: 72–78.

Pokorný, J. and Schmidt, Š. (2010). Phospholipids. In: *Chemical, Biological, and Functional Aspects of Food Lipids* (ed. Z.E. Sikorski and A. Kolakowska), 97–112. CRC Press.

Poudel, A., Gachumi, G., Wasan, K.M. et al. (2019). Development and characterization of liposomal formulations containing phytosterols extracted from canola oil deodorizer distillate along with Tocopherols as food additives. *Pharmaceutics* 11 (4): 185.

Rafiee, Z., Barzegar, M., Sahari, M.A., and Maherani, B. (2018). Nanoliposomes containing pistachio green hull's phenolic compounds as natural bio-preservatives for mayonnaise. *European Journal of Lipid Science and Technology* 120 (9): 1800086.

Rasti, B., Erfanian, A., and Selamat, J. (2017). Novel nanoliposomal encapsulated omega-3 fatty acids and their applications in food. *Food Chemistry* 230: 690–696.

Ren, J., Fang, Z., Jiang, L., and Du, Q. (2017). Quercetin-containing self-assemble proliposome preparation and evaluation. *Journal of Liposome Research* 27 (4): 335–342.

Reza Mozafari, M., Johnson, C., Hatziantoniou, S., and Demetzos, C. (2008). Nanoliposomes and their applications in food nanotechnology. *Journal of Liposome Research* 18 (4): 309–327.

Rezk, B.M., Haenen, G.R., van der Vijgh, W.J., and Bast, A. (2004). The extraordinary antioxidant activity of vitamin E phosphate. *Biochimica et Biophysica Acta (BBA)-Molecular and Cell Biology of Lipids* 1683 (1–3): 16–21.

Rezk, B.M., van der Vijgh, W., Bast, A., and Haenen, G. (2007). Alpha-tocopheryl phosphate is a novel apoptotic agent. *Frontiers of Bioscience* 12: 2013–2019.

Robert, C., Couëdelo, L., Vaysse, C., and Michalski, M.-C. (2020). Vegetable lecithins: a review of their compositional diversity, impact on lipid metabolism and potential in cardiometabolic disease prevention. *Biochimie* 169: 121–132.

Scholfield, C. (1981). Composition of soybean lecithin. *Journal of the American Oil Chemists' Society* 58 (10): 889–892.

Sebaaly, C., Charcosset, C., Stainmesse, S. et al. (2016a). Clove essential oil-in-cyclodextrin-in-liposomes in the aqueous and lyophilized states: from laboratory to large scale using a membrane contactor. *Carbohydrate Polymers* 138: 75–85.

Sebaaly, C., Greige-Gerges, H., Agusti, G. et al. (2016b). Large-scale preparation of clove essential oil and eugenol-loaded liposomes using a membrane contactor and a pilot plant. *Journal of Liposome Research* 26 (2): 126–138.

Sebaaly, C., Greige-Gerges, H., Stainmesse, S. et al. (2016c). Effect of composition, hydrogenation of phospholipids and lyophilization on the characteristics of eugenol-loaded liposomes prepared by ethanol injection method. *Food Bioscience* 15: 1–10.

Seth, A.K. and Misra, A. (2002). Mathematical modelling of preparation of acyclovir liposomes: reverse phase evaporation method. *Journal of Pharmacy and Pharmaceutical Sciences* 5 (3): 285–291.

Shi, N.-Q. and Qi, X.-R. (2018). Preparation of drug liposomes by reverse-phase evaporation. In: *Liposome-Based Drug Delivery Systems, Biomaterial Engineering* (ed. W.-L. Lu and X.-R. Qi), 1–10. Germany: Springer-Verlag GmbH https://doi.org/10.1007/978-3-662-49231-4_3-1.

Shishir, M.R.I., Karim, N., Gowd, V. et al. (2019). Pectin-chitosan conjugated nanoliposome as a promising delivery system for neohesperidin: characterization, release behavior, cellular uptake, and antioxidant property. *Food Hydrocolloids* 95: 432–444.

Silva-Weiss, A., Quilaqueo, M., Venegas, O., Ahumada, M., Silva, W., Osorio, F., & Giménez, B. (2018). Design of dipalmitoyl lecithin liposomes loaded with quercetin and rutin and their release kinetics from carboxymethyl cellulose edible films. *Journal of Food Engineering,* 224, 165–173.

Stamler, C.J., Breznan, D., Neville, T.A. et al. (2000). Phosphatidylinositol promotes cholesterol transport in vivo. *Journal of Lipid Research* 41 (8): 1214–1221.

Szejtli, J. (1997). Utilization of cyclodextrins in industrial products and processes. *Journal of Materials Chemistry* 7 (4): 575–587.

Szoka, F. and Papahadjopoulos, D. (1978). Procedure for preparation of liposomes with large internal aqueous space and high capture by reverse-phase evaporation. *Proceedings of the National Academy of Sciences* 75 (9): 4194–4198.

Szoka, F., Olson, F., Heath, T. et al. (1980). Preparation of unilamellar liposomes of intermediate size (0.1–0.2 μm) by a combination of reverse phase evaporation and extrusion through polycarbonate membranes. *Biochimica et Biophysica Acta (BBA)-Biomembranes* 601: 559–571.

Tometri, S.S., Ahmady, M., Ariaii, P., and Soltani, M.S. (2020). Extraction and encapsulation of *Laurus nobilis* leaf extract with nano-liposome and its effect on oxidative, microbial, bacterial and sensory properties of minced beef. *Journal of Food Measurement and Characterization* 14 (6): 3333–3344.

Toniazzo, T. and Pinho, S.C. (2016). Lyophilized liposomes for food applications: Fundamentals, processes, and potential applications. In: *Encapsulation and Controlled Release Technologies in Food Systems* (ed. J.M. Lakkis), 78–96. Wiley Blackwell.

Toniazzo, T., Berbel, I.F., Cho, S. et al. (2014). β-Carotene-loaded liposome dispersions stabilized with xanthan and guar gums: physico-chemical stability and feasibility of application in yogurt. *LWT-Food Science and Technology* 59 (2): 1265–1273.

Trucillo, P., Campardelli, R., and Reverchon, E. (2019a). Antioxidant loaded emulsions entrapped in liposomes produced using a supercritical assisted technique. *The Journal of Supercritical Fluids* 154: 104626.

Trucillo, P., Campardelli, R., and Reverchon, E. (2019b). A versatile supercritical assisted process for the one-shot production of liposomes. *The Journal of Supercritical Fluids* 146: 136–143.

Verma, M.L. (2017). Nanobiotechnology advances in enzymatic biosensors for the agri-food industry. *Environmental Chemistry Letters* 15 (4): 555–560.

Waghule, T., Rapalli, V.K., Singhvi, G. et al. (2020). Design of temozolomide-loaded proliposomes and lipid crystal nanoparticles with industrial feasible approaches: comparative assessment of drug loading, entrapment efficiency, and stability at plasma pH. *Journal of Liposome Research* 31 (2): 158–168.

Wagner, A. and Vorauer-Uhl, K. (2011). Liposome technology for industrial purposes. *Journal of Drug Delivery* 2011: 591325.

Wang, Q., Wei, Q., Yang, Q. et al. (2018). A novel formulation of [6]-gingerol: proliposomes with enhanced oral bioavailability and antitumor effect. *International Journal of Pharmaceutics* 535 (1–2): 308–315.

Weissig, V. (2010). Methods and protocols: pharmaceutical nanocarriers, ch. 2. In: *Liposomes*, vol. 1. Springer.

Yasufuku, K., Okafuji, H., Hasegawa, M., and Haga, N. (1988). Margarine containing fish oil. Google Patents US 4764392A, United States.

Zarrabi, A., Alipoor Amro Abadi, M., Khorasani, S. et al. (2020). Nanoliposomes and tocosomes as multifunctional nanocarriers for the encapsulation of nutraceutical and dietary molecules. *Molecules* 25 (3): 638.

Zasadzinski, J.A., Wong, B., Forbes, N. et al. (2011). Novel methods of enhanced retention in and rapid, targeted release from liposomes. *Current opinion in colloid & interface science 16* (3): 203–214.

Zhang, H. (2017). Thin-film hydration followed by extrusion method for liposome preparation. In: *Liposomes: Methods and Protocols*, Methods in Molecular Biology, vol. 1522 (ed. G.G.M. D'Souza), 17–22. Humana Press.

Zingg, J.-M. (2018). Water-soluble vitamin E—tocopheryl phosphate. *Advances in Food and Nutrition Research* 83: 311–363.

Index